Nutrition and Physical Activity in Inflammatory Diseases

Nutrition and Physical Activity in Inflammatory Diseases

Edited by

Manohar L. Garg

Nutraceuticals Research Group
University of Newcastle, Australia

and

Lisa G. Wood

Centre for Asthma & Respiratory Diseases
School of Biomedical Sciences & Pharmacy
University of Newcastle, Australia

www.cabi.org

CABI is a trading name of CAB International

CABI
Nosworthy Way
Wallingford
Oxfordshire OX10 8DE
UK

Tel: +44 (0)1491 832111
Fax: +44 (0)1491 833508
E-mail: info@cabi.org
Website: www.cabi.org

CABI
38 Chauncey Street
Suite 1002
Boston, MA 02111
USA

Tel: +1 800 552 3083 (toll free)
Tel: +1 (0)617 395 4051
E-mail: cabi-nao@cabi.org

A catalogue record for this book is available from the British Library, London, UK.

Library of Congress Cataloging-in-Publication Data

Nutrition & physical activity in inflammatory diseases/[edited by] Manohar L. Garg and Lisa G. Wood.
p. ; cm.
Nutrition and physical activity in inflammatory diseases
Includes bibliographical references and index.
ISBN 978-1-84593-910-6 (alk. paper)
I. Garg, Manohar L. II. Wood, Lisa G. III. C.A.B. International. IV. Title: Nutrition and physical activity in inflammatory diseases.
[DNLM: 1. Inflammation--physiopathology. 2. Nutritional Physiological Phenomena. 3. Physical Exertion--physiology. 4. Stress, Physiological. QZ 150]

616'.0473--dc23

2012021014

ISBN-13: 978 1 84593 910 6

Commissioning editor: Rachel Cutts
Editorial assistant: Alexandra Lainsbury
Production editor: Shankari Wilford

Typeset by SPi, Pondicherry, India.
Printed and bound in the UK by the MPG Books Group.

Contents

Preface

This book presents recent developments and discoveries in the vital areas of inflammation and related chronic diseases to stimulate further research and to translate such discoveries rapidly to the interested parties. The information presented in this book includes: an introduction to inflammation, with special reference to aspects that can be modified by nutrition and physical activity interventions; a description of how various nutrients affect inflammatory process; a summary of the impact of aerobic and strength training on inflammatory mediators; and a comprehensive review of how nutrition and physical activity interventions can be used to modulate inflammation to prevent the development and progression of chronic diseases including obesity, diabetes mellitus, cardiovascular disease, eye disease, inflammatory bowel disease, asthma and arthritis.

Inflammatory mediators originating in a single organ can spill over into the circulation and influence functioning of other organs. As a result, chronic inflammatory diseases often cluster together in individuals and are likely to be linked together via the common element, inflammation. Literature describing nutrition and physical activity as modifiers of inflammation highlights the potential for behavioural interventions to modify a broad range of diseases using non-pharmacological approaches. This presents an opportunity for multidisciplinary approaches to be used to tackle the multi-organ perspectives of inflammatory diseases, involving clinicians, nutritionists, food scientists and exercise physiologists.

Our experience with our own research has been that interventions targeting a specific disease process are relevant for a variety of other indications. The intention of the book is to compile knowledge and recent developments that demonstrate the multi-organ effects of chronic inflammation and the nutritional and physical activity approaches that can be used to reduce inflammation, particularly when pharmacological approaches alone have struggled to deliver safe and efficacious disease management.

Manohar L. Garg
Lisa G. Wood

Contributors

Tyler Barker, The Orthopedic Specialty Hospital, Murray, Utah, USA. E-mail: tyler.barker@imail.org

Kim Bell-Anderson, Discipline of Nutrition & Metabolism, School of Molecular Bioscience, University of Sydney, Sydney, New South Wales, Australia.

Jenney Brand-Miller, School of Molecular Bioscience, Boden Institute of Obesity, Nutrition and Exercise, University of Sydney, Sydney, New South Wales, Australia. E-mail: jennie.brandmiller@sydney.edu.au

Mònica Bulló, Human Nutrition Unit, Faculty of Medicine & Health Sciences, University Rovira i Virgili, Reus, Tarragona, Spain. E-mail: monica.bullo@urv.cat

Anette E. Buyken, Research Institute of Child Nutrition, Rheinische Friedrich-Wilhelms-Universität Bonn, Dortmund, Germany. E-mail: buyken@fke-do.de

Philip C. Calder, Human Development and Health Academic Unit, Faculty of Medicine, University of Southampton, Southampton General Hospital, Southampton, UK. E-mail: p.c.calder@soton.ac.uk

David Cameron-Smith, Centre for Physical Activity and Nutrition Research, School of Exercise and Nutrition Sciences, Deakin University, Burwood, Victoria, Australia and Liggins Institute, University of Auckland, New Zealand.

David Cheung, Department of Agricultural, Food & Nutritional Science, Alberta Diabetes Institute, University of Alberta, Faculty of Medicine & Dentistry, Edmonton, Alberta, Canada.

Jeff Coombes, School of Human Movement Studies, University of Queensland, Brisbane, Queensland, Australia. E-mail: jcoombes@hms.uq.edu.au

Trevor Day, School of Biomedical Sciences & Pharmacy, University of Newcastle, Newcastle, New South Wales, Australia. E-mail: trevor.day@newcastle.edu.au

Lynnette Ferguson, Department of Nutrition, School of Medical Sciences, University of Auckland, Auckland, New Zealand. E-mail: l.ferguson@auckland.ac.nz

Catherine Field, Department of Agricultural, Food & Nutritional Science, Alberta Diabetes Institute, University of Alberta, Faculty of Medicine & Dentistry, Edmonton, Alberta, Canada. E-mail: catherine.field@ualberta.ca

Meika Foster, Discipline of Nutrition & Metabolism, School of Molecular Bioscience, University of Sydney, Sydney, New South Wales, Australia.

Mar Garcia-Aloy, Human Nutrition Unit, Faculty of Medicine & Health Sciences, University Rovira i Virgili, Reus, Tarragona, Spain.

Manohar Garg, School of Biomedical Sciences & Pharmacy, University of Newcastle, Newcastle, New South Wales, Australia. E-mail: manohar.garg@newcastle.edu.au

Peter Gibson, School of Medicine & Public Health, University of Newcastle, Newcastle, New South Wales, Australia. E-mail: peter.gibson@hnehealth.nsw.gov.au

Blanka Golebiowski, School of Optometry and Vision Science, University of New South Wales, Sydney, New South Wales, Australia.

Jessica A. Grieger, Nutrition and Dietetics, Flinders University, Bedford Park, South Australia, Australia.

Brianna Hawkins, Department of Agricultural, Food & Nutritional Science, Alberta Diabetes Institute, University of Alberta, Faculty of Medicine & Dentistry, Edmonton, Alberta, Canada.

Alison Heather, School of Medical and Molecular Biosciences, University of Technology, Sydney, New South Wales, Australia. E-mail: Alison.Heather@uts.edu.au

David Heber, UCLA Center for Human Nutrition, David Geffen School of Medicine, Los Angeles, California, USA. E-mail: DHeber@mednet.ucla.edu

Angela Hofstra, Department of Agricultural, Food & Nutritional Science, Alberta Diabetes Institute, University of Alberta, Faculty of Medicine & Dentistry, Edmonton, Alberta, Canada.

Isabelle Jalbert, School of Optometry and Vision Science, University of New South Wales, Sydney, New South Wales, Australia.

Elizabeth J. Kovacs, Department of Surgery, Burn & Shock Trauma Institute, Alcohol Research Program, Loyola University Medical Centre, Maywood, Illinois, USA. E-mail: ekovacs@lumc.edu

Marlena Kruger, Institute of Food, Nutrition & Human Health, Riddett Institute, Massey University, Palmerston North, New Zealand. E-mail: M.C.Kruger@massey.ac.nz

Jessica Lieffers, Department of Agricultural, Food & Nutritional Science, Alberta Diabetes Institute, University of Alberta, Faculty of Medicine & Dentistry, Edmonton, Alberta, Canada.

Carla Lopes, Department of Clinical Epidemiology, Predictive Medicine and Public Health, University of Porto Medical School and Public Health Institute, University of Porto, Porto, Portugal.

Michele Madigan, School of Optometry and Vision Science, University of New South Wales, Sydney, New South Wales, and Save Sight Institute, Sydney Medical School, University of Sydney, Australia. E-mail: m.madigan@unsw.edu.au

Linda McCargar, Department of Agricultural, Food & Nutritional Science, Alberta Diabetes Institute, University of Alberta, Faculty of Medicine & Dentistry, Edmonton, Alberta, Canada.

Kristine McGrath, School of Medical and Molecular Biosciences, University of Technology, Sydney, New South Wales, Australia.

Robert K. McNamara, Department of Psychiatry, University of Cincinnati, College of Medicine, Cincinnati, Ohio, USA. E-mail: robert.mcnamara@uc.edu

Eugene Nalivaiko, School of Biomedical Sciences & Pharmacy, University of Newcastle, Newcastle, New South Wales, Australia. E-mail: eugene.nalivaiko@newcastle.edu.au

Caryl Nowson, Centre for Physical Activity and Nutrition Research, School of Exercise and Nutrition Sciences, Deakin University, Burwood, Victoria, Australia. E-mail: nowson@deakin.edu.au

Helen O'Connor, Discipline of Exercise & Sport Science, Faculty of Health Sciences, University of Sydney, Sydney, New South Wales, Australia.

Andreia Oliveira, Department of Clinical Epidemiology, Predictive Medicine and Public Health, University of Porto Medical School and Public Health Institute, University of Porto, Porto, Portugal. E-mail: acmatos@med.up.pt

Goran Paulsen, Norwegian School of Sports Science, Oslo, Norway. E-mail: Goran.Paulsen@nih.no

Jonathan Peake, School of Human Movement Studies, University of Queensland, Centre for Military and Veterans' Health, University of Queensland, and Centre of Excellence for Applied Sport Science Research, Queensland Academy of Sport, Brisbane, Queensland, Australia. E-mail: jpeake@hms.uq.edu.au

Samir Samman, Discipline of Nutrition & Metabolism, School of Molecular Bioscience, University of Sydney, Sydney, New South Wales, Australia. E-mail: samir.samman@sydney.edu.au

Hayley Scott, School of Medicine & Public Health, University of Newcastle, Newcastle, New South Wales, Australia. E-mail: hayley.scott@newcastle.edu.au

Fiona Stapleton, School of Optometry and Vision Science, University of New South Wales, Sydney, New South Wales, Australia.

F. Rohan Walker, School of Biomedical Sciences & Pharmacy, University of Newcastle, Newcastle, New South Wales, Australia. E-mail: Rohan.walker@newcastle.edu.au

Lisa Wood, School of Biomedical Sciences & Pharmacy, University of Newcastle, Newcastle, New South Wales, Australia. E-mail: lisa.wood@newcastle.edu.au

Inflammation: An Introduction

P.C. Calder*
Human Development and Health Academic Unit, University of Southampton, Southampton, UK

Introduction

Inflammation is a physiological response to infection, injury or irritants. It is part of the host's defence mechanism, acting to initiate pathogen killing. Inflammation also plays a role in tissue repair processes so helping to restore homeostasis at infected or damaged sites. Thus, in its physiological context, inflammation is protective. It is considered to be part of the innate immune system, being initiated by pathogens and being an essential component of the host

* Author, p.c.calder@soton.ac.uk

response aimed at eliminating pathogens. Inflammation involves interactions amongst many cell types and the production of, and responses to, a number of chemical mediators. Without inflammation, pathogens would not be efficiently eliminated and wounds and infections would not heal. Chronic inflammation can, however, damage host tissues and is a central element in a number of diseases, such as rheumatoid arthritis, Crohn's disease, ulcerative colitis, asthma, dermatitis and even atherosclerosis and cancer. Because of its potential to cause damage, it is important that inflammation is closely regulated.

The five classical signs of inflammation are pain (dolour), heat (calor), redness (rubor), swelling (tumour) and loss of function (functio laesa). The first four signs were described by Celsus 2000 years ago, whereas loss of function was recognized and added later. Redness and heat are due to increased blood flow to the inflamed site; swelling is caused by accumulation of fluid at that site; pain is due to release of chemicals that stimulate nerve endings. Inflammation may be classified as acute or chronic (Table 1.1).

Acute and Chronic Inflammation

Acute inflammation is the initial response of the body to harmful stimuli. It is a short-term process, usually appearing within a few minutes or hours and ceasing upon the removal of the injurious stimulus. Acute inflammation is initiated by cells already present in tissues prior to the arrival of the causative agent. These cells include macrophages, dendritic cells and mast cells and they express on their surface receptors known as pattern recognition receptors (PRRs). These recognize molecules that are general features of pathogens but not the host; these molecules are termed microbe-associated molecular patterns (MAMPs). An example of a PRR is toll-like receptor (TLR) 4 and an example of a MAMP is the lipopolysaccharide (LPS) structure that is a component of the cell wall of Gram-negative bacteria (Aderem and Ulevitch, 2000); LPS is sometimes called bacterial endotoxin. Upon exposure to an infectious microbe or as the result of another insult (e.g. a burn, exposure to ultraviolet irradiation or a penetrating injury) a PRR will recognize a MAMP and the cell expressing the PRR becomes activated. As a result, the cell releases chemicals termed inflammatory mediators. It is these mediators that are responsible for the clinical signs of inflammation. Vasodilation and the increase in blood flow that results causes the redness and heat. An increased permeability of blood vessels results in leakage of plasma fluid and proteins into the inflamed site causing a local oedema seen as swelling. Some of mediators that are released, e.g. bradykinin, play a role in causing pain, whereas some cause an increase in permeability across the blood vessel wall allowing the migration of leucocytes (these are the white blood cells) from the bloodstream into the tissue. These cells are attracted to the site of inflammation as a result of specific mediators, termed

Table 1.1. General features of acute and chronic inflammation.

	Acute	Chronic
Causative agent	Pathogens, injured tissues, irradiation, irritants	Persistent inflammation owing to pathogens or other foreign bodies, autoimmune reactions
Major cells involved	Neutrophils and other granulocytes, mononuclear cells (monocytes, macrophages)	Mononuclear cells (monocytes, macrophages, T lymphocytes, B lymphocytes)
Primary mediators	Vasoactive amines, eicosanoids, granule peptides	Cytokines, eicosanoids, growth factors, reactive oxygen species, hydrolytic enzymes
Onset	Immediate	Delayed
Duration	Hours to a few days	Up to months or years
Outcomes	Resolution, chronic inflammation	Tissue destruction, fibrosis, necrosis

chemoattractants, being released at that site; in the process called chemotaxis, leucocytes move along a concentration gradient of the chemoattractant. These events are depicted in Fig. 1.1 (Calder *et al.*, 2009).

In addition to the activation of cells and the production of chemical mediators by those cells, several biochemical cascade systems not involving cells are initiated in parallel with the above events. These cascade systems involve proteins existing initially in the bloodstream in an inactive state that become activated and then go on to activate other proteins. These cascade systems include the complement, kinin, coagulation and fibrinolytic systems. The complement system is activated by bacteria and acts to neutralize and then destroy bacteria. The kinin system acts to sustain inflammatory activities such as vasodilation at the blood vessel wall. The coagulation system promotes blood clotting, whereas the fibrinolytic system acts to inhibit it.

Through the localized cellular responses involved and through the effective action of the cascade systems, acute inflammation serves to neutralize the pathogen, injury or irritant and, if necessary, to initate the acquired immune response. The acute inflammatory response requires constant stimulation to be sustained. Inflammatory mediators have short half lives and are quickly degraded. Therefore once the initiating stimulus has been removed, acute inflammation ceases. The exact processes by which inflammation is terminated (called resolution) are rather poorly understood. Resolution is, however, important to prevent unnecessary damage to host tissues that might go on to become chronic. This self-regulation of inflammation involves the activation of negative-feedback mechanisms including the production of pro-resolving mediators, inhibition of pro-inflammatory signalling cascades, shedding of receptors for inflammatory mediators and activation of regulatory cells. Pathological chronic inflammation involves a loss of these regulatory processes and where this becomes excessive, irreparable damage to host tissues and disease can occur. Chronic inflammation leads to a progressive shift in the type of cells

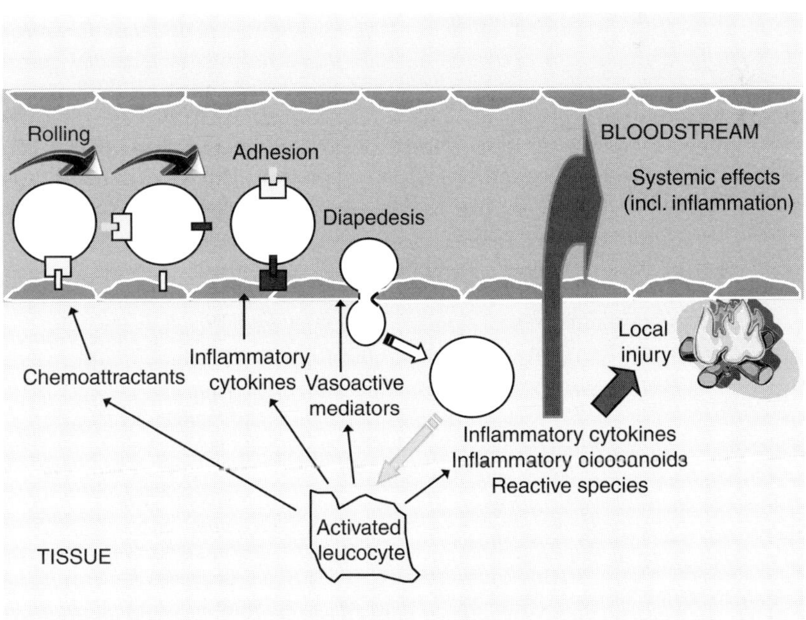

Fig. 1.1. Generalized view of inflammation. (Reproduced with permission from Calder *et al.*, 2009.)

present at the site of inflammation away from granulocytes (neutrophils, eosinophils and mast cells) to mononuclear cells (monocytes and lymphocytes).

Physiological Role of Principal Cells Involved in Inflammation

Neutrophils

Neutrophils (sometimes called polymorphonuclear neutrophils) are the most abundant leucocytes (white blood cells) typically accounting for about 70% of leucocytes in an adult human. They are a type of granulocyte; the other granulocytes are eosinophils and basophils (together neutrophils, eosinophils and basophils are termed polymorphonuclear cells). The principal roles of neutrophils are phagocytosis and bacterial killing (Witko-Sarset *et al.*, 2000; Segal, 2005; Nathan, 2006; Hickey and Kubes, 2009). They are highly granular. The average lifespan of a human neutrophil in the circulation is about 5 days. Neutrophil numbers in the bloodstream are increased during bacterial infection and acute inflammation; this is termed neutrophilia. Neutropenia, a decreased number of neutrophils in the bloodstream can occur with viral infections and after radiotherapy and chemotherapy. Neutrophils are typically the earliest responding inflammatory cells and early infectious or inflammatory foci are dominated by neutrophils. When the endothelium is activated, its expression of certain adhesion molecules is up-regulated. These adhesion molecules cause neutrophils to marginate (position themselves adjacent to the blood vessel endothelium) and they are then captured by and adhere to the endothelium (see the section on Leucocyte–Endothelium Interaction in Inflammation). They then migrate into the tissue and move towards sites of infection or inflammatory activity by the process of chemotaxis in response to chemotactic signals such as interleukin (IL)-8, leukotriene (LT) B_4, C5a or certain bacterial peptides. The chemoattractants are recognised by specific receptors (usually G-protein coupled receptors) on the neutrophil surface; the same process of chemotaxis is involved in the movement of other leucocytes to sites of infection and of inflammatory activity. Neutrophils survive within tissues for one or two days. They are the predominant cell type in pus. Within the bloodstream, unactivated neutrophils are spherical in shape but once activated they undergo shape change, forming projections that 'hunt' for bacteria.

Neutrophils produce a wide range of inflammatory mediators. Some of these mediators target bacteria directly, whereas others, particularly cytokines, act on other cell types to amplify the inflammatory response. Amongst the cytokines released by neutrophils are tumour necrosis factor (TNF), IL-1β, IL-8 and transforming growth factor (TGF)-β1, although the amounts released by neutrophils are typically much less than those produced by monocytes and macrophages. Neutrophils are also able to form eicosanoids from arachidonic acid; although neutrophils produce cyclooxygenase (COX) metabolites such as prostaglandin (PG) D_2, they typically produce greater amounts of 5-lipoxygenase (LOX) products, especially LTB_4. LTB_4 is a potent chemoattractant, serving to promote leucocyte movement to sites of inflammatory activity, so amplifying the response. The three antibacterial actions of neutrophils are phagocytosis, release of antimicrobial agents, and generation of extracellular 'traps' (Segal, 2005; Nathan, 2006; Hickey and Kubes, 2009).

Phagocytosis is the process of ingestion of microorganisms or particles. For targets to be recognized, they must be coated in so-called opsonins (the process is called opsonization and opsonins are commonly complement proteins or antibodies). The recognition of the opsonized target is receptor mediated. Important receptors involved in phagocytosis include some of the complement receptors (CR) such as CR3 (also known as Mac-1) and CR4 and antibody-binding receptors such as FcγRII. Once internalized, the microbe is killed within the internalized phagosome into which reactive oxygen species and hydrolytic enzymes are released. Because this process increases the rate of oxygen consumption by the phagocyte, the generation of reactive oxygen species is termed the respiratory burst. The respiratory burst involves the activation of the enzyme NADPH oxidase, which produces large quantities of superoxide, one of the reactive oxygen species. Superoxide is converted via the superoxide dismutase enzymes to hydrogen peroxide, which is in turn converted to hypochlorous acid by myeloperoxidase enzymes. Superoxide, hydrogen peroxide and hypochlorous acid are all toxic to bacteria.

Neutrophils also release an assortment of proteins by a process called degranulation. These proteins include lactoferrin, lysozyme, myeloperoxidase, elastase, cathepsin G and gelatinase. Many of these proteins are proteases capable of degrading bacteria.

The third mechanism of bacterial killing by neutrophils is the release of structures termed neutrophil extracellular traps. These are fibrous structures composed of DNA and proteases that trap and kill microbes extracellularly. These traps may provide a high local concentration of antimicrobial components and bind, disarm and kill microbes independent of phagocytic uptake.

Eosinophils

Eosinophils normally constitute 1–5% of the peripheral blood leucocytes. Eosinophils are also commonly located within many tissues including the lower gastrointestinal tract, but they are not normally present in the lungs or skin. Their main role is in protection against parasitic infections (Rothenberg and Hogan 2006; Hogan *et al.*, 2008). The numbers of eosinophils in the blood (eosinophilia) can be elevated with parasitic infections or in people with allergic diseases and asthma. Their lifetime in the blood stream is short (8–12 h), but they can survive in tissues for as long as 12 days in the absence of stimulation.

As they develop, eosinophils produce and store many proteins in cytosolic granules. After maturation, eosinophils circulate in the bloodstream and migrate to parasite-infected or inflammatory sites in tissues. The migration is promoted by chemoattractant chemokines such as eotaxin-1 (chemokine (C–C motif) ligand (CCL) 11), eotaxin-2 (CCL24), Regulated on Activation, Normal T Expressed and Secreted (RANTES; CCL5), and monocyte chemoattractant peptide (MCP)-1 and leukotrienes, especially LTB_4. At infected or inflamed sites, eosinophils are activated by type 2 cytokines released from a specific subset of helper T cells (Th2 cells); the key cytokines involved in eosinophil activation are IL-5, IL-13 and granulocyte macrophage colony stimulating factor (GM-CSF). Following activation, eosinophils produce a range of inflammatory mediators including: cytotoxic cationic granule proteins such as major basic protein, eosinophil cationic protein, eosinophil peroxidase and eosinophil-derived neurotoxin; elastase; reactive oxygen species (superoxide, hydrogen peroxide and hypobromous acid); eicosanoids including COX-derived PGE_2 and 5-LOX-derived cysteinyl LTs (LTC_4, LTD_4, LTE_4); growth factors including vascular endothelial growth factor (VEGF) and platelet-derived growth factor (PDGF); and cytokines including TNF, IL-1, IL-2, IL-4, IL-5, IL-6, IL-8, IL-13 and TGF-β (Bandeira-Melo *et al.*, 2002; Rothenberg and Hogan, 2006; Hogan *et al.*, 2008). Major basic protein, eosinophil peroxidase and eosinophil cationic protein are toxic, whereas eosinophil cationic protein and eosinophil-derived neurotoxin have antiviral activity. Major basic protein induces mast cell and basophil degranulation. Eosinophil cationic protein creates toxic pores in the membranes of target cells allowing the potential entry of other cytotoxic molecules to the cell. It can also induce degranulation of mast cells and stimulate fibroblast cells to secrete mucus.

Basophils

Basophils are the least common of the granulocytes, comprising only 0.01% to 0.3% of leucocytes. They are granular cells containing preformed histamine and heparin and they can be recruited into tissues. Like eosinophils, basophils play a role in both defence against parasitic infections and in allergic reactions (Schroeder, 2009; Nakanishi, 2010). Basophils express the high-affinity immunoglobulin (Ig) E receptor, FcεRI, meaning that they are IgE coated and degranulate in the presence of allergens. When activated, basophils degranulate to release histamine, heparin and chondroitin, and proteolytic enzymes such as elastase. They also produce eicosaoids including cysteinyl-LTs and several cytokines, in particular IL-4.

Mast cells

Mast cells (also known as mastocytes) are resident in many tissues. They are granular cells with the granules being rich in histamine and heparin. They are involved in defence against some pathogens and in wound healing, and also in allergy and anaphylaxis (Metcalfe *et al.*, 1997). Despite being similar, mast cells and basophils have a distinct precursor. Mast cells circulate in an immature form, only maturing once in a tissue site. Two types of mast cell have been identified: one is resident in connective tissue and the other is found at mucosal sites (skin, lungs, mouth, gastrointestinal tract). The latter are regulated by T lymphocytes. When activated, mast cells release the contents of their granules and also produce various inflammatory mediators. Mast cell degranulation is promoted by physical or chemical injury, cross-linking of IgE receptors (high-affinity FcεRI) on the surface, or certain complement proteins. It is the presence of the high-affinity IgE receptors to which IgE is bound that links mast cells with allergy. Binding of two or more IgE molecules (cross-linking) is required to activate the mast cell. Although this reaction is most well understood in terms of allergy, it seems to be involved in defence against intestinal parasitic worm infections. The mediators released from activated mast cells include histamine, serine proteases such as tryptase, serotonin, and heparin, all preformed and released from granules, and newly formed lipid mediators including PGD_2, TXA_2, LTC_4 and platelet-activating factor (PAF), eosinophil chemotactic factor, and cytokines including TNF. Histamine dilates post-capillary venules, activates the endothelium, and increases blood vessel permeability. This leads to local oedema, heat and redness, and to the attraction of other inflammatory cells. Histamine also irritates nerve endings causing itching or pain. Body-wide degranulation of mast cells can cause anaphylaxis. The complete role of mast cells in host immune defences is poorly understood.

Mononuclear phagocytes (monocytes and macrophages)

The principal mononuclear phagocytes are monocytes and macrophages (Ziegler-Heitbrock, 2007; Mosser and Edwards, 2008). Monocytes circulate in the bloodstream where their lifetime is a few days. In response to infection or an inflammatory stimulus, monocytes migrate to the site of the immuno-inflammatory activity where they differentiate into macrophages. Thus, macrophages do not circulate in the bloodstream but are found in tissues including secondary lymphoid organs such as the spleen and lymph nodes. Tissue macrophages are sometimes given site-specific names such as Kupffer cells in the liver, alveolar macrophages in the lungs and microglial cells in the brain. Tissue macrophages can survive for months or even years. The mononuclear phagocyte system has an important role in host defence against microorganisms and in the removal of senescent erythrocytes, leucocytes and megakaryocytes. Their primary modes of action are phagocytosis and subsequent digestion, as described earlier for neutrophils, antigen presentation and cytokine production. Mononuclear phagocytes can perform phagocytosis of opsonized microbes or via binding of PRRs to MAMPs. Microbial fragments that remain after digestion can serve as antigen. The fragments can be incorporated into major histocompatibility complex (MHC) molecules and then traffic to the cell surface of the phagocyte. This process is called antigen presentation and it leads to the activation of T lymphocytes, which then mount a specific immune response against the source of the antigen. Microbial products can directly activate mononuclear phagocytes leading to the production of pro-inflammatory cytokines; production of anti-inflammatory cytokines can follow later. Typical cytokines produced by monocytes and macrophages include TNF, IL-1, IL-6, IL-12 and IL-10. Macrophages have been classified as M1 or M2 macrophages. M1 macrophages are aggressive against microbes and can readily engulf and digest target cells; they produce many pro-inflammatory mediators. M2 macrophages are involved in wound healing and tissue repair, and have anti-inflammatory and immunosuppressive effects; they produce anti-inflammatory mediators such as IL-10.

Lymphocytes

Lymphocytes can be described as large or small; large granular lymphocytes include natural killer cells (NK cells), whereas small lymphocytes consist of T cells and B cells. T cells (thymus-derived cells) and B cells (bursa-derived cells) are the major cellular components of the adaptive immune response. T cells are involved in cell-mediated immunity, whereas B cells are primarily responsible for humoral (antibody-mediated) immunity. T and B cells have a lifetime of weeks to many months. Their function is to recognize specific 'non-self' antigens presented to them by antigen-presenting cells (e.g. macrophages, dendritic cells). Once activated, they mount specific responses that are tailored to maximally eliminate specific pathogens or pathogen-infected cells. B cells respond to pathogens by producing large quantities of antibodies that then neutralize foreign objects such as bacteria and viruses. In response to pathogens, some T cells, called T helper cells, produce cytokines that direct the immune response by regulating the function of other cell types, whereas other T cells, called cytotoxic T cells, produce toxic granules that contain powerful enzymes which induce the death of pathogen-infected cells. Once the source of the antigen is eliminated, some of the specific B cells and T cells remain as memory cells; the consequence of this is that a strong and rapid response can be mounted if the pathogen is detected again.

The most common way to distinguish the different types of lymphocyte is on the basis of cell-surface markers. NK cells express CD16 and CD56 but not CD3. T cells express the T-cell receptor and CD3; T helper cells also express CD4, whereas cytotoxic T cells express CD8.

T helper cells regulate the activity of other immune cells, for example by promoting the differentiation of B cells into antibody-producing cells or activating macrophages. They are mainly involved in defence against bacteria. Once activated, T helper cells differentiate, divide and produce cytokines. The cytokine profiles produced characterize the T helper cell subtype described as Th1, Th2, Th3 or Th17. It is the precise nature of the interaction with the antigen-presenting cell and the cytokines produced during that interaction that determine the subtype of helper T cell that is produced (McGeachy and Cua, 2008; Zhou *et al.*, 2009). Cytotoxic T cells destroy virally infected cells and tumour cells. Regulatory T cells (T_{reg} cells), formerly known as suppressor T cells, are important to maintain immunological tolerance (Steinman, 2007; Sakaguchi *et al.*, 2010). Their major role is to shut down T-cell-mediated immunity towards the end of an immune reaction and to suppress auto-reactive T cells.

Leucocyte–Endothelium Interactions in Inflammation

Movement of leucocytes from the bloodstream to sites of infection or inflammatory activity involves their interaction with and adhesion to the walls of blood vessels running through the affected tissue (Muller, 2011; Schmidt *et al.*, 2011). These adhesive interactions are a highly regulated process, as damage can result from adhesion to the wrong tissue. The molecules involved in mediating adhesive interactions between leucocytes and the luminal side of the endothelium are termed adhesion molecules; typically these act in pairs, with one half of each pair being expressed on the leucocyte and the other half on the endothelium. There are two phases of adhesion: the first (rolling) depends upon selectins and the second (migration) on β2 integrins.

The process of leucocyte adhesion begins with so-called 'rolling', whereby the leucocyte carried by blood flow rolls along the endothelium making weak and reversible interactions. Rolling allows the leucocyte to interact with the endothelium via L-selectin, which is constitutively expressed on non-activated leucocytes. L-selectin binds to endothelial glycoproteins termed glyCAMs or vascular addressins. Rolling is increased by inflammation because some chemical mediators, including TNF, IL-1β and C5a, as well as bacterial LPS, up-regulate P-selectin (platelet activation-dependent granule external membrane protein, PADGEM) and at a later timepoint E-selectin (endothelial–leucocyte adhesion molecule-1, ELAM-1) expression on the endothelium. This increased rolling is sometimes termed margination. Both P-selectin and E-selectin bind leucocyte surface glycoproteins (gp150-Lewis X (CD15) and sialo-Lewis X, respectively).

Diapedesis is the term used to describe the migration of the leucocyte between the endothelial cells; diapedesis is initiated by the integrin-dependent phase of adhesion. To enable this, L-selectin must be shed from the leucocyte. This is promoted by the release of certain factors including IL-8 and PAF from the endothelial cells involved in the interaction. At the same time the leucocyte upregulates expression of β2 integrins. The three major leucocyte integrins are leucocyte function-associated antigen (LFA)-1 (a dimer composed of CD11a/CD18), Mac-1 (CD11b/CD18 or CR3), and p150,95 (CD11c/CD18 or CR4). LFA-1 binds the immunoglobulin superfamily molecules intercellular adhesion molecule (ICAM)-1 and ICAM-2 and the leucocyte begins to search for the boundaries between two endothelial cells. Another immunoglobulin superfamily cell adhesion molecule, CD31 (platelet–endothelial cell adhesion molecule-1, PECAM-1), expressed on both the endothelium and the leucocyte seems to play a role in this stage of transendothelial migration.

Characteristics of Chronic Inflammatory Conditions

Despite its key role in host defence, chronic inflammation is a recognized contributor to the pathology of many conditions. In some cases, such as rheumatoid arthritis (RA), inflammatory bowel diseases (IBD), asthma and psoriasis, the central role of inflammation to the pathology is well recognized. Patients with these conditions have a heavy infiltration of inflammatory cells at the site of disease activity (e.g. the joints, the intestinal mucosa, the lungs and the skin) and they have elevated concentrations of inflammatory mediators at those sites and in the systemic circulation (Calder *et al.*, 2009). They might suffer secondary inflammatory complications at sites distant from the principal inflammatory lesion owing to the effects of the systemic inflammatory mediators. These conditions are treated with varying levels of success by anti-inflammatory drugs. In other cases, such as atherosclerosis and obesity, the role of inflammation has emerged more recently and its contribution to the pathology alongside the many other factors involved is less clear. Patients with these conditions show infiltration of inflammatory cells at the site of disease activity (e.g. the blood vessel wall and adipose tissue) and have moderately elevated levels of inflammatory mediators in the systemic circulation (Calder *et al.*, 2011). These conditions are not traditionally treated with anti-inflammatory drugs.

Chronic inflammation of the joints: rheumatoid arthritis (RA)

RA is a common autoimmune disease characterized by chronic inflammation of the synovium of the joints (Lee and Weinblatt, 2001). It can lead to long-term joint damage, resulting in chronic pain, loss of function and disability. The main risk factors for the disease include genetic susceptibility, sex (it is two to three times more common in women than in men), age, smoking and certain infectious agents. The main predisposing genetic factor is human leucocyte antigen (HLA)-DR4, which is involved in antigen presentation, although other genetic factors have been discovered, such as polymorphisms in the gene encoding lymphoid protein tyrosine phosphatase (Firestein, 2003) which result in altered

T lymphocyte reactivity. In RA, the synovium (or synovial membrane) becomes hypertrophic and oedematous. Angioneogenesis, recruitment of inflammatory cells due to production of chemokines, local retention of those cells and their proliferation contribute to the accumulation of cells in the inflamed synovium. Locally expressed matrix metalloproteinases digest the extracellular matrix and destroy articular structures. The synovial membrane is known as pannus. It actively invades and destroys the periarticular bone and cartilage at the margin between synovium and bone. T cells are actively involved in the pathogenesis of RA: activated T cells are present in high numbers in the inflamed joints of RA patients and these cells can stimulate other cells (e.g. B cells, macrophages and fibroblast-like synoviocytes; Panayi *et al.*, 1992). Thus, the T cells participate in the cell- and mediator-driven events that lead to amplified inflammation and joint destruction. B cells are the source of autoantibodies being produced in RA and contribute to immune complex formation and complement activation in the joints (Weyrand *et al.*, 2005). The major effector cells in the pathogenesis of arthritis are synovial macrophages and fibroblasts. Activated macrophages are critical in RA, in part owing to the production of cytokines (in particular TNF and IL-1β) in the synovial compartments. There is evidence for the proliferation and expression of inflammatory cytokines and chemokines by fibroblast-like synovial cells in inflamed synovia. Lipid mediators such as PGE_2 produced by macrophages are also recognized to have a key role in the inflammation seen in RA.

Chronic inflammation of the gastrointestinal mucosa: inflammatory bowel diseases

Ulcerative colitis (UC) and Crohn's disease (CD) are the two main forms of IBD. CD can affect any part of the gastrointestinal tract, whereas UC primarily affects the colon (Farrell and Peppercorn, 2002; Shanahan, 2002). A mutation in the NOD2/CARD-15 (called IBD-1) gene has been found in 30% of patients with CD (Ogura *et al.*, 2001). NOD2 is a cytoplasmic PRR for certain peptides found in bacterial cell walls. CD patients with this mutation may have a reduced ability to clear invasive bacteria. Indeed, there is evidence for microbial involvement in both forms of IBD, with a disturbed interaction between the mucosal immune system and the commensal gut microbiota being evident (Duchmann *et al.*, 1995). In both forms of IBD, there are large infiltrates of neutrophils in the inflamed gut mucosal tissue. The T-cell-response profiles associated with UC and CD are different: a Th1 pattern of cytokine formation develops in CD with increased production of TNF, interferon (IFN)-γ, IL-12, IL-6 and IL-1β, whereas UC more resembles a modified Th2 profile, where cytokines including IL-5 are upregulated, although IL-4 is not. In addition to this change in cytokine profile, intestinal B lymphocytes produce large amounts of IgG. TNF is expressed in the intestinal mucosa of patients with IBD and triggers inflammation via a nuclear factor kappa B (NFκB)-dependent signalling cascade. Many of the cytokines involved act on the signal transducers and activators of transcription (STAT) family. STAT-3 signalling has been found in UC and CD where it has been shown to be confined to areas of active inflammation, infiltrating macrophages and T cells. STAT-3 induces transcription of the pro-inflammatory cytokine IL-6, which can increase resistance of T cells to apoptosis, lengthening the chronicity of CD owing to the accumulation of reactive T cells. Other factors implicated in CD include the generation of matrix metalloproteinases, which can degrade extracellular matrices, causing ulceration and tissue destruction.

Chronic inflammation of the airways: asthma

Asthma is a chronic inflammatory disease of the lungs; it is classified into allergic and non-allergic asthma. Allergic asthma is the most common form in children, whereas in adults asthma without known allergen triggers is more common. The distinction can, however, be somewhat unclear. The prominent symptoms of asthma are chest tightness, wheeze, cough and dyspnoea. It is functionally characterized as reversible bronchial obstruction, caused by contraction of the smooth muscle layer in the mucosa of the bronchi, by mucus production, mucosal oedema and mucosal inflammation. Airway hyper-responsiveness (over-sensitivity and over-reactivity to stimuli) is typically present in asthma. Eosinophils have a central role, as do lymphocytes, and granulocytes other than eosinophils might be present to varying degrees. The inflammation might lead to destruction and shedding of the epithelial cell layer. Over time, structural changes take place in asthma, so-called airways remodelling; inflammation can become permanent and more severe, and reversibility of the airways obstruction is less complete. Variants in a number of genes have been implicated in asthma, including *ADAM33* (van Eerdewegh *et al.*, 2002). It is estimated that more than a dozen polymorphic genes regulate features of asthma like the inflammatory response, IgE synthesis, cytokine and chemokine production, airway remodelling and airway function (Fahy *et al.*, 2000). At the heart of the allergic reaction is the interaction between IgE molecules bound to specific receptors on mast cells and their corresponding allergens. When the IgE molecules are cross-linked by allergen, the mast cell is triggered to release the potent inflammatory mediators contained in its cytoplasmic granules and the allergic inflammatory response develops. This response has two phases, an early virtually immediate reaction, and a late response developing after several hours. Mast cells are the key cells in the early response, whereas eosinophils are the predominant cell in the late response. Increased levels of the Th2-cytokines IL-4, IL-5, IL-9 and IL-13 have been demonstrated in the asthmatic airway (Ray and Cohn, 1999). This Th2-driven inflammation has two arms, one via B cells activated by IL-4 to produce IgE, which triggers the mast-cell-mediated allergic inflammation, the other via IL-4-mediated, but mainly via IL-13-mediated, direct effects on epithelium and bronchial smooth muscle (Barrios *et al.*, 2006). TNF and 4-series LTs have also been reported to play an important role in severe asthma (van Oosterhout *et al.*, 2005).

Chronic inflammation of the skin: psoriasis

Psoriasis is a common inflammatory disease of the skin, although joint symptoms can also be a feature. There is a genetic susceptibility and associations with other inflammatory conditions. Streptococcal infections and physical trauma to the skin may also be involved. The pathophysiology involves an interaction between the immune system and the skin. There is an infiltrate of T lymphocytes into the dermis, formation of clusters of neutrophils in the epidermis, involvement of two or three layers of the epidermis in proliferation and a greatly accelerated but incomplete differentiation. Activation of the innate immune system by streptococcal products and, most likely, as yet unidentified factors, induces the release of cytokines including IFN-α and -γ. The cellular source of these cytokines is unclear but might be dendritic cells. These cytokines activate keratinocytes to proliferate and to produce angiogenic factors that induce proliferation of dermal microvessels.

Chronic inflammation of the vascular wall: atherosclerosis

Atherosclerosis, or 'hardening (or narrowing) of the arteries' is the major cause of cardiovascular disease. Endothelial dysfunction is the key underlying event and this is characterized by altered endothelial function, enhanced adhesion molecule expression and impaired endothelium-dependent vasodilator responses. Leucocytes become attached to the dysfunctional endothelium and subsequently accumulate within the sub-endothelial space. Monocyte-derived macrophages are converted to lipid-laden foam cells within the artery wall, giving rise to a lesion termed the fatty streak. The conversion of the fatty streak into a fibrous atheroscleritic plaque necessitates the recruitment and proliferation of vascular smooth muscle cells (Ross, 1999).

Atherosclerosis is now considered to be a chronic inflammatory disease, and at every stage of its evolution is characterized by monocyte/macrophage and T lymphocyte infiltration (Hallenbeck *et al.*, 2005; Hansson, 2005). The possible stimuli to this inflammatory process include oxidized low-density lipoproteins, homocysteine, free radicals generated from cigarette smoking and infectious microorganisms. The T-cell infiltrates are predominantly helper (i.e. $CD4^+$) cells and cells derived from human lesions react to antigens derived from oxidized low-density lipoproteins, heat-shock proteins and microorganisms (Hansson, 2005). The cytokine milieu within atherosclerotic lesions is thought to promote a Th1-dominated response associated with macrophage activation and the production of IFN-γ and IL-1β. The ongoing inflammation involves various growth factors and cytokines, which lead to intimal thickening by stimulating smooth muscle cell migration, proliferation and extracellular matrix generation.

Chronic inflammation of adipose tissue: obesity

Obesity is characterized by an expansion of the mass of adipose tissue and dramatic changes in its distribution in the body. A link between obesity and low-grade inflammation was first proposed by Hotamisligil *et al.* (1993) who showed that white adipose tissue synthesizes and releases TNF. The range of inflammatory proteins produced by adipose tissue is now known to be extremely wide and includes leptin, adiponectin, some acute phase proteins, cytokines (including IL-1, IL-6 and TNF), chemokines (including IL-8, MCP-1, RANTES (now known as chemokine (C-C motif) ligand (CCL) 5), and macrophage inflammatory protein-1α and -1β (now known as CCL3 and CCL4, respectively)), and complement factors (including C3) (Calder *et al.*, 2011). Obesity is associated with a chronic elevation of the circulating concentrations of inflammatory proteins including several acute-phase inflammatory proteins such as C-reactive protein (CRP), pro- and anti-inflammatory cytokines, and soluble adhesion molecules (Calder *et al.*, 2011).

Adipose tissue is a heterogeneous tissue composed of several cell types: mature adipocytes, pre-adipocytes, fibroblasts, endothelial cells, mast cells, granulocytes, lymphocytes and macrophages are all present. Because of the heterogeneity of cells in the adipose tissue, the cellular source of the inflammatory factors secreted by the tissue into the circulation remains unknown; however, both adipocytes and classic inflammatory cells, especially macrophages, seem likely to be involved. T lymphocytes seem to play a key early role in adipose tissue inflammation (Kintscher *et al.*, 2008). Many mediators synthesized by the adipose tissue are candidates to attract inflammatory cells. Leptin induces adhesion proteins, facilitating the migration of monocytes. Conversely, adiponectin may inhibit this process. MCP-1 is a strong chemoattractant and is thought to be a major player in macrophage accumulation within the adipose tissue. Local hypoxia could also play an important role in the attraction and retention of macrophages within the adipose tissue.

Common Features of Chronic Inflammatory Conditions and Mediators Involved

Although inflammation-induced tissue damage occurs in an organ-specific manner (joints, gut, lungs, skin, blood vessel wall, adipose tissue) in different diseases or conditions, there is some commonality amongst the responses seen in the different organs (summarized in Table 1.2). In general, the inflammatory response observed is normal but it occurs in the wrong context, which relates to inappropriate barrier function (epithelial or endothelial), inappropriate triggering (i.e. a response to a normally benign stimulus equivalent to a loss of immunological tolerance), lack of down-regulation to control the response and tissue destruction with a loss of function. In some cases, the inflammation is the result of exogenous triggers such as allergens or microbes. In other cases, it is due to tissue damage caused by endogenous

Table 1.2. A summary of the characteristics of selected inflammatory disease states. Modified with permission from Calder *et al.* (2009).

	Rheumatoid arthritis	Crohn's disease	Ulcerative colitis	Asthma	Psoriasis	Atherosclerosis	Obesity
Organ affected	Joints	Entire gastro-intestinal tract	Colon and rectum	Lungs	Skin	Vascular wall	Adipose tissue
Predisposing genetic factors	HLA-DR4 subtypes	NOD2, IBD locus	IBD locus, MUC-3, perhaps HLA-DR subtypes	ADAM33, Th2 gene cluster	PSORS1	Several	Not clear
Triggering factor(s)	Not known	Commensal gut microbes	Commensal gut microbes	Allergens, irritants	Skin streptococci	Endothelial injury, oxidized low-density lipoprotein	Energy intake in excess of expenditure
Clinical features	Joint swelling, pain and erosion	Gut ulceration, diarrhoea, abdominal pain, weight loss, malaise	Gut ulceration, bloody diarrhoea, abdominal pain	Wheeze, mucus, breathlessness, impaired lung function	Dry skin	Plaque formation – ultimately myocardial infarction, stroke etc. due to plaque rupture	Weight gain, insulin resistance
Cells involved	Th1 cells, fibroblasts, B cells, macrophages, synoviocytes	Th1 cells	Th1 and Th2 cells (Th2 dominant), granulocytes	Th2 cells, mast cells, eosinophils	Th1 cells, NK cells, granulocytes, keratinocytes	Macrophages, T cells, platelets, endothelial cells	Adipocytes, macrophages, T cells
Mediators involved	TNF, IL-1β, IL-6, IL-17, PGs, LTB_4, MMPs	TNF, IL-6, IL-12, PGs, MMPs	TNF, IL-5, IL-13, PGs	TNF, IL-5, IL-13, cysLTs	Th1 type cytokines, LTB_4, angiogenic factors	MCP-1 in plaque formation, MMPs in plaque rupture	MCP-1

Abbreviations: cysLTs, cysteinyl leukotrienes; HLA, human leucocyte antigen; IBD, inflammatory bowel disease; IL, interleukin; LT, leukotriene; MCP, monocyte chemoattractant protein; MMP, matrix metalloproteinase; PG, prostaglandin; Th, helper T cell; TNF, tumour necrosis factor.

molecules such as oxidized low-density lipoprotein. The involvement of different triggers is also reflected in the distinct associations with polymorphisms in receptors involved in 'pattern' recognition such as NOD2 in CD or with other molecules involved in specific adaptive immune responses such as HLA-DR subtypes in UC and RA (Table 1.2). Although trigger, localization and resulting clinical symptoms are different, many of the processes, cells and molecules involved in the actual inflammatory response are remarkably similar (Tables 1.2 and 1.3). Most, if not all, of the chronic inflammatory diseases are characterized by overproduction of cytokines (TNF, IL-1β, IL-6 and IFN-γ), chemokines (IL-8 and MCP-1), eicosanoids (PGE_2 and 4-series LTs) and matrix metalloproteinases. Elevated levels of these mediators act to amplify the inflammatory process (e.g. by attracting further inflammatory cells to the site) and contribute to tissue destruction (Fig. 1.1) and to the clinical symptoms observed. Many of these mediators are positively regulated through the transcription factor NFκB. The entry of inflammatory cells to sites of inflammatory activity is facilitated by the upregulation of adhesion molecules on the endothelium (see the Leucocyte–Endothelium Interactions in Inflammation section), a process that is promoted by inflammatory cytokines and by a range of inflammatory triggers, frequently acting through NFκB. The continuous process of tissue injury, healing and repair, owing to the release of cytokines, chemokines and growth factors by infiltrating inflammatory cells as well as resident tissue cells, results in tissue remodelling.

Why resolution of inflammation is absent or abnormal in so many pathophysiological processes remains largely unknown, although there are a number of mechanisms that might be involved. Firstly, persistent insult (i.e. chronic infection, continued exposure to triggering stimuli) could provide a continued pro-inflammatory stimulus. Secondly, the inflammatory response results in tissue damage and the consequent loss of barrier function may result in exposure to antigens and loss of tolerance to autoantigens or to components of the microbiota, which then provide a trigger to drive prolonged inflammation. Thirdly, local overproduction of survival factors such as IL-5, GM-CSF and IL-1β may result in prolonged survival and activity of granulocytes. Finally, there may be a deficiency in negative-feedback (control) mechanisms that leads to a loss of inflammatory control.

How to Measure Chronic Inflammation

Classic chronic inflammatory diseases such as RA, UC, CD, psoriasis and asthma are diagnosed on the basis of clinical history, examination or investigation of the likely affected region (where that is possible) and, in some cases, identification of general or specific inflammatory features. In most cases, a classification of disease severity can be made on the basis of a clinically accepted and validated scoring system. Thus, for diagonosis of RA, an examination of the joints and an evaluation of the number of swollen and tender joints and the extent of the swelling and tenderness and of the resulting loss of function (e.g. by measuring grip strength and duration of morning stiffness) can be made, along with X-rays of joints. The various data can be combined into scoring systems such as Ritchie's articular index and the American College of Rheumatology classification. For the diagnosis of IBD, information on abdominal pain and on bowel habit and stool appearance is collected, endoscopic examination of the intestinal mucosa performed, and assessment of secondary symptoms such as joint pain made; scoring systems such as Crohn's Disease Activity Index combine some of these using an algorithm that provides different weightings to each observation. For the diagnosis of asthma, a history of symptoms (e.g. shortness of breath, wheezing) is taken and lung function is measured by spirometry. Skin prick tests may be made to identify immune sensitization to suspected allergic triggers, lung function in response to a challenge may be performed, and, where a food trigger is suspected, blinded food challenges may be performed. As well as being diagnostic, in many cases these approaches are used to identify the efficacy of any therapeutic

Table 1.3. A selection of inflammatory mediators. (Note that neither the listing nor the characteristics are exhaustive.)

Type of mediator	Example(s)	Important source(s)	Major role(s)
Amino acid metabolite	Histamine	Basophils, mast cells	Bronchoconstriction, bronchial smooth muscle contraction, vasodilation, separation of endothelial cells, pain and itching, runny nose
Reactive oxygen species	Superoxide	Neutrophils, eosinophils, monocytes, macrophages	Bacterial killing
	Hydrogen peroxide	Neutrophils, eosinophils, monocytes, macrophages	Bacterial killing
Chemokines and cytokines	IL-1β	Mononuclear phagocytes	Fever, neutrophil activation, Th1 cell activation, muscle proteolysis, adipose lipolysis, hepatic acute phase protein synthesis
	IL-2	Th1 cells	Th1 cell proliferation, inhibition of Th2 proliferation
	IL-4	Th2 cells	IgE class switching in B cells
	IL-5	Th2 cells	Eosinophil activation
	IL-6	Mononuclear phagocytes, endothelial cells, T cells	Fever, neutrophil activation, T-cell activation, muscle proteolysis, adipose lipolysis, hepatic acute phase protein synthesis, inhibition of TNF and IL-1β synthesis
	IL-8 (CXCL8)	Endothelial cells	Neutrophil and basophil recruitment
	IL-10	Mononuclear phagocytes, T cells	Inhibition of antigen presentation, inhibition of TNF and IL-1β production, inhibition of Th1 cell activation
	IL-12	Mononuclear phagocytes	Th1 cell activation
	IL-17	Th17 cells	Cytokine and chemokine release
	IL-18	Macrophages	Th1 cell activation
	IL-23	Macrophages, dendritic cells	Promotes Th17 cell development
	IFN-γ	Th1 cells	Macrophage activation, promotes antigen presentation, Th1 cell proliferation, inhibition of Th2 proliferation
	TNF	Mononuclear phagocytes, Th1 cells	Fever, Th1 cell activation, muscle proteolysis, adipose lipolysis, hepatic acute phase protein synthesis
	TGF-β	Many cell types	Inhibits T cell and macrophage activity
	MIP-1α (CCL3)	Macrophages	Neutrophil recruitment and activation
	MCP-1 (CCL2)	Monocytes, macrophages, dendritic cells	Monocyte recruitment
	IP-10 (CXCL10)	Monocytes, endothelial cells, fibroblasts	Monocyte, macrophage, T cell, NK cell and dendritic cell recruitment

Continued

Table 1.3. Continued.

Type of mediator	Example(s)	Important source(s)	Major role(s)
	RANTES (CCL5)	T cells, fibroblasts	Eosinophil, basophil and T cell recruitment
Lipid mediators	PGE_2	Mononuclear phagocytes	Fever, pain, vasodilation, inhibition of TNF and IL-1β production, inhibition of Th1 cell activity, promotes IgE production by B cells
	PGD_2	Neutrophils, mast cells	Eosinophil, basophil and Th2 cell recruitment, vasodilation, bronchoconstriction
	LTB_4	Many leucocytes	Neutrophil and monocyte recruitment, promotes release of reactive oxygen species, promotes production of TNF and IL-1β
	Cysteinyl LTs (LTC_4, LTD_4, LTE_4)	Many leucocytes	Mast cell and eosinophil activation, bronchoconstriction, vasodilation, mucous production
	Platelet-activating factor	Many leucocytes, platelets, endothelial cells	Bronchoconstriction, vascular permeability, leucocyte recruitment, promotes release of reactive oxygen species
Acute phase proteins	C-reactive protein	Liver	Activates complement system
	Serum amyloid A	Liver	Leucocyte recruitment
	Fibrinogen	Liver	Coagulation
Soluble adhesion molecules	sVCAM-1	Endothelial cells	
	sICAM-1	Endothelial cells, leucocytes	
	sE-selectin	Endothelial cells	
	sP-selectin	Platelets	
Antibodies	IgE	B cells	Degranulation of mast cells and eosinophils

Abbreviations: CCL, chemokine (C-C motif) ligand; CXCL, chemokine (C-X-C motif) ligand; ICAM, intercellular adhesion molecule; IFN, interferon; IgE, immunoglobulin E; IL, interleukin; IP10, interferon gamma induced protein 10; LT, leukotriene; MCP, monocyte chemoattractant peptide; MIP, macrophage inflammatory peptide; NK, natural killer; PG, prostaglandin; RANTES, Regulated on Activation, Normal T Expressed and Secreted; TGF, transforming growth factor; Th; helper T cell; TNF, tumor necrosis factor; VCAM, vascular cell-adhesion molecule.

intervention. As such, these measures may be useful to examine the anti-inflammatory, or indeed therapeutic, activity of lifestyle interventions including changes in diet or use of nutritional supplements. However, these assessments focus upon the pathological end result of chronic inflammation at the specific site of inflammatory activity (e.g. the joints in RA, the gastrointestinal mucosa in IBD and the lungs in asthma) rather than upon the inflammation itself. To assess the inflammation either for diagnostic purposes or for evaluating the effect of an intervention, investigations can be made in blood and in material taken from the site of inflammation, which is usually more difficult to acquire. The measurements made may be of generic markers of inflammation or of some marker specific to the inflammatory condition.

Chronic inflammatory conditions typically result in an elevation in the total number of leucocytes in the bloodstream (leukocytosis) and in the numbers of specific subsets of leucocytes (e.g. neutrophils, eosinophils). There are established normal ranges for blood leucocyte numbers and 'leucocyte counts and differentials' are routinely performed in clinical laboratories and are used as a diagnostic tool. The presence and level of activation markers on the surface of various leucocyte subsets are modified with chronic inflammation and can be monitored as readouts of inflammatory drive. Chronic inflammatory conditions also result in elevated concentrations of various inflammatory mediators in the bloodstream, largely as 'spill-over' from the sites of inflammatory activity. Thus, elevated plasma concentrations of several inflammatory cytokines such as TNF and IL-6, of chemokines such as IL-8 and MCP-1, and of shed (soluble) adhesion molecules such as vascular cell adhesion molecule (VCAM)-1, ICAM-1 and E-selectin are typically seen. Because cytokines like TNF and IL-6 regulate hepatic acute phase protein synthesis, in chronic inflammatory conditions the plasma concentrations of positive acute phase proteins such as CRP, serum amyloid A and fibrinogen are elevated above normal, whereas the concentrations of negative acute phase proteins such as albumin and ceruloplasmin are decreased. The leucocytes, leucocyte subsets and inflammatory mediators that are elevated in the bloodstream are generic markers of inflammation and are, in general, not specific to inflammation at a particular body location or to a specific inflammatory condition. There may, however, be some more specific assocations such as elevated eosinophils and the presence of allergen-specific IgE with asthma. Furthermore, there are some blood markers that are fairly disease specific. Examples are autoantibodies termed rheumatoid factor seen in many, though not all, patients with RA and anti-*Saccharomyces cerevisae* antibodies seen in many patients with CD. Thus, it is evident that chronic inflammatory conditions result in elevated numbers of leucocytes in the bloodstream and in elevated protein concentrations in the blood plasma. The increase in fibrinogen concentration affects erythrocytes (red blood cells); fibrinogen causes erythrocytes to clump together. As a result, the rate at which erythrocytes settle (called the erythrocyte sedimentation rate) when blood is left standing is increased. Thus, erythrocyte sedimentation rate can be used as a measure of inflammation.

Obviously, in a chronic inflammatory condition, the major site of activity is at the inflammatory foci and as indicated earlier at these sites there is significant leucocyte infiltration, with the presence of activated leucocytes and of high concentrations of inflammatory mediators including some not so readily measured in the circulation such as lipid mediators and reactive oxygen species. Biopsies of these affected sites reveal significant information about the nature of the inflammatory activity. Examples of measurements that can be made, often for research purposes rather than as part of clinical diagnosis or monitoring, are thymic stromal lymphopoietin in skin lesions in atopic dermatitis; inflammatory cytokines such as TNF and IL-6 and inflammatory eicosanoids such as PGE_2 in synovial fluid in RA; eosinophils, tell-tale Th2-type cytokines such as IL-5, and cysteinyl-LTs in bronchoalveolar lavage fluid in asthma; and inflammatory cytokine messenger RNA in gut mucosal biopsies in IBD. In terms of monitoring inflammation, another useful feature of gastrointestinal inflammation such as seen in IBD or in food allergy, is the appearance of inflammatory mediators in faecal matter. Thus, in such conditions, markers such as calprotectin and eotaxin, emanating from mucosal inflammation, can be measured in aqueous faecal extracts.

Atherosclerosis and obesity represent conditions of weak (so-called 'low-grade') but chronic inflammation, as opposed to the 'high-grade' chronic inflammation seen in diseases like RA, IBD, asthma and psoriasis where the inflammation is central to the pathological tissue damage and directly results in the clinical signs and symptoms. Nevertheless, elevated numbers of leucocytes in the bloodstream, elevated plasma concentrations of inflammatory mediators such as cytokines, chemokines and soluble adhesion molecules, and elevated plasma concentrations of positive acute phase proteins such as CRP are seen in both atherosclerosis and obesity. Large population studies have demonstrated that the concentrations of CRP, IL-6 and sICAM-1 are predictive of the development of future cardiovascular disease, of having a cardiovascular event, and of cardiovascular mortality (Hwang *et al.*, 1997; Ridker *et al.*, 1998, 2000, 2001; Blake and Ridker, 2001). Although the concentrations of a range of cytokines, chemokines, soluble adhesion molecules, acute phase proteins and adipose-derived inflammatory proteins called adipokines increase with increasing body mass index, they differ according to adipose tissue distribution (Calder *et al.*, 2011). This is probably because visceral adipose tissue seems to release higher concentrations of inflammatory mediators than subcutaneous. Adipose tissue biopsies can be used to assess inflammation in the context of obesity: there is increased macrophage infiltration and increased inflammatory gene expression in biopsy material from obese compared with normal-weight persons.

Thus, there are many approaches to assessing inflammation. Most often these rely upon measuring cell numbers or activation state in the bloodstream or the concentrations of generic inflammatory mediators, usually proteins, in the blood plasma (or serum). There are some disease-specific markers that can be measured in the bloodstream, whereas both generic and disease-specific inflammatory markers can be measured in biopsy material taken from the site of inflammatory activity in persons with a chronic inflammatory condition.

Factors Affecting Inflammation

As indicated earlier, high-grade chronic inflammatory conditions seem to result from the co-incidence of genetic and environmental factors. For example, in CD these may be a mutation in NOD2 and breakdown in the gastrointestinal epithelium, exposing the immune system to normally benign commensal bacteria. There follows an inability to dampen the resulting immune reaction and, ultimately, this uncontrolled immune response translates into an ongoing state of inflammation with infiltrating leucocytes and their activation products within the gastrointestinal mucosa causing tissue damage and breakdown. For most, perhaps all, chronic inflammatory conditions neither the predisposing genetic factors nor the environmental factors are fully understood. Nevertheless, it makes sense that those without the genetic predisposition but with the environmental factor(s) or those without the environmental factor(s) but with the genetic predisposition might not develop the condition or might develop only a mild form. Furthermore, those without either the genetic predisposition or the environmental factor(s) would not be likely to develop the condition at all. High-grade chronic inflammatory diseases are treated with anti-inflammatory therapies. Obviously these therapies target the inflammatory processes involved in the disease and where the therapies work they reduce the inflammation and improve the pathology and the clinical signs. For example, corticosteroids reduce joint pain in patients with RA. In some conditions the environmental factor is a specific trigger to the inflammation. As an example, allergic asthma is due to, and is induced by, exposure to a specific allergen such as those present in pollen, house dust mites or peanuts. In this case, the inflammation and the exaggeration of the major disease symptom (airways dysfunction) can be prevented by avoiding the allergic trigger.

Amongst the chronic inflammatory conditions, the extent of the inflammation and of the pathological tissue damage and the severity of the clinical signs vary amongst patients. This probably relates to variations in the underlying genetic predisposing factor and/or in the exposure to the environmental factor(s) that may be a trigger, as in allergic asthma, or may be 'permissive' as for epithelial breakdown and exposure and reaction to commensal bacteria in IBD. There may also be some factors that are able to modify high-grade chronic inflammatory responses; these might include coincident oxidative stress, perhaps as a result of smoking or low dietary intake of antioxidants, ageing and the presence of certain infectious agents. A further modifying factor may be variations in the genes encoding proteins involved in the inflammatory response itself. Thus, the combination of genetic predisposition and environmental factor(s) results ultimately in a poorly controlled inflammatory response; the extent of certain aspects of this response is determined in part by variations, often single nucleotide polymorphisms (SNPs), in the genes encoding the inflammatory proteins involved in the response. SNPs are variations in DNA sequence at a single nucleotide that occur in at least 1% of the population. They can occur in both coding and non-coding regions of the genome. It is estimated that the human genome contains 3 million SNPs. Genotype is a description of the allele pair present at a given site in the genome, and typically there will be three possible genotypes (e.g. AA, AG and GG). There are variations in allele frequencies and genotypes among different human populations because certain alleles and genotypes might have offered an evolutionary advantage in one geographical region and not in another. SNPs within the coding sequence may produce a protein with a different amino acid sequence and so function. SNPs that are not in protein-coding regions may affect transcription-factor binding or gene splicing or the sequence of non-coding RNA and as a result the gene expression, and hence the level of the encoded protein, may differ among individuals with different genotypes. It is likely that SNPs occur frequently in regions of the genome encoding inflammatory proteins (e.g. cytokines, chemokines, adhesion molecules, acute phase proteins and receptors), encoding enzymes responsible for the synthesis of non-peptide inflammatory mediators (e.g. COX and LOX enzymes, and NADPH oxidase) and encoding regulatory proteins such as transcription factors. A number of these SNPs will be of functional significance, meaning that individuals with different genotypes will produce different levels of a particular inflammatory mediator in response to a given stimulus or trigger than other individuals (Jacob *et al.*, 1990; Messer *et al.*, 1991; Fishmann *et al.*, 1998; Santilla *et al.*, 1998). Thus genotype can influence the plasma concentration of inflammatory markers (Stuber *et al.*, 1996; Fishmann *et al.*, 1998; Kelbermann *et al.*, 2004). For example, the polymorphism at the +252 position of the TNFB gene significantly affected plasma TNF concentrations in patients with sepsis (Stuber *et al.*, 1996). The genotype of certain inflammatory genes has been associated with risk or severity of outcome in inflammatory disease (Wilson *et al.*, 1994, 1995).

Low-grade chronic inflammation is influenced by a number of factors, the most obvious perhaps being the presence of excess adipose tissue or of cardiovascular disease. Thus, the plasma concentrations of cytokines, chemokines, soluble adhesion molecules and positive acute phase proteins increase with body mass index, are higher in obese than normal-weight people, decrease with weight loss through either surgery or lifestyle change and are higher in those with cardiovascular disease (Calder *et al.*, 2009, 2011). As indicated above, genotype influences plasma concentrations of inflammatory mediators: for example, the G to C polymorphism at the -174 position of the IL-6 gene was reported to influence significantly the plasma IL-6 concentrations (Fishmann *et al.*, 1998). Other factors identified to affect low-grade inflammation are:

- Sex, with some studies reporting differences in inflammatory responses between men and women;
- Age, with increased plasma concentrations of inflammatory mediators with increasing age;
- Being physically fit, which results in lower plasma concentrations of inflammatory mediators;
- Cigarette smoking, with higher plasma concentrations of inflammatory mediators seen in smokers than in non-smokers;
- Diet, with a number of dietary factors modifying inflammatory mediator concentrations through different mechanisms including altering oxidative stress, regulating inflammatory signalling pathways and providing substrates for synthesis of mediators (Calder *et al.*, 2009, 2011).

Finally, there is increasing evidence that there is an influence of the gut microbiota on inflammatory processes, particularly within the gastrointestinal tract (e.g. as in IBD), but perhaps also systemically (Lomax and Calder, 2009; Chow *et al.*, 2011). Studies have revealed that differences in gut microbiota occur in atopic dermatitis and in obese people (Ley *et al.*, 2006; Penders *et al.*, 2007; Chow *et al.*, 2011; Delzenne and Cani, 2011). The precise causal role of the altered bacterial profile and the mechanisms involved remain to be established, however. Figure 1.2 depicts

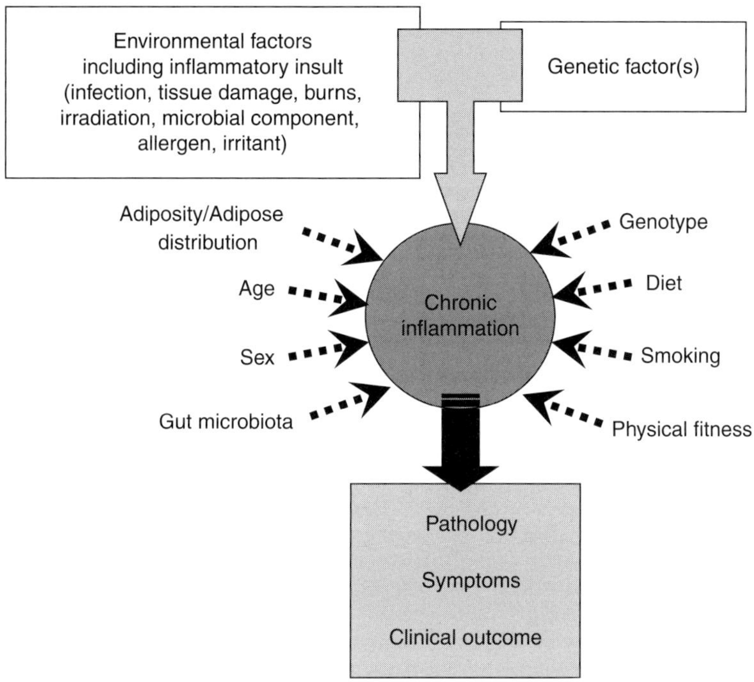

Fig. 1.2. The triggering and modifying factors of chronic inflammation. The key predisposing factors are shown in the upper two boxes. The modifying factors are shown with dotted arrows. The importance of the different factors will vary between different situations.

the various predisposing and modifying factors of chronic inflammation.

Summary and Conclusions

Inflammation is a stereotypical physiological response to infections and tissue injury; it initiates pathogen killing as well as tissue repair processes and helps to restore homeostasis at infected or damaged sites. Acute inflammatory reactions are usually self-limiting and resolve rapidly. This involves the activation of negative feedback mechanisms such as the secretion of immunoregulatory cytokines (e.g. IL-10 and TGF-β), inhibition of pro-inflammatory signalling cascades, receptor shedding and activation of regulatory cells. Inflammatory responses that fail to regulate themselves can become chronic and contribute to the perpetuation and progression of disease. Characteristics typical of chronic inflammatory responses include loss of barrier function, responsiveness to a normally benign stimulus, infiltration of inflammatory cells into compartments where they are not normally found in such high numbers, and overproduction of oxidants, cytokines, chemokines, eicosanoids and matrix metalloproteinases. The levels of these mediators amplify the inflammatory response, are destructive and contribute to the clinical symptoms. Irrespective of the nature of the stimulus and the site of the inflammatory activity, common cells, principally originating as blood leucocytes, and chemical mediators are produced. These mediators include amino acid derivatives, reactive oxygen specices, chemokines, cytokines, adhesion molecules, proteases, acute phase proteins, eicosanoids, resolvins and others. Markers of inflammation can be measured in blood and in biopsy material taken from the site of inflammatory activity. A number of factors, in addition to predisposing genetic factors and the inflammatory stimulus or insult, determine the extent of the inflammatory response and the nature and severity of the tissue damage caused.

References

Aderem, A. and Ulevitch, R.J. (2000) Toll-like receptors in the induction of the innate immune response. *Nature* 406, 782–787.

Bandeira-Melo, C., Bozza, P.T. and Weller, P.F. (2002) The cellular biology of eosinophil eicosanoid formation and function. *Journal of Allergy and Clinical Immunology* 109, 393–400.

Barrios, R.J., Kheradmand, F., Batts, L. and Corry, D.B. (2006) Asthma: pathology and pathophysiology. *Archives of Pathology and Laboratory Medicine* 130, 447–451.

Blake, G.J. and Ridker, P.M. (2001) Novel clinical markers of vascular wall inflammation. *Circulation Research* 89, 763–771.

Calder, P.C., Albers, R., Antoine, J.M., Blum, S., Bourdet-Sicard, R., *et al.* (2009) Inflammatory disease processes and interactions with nutrition. *British Journal of Nutrition* 101 Suppl 1, S1–S45.

Calder, P.C., Ahluwalia, N., Brouns, F., Buetler, T., Clement, K., *et al.* (2011) Dietary factors and low-grade inflammation in relation to overweight and obesity. *British Journal of Nutrition* 106 Suppl 3, S5–S78.

Chow, J., Tang, H. and Mazmanian, S.K. (2011) Pathobionts of the gastrointestinal microbiota and inflammatory disease. *Current Opinion in Immunology* 23, 470–480.

Delzenne, N.M. and Cani, P.D. (2011) Interaction between obesity and the gut microbiota: relevance in nutrition. *Annual Review in Nutrition* 31, 15–31.

Duchmann, R., Kaiser, I., Hermann, E., Mayet, W., Ewe, K. *et al.* (1995) Tolerance exists towards resident intestinal flora but is broken in active inflammatory bowel disease (IBD). *Clinical and Experimental Immunology* 102, 448–455.

Fahy, J.V., Corry, D.B. and Boushey, H.A. (2000) Airway inflammation and remodeling in asthma. *Current Opinion in Pulmonary Medicine* 6, 15–20.

Farrell, R.J. and Peppercorn, M.A. (2002) Ulcerative colitis. *Lancet* 359, 331–340.

Firestein, G.S. (2003) Evolving concepts of rheumatoid arthritis. *Nature* 423, 356–361.

Fishmann, D., Faulds, G., Jeffery, R., Mohamed-Ali, V., Yudkin, J.S., *et al.* (1998) The effect of novel polymorphisms in the interleukin-6 (IL-6) gene on IL-6 transcription and plasma IL-6 levels, and an association with systemic-onset juvenile chronic arthritis. *Journal of Clinical Investigation* 102, 1369–1376.

Hallenbeck, J.M., Hansson, G.K. and Becker, K.J. (2005) Immunology of ischemic vascular disease: plaque to attack. *Trends in Immunology* 26, 550–556.

Hansson, G.K. (2005) Inflammation, atherosclerosis, and coronary heart disease. *New England Journal of Medicine* 352, 1685–1695.

Hickey, M.J. and Kubes, P. (2009) Intravascular immunity: the host-pathogen encounter in blood vessels. *Nature Reviews Immunology* 9, 364–375.

Hogan, S.P., Rosenberg, H.F., Moqbel, R., Phipps, S., Foster, P.S., *et al.* (2008) Eosinophils: biological properties and role in health and disease. *Clinical and Experimental Allergy* 38, 709–750.

Hotamisligil, G.S., Shargill, N.S. and Spiegelman, B.M. (1993) Adipose expression of tumor necrosis factor-alpha: direct role in obesity-linked insulin resistance. *Science* 259, 87–91.

Hwang, S.J., Ballantyne, C.M., Sharrett, A.R., Smith, L.C., Davis, C.E., *et al.* (1997) Circulating adhesion molecules VCAM-1, ICAM-1, and E-selectin in carotid atherosclerosis and incident coronary heart disease cases: the Atherosclerosis Risk in Communities (ARIC) study. *Circulation* 96, 4219–4225.

Jacob, C.O., Fronek, Z., Lewis, G.D., Koo, M., Hansen, J.A., *et al.* (1990) Heritable major histocompatibility complex class II-associated differences in production of tumor necrosis factor alpha: relevance to genetic predisposition to systemic lupus erythematosus. *Proceedings of the National Academy of Sciences of the USA* 87, 1233–1237.

Kelberman, D., Fife, M., Rockman, M.V., Brull, D.J., Woo, P., *et al.* (2004) Analysis of common IL-6 promoter SNP variants and the AnTn tract in humans and primates and effects on plasma IL-6 levels following coronary artery bypass graft surgery. *Biochimica et Biophysica Acta* 1688, 160–167.

Kintscher, U., Hartge, M., Hess, K., Foryst-Ludwig, A., Clemenz, M., *et al.* (2008) T-lymphocyte infiltration in visceral adipose tissue: a primary event in adipose tissue inflammation and the development of obesity-mediated insulin resistance. *Arteriosclerosis Thrombosis and Vascular Biology* 28, 1304–1310.

Lee, D.M. and Weinblatt, M.E. (2001) Rheumatoid arthritis. *Lancet* 358, 903–911.

Ley, R.E., Turnbaugh, P.J., Klein, S. and Gordon, J.I. (2006) Microbial ecology: human gut microbes associated with obesity. *Nature* 444, 1022–1023.

Lomax, A.R. and Calder, P.C. (2009) Probiotics, immune function, infection and inflammation: a review of the evidence from studies conducted in humans. *Current Pharmaceutical Design* 15, 1428–1518.

McGeachy, M.J. and Cua, D.J. (2008) Th17 cell differentiation: the long and winding road. *Immunity* 28, 445–453.

Messer, G., Spengler, U., Jung, M.C., Honold, G., Blömer, K., *et al.* (1991) Polymorphic structure of the tumor necrosis factor (TNF) locus: an NcoI polymorphism in the first intron of the human TNF-beta gene correlates with a variant amino acid in position 26 and a reduced level of TNF-beta production. *Journal of Experimental Medicine* 173, 209–219.

Metcalfe, D.D., Baram, D. and Mekori, Y.A. (1997) Mast cells. *Physiological Reviews* 77, 1033–1079.

Mosser, D.M. and Edwards, J.P. (2008) Exploring the full spectrum of macrophage activation. *Nature Reviews Immunology* 8, 958–969.

Muller, W.A. (2011) Mechanisms of leukocyte transendothelial migration. *Annual Review in Pathology* 6, 323–344.

Nakanishi, K. (2010) Basophils as APC in Th2 response in allergic inflammation and parasite infection. *Current Opinion in Immunology* 22, 814–820.

Nathan, C. (2006) Neutrophils and immunity: challenges and opportunities. *Nature Reviews Immunology* 6, 173–182.

Ogura, Y., Bonen, D.K., Inohara, N., Nicolae, D.L., Chen, F.F., *et al.* (2001) A frameshift mutation in NOD2 associated with susceptibility to Crohn's disease. *Nature* 411, 603–606.

Panayi, G.S., Lanchbury, J.S. and Kingsley, G.H. (1992) The importance of the T cell in initiating and maintaining the chronic synovitis of rheumatoid arthritis. *Arthritis and Rheumatism* 35, 729–735.

Penders, J., Stobberingh, E.E., van den Brandt, P.A. and Thijs, C. (2007) The role of the intestinal microbiota in the development of atopic disorders. *Allergy* 62, 1223–1236.

Ray, A. and Cohn, L. (1999) Th2 cells and GATA-3 in asthma: new insights into the regulation of airway inflammation. *Journal of Clinical Investigations* 104, 985–993.

Ridker, P.M., Hennekens, C.H., Roitman-Johnson, B., Stampfer, M.J. and Allen, J. (1998) Plasma concentration of soluble intercellular adhesion molecule 1 and risks of future myocardial infarction in apparently healthy men. *Lancet* 351, 88–92.

Ridker, P.M., Rifai, N., Stampfer, M.J. and Hennekens, C.H. (2000) Plasma concentration of interleukin-6 and the risk of future myocardial infarction among apparently healthy men. *Circulation* 101, 1767–1772.

Ridker, P.M., Buring, J.E. and Rifai, N.I. (2001) Soluble P-selectin and the risk of future cardiovascular events. *Circulation* 103, 491–495.

Ross, R. (1999) Mechanisms of disease – atherosclerosis – an inflammatory disease. *New England Journal of Medicine* 340, 115-126.

Rothenberg, M.E. and Hogan, S.P. (2006) The eosinophil. *Annual Review in Immunology* 24, 147–174.

Sakaguchi, S., Miyara, M., Costantino, C.M. and Hafler, D.A. (2010) FOXP3+ regulatory T cells in the human immune system. *Nature Reviews Immunology* 10, 490–500.

Santtila, S., Savinainen, K. and Hurme, M. (1998) Presence of the IL-1RA allele 2 (IL1RN*2) is associated with enhanced IL-1beta production in vitro. *Scandinavian Journal of Immunology* 47, 195–198.

Schmidt, E.P., Lee, W.L., Zemans, R.L., Yamashita, C. and Downey, G.P. (2011) On, around, and through: neutrophil-endothelial interactions in innate immunity. *Physiology* 26, 334–347.

Schroeder, J.T. (2009) Basophils beyond effector cells of allergic inflammation. *Advances in Immunology* 101, 123–161.

Segal, A.W. (2005) How neutrophils kill microbes. *Annual Review in Immunology* 23, 197–223.

Shanahan, F. (2002) Crohn's disease. *Lancet* 359, 62–69.

Steinman, L. (2007) A brief history of T(H)17, the first major revision in the T(H)1/T(H)2 hypothesis of T cell-mediated tissue damage. *Nature Medicine* 13, 139–145.

Stuber, F., Petersen, M., Bokelmann, F. and Schade, U. (1996) A genomic polymorphism within the tumor necrosis factor locus influences plasma tumor necrosis factor-alpha concentrations and outcome of patients with severe sepsis. *Critical Care Medicine* 24, 381–384.

Van Eerdewegh, P., Little, R.D., Dupuis, J., Del Mastro, R.G., Falls, K., *et al.* (2002) Association of the ADAM33 gene with asthma and bronchial hyperresponsiveness. *Nature* 418, 426–430.

van Oosterhout, A.J. and Bloksma, N. (2005) Regulatory T-lymphocytes in asthma. *European Respiratory Journal* 26, 918–932.

Weyand, C.M., Seyler, T.M. and Goronzy, J.J. (2005) B cells in rheumatoid synovitis. *Arthritis Research and Therapeutics* 7, Suppl. 3, S9–S12.

Wilson, A.G., Gordon, C., di Giovine, F.S., de Vries, N., van de Putte, L.B., *et al.* (1994) A genetic association between systemic lupus erythematosus and tumor necrosis factor alpha. *European Journal of Immunology* 24, 191–195.

Wilson, A.G., di Giovine, F.S. and Duff, G.W. (1995) Genetics of tumour necrosis factor-alpha in autoimmune, infectious, and neoplastic diseases. *Journal of Inflammation* 45, 1–12.

Witko-Sarsat, V., Rieu, P., Descamps-Latscha, B., Lesavre, P. and Halbwachs-Mecarelli, L. (2000) Neutrophils: molecules, functions and pathophysiological aspects. *Laboratory Investigations* 80, 617–653.

Zhou, L., Chong, M.M. and Littman, D.R. (2009) Plasticity of CD4+ T cell lineage differentiation. *Immunity* 30, 646–655.

Ziegler-Heitbrock, L. (2007) The CD14+ CD16+ blood monocytes: their role in infection and inflammation. *Journal of Leukocyte Biology* 81, 584–592.

2 Dietary Fats and Inflammation

P.C. Calder*
Human Development and Health Academic Unit,
University of Southampton, UK

Introduction

Long-chain fatty acids have hydrocarbon chain lengths of 12 or more carbons. They are naturally occurring in the human diet; they circulate in the bloodstream either as components of more complex lipids within lipoproteins or 'free'; they are stored within adipose tissue and they are present in cell membranes, playing an important structural and functional role (Calder and Burdge, 2004). The diet, bloodstream, adipose tissue and cell membranes contain a number of different fatty acids, each present in different concentrations and relative amounts (Table 2.1).

* Author, p.c.calder@soton.ac.uk

Table 2.1. Long chain fatty acid nomenclature and common sources.

Systematic name	Trivial name	Shorthand notation	Abbreviation	Common sources
Dodecanoic	Lauric	12:0		Milk, coconut oil
Tetradecanoic	Myristic	14:0		Milk
Hexadecanoic	Palmitic	16:0		Milk, eggs, animal fats, meat, cocoa butter, palm oil (other vegetable oils contain lesser amounts, fish oils
Octadecanoic	Stearic	18:0		Milk, eggs, animal fats, meat, cocoa butter
cis 9-Hexadecenoic	Palmitoleic	16:1n-7		Desaturation of palmitic acid, fatty fish, fish oils
cis 9-Octadecenoic	Oleic	18:1n-9		Desaturation of stearic acid, milk, eggs, animal fats, meat, cocoa butter, most vegetable oils especially olive oil
trans 9-Octadecenoic	Elaidic	-		Biohydrogenation of vegetable oils
trans 11-Octadecenoic	*Trans* Vaccenic	-		Milk (ruminant), animal (ruminant) fats
cis 9, *cis* 12-Octadecadienoic	Linoleic	18:2n-6		Cannot be synthesized in animals, some milks, eggs, animal fats, meat, most vegetable oils especially corn, sunflower, safflower and soybean oils, green leaves
cis 9, *trans* 11-Octadecadienoic	9, 11 Conjugated linoleic acid	-	CLA	Milk (ruminant), meat (ruminant)
All *cis* 9, 12, 15-Octadecatrienoic	α-Linolenic	18:3n-3	ALNA	Cannot be synthesized in animals, green leaves, some vegetable oils especially rapeseed, soybean and flaxseed oils, flaxseeds, some nuts
All *cis* 6, 9, 12-Octadecatrienoic	γ-Linolenic	18:3n-6	GLA	Synthesized from linoleic acid, borage and evening primrose oils
All *cis* 6, 9, 12, 15-Octatetraenoic	Stearidonic acid	18:4n-3		Synthesized from ALNA, echium oil, genetically modified soybean oil
All *cis* 8, 11, 14-Eicosatrienoic	Dihomo-γ-linolenic	20:3n-6	DGLA	Synthesized from GLA
All *cis* 5, 8, 11, 14-Eicosatetraenoic	Arachidonic	20:4n-6	ARA	Synthesized from linoleic acid via GLA and DGLA, meat, milk, some algal oils, fish oils
All *cis* 5, 8, 11, 14, 17-Eicosapentaenoic	Eicosapentaenoic	20:5n-3	EPA	Synthesized from ALNA, seafood especially fatty fish, fish oils
All *cis* 7, 10, 13, 16, 19-Docosapentaenoic	Docosapentaenoic	22:5n-3	DPA	Synthesized from ALNA via EPA, seafood especially fatty fish, fish oils
All *cis* 4, 7, 10, 13, 16, 19-Docosahexaenoic	Docosahexaenoic	22:6n-3	DHA	Synthesized from ALNA via EPA and DPA, seafood especially fatty fish, fish oils, some algal oils

Fatty acids within the body can come intact from the diet or can be synthesized within the body from non-lipid or lipid precursors (Fig. 2.1). Although all fatty acids have a generic structure (a hydrocarbon chain terminated by a methyl group at one end of the chain and a carboxyl group at the other), there are several fatty acid families distinguished by structural characteristics. Their characteristics are:

- The absence or presence of double bonds within the hydrocarbon chain (distinguishing saturated and unsaturated fatty acids);
- The presence of a single or multiple double bonds within the hydrocarbon chain (distinguishing monounsaturated and polyunsaturated fatty acids);
- The configuration of the double bonds within the hydrocarbon chain (distinguishing *cis* and *trans* fatty acids);
- The position of the double bonds within the hydrocarbon chain (distinguishing omega (n-)9, n-6 and n-3 fatty acids; the omega classification refers to the carbon on which the first double bond is found, counting the methyl terminus carbon as number 1).

Fatty acids have systematic and common names, but are frequently described by a shorthand nomenclature that denotes the number of carbons and double bonds in the hydrocarbon chain and, in the case of unsaturated fatty acids, the omega classification (Table 2.1). Figure 2.1 shows the metabolic relationships among the different long chain fatty acids, whereas Table 2.1 lists typical dietary sources. Two fatty acids, linoleic (18:2n-6) and α-linolenic (18:3n-3; ALNA), cannot be synthesized in humans and are termed essential fatty acids. Because the composition of the diet differs amongst different people, there is significant variation in the intake of individual fatty acids within the population. However, typically, saturated fatty acids and oleic acid (18:1n-9) are consumed in the greatest amounts (several tens of grams per day), followed by linoleic acid (about 10g/day) and then ALNA (about 1g/day). Very long chain (i.e. ≥20 carbon) highly unsaturated fatty acids are consumed in much lower amounts, typically tens to hundreds of milligrams per day.

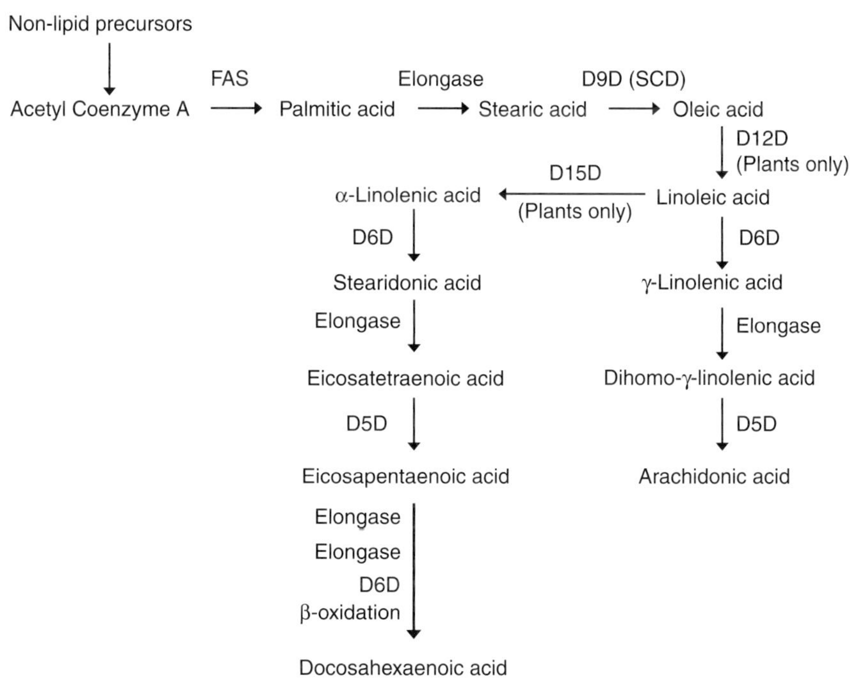

Fig. 2.1. The pathway of biosynthesis of fatty acids. DXD, delta-X desaturase; FAS, fatty acid synthase; SCD, stearoyl CoA desaturase.

Low versus High Fat Diets and Inflammation

It is considered that a high-fat diet will increase inflammation. This is well described in studies of laboratory rodents. However, a high-fat diet can lead to obesity, which itself is associated with inflammatory cell infiltration into adipose tissue and the liver. This results in higher concentrations of inflammatory markers in these tissues and in the bloodstream (Calder *et al.*, 2011). Thus, it is difficult to disentangle the effects of a high-fat diet per se and of high-fat-induced obesity on inflammation. Furthermore, high-fat diets are often rich in saturated fatty acids. As described below, these fatty acids may directly induce inflammatory responses via activation of pro-inflammatory signaling pathways. Therefore a pro-inflammatory effect of a high-fat diet rich in saturated fat may be due to the saturated fatty acid burden rather than the fat quantity. Thus, the effect of a high-fat diet on inflammation may very much depend upon its fatty acid composition, and it is possible that a high-fat diet could have a non-inflammatory fatty acid profile. Indeed, a 6-month intervention in obese subjects showed no difference in the effect of a low-fat diet (20–30% energy from fat) or a high monounsaturated fat diet (35–45% energy from fat with at least 20% energy from monounsaturated fatty acids) on plasma C-reactive protein (CRP) and interleukin (IL)-6 concentrations (Bladbjerg *et al.*, 2011). In an earlier 3-month intervention in obese subjects, a low-fat diet did not alter CRP or IL-6 concentration and actually increased the concentrations of soluble intercellular adhesion molecule (sICAM)-1 and soluble vascular cell adhesion molecule (sVCAM)-1 (Estruch *et al.*, 2006).

In a study of more than 5000 non-diabetic human subjects a dietary pattern described as a 'fats and processed meats pattern' (high use of fats, oils, processed meats, fried potatoes, salty snacks and desserts) was positively associated with circulating CRP and IL-6 concentrations (Nettleton *et al.*, 2006). Whether this is an effect of high-fat consumption or of specific fats or of other dietary components is not clear. An intervention in a small number of overweight middle-aged humans evaluated the effect of 2 weeks on a diet providing 35% of energy as fat and 45% as carbohydrate compared with an isocaloric diet providing 15% of energy as fat and 65% as carbohydrate in the same subjects (Koren *et al.*, 2006). The subjects' weight was stable during this 4-week period. There was no difference on plasma CRP concentration at the end of each diet period, suggesting that an isocaloric, weight-maintaining low-fat diet does not reduce inflammation (or at least CRP concentration) compared with a higher fat diet. The subjects then consumed the 15% energy as fat diet ad libitum for 12 weeks. During this period the subjects lost weight, and plasma CRP concentration decreased. The study confirms that weight loss decreases CRP concentration, and suggests that a decrease in dietary fat (from 35% to 15% of energy) without weight loss does not impact inflammation. Other studies report that using a low-fat diet in combination with exercise reduces inflammation. For example, 3 weeks of a low-fat, high-fibre diet and a daily aerobic exercise programme in obese subjects resulted in weight loss and a decrease in circulating CRP, sICAM-1, soluble P-selectin, macrophage inflammatory protein-1α and matrix metalloproteinase-9 concentrations (Roberts *et al.*, 2006). The contribution of the low-fat diet to the effects seen is not possible to specify.

In the hours after consuming a meal there is an elevation in the plasma concentrations of several pro-inflammatory mediators including tumour necrosis factor-alpha (TNF-α), IL-6 and several soluble adhesion molecules (Burdge and Calder, 2005). This is sometimes referred to as 'post-prandial inflammation'. The origin of the mediators is not entirely clear, but endothelial cells, circulating inflammatory cells and adipose tissue are all likely to be involved (Burdge and Calder, 2005). Post-prandial inflammation seems to be especially induced by a high-fat meal (Nappo *et al.*, 2002), although, once again, variation in what constitutes the fat component of the meal influences the magnitude of the effect seen. For example, Bellido *et al.* (2004) reported a much reduced post-prandial inflammatory response if olive oil was used instead of butter in the test meal. Thus, it seems that a high-fat meal does induce post-prandial inflammation but that the magnitude of the effect is determined by the composition of the fat. This conclusion means that attention should be focused on the influence of individual fatty acids on inflammatory processes.

Importance of Fatty Acid Composition for Function of Cells Involved in Inflammation

Fatty acids are key structural and functional components of phospholipids in all cell membranes. They contribute to the physical state of the membrane, ensuring the appropriate environment for the function of membrane proteins that include receptors, transport proteins, ion channels, enzymes and so on. A change in the physical state of the membrane that may accompany a change in its fatty acid composition can impact on the membrane protein function (Brenner, 1984; Stubbs and Smith, 1984; Murphy, 1990). Membrane structures, termed rafts, form upon cell stimulation, and bring together proteins involved in the relevant signal transduction pathway, so forming signalling platforms (Simons and Toomre, 2000; Pike, 2003). It seems that the fatty acid composition of the cell membrane can influence raft formation and so can influence signalling processes (Yaqoob, 2009; Yaqoob and Shaikh, 2010). Several membrane phospholipids are precursors of molecules involved in signal transduction, such as diacylglycerols, and the fatty acid composition of the signalling molecule, which reflects that of the parent phospholipid, can modify its biological potency (Miles and Calder, 1998). Fatty acids released from cell membrane phospholipids are precursors for mediators involved in inflammation such as prostaglandins (PGs), leukotrienes (LTs) and endocannabinoids. Thus, there are a number of mechanisms by which altering the fatty acid composition of the membranes of cells involved in inflammation can influence the functional responses of those cells.

Fatty acid composition of cells involved in inflammation

The phospholipids in monocytes, neutrophils and lymphocytes taken from the blood of humans consuming typical Western diets contain a lot of palmitic (16:0), oleic and linoleic acids, about 1–2% of fatty acids as dihomo-γ-linoleic acid (20:3n-6; DGLA), 10–20% as arachidonic acid (20:4n-6; ARA), with about 0.5–1% eicosapentaenoic acid (20:5n-3; EPA) and about 1.5–3% docosahexaenoic acid (22:6n-3; DHA) (Lee *et al.*, 1985; Endres *et al.*, 1989; Sperling *et al.*, 1993; Caughey *et al.*, 1996; Healy *et al.*, 2000; Yaqoob *et al.*, 2000; Kew *et al.*, 2003, 2004; Rees *et al.*, 2006). There are, however, marked differences in fatty acid contents of the different phospholipid classes (Sperling *et al.*, 1993).

Modification of the fatty acid composition of cells involved in inflammation

The fatty acid composition of human inflammatory cells can be modified as a result of changed intakes of various n-6 and n-3 fatty acids. γ-Linolenic acid (18:3n-6; GLA) does not accumulate in significant amounts in inflammatory cell membranes, even when it is provided in the diet (Johnson *et al.*, 1997; Rosetti *et al.*, 1997; Yaqoob *et al.*, 2000). Instead the content of its derivative DGLA is increased (Johnson *et al.*, 1997; Rosetti *et al.*, 1997; Yaqoob *et al.*, 2000). An increased intake of ARA results in increased ARA in blood mononuclear cells, a mixture of lymphocytes and monocytes (Thies *et al.*, 2001a). An increased intake of ALNA results in increased EPA in mononuclear cells (Kelley *et al.*, 1993; Caughey *et al.*, 1996; Kew *et al.*, 2003) and neutrophils (Mantzioras *et al.*, 1994; Healy *et al.*, 2000). The ALNA derivative stearidonic acid also results in increased EPA in mononuclear cells (Miles *et al.*, 2004). Several studies have demonstrated that an increased intake of EPA + DHA, usually from fish oil supplements, results in a higher content of EPA and DHA in mononuclear cells and neutrophils (Lee *et al.*, 1985; Endres *et al.*, 1989; Chilton *et al.*,

1993; Sperling *et al.*, 1993; Caughey *et al.*, 1996; Healy *et al.*, 2000; Yaqoob *et al.*, 2000; Thies *et al.*, 2001a; Kew *et al.*, 2003, 2004; Rees *et al.*, 2006). The increased content of EPA and DHA is associated with a decreased content of n-6 fatty acids, especially ARA. Time-course studies suggest that the net incorporation of EPA and DHA into human inflammatory cells begins within days and reaches its peak within a few weeks (Healy *et al.*, 2000; Yaqoob *et al.*, 2000; Thies *et al.*, 2001a; Rees *et al.*, 2006; Faber *et al.*, 2011). Studies that have used multiple doses of fish oil show that the incorporation of EPA and DHA occurs in a dose–response manner (Healy *et al.*, 2000; Rees *et al.*, 2006).

Lipid Mediators Produced from n-6 and n-3 Fatty Acids

Arachidonic acid and eicosanoids

Eicosanoids are a family of lipid mediators synthesized from 20-carbon polyunsaturated fatty acids. They include PGs, thromboxanes and LTs. Because of its high content in membrane phospholipids, ARA is the usual precursor for eicosanoid synthesis (Fig. 2.2). ARA is released from the phospholipids through the action of phospholipase A_2 enzymes, which are activated by inflammatory stimuli. The free ARA then acts as a substrate for cyclooxygenase (COX), lipoxygenase (LOX) or cytochrome P450 enzymes. COX enzymes lead to PGs and thromboxanes, LOX enzymes lead to LTs, and cytochrome P450 enzymes to hydroxyeicosatetraenoic and epoxyeicosatrienoic acids (Fig. 2.2). ARA yields the 2-series PGs and the 4-series LTs. These eicosanoids are long recognized as key mediators and regulators of inflammation (Lewis *et al.*, 1990; Tilley *et al.*, 2001; Kroetz and Zeldin, 2002) acting via specific receptors, usually G-protein-coupled receptors. Their synthesis and action are targets for a range of non-specific and specific pharmaceuticals. For example, PGE_2 increases vascular permeability, vasodilation, blood flow and local pyrexia, and potentiates pain caused by other agents. It also promotes the production of some matrix metalloproteinases that can cause local tissue damage and destruction (e.g. to bone in rheumatoid arthritis). LTB_4 increases vascular permeability, enhances local blood flow, is a potent chemotactic agent

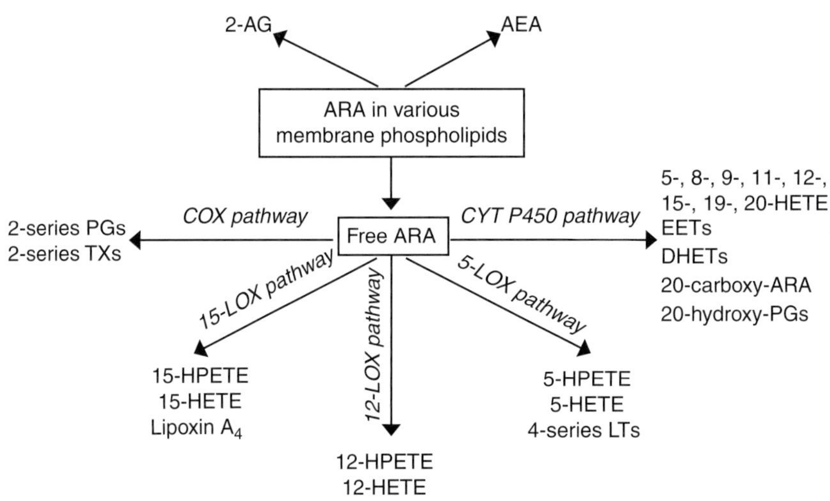

Fig. 2.2. Outline of the pathways of eicosanoid synthesis from arachidonic acid. AEA, arachidonoyl ethanolamine (anandamide); 2-AG, 2-arachidonoyl glycerol; ARA, arachidonic acid; COX, cyclooxygenase; CYT P450, cytochrome P450 enzymes; DHETs, dihydroxyeicosatrienoic acids; EETs, epoxyeicosatrienoic acids; HETE, hydroxyeicosatetraenoic acid; HPETE, hydroperoxyeicosatetraenoic acid; LOX, lipoxygenase; LTs, leukotrienes; PGs, prostaglandins; TXs, thromboxanes.

for leucocytes, induces release of lysosomal enzymes and enhances the release of reactive oxygen species and inflammatory cytokines.

Endocannabinoids are complex eicosanoids produced by cleavage of phospholipids by phospholipases (Di Marzo, 2008). The two major ARA-containing endocannabinoids are arachidonoyl ethanolamide (AEA), also known as anandamide, and 2-arachidonoyl glycerol (2-AG). AEA is formed by a pair of reactions involving the conversion of phosphatidylethanolamine to *N*-acyl-phosphatidylethanolamine followed by the action of phospholipase D. 2-AG is formed as a result of the sequential actions of phospholipase C and a diacylglycerol lipase. AEA and 2-AG act via the CB1 and CB2 receptors (Di Marzo, 2008).

Although it is generally considered that eicosanoids derived from ARA are pro-inflammatory, this is an over-simplification (Calder, 2009). For example, PGE_2 inhibits the production of two of the classic pro-inflammatory cytokines, TNF and IL-1, by monocytes and macrophages (Calder, 2009). Furthermore, in more recent years it has been discovered that PGE_2 inhibits 5-LOX and so decreases production of the inflammatory 4-series LTs (Levy *et al.*, 2001) and induces 15-LOX so promoting the formation of lipoxins (Levy *et al.*, 2001; Vachier *et al.*, 2002) that have been found to have anti-inflammatory effects (Gewirtz *et al.*, 2002). These findings show that PGE_2 possesses both pro- and anti-inflammatory actions; this may apply to other eicosanoids too. There may be a temporal change in the role of PGE_2 with an initial pro-inflammatory effect followed by a role in resolution of inflammation through inhibition of 5-LOX and induction of lipoxin production.

Dihomo-γ-linolenic acid and eicosanoids

DGLA is a substrate for COX giving rise to 1-series PGs, for 5-LOX giving rise to 3-series LTS and for 15-LOX giving rise to 15-hydroxy-DGLA. PGE_1 has several anti-inflammatory effects including inhibition of TNF, IL-1 and IL-6 production by macrophages (see Calder and Zurier, 2001). 15-Hydroxy-DGLA is an inhibitor of 5-LOX and 12-LOX and so can decrease the synthesis of mediators from ARA. Supplementing the human diet with GLA (more than about 2.5 g/day) increased PGE_1 production and decreased PGE_2, LTB_4 and LTC_4 production (Johnson *et al.*, 1997; Wu *et al.*, 1999).

n-3 Fatty acids and eicosanoids

Numerous studies have shown a decreased production of PGE_2 and 4 series-LTs by human inflammatory cells following the use of fish oil supplements for a period of weeks to months (Lee *et al.*, 1985; Endres *et al.*, 1989; Meydani *et al.*, 1991; Sperling *et al.*, 1993; von Schacky *et al.*, 1993; Caughey *et al.*, 1996). These studies have usually used fairly high intakes of the marine n-3 polyunsaturated fatty acids (PUFAs), most often several grams per day. A dose–response study in healthy volunteers reported that an EPA intake of 1.35 g/day for 3 months was not sufficient to influence *ex vivo* PGE_2 production by lipopolysaccharide (LPS)-stimulated mononuclear cells, whereas an EPA intake of 2.7 g/day did significantly decrease PGE_2 production (Rees *et al.*, 2006), giving an indication of the threshold dose of EPA required to exert an anti-inflammatory effect. Kelley *et al.* (1999) demonstrated that high-dose DHA (6 g/day) decreased PGE_2 and LTB_4 production by LPS-stimulated mononuclear cells. A diet rich in ALNA also results in decreased production of ARA-derived eicosanoids (Caughey *et al.*, 1996), probably because ALNA can be converted to EPA resulting in a higher EPA and lower ARA content of eicosanoid-producing cells.

Because EPA is a 20-carbon highly unsaturated fatty acid it is also a substrate for the COX, LOX and cytochrome P450 enzymes that produce eicosanoids, and EPA- and DHA-containing phospholipids are substrates for the synthesis of endocannabinoids. The mediators produced have, however, a different structure from those made from ARA (e.g. PGE_3 rather than PGE_2 and LTB_5 rather than LTB_4). The functional significance of the generation of eicosanoids from n-3 fatty acids is that they are often much less biologically active than those produced from ARA (Goldman *et al.*, 1983; Lee *et al.*, 1984; Bagga *et al.*, 2003). One reason for this reduced biological potency is that eicosanoid receptors typically have a much lower affinity for the EPA-derived mediator than for the ARA-derived one (Wada *et al.*, 2007). Thus, EPA results in a decreased production of potent eicosanoids from ARA and an increased production of weak eicosanoids. EPA- and DHA-containing endocannabinoids have marked anti-inflammatory properties in cell culture systems (Balvers *et al.*, 2010; Meijerink *et al.*, 2011).

n-3 Fatty acids and resolvins and protectins

In the past ten years or so new families of lipid mediators produced from marine n-3 fatty acids have been discovered. These include the resolvins produced from EPA (E-series) and DHA (D-series) and protectins produced from DHA (also referred to as neuroprotectins when generated within neural tissue). The synthesis of resolvins and protectins involves the COX and LOX pathways, with different epimers being produced in the presence and absence of aspirin (Serhan *et al.*, 2000a, 2000b, 2002, 2008). The biological effects of resolvins and protectins have been examined extensively in cell culture and animal models of inflammation. These models have shown them to be anti-inflammatory and inflammation resolving. For example, resolvin E1, resolvin D1 and protectin D1 all inhibited transendothelial migration of neutrophils, so preventing the infiltration of neutrophils into sites of inflammation; resolvin D1 inhibited IL-1β production; and protectin D1 inhibited TNF and IL-1β production (Serhan *et al.*, 2000a, 2000b, 2002, 2008). Resolvins reduce inflammation and protect experimental animals in models of inflammatory disease including arthritis (Lima-Garcia *et al.*, 2011), colitis (Arita *et al.*, 2005a), and asthma (Aoki *et al.*, 2008; Haworth *et al.*, 2008). The biological activities of resolvins are mediated via specific G-protein-coupled receptors (Arita *et al.*, 2005b, 2007; Yin *et al.*, 2009; Krishnamoorthy *et al.*, 2010).

Effects of Specific Fatty Acids on Inflammation

As indicated above the fatty acid composition of cells involved in inflammation can be modified by increased oral intake of various polyunsaturated fatty acids. The altered membrane composition can influence the function of membrane proteins, the assembly of signalling platforms within raft regions, the structure and activity of phospholipid-derived signalling molecules, and the mix of lipid mediators produced upon cellular stimulation. In turn, these altered intracellular and extracellular signals can influence other aspects of the inflammatory response including chemotaxis, adhesive interactions between cells, and inflammatory cytokine, oxidant and protease production. Thus, fatty acids can potentially affect all aspects of inflammatory cell responses. These effects can be studied in model systems such as in cell culture or in experimental animals. Such approaches involve highly controlled experimental settings and allow for detailed examination of mechanisms underpinning functional effects of fatty acids. The conditions used, however, are often not physiological, so limiting translation to human health and disease. In this section, human studies investigating the impact of altered fatty acid exposures on markers of inflammation will be summarized. These studies have used two different general approaches. The first is to examine the relationship between intake or status of a particular fatty acid and the inflammatory marker. The second approach has been to increase the intake of the fatty acid under study and to identify the effect of changed intake or status. This approach often uses fatty acids supplied as supplements, usually in capsules. The markers of inflammation studied in these investigations have fallen into two types. The first is blood markers of inflammation such as white cell count, white cell activation state, or serum or plasma concentrations of acute phase proteins, cytokines or soluble adhesion molecules. The second is the response of white cells to an *ex vivo* stimulus such as bacterial endotoxin (LPS); the outcome here would be production of one or more mediators involved in inflammation (e.g. TNF). Findings from such *ex vivo* cultures can be influenced by differences in protocol such as cell concentration, type of stimulant and its concentration, source and concentration of plasma or serum, culture duration, and type of assay used to measure the inflammatory marker. Studies in patients with an inflammatory condition can also investigate outcomes more closely related to the pathology caused by the inflammatory response.

Saturated fatty acids

In vitro studies have suggested that monocytes and dendritic cells can be activated directly by saturated fatty acids, especially lauric acid (12:0), in a process involving the LPS receptor, toll-like receptor (TLR)-4 and subsequent activation of the pro-inflammatory transcription factor nuclear factor kappa B (NFκB) (Lee *et al.*, 2001; Weatherill *et al.*, 2005). Two observational studies have investigated the relationship between saturated fatty acid exposure and circulating markers of inflammation (Fernandez-Real *et al.*, 2003; Klein-Platat *et al.*, 2005). Fernandez-Real *et al.* (2003) did not see any relationship between serum saturated fatty acids and CRP or IL-6 concentrations in lean individuals, whereas in overweight individuals serum saturated fatty acids were positively associated with IL-6 concentration and the ratio of saturated fatty acids to n-6 or n-3 fatty acids was positively associated with IL-6 and CRP concentrations, respectively. A study in overweight adolescents showed positive relationships between total saturated fatty acids in plasma phospholipids or cholesteryl esters and IL-6, but not CRP, concentration (Klein-Platat *et al.*, 2005). Thus, there is general agreement between two studies in overweight subjects that saturated fatty acid exposure is associated with higher IL-6 concentration, but lean individuals did not show this. An intervention study feeding diets rich in stearic acid (18:0) or in the combination of lauric, myristic (14:0) and palmitic acids to men for 5 weeks showed higher concentrations of CRP, fibrinogen, IL-6 and soluble E-selectin (sE-selectin) compared with a diet enriched in oleic acid (Baer *et al.*, 2004). There are few other intervention studies chronically increasing saturated fatty acid intake in humans and reporting inflammatory markers. The data that exists from two observational and one intervention study indicate, however, that saturated fatty acids may increase inflammation.

Trans fatty acids

There were positive relationships between dietary *trans* fatty acid intake and concentrations of six inflammatory markers, including CRP, IL-6 and three soluble adhesion molecules, in the Nurses' Health Study (Lopez-Garcia *et al.*, 2005). In a 5-week intervention study in healthy men, a *trans* fatty acid enriched diet resulted in higher CRP and IL-6 concentrations than diets rich in oleic acid, stearic acid or the combination of lauric, myristic and palmitic acids (Baer *et al.*, 2004). Furthermore, the concentration of sE-selectin was higher than in all other dietary groups including the stearic acid and lauric + myristic + palmitic groups. Thus, one association study and one intervention study both suggest that dietary *trans* fatty acids elevate the concentrations of a range of inflammatory markers including CRP, IL-6 and adhesion molecules, and that *trans* fatty acids may be more 'pro-inflammatory' than saturated fatty acids.

Conjugated linoleic acids

In vitro and animal-feeding studies have suggested marked effects of conjugated linoleic acids (CLAs) on inflammation (Li *et al.*, 2005, 2006; Moloney *et al.*, 2007). Human studies using CLA-rich capsules provide mixed findings, however (Riserus *et al.*, 2002; Tricon *et al.*, 2004; Nugent *et al.*, 2005; Ramakers *et al.*, 2005; Smedman *et al.*, 2005; Song *et al.*, 2005; Mullen *et al.*, 2007). Two studies reported that CLAs, especially the *trans*-10, *cis*-12 isomer, increase

CRP concentration, but not the concentrations of several cytokines or soluble adhesion molecules (Riserus *et al.* 2002, Smedman *et al.*, 2005). However, a number of other studies has failed to show an effect of CLA on CRP concentration (Tricon *et al.*, 2004; Ramakers *et al.*, 2005; Mullen *et al.*, 2007). Most studies have used mixtures of CLA isomers in different proportions, and this may explain the discrepancy in the literature because the precise dose of the more potent isomer (perhaps the *trans*-10, *cis*-12 isomer) differs amongst these studies. The two studies showing increased CRP with CLA provided 2.1 g/day (Smedman *et al.*, 2005) and 2.7 g/day (Riserus *et al.*, 2002) *trans*-10, *cis*-12 CLA. The four studies showing no effect of CLA on CRP used between 0.4 g/day and 2.5 g/day of this isomer (Tricon *et al.*, 2004; Ramakers *et al.*, 2005; Mullen *et al.*, 2007). Studies investigating the effect of several weeks of intake of CLA on *ex vivo* inflammatory cytokine production by mononuclear cells report little or no effect (Albers *et al.*, 2001; Kelley *et al.*, 2001; Nugent *et al.*, 2005; Ramakers *et al.*, 2005). Thus, it is not yet clear whether CLAs per se, or whether specific CLA isomers, increase inflammation.

Linoleic acid

Because of the role of linoleic acid as the precursor of ARA, which is, in turn, the substrate for the synthesis of inflammatory eicosanoids such as PGE_2 and 4-series LTs, it is often stated that elevated n-6 and low n-3 fatty acids (i.e. a high n-6 to n-3 fatty acid ratio) in the diet will promote inflammation. Available evidence does not seem to support this contention, however. Dietary intakes of linoleic acid were not associated with CRP or IL-6 concentrations in subgroups of the Physicians' Health Study and the Nurses' Health Study (Pischon *et al.*, 2003), whereas the concentration of linoleic acid in blood lipids (Klein-Platat *et al.*, 2005; Ferrucci *et al.*, 2006) or granulocytes (Madsen *et al.*, 2001) was not associated with CRP or IL-6 concentration. In contrast, a large Swedish study reported an inverse association between linoleic acid in cholesteryl esters and CRP concentration (Petersson *et al.*, 2008). Total n-6 fatty acids in serum fatty acids in overweight, but not in lean, subjects were inversely associated with IL-6, but not CRP, concentration (Fernandez-Real *et al.*, 2003). The ratio of saturated fatty acids to n-6 fatty acids in serum lipids or in plasma phospholipids was positively associated with IL-6, but not CRP, in overweight subjects (Fernandez-Real *et al.*, 2003; Klein-Platat *et al.*, 2005). This suggests that decreasing saturated fatty acid status while increasing n-6 fatty acid status might reduce inflammation.

Several intervention studies with ALNA (see the α-linolenic acid section below) have involved a group consuming a high intake of linoleic acid, frequently as the control for the high α-linolenic acid intake. These studies provide some information about the impact of linoleic acid on inflammation. Studies by Rallidis *et al.* (2003, 2004) and Paschos *et al.* (2007) provided 11 g/day of linoleic acid to subjects with a habitual intake of about 11 g/day, approximately doubling linoleic acid intake. This did not alter the concentrations of CRP, TNF, IL-6, serum amyloid A, sICAM-1 or sE-selectin, but the concentration of sVCAM-1 was decreased. In the study of Yaqoob *et al.* (2000), one group of subjects consumed about 6 g/day linoleic acid from safflower oil capsules for 12 weeks; dietary intake was not reported but average habitual intake of linoleic acid among adults in the UK is about 11 g/day. Thus these individuals increased intake of linoleic acid by about 55%. There was no effect on the production of TNF, IL-1α or IL-1β or IL-6 by LPS-stimulated mononuclear cells. These studies did not alter any aspect of diet but required subjects to consume oil providing linoleic acid on top of the normal diet. They show that markedly increasing linoleic acid intake in those consuming on average about 11 g/day does not increase inflammation.

Arachidonic acid

ARA is the most prevalent n-6 fatty acid and polyunsaturated fatty acid in the membranes of inflammatory cells and other cells that might be involved in inflammation such as endothelial cells and platelets. This reflects the important functional role of ARA as a precursor of eicosanoids (see above). Because eicosanoids are classically associated with inflammatory processes and are targeted by common anti-inflammatory therapies, it is generally considered that ARA will enhance inflammation. However, observations that classical pro-inflammatory mediators such as PGE_2 can also exert anti-inflammatory effects and that ARA gives rise to anti-inflammatory mediators like lipoxin A_4, have started to challenge the earlier view (Calder, 2009). Several studies have examined the association between ARA status and markers of inflammation. There was no association between ARA in granulocytes and CRP concentration (Madsen *et al.*, 2001), whereas serum free ARA was not associated with sICAM-1 or sE-selectin concentrations and was actually inversely associated with sVCAM-1 concentration (Yli-Jama *et al.*, 2002). Ferrucci *et al.* (2006) reported no association between ARA in plasma and CRP, TNF, IL-1β, IL-10 and soluble IL-6 receptor (sIL-6R) concentrations, whereas there was an inverse association with IL-6 and IL-1 receptor antagonist concentrations and a positive association with transforming growth factor (TGF)-β concentration. These observations suggest either that plasma ARA has little impact on inflammation (does not affect CRP or TNF) or that it is anti-inflammatory (lowers IL-6; increases TGF-β). There are very few intervention studies with ARA reporting on inflammation. In an uncontrolled study, Kelley *et al.* (1997) reported higher granulocyte numbers in the blood of a small group of healthy men taking a supplement of 1.5 g/day ARA for 100 days. There was no effect on the production of TNF, IL-β or IL-6 by LPS-stimulated mononuclear cells. In another small, but controlled, study, older subjects consumed capsules providing 700 mg/day ARA acid for 12 weeks (Thies *et al.*, 2001b); there was no effect on plasma sVCAM-1, sICAM-1 or sE-selectin concentrations or on production of TNF, IL-β or IL-6 by LPS-stimulated mononuclear cells. Collectively these data suggest little impact of modest increases of ARA intake on inflammation. The effect of lowering ARA intake below habitual levels on inflammation has not been investigated.

α-Linolenic acid

Increased consumption of ALNA results in an increased content of EPA in the membranes of inflammatory cells (Kelley *et al.*, 1993; Mantzioras *et al.*, 1994; Caughey *et al.*, 1996; Healy *et al.*, 2000; Kew *et al.*, 2003) in parallel with a decreased content of ARA. This might be expected to affect inflammation. However dietary ALNA intake was not associated with CRP or IL-6 concentrations in one study on subgroups of the Physicians' Health Study and the Nurses' Health Study (Pischon *et al.*, 2003). In a second study on another subgroup of the Nurses' Health Study, ALNA intake was not associated with CRP, sICAM-1 or sE-selectin concentrations but was associated with lower IL-6 and sVCAM-1 concentrations (Lopez-Garcia *et al.*, 2004). The concentration of ALNA in blood lipids (Klein-Platat *et al.*, 2005; Petersson *et al.*, 2008) or granulocytes (Madsen *et al.*, 2001) was not associated with CRP or IL-6 concentration. In another study there was no association between ALNA in plasma fatty acids and several cytokines including IL-6 and TNF, but there was an inverse association with CRP (Ferrucci *et al.*, 2006). These association studies suggest a limited anti-inflammatory effect of ALNA.

Several intervention studies have involved high ALNA intakes usually by providing flaxseed oil in capsules or in liquid form or foodstuffs made using flaxseed oil. Frequently these studies have used a control group with a high intake of linoleic acid, with the comparison essentially being the replacement of linoleic acid with α-linolenic acid. These studies have produced inconsistent findings with some identifying effects of ALNA on some markers and not others (Thies *et al.*, 2001b; Rallidis *et al.*, 2003, 2004; Bemelmans *et al.*, 2004; Paschos *et al.*, 2004; Zhao *et al.*, 2004), and some studies finding no effects (Junker *et al.*, 2001; Paschos *et al.*, 2007). However, what is apparent is that a substantial increase in intake of ALNA can decrease inflammation as indicated by circulating

CRP, IL-6 or soluble adhesion molecules (Thies *et al.*, 2001b; Rallidis *et al.*, 2003, 2004; Bemelmans *et al.*, 2004; Paschos *et al.*, 2004; Zhao *et al.*, 2004).

Caughey *et al.* (1996) reported that 13.7 g/day ALNA for 4 weeks resulted in a decreased production of TNF and IL-1β by LPS-stimulated mononuclear cells by 27% and 30%, respectively. By comparison, fish oil providing 2.7 g/day EPA + DHA decreased the production of these inflammatory cytokines by 70% and 78%, respectively (Caughey *et al.*, 1996). Thus, on a gram per day basis, marine n-3 fatty acids are about ten times more potent than ALNA. In contrast to the observations of Caughey *et al.* (1996), several studies using lower intakes of ALNA (2–9.5 g/day) did not find effects on neutrophil chemotaxis, neutrophil or monocyte respiratory burst, or TNF, IL-1β and IL-6 production by LPS-stimulated mononuclear cells (all studied *ex vivo*), or on soluble adhesion molecule concentrations (Healy *et al.*, 2000; Thies *et al.*, 2001b; Kew *et al.*, 2003; Wallace *et al.*, 2003). Taken together, these data suggest that a marked increase in ALNA intake is required in order for anti-inflammatory effects to be seen. Even then, the effects will be much more modest than those exerted by marine n-3 PUFAs. The observed effects of high intakes of ALNA on inflammation seem to be due to its derivative EPA rather than to ALNA itself (Zhao *et al.*, 2004). Thus, the likely explanation for the lack of anti-inflammatory effect of ALNA at modest, and even at rather high, intakes is that there has been insufficient conversion to the more active EPA.

Marine n-3 fatty acids

The incorporation of EPA and DHA into inflammatory cells is partly at the expense of ARA, resulting in less substrate available for the synthesis of the classic inflammatory eicosanoids. Through altered eicosanoid production, marine n-3 fatty acids could affect inflammation and inflammatory processes, although they also exert non-eicosanoid mediated actions on cell signalling and gene expression (Fig. 2.3). These actions include modification of formation of signalling platforms termed rafts in the cell membrane, activation of the anti-inflammatory transcription factor peroxisome proliferator activated receptor (PPAR)-γ and inhibition of activation of the pro-inflammatory transcription factor NFκB (Calder, 2011, 2012). Recent studies indicate a membrane-bound G-protein-coupled receptor called GPR120 that is important for the anti-inflammatory effects of DHA in macrophages (Oh *et al.*, 2010). The effects of marine n-3 fatty acids have been examined in many model systems and findings from cell culture systems and from animal models are generally consistent in identifying anti-inflammatory actions (Calder, 2003). Furthermore, clinical trials have demonstrated anti-inflammatory effects and some clinical benefit from fish oil administration in diseases with a frank inflammatory basis including rheumatoid arthritis (RA), inflammatory bowel diseases (IBD) and childhood asthma (Calder, 2006).

Cross-sectional studies consistently show an inverse association between intake or status of marine n-3 fatty acids and markers of inflammation. Data from subgroups of the Physicians' Health Study and the Nurses' Health Study showed inverse associations between dietary intake of EPA + DHA and concentrations of CRP (Pischon *et al.*, 2003) and CRP, sICAM-1, sVCAM-1 and sE-selectin (Lopez-Garcia *et al.*, 2004). The concentration

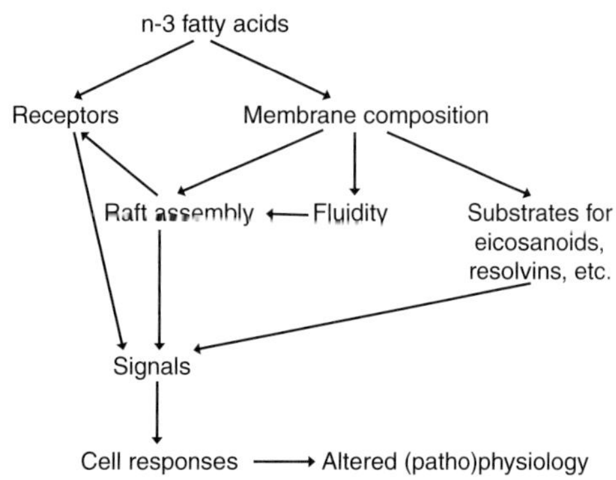

Fig. 2.3. Overview of the mechanisms by which n-3 fatty acids can influence inflammation. (Modified from Calder, 2011, with permission from Elsevier.)

of either EPA or DHA in granulocyte membranes was inversely associated with CRP concentration in one study (Madsen *et al.*, 2001); the effect of DHA was stronger than that of EPA. Serum non-esterified EPA and DHA were both inversely associated with concentrations of sVCAM-1 and sICAM-1 in patients at risk of coronary heart disease (Yli-Jama *et al.*, 2002); EPA was also inversely associated with sE-selectin concentration. Plasma cholesteryl ester EPA was inversely associated with CRP concentration in overweight subjects (Klein-Platat *et al.*, 2005). In an elderly Italian population, plasma EPA was inversely associated with IL-6 concentration and positively associated with the concentrations of the anti-inflammatory cytokines IL-10 and TGF-β (Ferrucci *et al.*, 2006). Furthermore plasma DHA was inversely associated with IL-6 and TNF concentrations and was also positively associated with the concentrations of IL-10 and TGF-β (Ferrucci *et al.*, 2006). Thus, observational studies suggest that both EPA and DHA are anti-inflammatory.

The ready availability of fish oil capsules has facilitated numerous supplementation studies of marine n-3 fatty acids in various subject and patient groups. Studies have shown that these fatty acids lower the concentrations of CRP (Ciubotaru *et al.*, 2003; Browning *et al.*, 2007; Rasic-Milutinovic *et al.*, 2007), IL-6 (Ciubotaru *et al.*, 2003; Browning *et al.*, 2007; Rasic-Milutinovic *et al.*, 2007), TNF (Rasic-Milutinovic *et al.*, 2007), IL-18 (Troseid *et al.*, 2009), sICAM-1 (Eschen *et al.*, 2004; Hjerkinn *et al.*, 2005; Yamada *et al.*, 2008; Yusof *et al.*, 2008), sVCAM-1 (Thies *et al.*, 2001b; Yamada *et al.*, 2008), and sE-selectin (Abe *et al.*, 1998). Both EPA and DHA (4 g/day for 6 weeks) decreased plasma TNF-α concentrations in type 2 diabetics, although DHA was more potent (Mori *et al.*, 2003).

A number of dietary supplementation studies that used between 3.1 g/day and 14.4 g/day EPA + DHA have demonstrated a time-dependent decrease in chemotaxis of human neutrophils and monocytes towards various chemoattractants (Lee *et al.*, 1985; Endres *et al.*, 1989; Schmidt *et al.*, 1989, 1991, 1992; Luostarinen *et al.*, 1992; Sperling *et al.*, 1993). One study reported a decreased expression of ICAM-1 on the surface of monocytes after an intake of 1.5 g/day EPA + DHA for several weeks (Hughes *et al.*, 1996). Supplementation studies providing 3.1–8.4 g/day EPA + DHA have reported decreased production of oxidants, including superoxide or hydrogen peroxide, by stimulated human neutrophils and monocytes (Fisher *et al.*, 1990; Thompson *et al.*, 1991; Varming *et al.*, 1995; Luostarinen and Saldeen, 1996). Supplementation of the diet of human volunteers with fish oil providing more than 2 g/day EPA + DHA has been shown to decrease production of TNF, IL-1 and IL-6 by mononuclear cells in some studies (Endres *et al.*, 1989; Meydani *et al.*, 1991; Caughey *et al.*, 1996; Trebble *et al.*, 2003). Caughey *et al.* (1996) reported a significant inverse correlation between the EPA content of mononuclear cells and the ability of those cells to produce TNF and IL-1β in response to LPS. Kelley *et al.* (1999) showed that 6 g/day DHA for 12 weeks decreased production of TNF and IL-1β by LPS-stimulated mononuclear cells. There are, however, a number of such studies reporting no effects of EPA + DHA on *ex vivo* cytokine production (see Calder, 2006).

Thus, the overwhelming view is that EPA + DHA given at sufficient doses are anti-inflammatory. However, study findings are not entirely consistent. The lack of consistency may be related to differences in: duration of treatment; sample size; characteristics of the populations studied (e.g. age, healthy versus diseased, type of disease, smokers versus non-smokers); background diet; dose of EPA + DHA used; relative contribution of EPA and DHA, because they may have different anti-inflammatory potencies; chemical formulation (e.g. triglyceride versus ethyl ester); and degree of oxidative stress present. One other factor that has been recently identified is genetic differences among individuals, which might have an impact on the ability of n-3 fatty acids to exert an anti-inflammatory effect. This was first identified by Grimble *et al.* (2002) who showed that the ability of fish oil to lower the LPS-stimulated production of TNF by blood mononuclear cells was determined in part by polymorphisms within the TNF and lymphotoxin genes.

The ability of marine n-3 fatty acids to down-regulate several aspects of inflammation suggests that these fatty acids might be important in determining the development and severity of inflammatory diseases and that they may be useful as a component of therapy. Amongst the classic inflammatory conditions, fish oil has been most thoroughly examined in RA (Calder 2008a). Animal models have demonstrated that marine n-3 fatty acids can delay the onset of arthritis, reduce its severity and improve joint pathology (Leslie *et al.*, 1985; Volker *et al.*, 2000; Ierna *et al.*, 2010). Cleland *et al.* (2006) found that RA patients using fish oil supplements were more likely to reduce use of non-steroidal anti-inflammatory drugs (NSAIDS) and to be in remission than those patients who did not use fish oil. Randomized controlled trials of fish oil in RA report improvements in several clinical outcomes including reduced duration of morning stiffness, reduced number of tender or swollen joints, reduced joint pain, reduced time to fatigue, increased grip strength and decreased use of NSAIDs (Calder, 2008a). The dose of n-3 fatty acids used in these trials has typically been high, between about 1 g/day and 7 g/day and averaging about 3.5 g/day. This dose would be difficult to achieve through the diet, but can be achieved through the use of supplements or liquid oil. A meta-analysis concluded that dietary fish oil supplementation for 3 months significantly reduced tender joint count and morning stiffness (Fortin *et al.*, 1995). A more recent meta-analysis concluded that fish oil reduces patient assessed joint pain, duration of morning stiffness, number of painful and/or tender joints, and consumption of NSAIDs (Goldberg and Katz, 2009). Thus there is fairly robust evidence of the efficacy of marine n-3 fatty acids in RA.

Animal models have demonstrated that marine n-3 fatty acids decrease chemically induced colonic damage and inflammation (see Calder, 2008b). The effects on disease severity were, in all cases, associated with a reduction in production of ARA-derived eicosanoids. A more recent study investigated chemically induced colitis in *fat-1* mice (Hudert *et al.*, 2006). The mice showed much less colonic damage and inflammation than wild-type mice and this was associated with a marked change in the pattern of inflammatory mediators present in colonic tissue. A study in IL-10 knock-out mice that spontaneously develop colitis, demonstrated reduced colonic inflammation if the mice were fed fish oil (Chapkin *et al.*, 2007). EPA and DHA are incorporated into the gut mucosal tissue of patients with IBD who supplement their diet with fish oil and this is associated with reduced inflammation (see Calder, 2008b). Some randomized controlled trials of fish oil in IBD have reported clinical benefits including improved clinical score, improved gut mucosal histology, improved sigmoidoscopic score, lower rate of relapse and decreased use of corticosteroids (see Calder, 2008b). The dose of EPA + DHA used in these trials has typically been high, between 2.5 and 6 g/day, averaging about 4 g/day. Several trials do not report benefits, however, and meta-analyses are not supportive of an effect (MacLean *et al.*, 2004; Turner *et al.*, 2007, 2009; De Ley *et al.*, 2007). Thus, despite some favourable studies, there is at best only weak evidence that marine n-3 fatty acids have clinical benefits in human IBD.

ARA-derived eicosanoids such as PGD_2, LTC_4, LTD_4 and LTE_4 are produced by the cells that mediate pulmonary inflammation in asthma and are believed to be major mediators of asthmatic bronchoconstriction. DHA reduced lung inflammation and improved lung function in a murine model of asthma (Yokoyama *et al.*, 2000). Epidemiologic data link high n-6 PUFA or low n-3 PUFA consumption with childhood asthma. Studies have reported anti-inflammatory effects of fish oil in patients with asthma, such as decreased production of 4-series LTs and reduced leucocyte chemotaxis (see Calder, 2006). However, randomized controlled trials of fish oil in adult asthma have reported no clinical benefit (Calder, 2006). Conversely, marine n-3 fatty acids may improve lung function in children with asthma (Hodge *et al.*, 1998; Nagakura *et al.*, 2000) and may improve disease activity (Nagakura *et al.*, 2000). A meta-analysis identified that there was no consistent effect of fish oil on lung function, asthma symptoms or asthma medication use, but stated that one study in children showed improved lung function and reduced asthma medication use (Thien *et al.*, 2002). Clearly, more needs to be done in this area, especially in children.

The hierarchy of effects of fatty acids on inflammation

The interrogation of the findings from studies of fatty acids and inflammation performed in humans as reported above allows a hierarchy of effects to be identified (Fig. 2.4). This is supported by animal feeding experiments, not discussed here, and by established and emerging mechanistic understandings. Amongst the more common dietary constituents, *trans* and saturated fatty acids enhance inflammation, with an indication (Baer *et al.*, 2004) that the effect of *trans* may be greater than that of saturated fatty acids. Replacing saturated fatty acids with polyunsaturated fatty acids or specifically with linoleic acid or ALNA decreases inflammation. High intakes of ALNA decrease inflammation when they replace linoleic acid or when they markedly lower the ratio of linoleic acid to ALNA taken orally. In turn, marine n-3 fatty acids (the combination of EPA plus DHA) are more potent than ALNA at reducing inflammation. It is important to note, however, that there are inconsistencies in the findings of observational and interventional studies. These probably relate to differences in duration of treatment in intervention studies; sample size; inherent characteristics of the populations studied such as age, health status, background diet and genetics; dose of the fatty acid used in intervention studies; whether the fatty acid replaced another or was simply added on top of the diet; and probably many other factors.

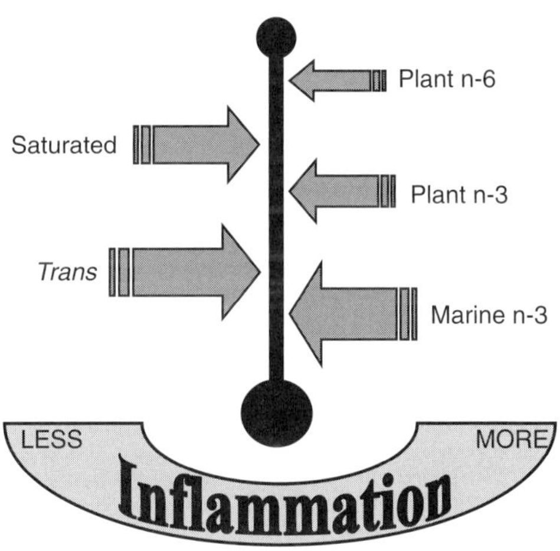

Fig. 2.4. Qualitative depiction of the relative effects of different types of fatty acid on inflammation. Saturated and *trans* fatty acids promote inflammation pushing the pendulum to the right. *Trans* fatty acids may have a greater impact than saturated fatty acids. Plant-derived n-6 fatty acids and n-3 fatty acids inhibit inflammation, pushing the pendulum to the left. n-3 Fatty acids have a greater impact than plant-derived n-6 fatty acids and within the n-3 fatty acid family marine-derived fatty acids (EPA and DHA) have a greater impact than plant-derived fatty acids (ALNA).

Summary and Conclusions

Fatty acids can influence inflammatory cell function and inflammation through a variety of mechanisms, including acting via cell-surface and intracellular receptors that control inflammatory cell signalling and gene expression patterns. Some effects of fatty acids on inflammatory processes involve lipid mediators generated from the fatty acids themselves. Often these fatty acids will be released from cell membrane phospholipids prior to their conversion to the bioactive mediators.

Cells involved in the inflammatory response are typically rich in the n-6 fatty acid ARA, which is a precursor to inflammatory eicosanoids. The membrane contents of ARA and of the n-3 fatty acids EPA and DHA can be altered through the oral administration of EPA and DHA. EPA also gives rise to eicosanoids and these often have differing properties from those of the ARA-derived analogues, typically being less potent. EPA and DHA give rise to resolvins, and DHA to protectins, which are anti-inflammatory and inflammation resolving. These relatively recently discovered mediators provide a novel mechanism by which n-3 fatty acids can influence inflammatory processes. Thus marine n-3 fatty acids reduce inflammation through a number of actions. The plant n-3 fatty acid ALNA can also reduce inflammation and its effects seem to relate to its conversion to EPA, explaining the lower potency of ALNA compared with marine n-3 fatty acids.

In contrast to the anti-inflammatory actions of n-3 fatty acids, saturated fatty acids enhance inflammation acting to increase NFκB activation and inflammatory gene expression. Interestingly, in cell culture models marine n-3 fatty acids, especially DHA, can prevent the effect of saturated fatty acids. Human studies demonstrate that *trans* fatty acids are pro-inflammatory, perhaps more so than saturated fatty acids. These considerations establish that *trans* and saturated fatty acids promote greater inflammatory responses and that n-3 fatty acids are anti-inflammatory with those of marine origin being more potent than the plant derived ALNA.

A consideration of the impact of n-6 fatty acids is more complex. Because ARA is the precursor to eicosanoids known to have a central role in inflammation and because drugs that target ARA metabolism have some efficacy as anti-inflammatories, the widely held view has been that n-6 fatty acids must, almost by definition, promote inflammation. This view is reinforced by knowledge that marine n-3 fatty acids are anti-inflammatory and that they work, at least in part, by interfering with ARA metabolism. However, the relationship of ARA and ARA-derived eicosanoids to inflammation is more complex than first realized, with anti-inflammatory and inflammation resolving effects being identified. This 'middle ground' occupied by n-6 fatty acids is borne out by human studies. Observational and interventional studies suggest that replacing saturated fatty acids with linoleic acid reduces inflammation; thus linoleic acid must be 'less inflammatory' than saturated fatty acids and could even be said to be 'anti-inflammatory' compared with saturated fatty acids. On the other hand, replacing linoleic acid with ALNA decreases inflammation indicating that linoleic acid is 'less anti-inflammatory' than ALNA and could therefore be considered to be 'pro-inflammatory' relative to ALNA. The difference between linoleic acid and marine n-3 fatty acids will be even stronger. If the aim is to reduce inflammation, then replacing *trans* and saturated fatty acids in the diet with polyunsaturated fatty acids would be one strategy. Amongst the polyunsaturated fatty acids there may be a place for linoleic acid, but it would be more important to increase intake of ALNA and even more importantly of EPA + DHA.

The multiple mechanisms involved in the interaction of fatty acids with inflammatory cells create a complex picture. Currently these multiple mechanisms of action are not fully integrated, but it seems likely that alterations in cell membrane composition are a key event because such alterations can influence lipid mediator profiles, membrane receptor function and cell signalling processes. It seems likely that future work will focus on defining the membrane structure–function interaction that is associated with different fatty acid compositions and on describing the biosynthesis and actions of novel lipid mediators such as resolvins and protectins and mechanisms that underlie their effects.

References

Abe, Y., El-Masri, B., Kimball, K.T., Pownall, H., Reilly, C.F., *et al.* (1998) Soluble cell adhesion molecules in hypertriglyceridemia and potential significance on monocyte adhesion. *Arteriosclerosis Thrombosis and Vascular Biology* 18, 723–731.

Albers, R., van der Wielen, R.P., Brink, E.J., Hendriks, H.F., Dorovska Taran, V.N. *et al* (2003) Effects of cis-9, trans-11 and trans-10, cis-12 conjugated linoleic acid (CLA) isomers on immune function in healthy men. *European Journal of Clinical Nutrition* 57, 595–603.

Aoki, H., Hisada, T., Ishizuka, T., Utsugi, M., Kawata, T., *et al.* (2008) Resolvin E1 dampens airway inflammation and hyperresponsiveness in a murine model of asthma. *Biochemical and Biophysical Research Communications* 367, 509–515.

Arita, M., Yoshida, M., Hong, S., Tjonahen, E., Glickman, J.N., *et al.* (2005a) Resolvin E1, an endogenous lipid mediator derived from omega-3 eicosapentaenoic acid, protects against 2,4,6-trinitrobenzene sulfonic acid-induced colitis. *Proceedings of the National Academy of Science USA* 102, 7621–7626.

Arita, M., Bianchini, F., Aliberti, J., Sher, A., Chiang, N., *et al.* (2005b) Stereochemical assignment, antiinflammatory properties, and receptor for the omega-3 lipid mediator resolvin E1. Journal of Experimental Medicine 201, 713–722.

Arita, M., Ohira, T., Sun, Y.P., Elangovan, S., Chiang, N. and Serhan, C.N. (2007) Resolvin E1 selectively interacts with leukotriene B4 receptor BLT1 and ChemR23 to regulate inflammation. *Journal of Immunology* 178, 3912–3917.

Baer, D.J., Judd, J.T., Clevidence, B.A. and Tracey, R.P. (2004) Dietary fatty acids affect plasma markers of inflammation in healthy men fed controlled diets: a randomized crossover study. *American Journal of Clinical Nutrition* 79, 969–973.

Bagga, D., Wang, L., Farias-Eisner, R., Glaspy, J.A. and Reddy, S.T. (2003) Differential effects of prostaglandin derived from ω-6 and ω-3 polyunsaturated fatty acids on COX-2 expression and IL-6 secretion. *Proceedings of the National Academy of Science USA* 100, 1751–1756.

Balvers, M.G., Verhoeckx, K.C., Plastina, P., Wortelboer, H.M., Meijerink, J. *et al.* (2010) Docosahexaenoic acid and eicosapentaenoic acid are converted by 3T3-L1 adipocytes to N-acyl ethanolamines with anti-inflammatory properties. *Biochimica et Biophysica Acta* 1801, 1107–1114.

Bellido, C., López-Miranda, J., Blanco-Colio, L.M., Pérez-Martínez, P., Muriana, F.J., *et al.* (2004) Butter and walnuts, but not olive oil, elicit postprandial activation of nuclear transcription factor kappaB in peripheral blood mononuclear cells from healthy men. *American Journal of Clinical Nutrition* 80, 1487–1491.

Bemelmans, W.J., Lefrandt, J.D., Feskens, E.J., van Haelst, P.L., Broer, J., *et al.* (2004) Increased alpha-linolenic acid intake lowers C-reactive protein, but has no effect on markers of atherosclerosis. *European Journal of Clinical Nutrition* 58, 1083–1089.

Bladbjerg, E.M., Larsen, T.M., Due, A., Stender, S., Astrup, A. *et al.* (2011) Effects on markers of inflammation and endothelial cell function of three ad libitum diets differing in type and amount of fat and carbohydrate: a 6-month randomised study in obese individuals. *British Journal of Nutrition* 106, 123–129.

Brenner, P.R. (1984) Effect of unsaturated fatty acids on membrane structure and enzymic kinetics. *Progress in Lipid Research* 23, 69–96.

Browning, L.M., Krebs, J.D., Moore, C.S., Mishra, G.D., O'Connell, M.A. *et al.* (2007) The impact of long chain n-3 polyunsaturated fatty acid supplementation on inflammation, insulin sensitivity and CVD risk in a group of overweight women with an inflammatory phenotype. *Diabetes Obesity and Metabolism* 9, 70–80.

Burdge, G.C. and Calder, P.C. (2005) Plasma cytokine response during the postprandial period: a potential causal process in vascular disease? *British Journal of Nutrition* 93, 3–9.

Calder, P.C. (2003) N-3 polyunsaturated fatty acids and inflammation: from molecular biology to the clinic. Lipids 38, 342–352.

Calder, P.C. (2006) N-3 polyunsaturated fatty acids, inflammation, and inflammatory diseases. *American Journal of Clinical Nutrition* 83,1505S–1519S.

Calder, P.C. (2008a) PUFA, inflammatory processes and rheumatoid arthritis. *Proceedings of the Nutrition Society* 67, 409–418.

Calder, P.C. (2008b) Polyunsaturated fatty acids, inflammatory processes and inflammatory bowel diseases. *Molecular Nutrition and Food Research* 52, 885–897.

Calder, P.C. (2009) Polyunsaturated fatty acids and inflammatory processes: new twists in an old tale. *Biochimie* 91, 791–795.

Calder, P.C. (2011) Fatty acids and inflammation: The cutting edge between food and pharma. *European Journal of Pharmacology* 668, S50–S58.

Calder, P.C. (2012) Mechanisms of action of (n-3) fatty acids. *Journal of Nutrition* 142, 592S–599S.

Calder, P.C. and Burdge, G.C. (2004) Fatty acids. In: Nicolaou, A. and Kafatos, G. (eds) *Bioactive Lipids.* The Oily Press, Bridgewater, UK, pp. 1–36.

Calder, P.C. and Zurier, R.B. (2001) Polyunsaturated fatty acids and rheumatoid arthritis. *Current Opinion in Clinical Nutrition and Metabolic Care* 4, 115–121.

Calder, P.C., Ahluwalia, N., Brouns, F., Buetler, T., Clement, K., *et al.* (2011) Dietary factors and low-grade inflammation in relation to overweight and obesity. *British Journal of Nutrition* 106 (Suppl 3), S5–S78.

Caughey, G.E., Mantzioris, E., Gibson, R.A., Cleland, L.G. and James, M.J. (1996) The effect on human tumor necrosis factor α and interleukin 1β production of diets enriched in n-3 fatty acids from vegetable oil or fish oil. *American Journal of Clinical Nutrition* 63, 116–122.

Chapkin, R.S., Davidson, L.A., Ly, L., Weeks, B.R., Lupton, J.R. *et al.* (2007) Immunomodulatory effects of (n-3) fatty acids: putative link to inflammation and colon cancer. *Journal of Nutrition* 137, 200S–204S.

Chilton, F.H., Patel, M., Fonteh, A.N., Hubbard, W.C. and Triggiani, M. (1993) Dietary n-3 fatty acid effects on neutrophil lipid composition and mediator production. Influence of duration and dosage. *Journal of Clinical Investigation* 91, 115–122.

Ciubotaru, I., Lee, Y.S. and Wander, R.C. (2003) Dietary fish oil decreases C-reactive protein, interleukin-6, and triacylglycerol to HDL-cholesterol ratio in postmenopausal women on HRT. *Journal of Nutritional Biochemistry* 14, 513–521.

Cleland, L.G., Caughey, G.E., James, M.J. and Proudman, S.M. (2006) Reduction of cardiovascular risk factors with longterm fish oil treatment in early rheumatoid arthritis. *Journal of Rheumatology* 33, 1973–1979.

De Ley, M., de Vos, R., Hommes, D.W. and Stokkers, P. (2007) Fish oil for induction of remission in ulcerative colitis. *Cochrane Database Systematic Reviews* 17, CD005986.

Di Marzo, V. (2008) The endocannabinoid system in obesity and type 2 diabetes. *Diabetologia* 51, 1356–1367.

Endres, S., Ghorbani, R., Kelley, V.E., Georgilis, K., Lonnemann, G., *et al.* (1989) The effect of dietary supplementation with n-3 polyunsaturated fatty acids on the synthesis of interleukin-1 and tumor necrosis factor by mononuclear cells. *New England Journal of Medicine* 320, 265–271.

Eschen, O., Christensen, J.H., De Caterina, R. and Schmidt, E.B. (2004) Soluble adhesion molecules in healthy subjects: a dose-response study using n-3 fatty acids. *Nutrition and Metabolism in Cardiovascular Disease* 14, 180–185.

Estruch, R., Martínez-González, M.A., Corella, D., Salas-Salvadó, J., Ruiz-Gutiérrez, V., *et al.*, PREDIMED Study Investigators (2006) Effects of a Mediterranean-style diet on cardiovascular risk factors: a randomized trial. *Annals of Internal Medicine* 145, 1–11.

Faber, J., Berkhout, M., Vos, A.P., Sijben, J.W., Calder, P.C., *et al.* (2011) Supplementation with a fish oil-enriched, high-protein medical food leads to rapid incorporation of EPA into white blood cells and modulates immune responses within one week in healthy men and women. *Journal of Nutrition* 141, 964–970.

Fernández-Real, J.M., Broch, M., Vendrell, J. and Ricart, W. (2003) Insulin resistance, inflammation, and serum fatty acid composition. *Diabetes Care* 26, 1362–1368.

Ferrucci, L., Cherubini, A., Bandinelli, S., Bartali, B., Corsi, A., *et al.* (2006) Relationship of plasma polyunsaturated fatty acids to circulating inflammatory markers. *Journal of Clinical Endocrinology and Metabolism* 91, 439–446.

Fisher, M., Levine, P.H., Weiner, B.H., Johnson, M.H., Doyle, E.M., *et al.* (1990) Dietary n-3 fatty acid supplementation reduces superoxide production and chemiluminescence in a monocyte-enriched preparation of leukocytes. *American Journal of Clinical Nutrition* 51, 804–808.

Fortin, P.R., Lew, R.A., Liang, M.H., Wright, E.A., Beckett, L.A., *et al.* (1995) Validation of a metaanalysis: The effects of fish oil in rheumatoid arthritis. *Journal of Clinical Epidemiology* 48, 1379–1390.

Gewirtz, A.T., Collier-Hyams, L.S., Young, A.N., Kucharzik, T., Guilford, W.J., *et al.* (2002) Lipoxin A4 analogs attenuate induction of intestinal epithelial proinflammatory gene expression and reduce the severity of dextran sodium sulfate-induced colitis. *Journal of Immunology* 168, 5260–5267.

Goldberg, R.J. and Katz, J. (2009) A meta-analysis of the analgesic effects of omega-3 polyunsaturated fatty acid supplementation for inflammatory joint pain. *Pain* 129, 210–233.

Goldman, D.W., Pickett, W.C. and Goetzl, E.J. (1983) Human neutrophil chemotactic and degranulating activities of leukotriene B_5 (LTB_5) derived from eicosapentaenoic acid. *Biochemical and Biophysical Research Communications* 117, 282–288.

Grimble, R.F., Howell, W.M., O'Reilly, G., Turner, S.J., Markovic, O., *et al.* (2002) The ability of fish oil to suppress tumor necrosis factor-α production by peripheral blood mononuclear cells in healthy men is associated with polymorphisms in genes that influence tumor necrosis factor α production. *American Journal of Clinical Nutrition* 76, 454–459.

Haworth, O., Cernadas, M., Yang, R., Serhan, C.N. and Levy, B.D. (2008) Resolvin E1 regulates interleukin 23, interferon-gamma and lipoxin A4 to promote the resolution of allergic airway inflammation. *Nature Immunology* 9, 873–879.

Healy, D.A., Wallace, F.A., Miles, E.A., Calder, P.C. and Newsholme, P. (2000) The effect of low to moderate amounts of dietary fish oil on neutrophil lipid composition and function. *Lipids* 35, 763–768.

Hjerkinn, E.M., Seljeflot, I., Ellingsen, I., Berstad, P., Hjermann, I., *et al.* (2005) Influence of long-term intervention with dietary counseling, long-chain n-3 fatty acid supplements, or both on circulating markers of endothelial activation in men with long-standing hyperlipidemia. *American Journal of Clinical Nutrition* 81, 583–589.

Hodge, L., Salome, C.M., Hughes, J.M., Liu-Brennan, D., Rimmer, J., *et al.* (1998) Effect of dietary intake of omega-3 and omega-6 fatty acids on severity of asthma in children. *European Respiratory Journal* 11, 361–365.

Hudert, C.A., Weylandt, K.H., Lu, Y., Wang, J., Hong, S., *et al.* (2006) Transgenic mice rich in endogenous omega-3 fatty acids are protected from colitis. *Proceedings of the National Academy of Science USA* 103, 11276–11281.

Hughes, D.A., Pinder, A.C., Piper, Z., Johnson, I.T. and Lund, E.K. (1996) Fish oil supplementation inhibits the expression of major histocompatibility complex class II molecules and adhesion molecules on human monocytes. *American Journal of Clinical Nutrition* 63, 267–272.

Ierna, M., Kerr, A., Scales, H., Berge, K. and Griinari, M. (2010) Supplementation of diet with krill oil protects against experimental rheumatoid arthritis. *BMC Musculoskeletal Disorders* 11, 136.

Johnson, M.M., Swan, D.D., Surette, M.E., Stegner, J., Chilton, T., *et al.* (1997) Dietary supplementation with gamma-linolenic acid alters fatty acid content and eicosanoid production in healthy humans. *Journal of Nutrition* 127, 1435–1444.

Junker, R., Pieke, B., Schulte, H., Nofer, R., Neufeld, M., *et al.* (2001) Changes in hemostasis during treatment of hypertriglyceridemia with a diet rich in monounsaturated and n-3 polyunsaturated fatty acids in comparison with a low-fat diet. *Thrombosis Research* 101, 355–366.

Kelley, D.S., Nelson, G.J., Love, J.E., Branch, L.B., Taylor, P.C., *et al.* (1993) Dietary alpha-linolenic acid alters tissue fatty acid composition, but not blood lipids, lipoproteins or coagulation status in humans. *Lipids* 28, 533–537.

Kelley, D.S., Taylor, P.C., Nelson, G.J., Schmidt, P.C., Mackey, B.E. *et al.* (1997) Effects of dietary arachidonic acid on human immune response. *Lipids* 32, 449–456.

Kelley, D.S., Taylor, P.C., Nelson, G.J., Schmidt, P.C., Ferretti, A., *et al.* (1999) Docosahexaenoic acid ingestion inhibits natural killer cell activity and production of inflammatory mediators in young healthy men. *Lipids* 34, 317–324.

Kelley, D.S., Simon, V.A., Taylor, P.C., Rudolph, I.L., Benito, P., *et al.* (2001) Dietary supplementation with conjugated linoleic acid increased its concentration in human peripheral blood mononuclear cells, but did not alter their function. *Lipids* 36, 669–674.

Kew, S., Banerjee, T., Minihane, A.M., Finnegan, Y.E., Muggli, R., *et al.* (2003) Lack of effect of foods enriched with plant- or marine-derived n-3 fatty acids on human immune function. *American Journal of Clinical Nutrition* 77, 1287–1295.

Kew, S., Mesa, M.D., Tricon, S., Buckley, R., Minihane, A.M. *et al.* (2004) Effects of oils rich in eicosapentaenoic and docosahexaenoic acids on immune cell composition and function in healthy humans. *American Journal of Clinical Nutrition* 79, 674–681.

Klein-Platat, C., Drai, J., Oujaa, M., Schlienger, J.L. and Simon, C. (2005) Plasma fatty acid composition is associated with the metabolic syndrome and low-grade inflammation in overweight adolescents. *American Journal of Clinical Nutrition* 82, 1178–1184.

Koren, M.S., Purnell, J.Q., Breen, P.A., Matthys, C.C., Callahan, H.S., *et al.* (2006) Plasma C-reactive protein concentration is not affected by isocaloric dietary fat reduction. *Nutrition* 22, 444–448.

Krishnamoorthy, S., Recchiuti, A., Chiang, N., Yacoubian, S., Lee, C.H., *et al.* (2010) Resolvin D1 binds human phagocytes with evidence for proresolving receptors. *Proceedings of the National Academy of Science USA* 107, 1660–1665.

Kroetz, D.L. and Zeldin, D.C. (2002) Cytochrome P450 pathways of arachidonic acid metabolism. *Current Opinion in Lipidology* 13, 273–283.

Lee, J.Y., Sohn, K.H., Rhee, S.H. and Hwang, D. (2001) Saturated fatty acids, but not unsaturated fatty acids, induce the expression of cyclooxygenase-2 through Toll-like receptor. *Journal of Biological Chemistry* 276, 16683–16689.

Lee, T.H., Mencia-Huerta, J.M., Shih, C., Corey, E.J., Lewis, R.A., *et al.* (1984) Characterization and biologic properties of 5,12-dihydroxy derivatives of eicosapentaenoic acid, including leukotriene-B5 and the double lipoxygenase product. *Journal of Biological Chemistry* 259, 2383–2389.

Lee, T.H., Hoover, R.L., Williams, J.D., Sperling, R.I., Ravalese, J. 3rd, *et al.* (1985) Effects of dietary enrichment with eicosapentaenoic acid and docosahexaenoic acid on in vitro neutrophil and monocyte leukotriene generation and neutrophil function. *New England Journal of Medicine* 312, 1217–1224.

Leslie, C.A., Gonnerman, W.A., Ullman, M.D., Hayes, K.C., Franzblau, C., *et al.* (1985) Dietary fish oil modulates macrophage fatty acids and decreases arthritis susceptibility in mice. *Journal of Experimental Medicine* 162, 1336–1339.

Levy, B.D., Clish, C.B., Schmidt, B., Gronert, K. and Serhan, C.N. (2001) Lipid mediator class switching during acute inflammation: signals in resolution. *Nature Immunology* 2, 612–619.

Lewis, R.A., Austen, K.F. and Soberman, R.J. (1990) Leukotrienes and other products of the 5-lipoxygenase pathway: biochemistry and relation to pathobiology in human diseases. *New England Journal of Medicine* 323, 645–655.

Li, G., Barnes, D., Butz, D., Bjorling, D. and Cook, M.E. (2005) 10t,12c-conjugated linoleic acid inhibits lipopolysaccharide-induced cyclooxygenase expression in vitro and in vivo. *Journal of Lipid Research* 46, 2134–2142.

Li, G., Dong, B., Butz, D.E., Park, Y., Pariza, M.W., *et al.* (2006) NF-kappaB independent inhibition of lipopolysaccharide-induced cyclooxygenase by a conjugated linoleic acid cognate, conjugated nonadecadienoic acid. *Biochimica et Biophysica Acta* 1761, 969–972.

Lima-Garcia, J.F., Dutra, R.C., da Silva, K., Motta, E.M., Campos, M.M., *et al.* (2011) The precursor of resolvin D series and aspirin-triggered resolvin D1 display anti-hyperalgesic properties in adjuvant-induced arthritis in rats. *British Journal of Pharmacology* 164, 278–293.

Lopez-Garcia, E., Schulze, M.B., Manson, J.E., Meigs, J.B., Albert, C.M., *et al.* (2004) Consumption of (n-3) fatty acids is related to plasma biomarkers of inflammation and endothelial activation in women. *Journal of Nutrition* 134, 1806–1811.

Lopez-Garcia, E., Schulze, M.B., Meigs, J.B., Manson, J.E., Rifai, N., *et al.* (2005) Consumption of trans fatty acids is related to plasma biomarkers of inflammation and endothelial dysfunction. *Journal of Nutrition* 135, 562–566.

Luostarinen, R. and Saldeen, T. (1996) Dietary fish oil decreases superoxide generation by human neutrophils: relation to cyclooxygenase pathway and lysosomal enzyme release. *Prostaglandins Leukotrienes and Essential Fatty Acids* 55, 167–172.

Luostarinen, R., Siegbahn, A. and Saldeen, T. (1992) Effect of dietary fish oil supplemented with different doses of vitamin E on neutrophil chemotaxis in healthy volunteers. *Nutrition Research* 12, 1419–1430.

MacLean, C.H., Mojica, W.A., Morton, S.C., Pencharz, J., Hasenfeld Garland, R., *et al.* (2004) Effects of omega-3 fatty acids on inflammatory bowel disease, rheumatoid arthritis, renal disease, systemic lupus erythematosus, and osteoporosis. Evidence report/technical Assessment no. 89. AHRQ Publication no. 04-E012-2, Agency for Healthcare Research and Quality, Rockville, MD. Available at http://www.ahrq.gov/clinic/tp/o3lipidtp.htm

Madsen, T., Skou, H.A., Hansen, V.E., Fog, L., Christensen, J.H., *et al.* (2001) C-reactive protein, dietary n-3 fatty acids, and the extent of coronary artery disease. *American Journal of Cardiology* 88, 1139–1142.

Mantzioris, E., James, M.J., Gibson, R.A. and Cleland, L.G. (1994) Dietary substitution with an alpha-linolenic acid-rich vegetable oil increases eicosapentaenoic acid concentrations in tissues. *American Journal of Clinical Nutrition* 59, 1304–1309.

Meijerink, J., Plastina, P., Vincken, J.P., Poland, M., Attya, M., *et al.* (2011) The ethanolamide metabolite of DHA, docosahexaenoylethanolamine, shows immunomodulating effects in mouse peritoneal and RAW264.7 macrophages: evidence for a new link between fish oil and inflammation. *British Journal of Nutrition* 105, 1789–1807.

Meydani, S.N., Endres, S., Woods, M.M., Goldin, B.R., Soo, C., *et al.* (1991) Oral (n-3) fatty acid supplementation suppresses cytokine production and lymphocyte proliferation: comparison between young and older women. *Journal of Nutrition* 121, 547–555.

Miles, E.A. and Calder, P.C. (1998) Modulation of immune function by dietary fatty acids. *Proceedings of the Nutrition Society* 57, 277–292.

Miles, E.A., Banerjee, T. and Calder, P.C. (2004) The influence of different combinations of γ-linolenic, stearidonic and eicosapentaenoic acids on the fatty acid composition of blood lipids and mononuclear cells in human volunteers. *Prostaglandins Leukotrienes and Essential Fatty Acids* 70, 529–538.

Moloney, F., Toomey, S., Noone, E., Nugent, A., Allan, B., *et al.* (2007) Antidiabetic effects of cis-9, trans-11-conjugated linoleic acid may be mediated via anti-inflammatory effects in white adipose tissue. *Diabetes* 56, 574–582.

Mori, T.A., Woodman, R.J., Burke, V., Puddey, I.B., Croft, K.D., *et al.* (2003) Effect of eicosapentaenoic acid and docosahexaenoic acid on oxidative stress and inflammatory markers in treated-hypertensive type 2 diabetic subjects. *Free Radicals in Biology and Medicine* 35, 772–781.

Mullen, A., Moloney, F., Nugent, A.P., Doyle, L., Cashman, K.D., *et al.* (2007) Conjugated linoleic acid supplementation reduces peripheral blood mononuclear cell interleukin-2 production in healthy middle-aged males. *Journal of Nutritional Biochemistry* 18, 658–666.

Murphy, M.G. (1990) Dietary fatty acids and membrane protein function. *Journal of Nutritional Biochemistry* 1, 68–79.

Nagakura, T., Matsuda, S., Shichijyo, K., Sugimoto, H. and Hata, K. (2000) Dietary supplementation with fish oil rich in omega-3 polyunsaturated fatty acids in children with bronchial asthma. *European Respiratory Journal* 16, 861–865.

Nappo, F., Esposito, K., Cioffi, M., Giugliano, G., Molinari, A.M., *et al.* (2002) Postprandial endothelial activation in healthy subjects and in type 2 diabetic patients: role of fat and carbohydrate meals. *Journal of the American College of Cardiology* 39, 1145–1150.

Nettleton, J.A., Steffen, L.M., Mayer-Davis, E.J., Jenny, N.S., Jiang, R., *et al.* (2006) Dietary patterns are associated with biochemical markers of inflammation and endothelial activation in the Multi-Ethnic Study of Atherosclerosis (MESA). *American Journal of Clinical Nutrition* 83, 1369–1379.

Nugent, A.P., Roche, H.M., Noone, E.J., Long, A., Kelleher, D.K., *et al.* (2005) The effects of conjugated linoleic acid supplementation on immune function in healthy volunteers. *European Journal of Clinical Nutrition* 59, 742–750.

Oh, D.Y., Talukdar, S., Bae, E.J., Imamura, T., Morinaga, H., *et al.* (2010) GPR120 is an omega-3 fatty acid receptor mediating potent anti-inflammatory and insulin-sensitizing effects. *Cell* 142, 687–698.

Paschos, G.K., Rallidis, L.S., Liakos, G.K., Panagiotakos, D., Anastasiadis, G., *et al.* (2004) Background diet influences the anti-inflammatory effect of alpha-linolenic acid in dyslipidaemic subjects. *British Journal of Nutrition* 92, 649–655.

Paschos, G.K., Zampelas, A., Panagiotakos, D.B., Katsiougiannis, S., Griffin, B.A., *et al.* (2007) Effects of flaxseed oil supplementation on plasma adiponectin levels in dyslipidemic men. *European Journal of Nutrition* 46, 315–320.

Petersson, H., Basu, S., Cederholm, T., *et al.* (2008) Serum fatty acid composition and indices of stearoyl-CoA desaturase activity are associated with systemic inflammation: longitudinal analyses in middle-aged men. *British Journal of Nutrition* 99, 1186–1189.

Pike, L.J. (2003) Lipid rafts: bringing order to chaos. *Journal of Lipid Research* 44, 655–667.

Pischon, T., Hankinson, S.E., Hotamisligil, G.S., Rifai, N., Willett, W.C., *et al.* (2003) Habitual dietary intake of n-3 and n-6 fatty acids in relation to inflammatory markers among US men and women. *Circulation* 108, 155–160.

Rallidis, L.S., Paschos, G., Liakos, G.K., Velissaridou, A.H., Anastasiadis, G., *et al.* (2003) Dietary alpha-linolenic acid decreases C-reactive protein, serum amyloid A and interleukin-6 in dyslipidaemic patients. *Atherosclerosis* 167, 237–242.

Rallidis, L.S., Paschos, G., Papaioannou, M.L., Liakos, G.K., Panagiotakos, D.B., *et al.* (2004) The effect of diet enriched with alpha-linolenic acid on soluble cellular adhesion molecules in dyslipidaemic patients. *Atherosclerosis* 174, 127–132.

Ramakers, J.D., Plat, J., Sebedio, J.L. and Mensink, R.P. (2005) Effects of the individual isomers cis-9,trans-11 vs. trans-10,cis-12 of conjugated linoleic acid (CLA) on inflammation parameters in moderately overweight subjects with LDL-phenotype B. *Lipids* 40, 909–918.

Rasic-Milutinovic, Z., Perunicic, G., Pljesa, S., Gluvic, Z., Sobajic, S., *et al.* (2007) Effects of N-3 PUFAs supplementation on insulin resistance and inflammatory biomarkers in hemodialysis patients. *Renal Failure* 29, 321–329.

Rees, D., Miles, E.A., Banerjee, T., Wells, S.J., Roynette, C.E., *et al.* (2006) Dose-related effects of eicosapentaenoic acid on innate immune function in healthy humans: a comparison of young and older men. *American Journal of Clinical Nutrition* 83, 331–342.

Riserus, U., Basu, S., Jovinge, S., *et al.* (2002) Supplementation with conjugated linoleic acid causes isomer-dependent oxidative stress and elevated C-reactive protein: a potential link to fatty acid-induced insulin resistance. *Circulation* 106, 1925–1929.

Roberts, C.K., Won, D., Pruthi, S., Kurtovic, S., Sindhu, R.K., *et al.* (2006) Effect of a short-term diet and exercise intervention on oxidative stress, inflammation, MMP-9, and monocyte chemotactic activity in men with metabolic syndrome factors. *Journal of Applied Physiology* 100, 1657–1665.

Rossetti, R.G., Seiler, C.M., DeLuca, P., Laposata, M. and Zurier, R.B. (1997) Oral administration of unsaturated fatty acids: effects on human peripheral blood T lymphocyte proliferation. *Journal of Leukocyte Biology* 62, 438–443.

Schmidt, E.B., Pedersen, J.O., Ekelund, S., Grunnet, N., Jersild, C., *et al.* (1989) Cod liver oil inhibits neutrophil and monocyte chemotaxis in healthy males. *Atherosclerosis* 77, 53–57.

Schmidt, E.B., Pedersen, J.O., Varming, K., Ernst, E., Jersild, C., *et al.* (1991) N-3 fatty acids and leukocyte chemotaxis: effects in hyperlipidemia, and dose-response studies in healthy males. *Arteriosclerosis and Thrombosis* 11, 429–435.

Schmidt, E.B., Varming, K., Pedersen, J.O., Lervang, H.H., Grunnet, N., *et al.* (1992) Long term supplementation with n-3 fatty acids, ii: Effect on neutrophil and monocyte chemotaxis. *Scandinavian Journal of Clinical and Laboratory Investigations* 52, 229–236.

Serhan, C.N., Clish, C.B., Brannon, J., Colgan, S.P., Chiang, N., *et al.* (2000a) Novel functional sets of lipid-derived mediators with antinflammatory actions generated from omega-3 fatty acids via cyclooxygenase 2-nonsteroidal antiinflammatory drugs and transcellular processing. *Journal of Experimental Medicine* 192, 1197–1204.

Serhan, C.N., Clish, C.B., Brannon, J., Colgan, S.P., Gronert, K., *et al.* (2000b) Anti-inflammatory lipid signals generated from dietary n-3 fatty acids via cyclooxygenase-2 and transcellular processing: a novel mechanism for NSAID and n-3 PUFA therapeutic actions. *Journal of Physiological Pharmacology* 4, 643–654.

Serhan, C.N., Hong, S., Gronert, K., Colgan, S.P., Devchand, P.R., *et al.* (2002) Resolvins: a family of bioactive products of omega-3 fatty acid transformation circuits initiated by aspirin treatment that counter pro-inflammation signals. *Journal of Experimental Medicine* 196, 1025–37.

Serhan, C.N., Chiang, N. and van Dyke, T.E. (2008) Resolving inflammation: dual anti-inflammatory and pro-resolution lipid mediators. *Nature Reviews Immunology* 8, 349–361.

Simons, K. and Toomre, D. (2000) Lipid rafts and signal transduction. *Nature Reviews Molecular Cell Biology* 1, 31–41.

Smedman, A., Basu, S., Jovinge, S., Fredrikson, G.N. and Vessby, B. (2005) Conjugated linoleic acid increased C-reactive protein in human subjects. *British Journal of Nutrition* 94, 791–795.

Song, H.J., Grant, I., Rotondo, D., Mohede, I., Sattar, N., *et al.* (2005) Effect of CLA supplementation on immune function in young healthy volunteers. *European Journal of Clinical Nutrition* 59, 508–517.

Sperling, R.I., Benincaso, A.I., Knoell, C.T., Larkin, J.K., Austen, K.F., *et al.* (1993) Dietary ω-3 polyunsaturated fatty acids inhibit phosphoinositide formation and chemotaxis in neutrophils. Journal of Clinical Investigation 91, 651–660.

Stubbs, C.D. and Smith, A.D. (1984) The modification of mammalian membrane polyunsaturated fatty acid composition in relation to membrane fluidity and function. *Biochimica et Biophysica Acta* 779, 89–137.

Thien, F.C.K., Woods, R., De Luca, S. and Abramson, M.J. (2002) Dietary marine fatty acids (fish oil) for asthma in adults and children. *Cochrane Database of Systematic Reviews* 2, CD001283.

Thies, F., Nebe-von-Caron, G., Powell, J.R., Yaqoob, P., Newsholme, E.A., *et al.* (2001a) Dietary supplementation with γ-linolenic acid or fish oil decreases T lymphocyte proliferation in healthy older humans. *Journal of Nutrition* 131, 1918–1927.

Thies, F., Miles, E.A., Nebe-von-Caron, G., Powell, J.R., Hurst, T.L., *et al.* (2001b) Influence of dietary supplementation with long chain n-3 or n-6 polyunsaturated fatty acids on blood inflammatory cell populations and functions and on plasma soluble adhesion molecules in healthy adults. *Lipids* 36, 1183–1193.

Thompson, P.J., Misso, N.L., Passarelli, M. and Phillips, M.J. (1991) The effect of eicosapentaenoic acid consumption on human neutrophil chemiluminescence. *Lipids* 26, 1223–1226.

Tilley, S.L., Coffman, T.M. and Koller, B.H. (2001) Mixed messages: modulation of inflammation and immune responses by prostaglandins and thromboxanes. *Journal of Clinical Investigation* 108, 15–23.

Trebble, T., Arden, N.K., Stroud, M.A., Wootton, S.A., Burdge, G.C., *et al.* (2003) Inhibition of tumour necrosis factor-α and interleukin-6 production by mononuclear cells following dietary fish-oil supplementation in healthy men and response to antioxidant co-supplementation. *British Journal of Nutrition* 90, 405–412.

Tricon, S., Burdge, G.C., Kew, S., Banerjee, T., Russell, J.J., *et al.* (2004) Effects of cis-9,trans-11 and trans-10,cis-12 conjugated linoleic acid on immune cell function in healthy humans. *American Journal of Clinical Nutrition* 80, 1626–1633.

Troseid, M., Arnesen, H., Hjerkinn, E.M. and Seljeflot, I. (2009) Serum levels of interleukin-18 are reduced by diet and n-3 fatty acid intervention in elderly high-risk men. *Metabolism* 58, 1543–1549.

Turner, D., Steinhart, T.H. and Griffiths, A.M. (2007) Omega 3 fatty acids (fish oil) for maintenance of remission in ulcerative colitis. *Cochrane Database of Systematic Reviews* 18, CD006443.

Turner, D., Zlotkin, S.H., Shah, P.S. and Griffiths, A.M. (2009) Omega 3 fatty acids (fish oil) for maintenance of remission in Crohn's disease. *Cochrane Database of Systematic Reviews* 21, CD006320.

Vachier, I., Chanez, P., Bonnans, C., Godard, P., Bousquet, J., *et al.* (2002) Endogenous anti-inflammatory mediators from arachidonate in human neutrophils. *Biochemical and Biophysical Research Communications* 290, 219–224.

Varming, K., Schmidt, E.B., Svaneborg, N., Møller, J.M., Lervang, H.H., *et al.* (1995) The effect of n-3 fatty acids on neutrophil chemiluminescence. *Scandinavian Journal of Clinical and Laboratory Investigation* 55, 47–52.

Volker, D.H., FitzGerald, P.E.B. and Garg, M.L. (2000) The eicosapentaenoic to docosahexaenoic acid ratio of diets affects the pathogenesis of arthritis in Lew/SSN rats. *Journal of Nutrition* 130, 559–565.

Von Schacky, C., Kiefl, R., Jendraschak, E. and Kaminski, W.E. (1993) N-3 fatty acids and cysteinyl-leukotriene formation in humans in vitro, ex vivo and in vivo. *Journal of Laboratory and Clinical Medicine* 121, 302–309.

Wada, M., DeLong, C.J., Hong, Y.H., Rieke, C.J., Song, I., *et al.* (2007) Enzymes and receptors of prostaglandin pathways with arachidonic acid-derived versus eicosapentaenoic acid-derived substrates and products. *Journal of Biological Chemistry* 282, 22254–22266.

Wallace, F.A., Miles, E.A. and Calder, P.C. (2003) Comparison of the effects of linseed oil and different doses of fish oil on mononuclear cell function in healthy human subjects. *British Journal of Nutrition* 89, 679–689.

Weatherill, A.R., Lee, J.Y., Zhao, L., Lemay, D.G., Youn, H.S., *et al.* (2005) Saturated and polyunsaturated fatty acids reciprocally modulate dendritic cell functions mediated through TLR4. *Journal of Immunology* 174, 5390–5397.

Wu, D., Meydani, M., Leka, L.S., Nightingale, Z., Handelman, G.J., *et al.* (1999) Effect of dietary supplementation with black currant seed oil on the immune response of healthy elderly subjects. *American Journal of Clinical Nutrition* 70, 536–543.

Yamada, H., Yoshida, M., Nakano, Y., Suganami, T., Satoh, N., *et al.* (2008) In vivo and in vitro inhibition of monocyte adhesion to endothelial cells and endothelial adhesion molecules by eicosapentaenoic acid. *Arteriosclerosis Thrombosis and Vascular Biology* 28, 2173–2179.

Yaqoob, P. (2009) The nutritional significance of lipid rafts. *Annual Review in Nutrition* 29, 257–282.

Yaqoob, P. and Shaikh, S.R. (2010) The nutritional and clinical significance of lipid rafts. *Current Opinion in Clinical Nutrition and Metabolic Care* 13, 156–166.

Yaqoob, P., Pala, H.S., Cortina-Borja, M., Newsholme, E.A. and Calder, P.C. (2000) Encapsulated fish oil enriched in α-tocopherol alters plasma phospholipid and mononuclear cell fatty acid compositions but not mononuclear cell functions. *European Journal of Clinical Investigation* 30, 260–274.

Yin, H., Chu, A., Li, W., Wang, B., Shelton, F., *et al.* (2009) Lipid G protein-coupled receptor ligand identification using beta-arrestin PathHunter assay. *Journal of Biological Chemistry* 284, 12328–12338.

Yli-Jama, P., Seljeflot, I., Meyer, H.E., Hjerkinn, E.M., Arnesen, H., *et al.* (2002) Serum non-esterified very long-chain PUFA are associated with markers of endothelial dysfunction. *Atherosclerosis* 164, 275–281.

Yokoyama, A., Hamazaki, T., Ohshita, A., Kohno, N., Sakai, K., *et al.* (2000) Effect of aerosolized docosahexaenoic acid in a mouse model of atopic asthma. *International Archives of Allergy and Immunology* 123, 327–332.

Yusof, H.M., Miles, E.A. and Calder, P.C. (2008) Influence of very long-chain n-3 fatty acids on plasma markers of inflammation in middle-aged men. *Prostaglandins Leukotrienes and Essential Fatty Acids* 78, 219–228.

Zhao, G., Etherton, T.D., Martin, K.R., West, S.G., Gillies, P.J., *et al.* (2004) Dietary alpha-linolenic acid reduces inflammatory and lipid cardiovascular risk factors in hypercholesterolemic men and women. *Journal of Nutrition* 134, 2991–2997.

3 Carbohydrates and Inflammation

A.E. Buyken,*,[1] and J. Brand-Miller[2]

[1]*Research Institute of Child Nutrition, Rheinische Friedrich-Wilhelms-Universität Bonn, Germany;* [2]*School of Molecular Bioscience, Boden Institute of Obesity, Nutrition and Exercise, University of Sydney, Australia*

Introduction

Chronic low-grade inflammation plays a recognized role in the development and the progression of both type 2 diabetes and cardiovascular disease (CVD) (Couzin-Frankel, 2010). Inflammation is also a likely intermediary between aspects of carbohydrate nutrition and chronic disease. In this chapter, we provide an overview of the available observational and clinical evidence linking dietary carbohydrates with inflammation, and summarize the potential mechanisms that suggest a causal, rather than coincidental, association.

Carbohydrates comprise a wide range of components that differ notably in both their chemical structure and their physiological properties. The terminology based on chemistry distinguishes monosaccharides (glucose, fructose and galactose), disaccharides (e.g. sucrose and lactose) and oligosaccharides as well as polysaccharides comprising both starches (e.g. amylose, amylopectin, modified starches) and non-starch polysaccharides (cellulose, hemicelluloses, pectin, β-glucan, etc.) (Cummings and Stephen, 2007). Digestible sugars and starches are also commonly termed 'available carbohydrates', whereas dietary

* Corresponding author, [illegible]

 Nutrition and Physical Activity in Inflammatory Diseases (eds M.L. Garg and L.G. Wood)

fibres, resistant starch, and low-digestibility sugars and oligosaccharides are not digested and absorbed (Englyst *et al.*, 2007).

On the basis of the observation that chemical composition of the carbohydrate cannot predict its postprandial blood glucose rise, Jenkins *et al.* (1981) proposed the glycaemic index (GI) as a system of ranking carbohydrate containing foods for their 'glycaemic potency'. The dietary GI is calculated as the blood glucose response to 50 g (or 25 g) of available carbohydrate from a food, expressed as a percentage of the same amount of available carbohydrate from a reference food (glucose or white bread) (Jenkins *et al.*, 1981). In 1997, Salmeron *et al.* (1987) introduced the concept of the glycaemic load (GL) to describe the absolute glucose response induced by a serving of a food. The GL corresponds to the quantity of carbohydrate multiplied by the respective GI and can be interpreted as a global indicator of the overall glucose response induced by the consumed amounts of foods.

Current controversy regarding the definition of dietary fibre relates to the question of whether fibre reflects the naturally occurring cell-wall polysaccharides of fruit, vegetables and whole grains or whether it should encompass all carbohydrates indigestible in the small intestine. The main argument against the latter relates to the fact that health benefits have been primarily demonstrated for naturally occurring fibre (Englyst *et al.*, 2007; Mann and Cummings, 2009). Similarly, debate surrounds the term 'whole grains'. The US Food and Drug Administration defined them as consisting of the 'intact, ground, cracked or flaked fruit of the grains whose principal components – the starchy endosperm, germ and bran – are present in the same relative proportions as they exist in the intact grain' (FDA, 2006), and considers whole-grain foods as those containing at least 51% whole grain (Cummings and Stephen, 2007). However, many studies use a broader meaning to define whole grains (e.g. additional consideration of bran or germ) (Cummings and Stephen, 2007; De Moura *et al.*, 2009). Whole-grain definitions do not generally differentiate between intact kernels and milled whole grains (e.g. 'whole-grain flour'), despite the fact that the postprandial glycaemic response is known to differ markedly between these physical forms of whole grains (Holt and Miller, 1994; Atkinson *et al.*, 2008).

Potential Underlying Mechanisms

Among the components of carbohydrates, specific mechanisms linking them to inflammation have been proposed for dietary glucose, meals with high GI and dietary fibre (Fig. 3.1).

Dietary glucose

Interest in the role of carbohydrate nutrition in inflammation can be traced to the observation that reactive oxygen species (ROS) and superoxide radicals are generated even in healthy people after a single 75 g glucose challenge (Ceriello, 2005; Dandona *et al.*, 2007). At the molecular level, Ceriello (2005) proposed that intracellular hyperglycaemia induces the overproduction of superoxide within mitochondria. Thus, as glucose is progressively oxidized, the mitochondrial proton gradient increases, electrons are transferred to oxygen and then to the superoxide anion. Under the influence of insulin, there is a simultaneous increase in nitric oxide (NO) generation. Subsequently, superoxide combines with NO to produce peroxynitrite, a reactive molecule that damages DNA and hence mitochondrial and cellular function. According to Ceriello's hypothesis, this is the first step in the development of both endothelial dysfunction and diabetes complications associated with postprandial hyperglycaemia (Ceriello and Motz, 2004; Ceriello, 2005). A single glucose challenge has also been shown to increase the activation of pro-inflammatory transcription factors, such as nuclear factor-kappaB (NFκB), and the expression of specific genes, particularly those associated with the expression of adhesion molecules (Dandona *et al.*, 2007).

Although oxidative stress and an increase in plasma levels of inflammatory markers occur in healthy, glucose-tolerant individuals, the effect is short lived. In contrast, in individuals with impaired glucose tolerance, obesity or persons with type 2 diabetes, the result is

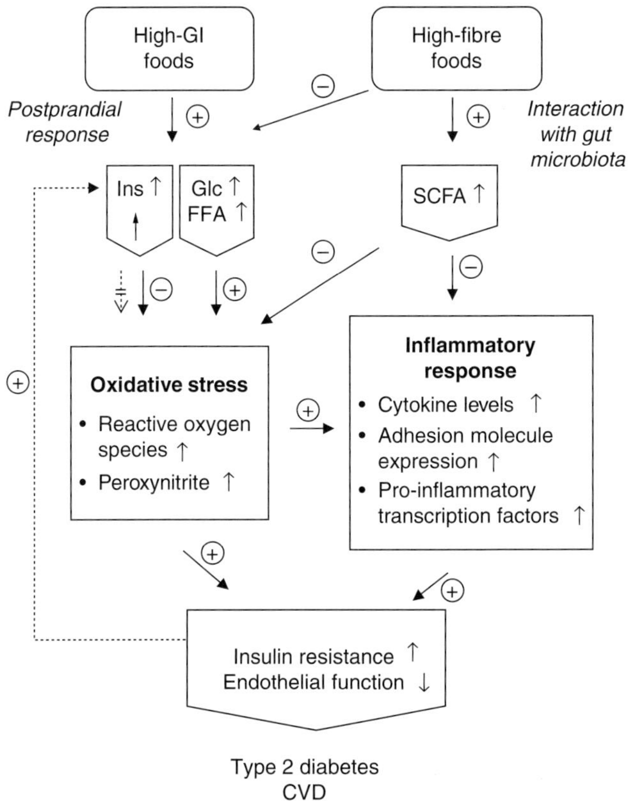

Fig. 3.1. Central to the proposed effects of foods with a high glycaemic index (GI) are the recurrent postprandially elevated blood glucose levels (Glc). Hyperglycaemia in the early postprandial phase as well as elevated levels of free fatty acids (FFA) in the late postprandial phase are considered to result in an overproduction of reactive free radical molecules and release of pro-inflammatory cytokines, which may in turn induce inflammation and vascular damage (Ceriello, 2005). In insulin-sensitive individuals, these effects are cancelled out by the anti-inflammatory effect of concurrent increases in postprandial insulin levels (Ins). Among insulin-resistant individuals (dashed line), the anti-inflammatory actions of insulin are diminished or even lacking (Dandona *et al.*, 2007). Dietary fibre intake may contribute to a reduction of both oxidative stress and the inflammatory response because short chain fatty acids (SFCA) are produced from fermentable fibre in interaction with the gut microbiota (Rodriguez-Cabezas *et al.*, 2002; Maslowski *et al.*, 2009). ↓ = decrease, ↑ = increase, CVD = cardiovascular disease.

more pronounced and lasts longer (>2–3 h) (Kempf *et al.*, 2006). Dandona *et al.* (2007) propose that the difference stems from the varying effects of insulin in insulin-sensitive versus insulin-resistant states. In insulin-sensitive individuals, insulin has clear dose-related, anti-inflammatory effects on endothelial cells and mononuclear leucocytes, resulting in vasodilatory and anti-thrombogenic effects that help to cancel out the pro-inflammatory effects of glucose. These beneficial effects arise because insulin directly stimulates nitric oxide synthase and the release of nitric oxide from the endothelium. Unlike glucose, insulin also suppresses ROS superoxide generation and NFκB binding, reducing plasma concentrations of pro-inflammatory cytokines (Dandona *et al.*, 2007).

Insulin-resistant individuals, however, present diminished anti-inflammatory effects of insulin (Dandona *et al.*, 2007). Because insulin resistance impairs the PI 3-kinase signalling pathway, compensatory hyperinsulinaemia becomes proatherogenic by over-stimulating both the MAP-kinase signalling pathway and excessive prenylation of Ras and Rho proteins (Wang *et al.*, 2004). Furthermore, exaggerated compensatory postprandial insulin excursions promote a mild 'reactive' hypoglycaemia, which results in increased secretion of counter-regulatory stress hormones and release of free fatty acids during the late postprandial phase (Ludwig, 2002). Higher levels of catecholamines and free fatty acids are believed to exaggerate the pro-inflammatory response to glucose (Dandona *et al.*, 2007; Kallio *et al.*, 2008).

Meals with a high glycaemic index (GI)

Postprandial glucose excursions and exaggerated insulin responses leading to mild hypoglycaemia are also known to occur in response to the consumption of high GI meals (Brand-Miller *et al.*, 2009). Indeed, in individuals with type 2 diabetes, glucose fluctuations during postprandial periods have a more specific triggering effect on oxidative stress than chronic sustained hyperglycaemia (Monnier *et al.*, 2006). Taken together, these findings suggest that consumption of high GI meals, particularly by insulin-resistant individuals, will promote oxidative stress. In these people, habitual consumption of meals with a high GI will exert greater demands on beta cell function. Because beta cells are particularly sensitive to oxidative stress this could eventually promote a more rapid development of type 2 diabetes (Fig. 3.2).

In a short-term metabolic ward study, the consumption of high GI foods has been directly linked to the creation of oxidative stress: in healthy lean adults, the consumption of 50 g of available carbohydrate as either glucose or white bread (a high GI food) resulted in three times greater activation of NFκB during the subsequent 3 h compared with the ingestion of 50 g of carbohydrate in the form of pasta. Nitrotyrosine generation was also significantly higher after bread, suggesting a higher production of peroxynitrite. Changes in NFκB paralleled the rise in postprandial glucose, rather than insulin levels, implying that the pro-inflammatory effects of glucose temporarily outpaced the anti-inflammatory effects of insulin even in insulin-sensitive individuals (Dickinson *et al.*, 2008).

Unfortunately, the science is not consistent. In healthy overweight women, Motton *et al.* (2007) reported significant increases in monocytes expressing TNF-α (an acute phase pro-inflammatory cytokine) at 3.5 h and 8 h following the consumption of *both* low and high GI meals. Although the authors speculate that only some individuals might be 'carbohydrate sensitive', it is also possible that differences existed in the responses within the first 3 h of consumption.

The presence of oxidative stress can also be detected by an acute decline in antioxidant concentrations in plasma following a meal. Botero *et al.* (2009) observed differences in fasting and postprandial total antioxidant capacity over the course of a 5-h observation period following 1 week on a low or high GI diet in overweight men. Plasma total antioxidant capacity in response to the GI of the diet may therefore be the first metabolic adaptation on the pathway linking carbohydrate nutrition and dietary GI to type 2 diabetes and/or CVD.

Meals rich in dietary fibre

A comparison of postprandial responses to a high-fat high-carbohydrate (HFHC) meal and to those following the ingestion of a meal rich in fibre and fruit in healthy lean subjects revealed increases in plasma endotoxin concentrations, the expression of toll-like receptors and suppressor of cytokine signalling-3 in mononuclear cells, after the HFHC only. Notably, the postprandial glucose excursion was markedly higher after the HFHC, whereas insulin responses were comparable. The authors attribute these differences mainly to the fruits and fibre provided in the intervention meal, which included foods with a low GI (oatmeal, milk, orange juice, raisins, English muffin) (Ghanim *et al.*, 2009).

There are additional mechanisms linking fibre intake per se to inflammatory responses. Maslowksi *et al.* (2009) propose that fibre intake and gut microbiota may be directly associated at the molecular level to inflammatory responses. In a study conducted in mice they showed that short-chain

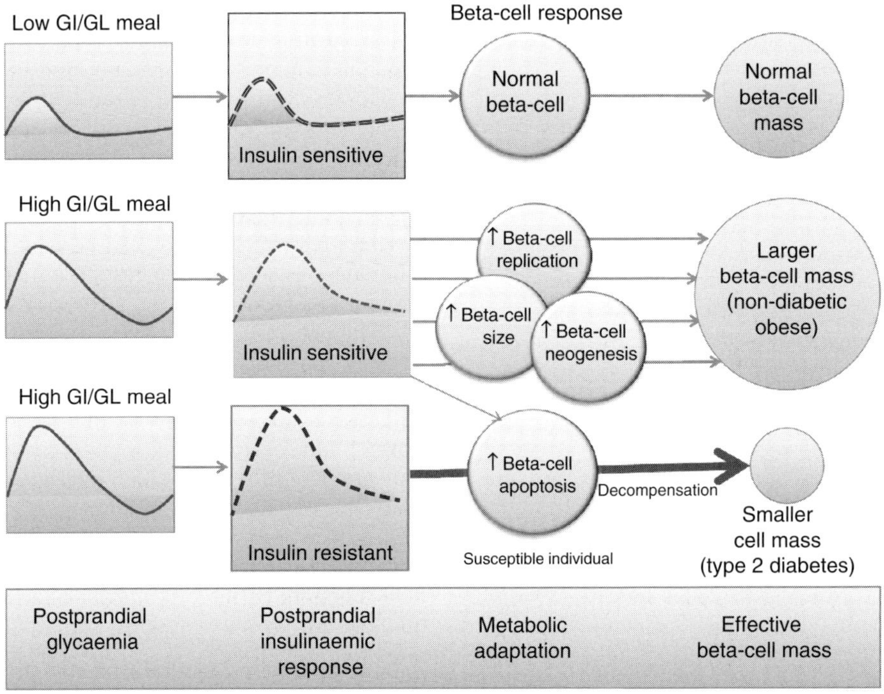

Fig. 3.2. A tenuous balance exists between insulin resistance and an effective beta-cell mass. For the most part, beta-cell mass adapts adequately to compensate for changes in the metabolic load. However, beta cells can be pushed too far in susceptible individuals. High-GI carbohydrates and high-GI diets can worsen insulin resistance and contribute to an overwhelming metabolic load. Eventually the beta-cell mass fails to compensate for insulin resistance and type 2 diabetes ensues. This failure may be caused by a marked increase in beta-cell apoptosis, probably induced by a combination of chronic postprandial hyperglycaemia and hyperlipidaemia, and/or certain cytokines that interfere with the signalling pathways that maintain normal beta-cell growth and survival. Of all tissues, the beta cells in particular are especially sensitive to endoplasmic reticulum stress and to oxidative stress caused by high throughput through the mitochondrial chain. The net effect is a reduction in functional beta-cell mass in the type 2 diabetic state. Information drawn from previously published work (Dickinson *et al.*, 2002; Rhodes, 2005). (From Buyken *et al.*, 2010b, with permission from Springer Science and Business Media.)

fatty acids (SCFAs) produced from fermentable fibre, bind to G-protein-coupled receptor 43 (GPR43). Because GPR43 is the sole functional receptor for SCFAs on neutrophils, it might be of particular relevance in the regulation of inflammatory responses by SCFAs (Maslowski *et al.*, 2009). In an experiment in rats with induced colitis, those supplemented with fibre (5% *Plantago ovata* seeds) for 1 week showed a significant decrease in colonic TNF-α levels compared with non-treated rats. Faecal butyrate and propionate levels that provide substrates to the colonocytes were also increased. In addition, colonic NOS activity was inhibited during fibre supplementation, which the authors attribute to the inhibitory effect exerted by butyrate on NOS induction (Rodriguez-Cabezas *et al.*, 2002).

Importantly, diets rich in fibre or whole grains are commonly higher in vitamins and phytonutrients representing other potentially relevant mechanisms linking fibre intake to inflammation (Fardet, 2010).

Carbohydrate Nutrition and Inflammatory Markers

A number of studies comparing high-carbohydrate, high-fibre diets with 'control' diets found significant improvements in inflammatory markers (Roberts *et al.*, 2006; Rankin and Turpyn, 2007; Keogh *et al.*, 2008). One intervention study in postmenopausal women suggested, however, that a low-fat, high-carbohydrate diet may only favourably affect inflammatory risk markers to the extent that it induces weight loss (Kasim-Karakas *et al.*, 2006). In line with this, Dansinger *et al.* (2005) reported that the use of Atkins, Zone, Weight Watcher and Ornish diets for 1 year resulted in similar changes in C-reactive protein (CRP) in line with the change in body weight (Dansinger *et al.*, 2005). Similarly, other longer-term weight-loss studies using either low-carbohydrate dietary approaches or high-protein regimens accompanied by a lower carbohydrate content reported these diets to be comparable to the conventionally used high-carbohydrate diets with respect to their effect on inflammatory markers (Brinkworth *et al.*, 2004; Seshadri *et al.*, 2004; Due *et al.*, 2005; O'Brien *et al.*, 2005; Tay *et al.*, 2008). Taken together, these studies imply that total carbohydrate intake may be of minor relevance for inflammation, but the quality of carbohydrate may be crucial.

Dietary glycaemic index or glycaemic load

Epidemiological evidence

Several cross-sectional analyses from different cohorts suggest an association between the dietary GI and/or dietary GL with levels of CRP or adiponectin (Liu *et al.*, 2002; Qi *et al.*, 2005; Qi *et al.*, 2006a; Qi *et al.*, 2006b; Du *et al.*, 2008; Levitan *et al.*, 2008) (Table 3.1). Liu was the first to report a relationship between dietary GL and GI and CRP levels for a random sample of 244 women selected from the Women's Health Study (Liu *et al.*, 2002). In this analysis, multivariable-adjusted CRP levels in the highest quintile were more than twofold that in the lowest quintile. A later analysis from the same study among 18,137 women confirmed an association for dietary GI only, with a multivariable-adjusted difference in CRP of 12% between the extreme quintiles (Levitan *et al.*, 2008). Similarly, dietary GI but not GL was cross-sectionally related to CRP levels in a Dutch population of 974 middle-aged men and women (Du *et al.*, 2008). Two further analyses of data from the Nurses' Health Study and the Health Professionals' Follow-up Study among participants with type 2 diabetes also support inverse associations between levels of CRP and TNF-R2 versus adiponectin (Qi *et al.*, 2005; Qi *et al.*, 2006a; Qi *et al.*, 2006b). Effect sizes were particularly pronounced for the association between dietary GI and CRP levels among women with type 2 diabetes, with a 32% difference between the highest and lowest quintile (Qi *et al.*, 2006b). However, the only prospective study published so far found no relationship between changes in dietary GI or GL and change of CRP levels during 1 year (Griffith *et al.*, 2008). Similarly, a small study in 136 middle-aged women and men enrolled in an exercise intervention trial did not find an independent cross-sectional association between dietary GI or GL and CRP levels (Huffman *et al.*, 2007).

Evidence from intervention studies

Several intervention studies conducted in very diverse populations (Pereira *et al.*, 2004b; Pittas *et al.*, 2006; Kallio *et al.*, 2008; Wolever *et al.*, 2008; Rhodes *et al.*, 2010) support a potential relevance of dietary GI or GL to inflammation, independent of potential effects on body weight. The longest study was performed in 162 patients with type 2 diabetes and optimal glycaemic control treated by diet alone, where a high-carbohydrate, low-GI diet consumed over a period of 1 year resulted in a sustained reduction in CRP levels in comparison to a high-carbohydrate high-GI diet (Wolever *et al.*, 2008). In a 6-month weight-loss trial, conducted in 34 young overweight or obese men and women, the percentage of participants experiencing a decrease in CRP levels was significantly larger among those on a low-GL diet compared with those on a high-GL diet, despite similar weight loss (Pittas *et al.*, 2006). Similarly, Pereira *et al.* (2004b), who conducted a weight-loss study in 39 overweight or obese men and women, reported a 48% CRP reduction after following a low-GL regimen for approximately 10 weeks, whereas CRP reduction was only 5% among those on a high-GL diet, despite similar changes in body composition. Kallio *et al.* (2008) compared the effects of foods inducing an exaggerated postprandial insulinaemic response to foods with low insulinaemic response among 47 overweight or obese individuals: during the 12-week intervention under weight-stable conditions, the two dietary groups differed with respect to changes in fasting levels of interleukin (IL)-1β and IL-6 and with respect to the gene expression of IL-10 receptor alpha, TNF-α in subcutaneous adipose tissue. In a recent pilot study conducted in 46 pregnant overweight women, consumption of a low-GL diet from the second or third trimester onwards resulted in a greater decrease of CRP levels until week 36 than the consumption of a low-fat diet (Rhodes *et al.*, 2010). Again, changes in weight or body-mass index (BMI) were comparable between the two study arms. However, two cross-over studies comparing 4 weeks each under a low- or high-GI regimen in 64 and 24 overweight or obese men, respectively, found no differences with respect to CRP or other inflammatory markers (Shikany *et al.*, 2009; Hartman *et al.*, 2010; Table 3.1).

Dietary fibre/whole-grain intake

Epidemiological evidence

Observational studies in US and European adults unanimously report that higher intakes of dietary fibre are related to lower levels of inflammatory markers or a reduced risk of elevated CRP (King *et al.*, 2003; Ajani *et al.*, 2004; Qi *et al.*, 2005; Bo *et al.*, 2006; Ma *et al.*, 2006; Qi *et al.*, 2006a,b; Ma *et al.*, 2008; Herder *et al.*, 2009; Wannamethee *et al.*, 2009). This evidence comes mostly from cross-sectional studies; however, two studies also found increases in fibre intake over the course of 1 year to be associated with decreases in CRP (Ma *et al.*, 2008; Herder *et al.*, 2009) and IL-6 levels (Herder *et al.*, 2009), independently of concurrent changes in BMI.

More detailed analyses available from US populations suggest that the beneficial effects of fibre intake could be primarily attributable to intakes in cereal fibre (Qi *et al.*, 2005, 2006a,b) or insoluble fibre (Ma *et al.*, 2008). In line with this, similar benefits for different inflammatory markers were observed in most (Qi *et al.*, 2006b; Lutsey *et al.*, 2007; Gaskins *et al.*, 2010; Masters *et al.*, 2010), but not all (Jensen *et al.*, 2006) of the more recent observational studies focusing on whole grains in place of fibre. Despite the general agreement of these data, it should be borne in mind, however, that the observed associations could be largely attributable to the fact that dietary fibre or whole grains reflect an overall healthier lifestyle (van Dam and Seidell, 2007) (see also Table 3.1).

Evidence from intervention studies

Data from intervention studies are much less conclusive, adding to the uncertainty about whether the dietary fibre or whole grains directly influence inflammation. King *et al.* (2007) found a reduction in CRP levels after 3 weeks on a high-fibre or fibre-supplemented diet, which was, however, confined to 18 lean normotensive participants, with no significant change among 17 obese hypertensive patients. In a subsequent randomized trial, psyllium fibre supplementation for 3 months did not significantly reduce CRP or IL-6 levels in 162 overweight or obese individuals (King *et al.*, 2008). Similarly, a 3-month supplementation with high-fibre cereal foods did not affect CRP levels in 23 people with diabetes (Jenkins *et al.*, 2002). In four recent studies comparing the consumption of whole-grain foods to that of refined grain alternatives by overweight, but otherwise healthy, individuals, no effects on inflammatory markers were observed after 3–16 weeks (Andersson *et al.*, 2007; Brownlee *et al.*, 2010; Giacco *et al.*, 2010; Tighe *et al.*, 2010). Only one study conducted in 50 obese individuals who presented with the metabolic syndrome found a decrease in CRP by 38% after 12 weeks among those advised to obtain all of their grain servings

Table 3.1. Quality of dietary carbohydrate intake in relation to inflammatory markers

Study type	Results from the studies	Methodological considerations[a]
GI/GL: Cohort studies		
6 Cross-sectional	5 of 6: Inflammatory marker(s) ↑ with GI/GL ↑[b] (Liu *et al.*, 2002; Qi *et al.*, 2005; Qi *et al.*, 2006a; Qi *et al.*, 2006b; Du *et al.*, 2008; Levitan *et al.*, 2008) 1 of 6: No association (Huffman *et al.*, 2007)	• Dietary assessment methods generally not designed to determine GI/GL. • Validity for GI/GL may be low in some studies. • Residual confounding by lifestyle related factors less likely. • GI/GL specific under-reporting unlikely
1 Prospective	1 of 1: No association (Griffith *et al.*, 2008)	
GI/GL: Intervention studies		
7 Studies: Duration, 4–52 weeks; 24–162 participants	5 of 7: Inflammatory marker(s) ↓ on low GI/GI/II diet[c] (Pereira *et al.*, 2004b; Pittas *et al.*, 2006; Kallio *et al.*, 2008; Wolever *et al.*, 2008; Rhodes *et al.*, 2010) 2 of 7: No difference[c] (Shikany *et al.*, 2009; Hartman *et al.*, 2010)	• Very diverse populations (see text). • Power considerations mostly based on other primary outcome measures
Dietary fibre: Cohort studies		
8 Cross-sectional	8 of 8: Inflammatory marker(s) ↓ with fibre ↑[b] (King *et al.*, 2003; Ajani *et al.*, 2004; Qi *et al.*, 2005; Bo *et al.*, 2006; Ma *et al.*, 2006; Qi *et al.*, 2006a; Qi *et al.*, 2006b; Wannamethee *et al.*, 2009)	• May be particularly prone to residual confounding by lifestyle or socioeconomic factors, which epidemiological studies cannot fully control for. • Fibre-specific over-reporting cannot be precluded
2 Prospective	2 of 2: Inflammatory marker(s) ↓ with fibre ↑[b] (Ma *et al.*, 2008; Herder *et al.*, 2009)	
Dietary fibre: Intervention studies		
3 Studies: Duration, 3–12 weeks; 23–158 participants	1 of 3: Inflammatory marker(s) ↓ on high fibre or fibre-supplemented diet[c] (King *et al.*, 2007) 2 of 3: No difference[c] (King *et al.*, 2008; Jenkins *et al.*, 2002)	• Studies use high-fibre diets and fibre supplementations. • Power considerations were mostly based on other primary outcome measures
Whole-grain intake: Cohort studies		
5 Cross-sectional	4 of 5: Inflammatory marker(s) ↓ with whole-grain intake↑[b] (Qi *et al.*, 2006b; Lutsey *et al.*, 2007; Gaskins *et al.*, 2010; Masters *et al.*, 2010) 1 of 5: No association (Jensen *et al.*, 2006)	• May be particularly prone to residual confounding. • Definition of whole-grain product varies between studies. • Ascertainment of whole-grain content is difficult. • Whole-grain-specific over-reporting cannot be precluded

Continued

Table 3.1. Continued.

Study type	Results from the studies	Methodological considerations[a]
Whole-grain intake: Intervention studies		
5 Studies: Duration, 3–16 weeks; 15–316 participants	1 of 5: Inflammatory marker(s) ↓ on whole-grain diet[c] (Katcher *et al.*, 2008) 4 of 5: No difference[c] (Andersson *et al.*, 2007; Brownlee *et al.*, 2010; Giacco *et al.*, 2010; Tighe *et al.*, 2010)	Studies used provision of whole grain foods or advise to obtain all grains from whole grains. Power considerations were mostly based on other primary outcome measures
Western food pattern[d]: Cohort studies		
6 Cross-sectional	6 of 6: Inflammatory marker(s) ↑ with Western dietary pattern[d] (Lopez-Garcia *et al.*, 2004; Heidemann *et al.*, 2005; Schulze *et al.*, 2005; Nettleton *et al.*, 2006; Nanri *et al.*, 2008; Liese *et al.*, 2009)	Food pattern depends on the population they were derived from. Specific under-reporting of these 'socially less desirable foods' cannot be precluded. Identifiable food groups are determined by the dietary assessment tool (mostly FFQ) used
5 Relating cross-sectionally identified patterns[e] to development of type 2 diabetes or CVD ('mediation')	5 of 5: Confirm relevance of patterns to development of type 2 diabetes or CVD[e] (Hoffmann *et al.*, 2004; Heidemann *et al.*, 2005; Schulze *et al.*, 2005; Liese *et al.*, 2009; Liese *et al.*, 2010)	

↓, Decrease; ↑, increase; FFQ, food frequency questionnaire; CVD, cardiovascular disease; GI, glycaemic index; GL, glycaemic load.
[a]Methodological considerations modified and extended from Buyken *et al.* (2010b).
[b]Highest quantile compared to lowest quantile.
[c]As compared to control diet.
[d]As compared to prudent dietary patterns (see text). Carbohydrate sources in 'Western pattern' comprised soft drinks, low-fibre breads and cereals or refined grains, fried potatoes/French fries, sweets.
[e]Patterns maximally explaining variations in inflammatory and haemostatic markers were extracted using reduced rank regression. These patterns were then related to disease outcomes confirming 'mediation' of inflammation in the association between these patterns and type 2 diabetes or CVD.

from whole grains. CRP remained unchanged in those advised to avoid whole grains (Katcher *et al.*, 2008). Hence, use of whole grains might be effective for reducing inflammatory responses only among high-risk populations (Table 3.1).

Dietary pattern

In this emerging field, separate appraisal of the evidence for fibre/whole grain and GI/GL can be helpful in differentiating mechanisms. None the less, in public-health terms, approaches that detect the different dietary *patterns* associated with disease could be much more important. Beneficial effects on inflammatory markers have been reported from interventional studies using a 'Mediterranean dietary pattern' as well as moderate carbohydrate diets rich in vegetable protein, e.g. 'Eco-Atkins' or Okinawan diet (O'Keefe *et al.*, 2008). Notably, these dietary approaches induce lower glycaemic and insulinaemic spikes, i.e. are lower in GI, and yet are relatively rich in dietary fibre, antioxidants and other micronutrients.

The benefits might not be limited to the *a priori* defined dietary pattern. In epidemiological studies from very different populations (including Asian and minorities in the USA) dietary pattern analyses were found to be closely associated with inflammatory markers. In these, carbohydrate sources identified as beneficial included rice, pasta, whole grains, fruits and legumes, whereas carbohydrate sources related to higher inflammatory markers comprised soft drinks, low-fibre bread and cereals, refined grains, fried potatoes/French fries, soy products and sweets (Schulze *et al.*, 2005; Nettleton *et al.*, 2006; Nanri *et al.*, 2008; Liese *et al.*, 2009) (Table 3.1) Overall, the choices associated with higher concentrations of inflammatory markers are generally known to be low in fibre and yield higher postprandial glucose spikes, whereas those associated with a lower risk are richer in fibre and/or elicit lower postprandial responses (Atkinson *et al.*, 2008).

Carbohydrate Nutrition and Inflammatory Diseases

Interest in the relationship between carbohydrate nutrition and inflammation is sparked mainly by links between inflammation and the development of type 2 diabetes and CVD.

Carbohydrate nutrition and type 2 diabetes or CVD

Dietary pattern analyses using reduced rank regression permit some insight into the extent to which inflammation may represent a 'mediator' in relation to type 2 diabetes or CVD. Using this approach, as a first step, food-intake patterns maximally explaining the variation of inflammatory and haemostatic markers have been extracted (see above). In a second step, these patterns were also found to be strongly related to the development of type 2 diabetes (Heidemann *et al.*, 2005; Schulze *et al.*, 2005; Liese *et al.*, 2009) or coronary artery disease (Hoffmann *et al.*, 2004; Liese *et al.*, 2010) (Table 3.1).

Numerous epidemiological studies have shown a higher risk of type 2 diabetes and CVD in those with lower (cereal) fibre intake (Pereira *et al.*, 2004a; Schulze *et al.*, 2007). Similarly, a higher dietary GI or GL was also associated with an increased risk of type 2 diabetes and CVD in different populations from the USA, Australia and Europe, although not all studies have confirmed this association (Liu and Chou, 2010). To date, only one epidemiological study has explicitly addressed 'mediation' by low-grade inflammation, showing that adjustment for the inflammatory markers IL-6 and tissue plasminogen activator (t-PA) notably attenuated the relationship between total or cereal fibre and the development of type 2 diabetes (Wannamethee *et al.*, 2009). Generally, the concept of 'mediation' can presently only be tested in observational studies, which are, however, hampered by potential residual confounding (Table 3.1). Although it seems plausible that inflammation and oxidative stress may represent major pathways for these diseases, direct evidence for a causal relation will remain difficult to obtain.

Carbohydrate and inflammatory disease mortality

Recent observations of an association between carbohydrate nutrition and death from inflammatory diseases provide some of the strongest evidence yet for direct links between carbohydrate consumption and inflammation. Jacobs *et al.* (2007) introduced this new categorization of mortality from non-CVD, non-cancer inflammatory diseases, explicitly focusing on diseases for which inflammation or oxidative stress is the predominant pathophysiological factor (Jacobs *et al.*, 2007). Among 27,312 women participating in the Iowa Women's Health Study, risk of death attributed to inflammatory disease during the 17-year follow-up was reduced by 35% among women reporting the highest intake of whole grains, i.e. a risk reduction larger than that previously reported for type 2 diabetes and CVD (Jacobs *et al.*, 2007). For 1490 women in the Blue Mountains Mountain Eye study, an almost threefold higher risk of inflammatory mortality during 13-year follow-up was observed among women in the highest GI tertile compared with those in the lowest GI tertile, which again considerably exceeds risk increases so far reported for other diseases linked to GI, including type 2 diabetes and CVD (Buyken *et al.*, 2010a).

Summary and Conclusions

Acute hyperglycaemia-induced oxidative stress contributing to a state of chronic low-grade inflammation has been proposed as the primary mechanism underlying adverse effects exerted by diets dominated by high-GI carbohydrate foods. Higher fibre intakes may beneficially interact with gut microflora, producing SCFAs which modulate cytokine and antibody production. Although the epidemiological and clinical studies available to date support the relevance of dietary GI and fibre for inflammatory diseases, the evidence should be judged as 'preliminary' at the present time. Most intervention studies suffer from small sample size because power considerations were based on other primary outcome measures. Further studies are needed to confirm the longer-term relevance of dietary patterns combining foods with a low GI and high-fibre content.

References

Ajani, U.A., Ford, E.S. and Mokdad, A.H. (2004) Dietary fiber and C-reactive protein: findings from national health and nutrition examination survey data. *Journal of Nutrition* 134, 1181–1185.

Andersson, A., Tengblad, S., Karlstrom, B., Kamal-Eldin, A., Landberg, R., *et al.* (2007) Whole-grain foods do not affect insulin sensitivity or markers of lipid peroxidation and inflammation in healthy, moderately overweight subjects. *Journal of Nutrition* 137, 1401–1407.

Atkinson, F.S., Foster-Powell, K. and Brand-Miller, J.C. (2008) International tables of glycemic index and glycemic load values: 2008. *Diabetes Care* 31, 2281–2283.

Bo, S., Durazzo, M., Guidi, S., Carello, M., Sacerdote, C., *et al.* (2006) Dietary magnesium and fiber intakes and inflammatory and metabolic indicators in middle-aged subjects from a population-based cohort. *American Journal of Clinical Nutrition* 84, 1062–1069.

Botero, D., Ebbeling, C.B., Blumberg, J.B., Ribaya-Mercado, J.D., Creager, M.A., *et al.* (2009) Acute effects of dietary glycemic index on antioxidant capacity in a nutrient-controlled feeding study. *Obesity (Silver Spring)* 17, 1664–1670.

Brand-Miller, J.C., Stockmann, K., Atkinson, F., Petocz, P. and Denyer, G. (2009) Glycemic index, postprandial glycemia, and the shape of the curve in healthy subjects: analysis of a database of more than 1,000 foods. *American Journal of Clinical Nutrition* 89, 97–105.

Brinkworth, G.D., Noakes, M., Keogh, J.B., Luscombe, N.D., Wittert, G.A., *et al.* (2004) Long-term effects of a high-protein, low-carbohydrate diet on weight control and cardiovascular risk markers in obese hyperinsulinemic subjects. *International Journal of Obesity Related Metabolic Disorders* 28, 661–670.

Brownlee, I.A., Moore, C., Chatfield, M., Richardson, D.P., Ashby, P., *et al.* (2010) Markers of cardiovascular risk are not changed by increased whole-grain intake: the WHOLEheart study, a randomised, controlled dietary intervention. *British Journal of Nutrition* 104, 125–134.

Buyken, A.E., Flood, V., Empson, M., Rochtchina, E., Barclay, A.W., *et al.* (2010a) Carbohydrate nutrition and inflammatory disease mortality in older adults. *American Journal of Clinical Nutrition* 92, 634–643.

Buyken, A.E., Mitchell, P., Ceriello, A. and Brand-Miller, J. (2010b) Optimal dietary approaches for prevention of type 2 diabetes: a life-course perspective. *Diabetologia* 53, 406–418.

Ceriello, A. (2005) Postprandial hyperglycemia and diabetes complications: is it time to treat? *Diabetes* 54, 1–7.

Ceriello, A. and Motz, E. (2004) Is oxidative stress the pathogenic mechanism underlying insulin resistance, diabetes, and cardiovascular disease? The common soil hypothesis revisited. *Arteriosclerosis, Thrombosis, and Vascular Biology* 24, 816–823.

Couzin-Frankel, J. (2010) Inflammation bares a dark side. *Science* 330, 1621.

Cummings, J.H. and Stephen, A.M. (2007) Carbohydrate terminology and classification. *European Journal of Nutrition* 61 Suppl 1, S5–S18.

Dandona, P., Chaudhuri, A., Mohanty, P. and Ghanim, H. (2007) Anti-inflammatory effects of insulin. *Current Opinion in Clinical Nutrition and Metabolic Care* 10, 511–517.

Dansinger, M.L., Gleason, J.A., Griffith, J.L., Selker, H.P. and Schaefer, E.J. (2005) Comparison of the Atkins, Ornish, Weight Watchers, and Zone diets for weight loss and heart disease risk reduction: a randomized trial. *Journal of the American Medical Association* 293, 43–53.

de Moura, F.F., Lewis, K.D. and Falk, M.C. (2009) Applying the FDA definition of whole grains to the evidence for cardiovascular disease health claims. *Journal of Nutrition* 139, 2220S–2226S.

Dickinson, S., Colagiuri, S., Faramus, E., Petocz, P. and Brand-Miller, J.C. (2002) Postprandial hyperglycemia and insulin sensitivity differ among lean young adults of different ethnicities. *Journal of Nutrition* 132, 2574–2579.

Dickinson, S., Hancock, D.P., Petocz, P., Ceriello, A. and Brand-Miller, J. (2008) High-glycemic index carbohydrate increases nuclear factor-kappaB activation in mononuclear cells of young, lean healthy subjects. *American Journal of Clinical Nutrition* 87, 1188–1193.

Du, H., van der, A.D., van Bakel, M.M., van der Kallen, C.J., Blaak, E.E., *et al.* (2008) Glycemic index and glycemic load in relation to food and nutrient intake and metabolic risk factors in a Dutch population. *American Journal of Clinical Nutrition* 87, 655–661.

Due, A., Toubro, S., Stender, S., Skov, A.R. and Astrup, A. (2005) The effect of diets high in protein or carbohydrate on inflammatory markers in overweight subjects. *Diabetes, Obesity and Metabolism* 7, 223–229.

Englyst, K.N., Liu, S. and Englyst, H.N. (2007) Nutritional characterization and measurement of dietary carbohydrates. *European Journal of Nutrition* 61 Suppl 1, S19–S39.

Fardet, A. (2010) New hypotheses for the health-protective mechanisms of whole-grain cereals: what is beyond fibre? *Nutrition Research Reviews* 23, 65–134.

FDA (2006) Guidance for industry and FDA staff: whole grain label statements [draft guidance]. Available at: http://www.fda.gov/Food/GuidanceComplianceRegulatoryInformation/GuidanceDocuments/FoodLabelingNutrition/UCM059088 (Accessed August 2011).

Gaskins, A.J., Mumford, S.L., Rovner, A.J., Zhang, C., Chen, L., *et al.* (2010) Whole grains are associated with serum concentrations of high sensitivity C-reactive protein among premenopausal women. *Journal of Nutrition* 140, 1669–1676.

Ghanim, H., Abuaysheh, S., Sia, C.L., Korzeniewski, K., Chaudhuri, A., *et al.* (2009) Increase in plasma endotoxin concentrations and the expression of Toll-like receptors and suppressor of cytokine signaling-3 in mononuclear cells after a high-fat, high-carbohydrate meal: implications for insulin resistance. *Diabetes Care* 32, 2281–2287.

Giacco, R., Clemente, G., Cipriano, D., Luongo, D., Viscovo, D., *et al.* (2010) Effects of the regular consumption of wholemeal wheat foods on cardiovascular risk factors in healthy people. *Nutrition, Metabolism and Cardiovascular Disease* 20, 186–194.

Griffith, J.A., Ma, Y., Chasan-Taber, L., Olendzki, B.C., Chiriboga, D.E., *et al.* (2008) Association between dietary glycemic index, glycemic load, and high-sensitivity C-reactive protein. *Nutrition* 24, 401–406.

Hartman, T.J., Albert, P.S., Zhang, Z., Bagshaw, D., Kris-Etherton, P.M., *et al.* (2010) Consumption of a legume-enriched, low-glycemic index diet is associated with biomarkers of insulin resistance and inflammation among men at risk for colorectal cancer. *Journal of Nutrition* 140, 60–67.

Heidemann, C., Hoffmann, K., Spranger, J., Klipstein-Grobusch, K., Mohlig, M., *et al.* (2005) A dietary pattern protective against type 2 diabetes in the European Prospective Investigation into Cancer and Nutrition (EPIC)–Potsdam Study cohort. *Diabetologia* 48, 1126–1134.

Herder, C., Peltonen, M., Koenig, W., Sutfels, K., Lindstrom, J., *et al.* (2009) Anti-inflammatory effect of lifestyle changes in the Finnish Diabetes Prevention Study. *Diabetologia* 52, 433–442.

Hoffmann, K., Zyriax, B.C., Boeing, H. and Windler, E. (2004) A dietary pattern derived to explain biomarker variation is strongly associated with the risk of coronary artery disease. *American Journal of Clinical Nutrition* 80, 633–640.

Holt, S.H. and Miller, J.B. (1994) Particle size, satiety and the glycaemic response. *European Journal of Nutrition* 48, 496–502.

Huffman, K.M., Orenduff, M.C., Samsa, G.P., Houmard, J.A., Kraus, W.E., *et al.* (2007) Dietary carbohydrate intake and high-sensitivity C-reactive protein in at-risk women and men. *American Heart Journal* 154, 962–968.

Jacobs, D.R., Jr., Andersen, L.F. and Blomhoff, R. (2007) Whole-grain consumption is associated with a reduced risk of noncardiovascular, noncancer death attributed to inflammatory diseases in the Iowa Women's Health Study. *American Journal of Clinical Nutrition* 85, 1606–1614.

Jenkins, D.J., Wolever, T.M., Taylor, R.H., Barker, H., Fielden, H., *et al.* (1981) Glycemic index of foods: a physiological basis for carbohydrate exchange. *American Journal of Clinical Nutrition* 34, 362–366.

Jenkins, D.J., Kendall, C.W., Augustin, L.S., Martini, M.C., Axelsen, M., *et al.* (2002) Effect of wheat bran on glycemic control and risk factors for cardiovascular disease in type 2 diabetes. *Diabetes Care* 25, 1522–1528.

Jensen, M.K., Koh-Banerjee, P., Franz, M., Sampson, L., Gronbaek, M., *et al.* (2006) Whole grains, bran, and germ in relation to homocysteine and markers of glycemic control, lipids, and inflammation. *American Journal of Clinical Nutrition* 83, 275–283.

Kallio, P., Kolehmainen, M., Laaksonen, D.E., Pulkkinen, L., Atalay, M., *et al.* (2008) Inflammation markers are modulated by responses to diets differing in postprandial insulin responses in individuals with the metabolic syndrome. *American Journal of Clinical Nutrition* 87, 1497–1503.

Kasim-Karakas, S.E., Tsodikov, A., Singh, U. and Jialal, I. (2006) Responses of inflammatory markers to a low-fat, high-carbohydrate diet: effects of energy intake. *American Journal of Clinical Nutrition* 83, 774–779.

Katcher, H.I., Legro, R.S., Kunselman, A.R., Gillies, P.J., Demers, L.M., *et al.* (2008) The effects of a whole grain-enriched hypocaloric diet on cardiovascular disease risk factors in men and women with metabolic syndrome. *American Journal of Clinical Nutrition* 87, 79–90.

Kempf, K., Rose, B., Herder, C., Kleophas, U., Martin, S. and Kolb, H. (2006) Inflammation in metabolic syndrome and type 2 diabetes: Impact of dietary glucose. *Annals of the New York Academy of Science* 1084, 30–48.

Keogh, J.B., Brinkworth, G.D., Noakes, M., Belobrajdic, D.P., Buckley, J.D., *et al.* (2008) Effects of weight loss from a very-low-carbohydrate diet on endothelial function and markers of cardiovascular disease risk in subjects with abdominal obesity. *American Journal of Clinical Nutrition* 87, 567–576.

King, D.E., Egan, B.M. and Geesey, M.E. (2003) Relation of dietary fat and fiber to elevation of C-reactive protein. *American Journal of Cardiology* 92, 1335–1339.

King, D.E., Egan, B.M., Woolson, R.F., Mainous, A.G., 3rd, Al-Solaiman, Y., *et al.* (2007) Effect of a high-fiber diet vs a fiber-supplemented diet on C-reactive protein level. *Archives of Internal Medicine* 167, 502–506.

King, D.E., Mainous, A.G., 3rd, Egan, B.M., Woolson, R.F. and Geesey, M.E. (2008) Effect of psyllium fiber supplementation on C-reactive protein: the trial to reduce inflammatory markers (TRIM). *Annals of Family Medicine* 6, 100–106.

Levitan, E.B., Cook, N.R., Stampfer, M.J., Ridker, P.M., Rexrode, K.M., *et al.* (2008) Dietary glycemic index, dietary glycemic load, blood lipids, and C-reactive protein. *Metabolism* 57, 437–443.

Liese, A.D., Weis, K.E., Schulz, M. and Tooze, J.A. (2009) Food intake patterns associated with incident type 2 diabetes: the Insulin Resistance Atherosclerosis Study. *Diabetes Care* 32, 263–268.

Liese, A.D., Nichols, M., Hodo, D., Mellen, P.B., Schulz, M., *et al.* (2010) Food intake patterns associated with carotid artery atherosclerosis in the Insulin Resistance Atherosclerosis Study. *British Journal of Nutrition* 103, 1471–1479.

Liu, S. and Chou, E.L. (2010) Dietary glycemic load and type 2 diabetes: modeling the glucose-raising potential of carbohydrates for prevention. *American Journal of Clinical Nutrition* 92, 675–677.

Liu, S., Manson, J.E., Buring, J.E., Stampfer, M.J., Willett, W.C., *et al.* (2002) Relation between a diet with a high glycemic load and plasma concentrations of high-sensitivity C-reactive protein in middle-aged women. *American Journal of Clinical Nutrition* 75, 492–498.

Lopez-Garcia, E., Schulze, M.B., Fung, T.T., Meigs, J.B., Rifai, N., *et al.* (2004) Major dietary patterns are related to plasma concentrations of markers of inflammation and endothelial dysfunction. *American Journal of Clinical Nutrition* 80, 1029–1035.

Ludwig, D.S. (2002) The glycemic index: physiological mechanisms relating to obesity, diabetes, and cardiovascular disease. *Journal of the American Medical Association* 287, 2414–2423.

Lutsey, P.L., Jacobs, D.R., Jr., Kori, S., Mayer-Davis, E., Shea, S., *et al.* (2007) Whole grain intake and its cross-sectional association with obesity, insulin resistance, inflammation, diabetes and subclinical CVD: The MESA Study. *British Journal of Nutrition* 98, 397–405.

Ma, Y., Griffith, J.A., Chasan-Taber, L., Olendzki, B.C., Jackson, E., *et al.* (2006) Association between dietary fiber and serum C-reactive protein. *American Journal of Clinical Nutrition* 83, 760–766.

Ma, Y., Hebert, J.R., Li, W., Bertone-Johnson, E.R., Olendzki, B., *et al.* (2008) Association between dietary fiber and markers of systemic inflammation in the Women's Health Initiative Observational Study. *Nutrition* 24, 941–949.

Mann, J.I. and Cummings, J.H. (2009) Possible implications for health of the different definitions of dietary fibre. *Nutrition, Metabolism and Cardiovascular Disease* 19, 226–229.

Maslowski, K.M., Vieira, A.T., Ng, A., Kranich, J., Sierro, F., *et al.* (2009) Regulation of inflammatory responses by gut microbiota and chemoattractant receptor GPR43. *Nature* 461, 1282–1286.

Masters, R.C., Liese, A.D., Haffner, S.M., Wagenknecht, L.E. and Hanley, A.J. (2010) Whole and refined grain intakes are related to inflammatory protein concentrations in human plasma. *Journal of Nutrition* 140, 587–594.

Monnier, L., Mas, E., Ginet, C., Michel, F., Villon, L., *et al.* (2006) Activation of oxidative stress by acute glucose fluctuations compared with sustained chronic hyperglycemia in patients with type 2 diabetes. *Journal of the American Medical Association* 295, 1681–1687.

Motton, D.D., Keim, N.L., Tenorio, F.A., Horn, W.F. and Rutledge, J.C. (2007) Postprandial monocyte activation in response to meals with high and low glycemic loads in overweight women. *American Journal of Clinical Nutrition* 85, 60–65.

Nanri, A., Yoshida, D., Yamaji, T., Mizoue, T., Takayanagi, R., *et al.* (2008) Dietary patterns and C-reactive protein in Japanese men and women. *American Journal of Clinical Nutrition* 87, 1488–1496.

Nettleton, J.A., Steffen, L.M., Mayer-Davis, E.J., Jenny, N.S., Jiang, R., *et al.* (2006) Dietary patterns are associated with biochemical markers of inflammation and endothelial activation in the Multi-Ethnic Study of Atherosclerosis (MESA). *American Journal of Clinical Nutrition* 83, 1369–1379.

O'Brien, K.D., Brehm, B.J., Seeley, R.J., Bean, J., Wener, M.H., *et al.* (2005) Diet-induced weight loss is associated with decreases in plasma serum amyloid a and C-reactive protein independent of dietary macronutrient composition in obese subjects. *Journal of Clinical Endocrinology and Metabolism* 90, 2244–2249.

O'Keefe, J.H., Gheewala, N.M. and O'Keefe, J.O. (2008) Dietary strategies for improving post-prandial glucose, lipids, inflammation, and cardiovascular health. *Journal of the American College of Cardiology* 51, 249–255.

Pereira, M.A., O'Reilly, E., Augustsson, K., Fraser, G.E., Goldbourt, U., *et al.* (2004a) Dietary fiber and risk of coronary heart disease: a pooled analysis of cohort studies. *Archives of Internal Medicine* 164, 370–376.

Pereira, M.A., Swain, J., Goldfine, A.B., Rifai, N. and Ludwig, D.S. (2004b) Effects of a low-glycemic load diet on resting energy expenditure and heart disease risk factors during weight loss. *Journal of the American Medical Association* 292, 2482–2490.

Pittas, A.G., Roberts, S.B., Das, S.K., Gilhooly, C.H., Saltzman, E., *et al.* (2006) The effects of the dietary glycemic load on type 2 diabetes risk factors during weight loss. *Obesity (Silver Spring)* 14, 2200–2209.

Qi, L., Rimm, E., Liu, S., Rifai, N. and Hu, F.B. (2005) Dietary glycemic index, glycemic load, cereal fiber, and plasma adiponectin concentration in diabetic men. *Diabetes Care* 28, 1022–1028.

Qi, L., Meigs, J.B., Liu, S., Manson, J.E., Mantzoros, C., *et al.* (2006a) Dietary fibers and glycemic load, obesity, and plasma adiponectin levels in women with type 2 diabetes. *Diabetes Care* 29, 1501–1505.

Qi, L., van Dam, R.M., Liu, S., Franz, M., Mantzoros, C., *et al.* (2006b) Whole-grain, bran, and cereal fiber intakes and markers of systemic inflammation in diabetic women. *Diabetes Care* 29, 207–211.

Rankin, J.W. and Turpyn, A.D. (2007) Low carbohydrate, high fat diet increases C-reactive protein during weight loss. *Journal of the American College of Nutrition* 26, 163–169.

Rhodes, C.J. (2005) Type 2 diabetes-a matter of beta-cell life and death? *Science* 307, 380–384.

Rhodes, E.T., Pawlak, D.B., Takoudes, T.C., Ebbeling, C.B., Feldman, H.A., *et al.* (2010) Effects of a low-glycemic load diet in overweight and obese pregnant women: a pilot randomized controlled trial. *American Journal of Clinical Nutrition* 92, 1306–1315.

Roberts, C.K., Won, D., Pruthi, S., Kurtovic, S., Sindhu, R.K., Vaziri, N.D. and Barnard, R.J. (2006) Effect of a short-term diet and exercise intervention on oxidative stress, inflammation, MMP-9, and monocyte chemotactic activity in men with metabolic syndrome factors. *Journal of Applied Physiology* 100, 1657–1665.

Rodriguez-Cabezas, M.E., Galvez, J., Lorente, M.D., Concha, A., Camuesco, D., Azzouz, S., Osuna, A., Redondo, L. and Zarzuelo, A. (2002) Dietary fiber down-regulates colonic tumor necrosis factor alpha and nitric oxide production in trinitrobenzenesulfonic acid-induced colitic rats. *Journal of Nutrition* 132, 3263–3271.

Salmeron, J., Manson, J.E., Stampfer, M.J., Colditz, G.A., Wing, A.L., *et al.* (1997) Dietary fiber, glycemic load, and risk of non-insulin-dependent diabetes mellitus in women. *Journal of the American Medical Association* 277, 472–477.

Schulze, M.B., Hoffmann, K., Manson, J.E., Willett, W.C., Meigs, J.B., *et al.* (2005) Dietary pattern, inflammation, and incidence of type 2 diabetes in women. *American Journal of Clinical Nutrition* 82, 675–684; quiz 714–675.

Schulze, M.B., Schulz, M., Heidemann, C., Schienkiewitz, A., Hoffmann, K., *et al.* (2007) Fiber and magnesium intake and incidence of type 2 diabetes: a prospective study and meta-analysis. *Archives of Internal Medicine* 167, 956–965.

Seshadri, P., Iqbal, N., Stern, L., Williams, M., Chicano, K.L., *et al.* (2004) A randomized study comparing the effects of a low-carbohydrate diet and a conventional diet on lipoprotein subfractions and C-reactive protein levels in patients with severe obesity. *American Journal of Medicine* 117, 398–405.

Shikany, J.M., Phadke, R.P., Redden, D.T. and Gower, B.A. (2009) Effects of low- and high-glycemic index/glycemic load diets on coronary heart disease risk factors in overweight/obese men. *Metabolism* 58, 1793–1801.

Tay, J., Brinkworth, G.D., Noakes, M., Keogh, J. and Clifton, P.M. (2008) Metabolic effects of weight loss on a very-low-carbohydrate diet compared with an isocaloric high-carbohydrate diet in abdominally obese subjects. *Journal of the American College of Cardiology* 51, 59–67.

Tighe, P., Duthie, G., Vaughan, N., Brittenden, J., Simpson, W.G., *et al.* (2010) Effect of increased consumption of whole-grain foods on blood pressure and other cardiovascular risk markers in healthy middle-aged persons: a randomized controlled trial. *American Journal of Clinical Nutrition* 92, 733–740.

van Dam, R.M. and Seidell, J.C. (2007) Carbohydrate intake and obesity. *European Journal of Nutrition* 61 Suppl 1, S75-S99.

Wang, C.C., Goalstone, M.L. and Draznin, B. (2004) Molecular mechanisms of insulin resistance that impact cardiovascular biology. *Diabetes* 53, 2735–2740.

Wannamethee, S.G., Whincup, P.H., Thomas, M.C. and Sattar, N. (2009) Associations between dietary fiber and inflammation, hepatic function, and risk of type 2 diabetes in older men: potential mechanisms for the benefits of fiber on diabetes risk. *Diabetes Care* 32, 1823–1825.

Wolever, T.M., Gibbs, A.L., Mehling, C., Chiasson, J.L., Connelly, P.W., *et al.* (2008) The Canadian Trial of Carbohydrates in Diabetes (CCD), a 1-y controlled trial of low-glycemic-index dietary carbohydrate in type 2 diabetes: no effect on glycated hemoglobin but reduction in C-reactive protein. *American Journal of Clinical Nutrition* 87, 114–125.

4 Alcohol and Inflammation

M.D. Bird* **and E.J. Kovacs**
Department of Surgery, Burn and Shock Trauma Institute, Loyola University Medical Center, Maywood, Illinois, USA

Introduction

Frequency of alcohol use

Alcohol use has been well described throughout human history, from ancient Mesopotamia to today. Currently, understanding the ill effects of alcoholism and abuse has led to the establishment of specific guidelines and definitions. For instance, acute or moderate drinking is generally defined as the occasional consumption of 1–2 drinks, whereas binge drinking is characterized as larger amounts of alcohol (5 or more drinks on one occasion for men and 4 for women) imbibed on multiple consecutive days with several days of sobriety or withdrawal in between drinking sessions (US Department of Health and Human Services and US Department of Agriculture, 2010). In contrast, chronic alcohol use is considered to be daily consumption of greater than 3–5 drinks for men and greater than 2 drinks for women (US Department of Health and Human Services and US Department

* Corresponding author, mbird12@jcc.edu

 Nutrition and Physical Activity in Inflammatory Diseases (eds M.L. Garg and L.G. Wood)

of Agriculture, 2010). A drink is defined as 12 ounces of beer, 5 ounces of wine, or 1.5 ounces of distilled spirits (80 proof) that contain 15 g of alcohol. Currently it is estimated that over half of the US adult population consumes alcohol, with only 5% drinking heavily and 15% binge drinking (Centers for Disease Control, 2011) (Fig. 4.1). These 'excessive' drinkers are more likely to incur health problems such as liver disease and injuries. According to the Centers for Disease Control (CDC), there were approximately 79,000 deaths annually from 2001 to 2005 that can be attributed to alcohol, making excessive alcohol use the third leading lifestyle-related cause of death in the USA (Centers for Disease Control, 2011). Worldwide, alcohol is responsible for 2.5 million deaths each year and is the third largest risk factor for premature mortality and disability (World Health Organization, 2010). Underage drinking is a significant health problem in the USA with alcohol being the most commonly used and abused drug among young persons. The majority (90%) of the alcohol consumed in this age group is in binge form and, on average, underage drinkers consume more alcoholic drinks per occasion than adults (Centers for Disease Control, 2011).

Outcomes of alcohol use and abuse

There is extensive evidence detailing the complex effects of alcohol consumption on human health (Rehm *et al.*, 2003), which are dependent on numerous factors such as sex, amount consumed and pattern of drinking behaviour (chronic versus moderate/acute). Chronic alcohol use is associated with a suppressed immune system and increased morbidity and mortality (Nelson and Kolls, 2002). Chronic alcoholics also show increased prevalence of disease including cardiomyopathy, stroke, high blood pressure and acute respiratory distress syndrome (Rehm *et al.*, 2003; Hanna *et al.*, 1997), and of course, alcoholic liver disease. In addition, consumption of alcohol is a major risk factor for all types of injuries, such as falls, fires, drowning, assaults, suicides and motor vehicle collisions (Driscoll *et al.*, 2004; Hingson, 2004; McDonald *et al.*, 2004). Almost half of alcohol-related deaths are due to injuries, with motor vehicle collisions being the leading cause of death in alcohol-related incidents (Mokdad *et al.*, 2004; Schermer, 2006). Additionally, excessive alcohol consumption is the third leading cause of preventable death

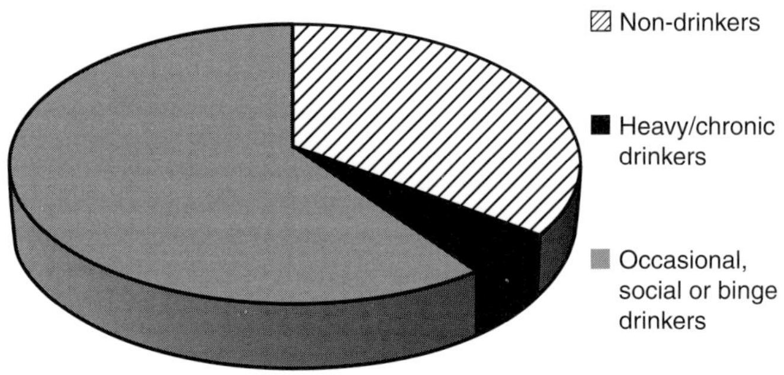

- Over half the adult population consumes alcohol*
    - 15% binge drinking
    - 5% heavy (chronic) drinking
- Excessive alcohol use = 3rd leading lifestyle-related cause of death (2.5 million deaths each year)*
    - 50% of these deaths are injury related**
    - $166 billion dollars annually in medical costs associated with excessive alcohol use***

Fig. 4.1. Alcohol consumption in the USA. *Centers for Disease Control, 2011; **Mokdad *et al.*, 2004; Schermer, 2006; ***Nelson and Krolls, 2002.

in the USA (Mokdad *et al.*, 2004). Alcohol is known to cause changes in the physiological response following trauma and injury leading to increased complications and mortality (Bird *et al.*, 2009). With alcohol's involvement in multiple disease states and injury, the medical costs associated with alcohol abuse in the USA is approximately US$166 billion/year, of which more than US$30 billion is for direct medical costs (Nelson and Kolls, 2002).

Modelling the effects of alcohol

Alcohol has long been known to exert opposite effects depending on the dose, a property known as hormesis. As such there exists a biphasic pattern in inflammation between chronic and acute alcohol, with acute alcohol being suppressive and chronic alcohol augmenting the inflammatory response (Table 4.1). To study the effect of alcohol in the laboratory, several *in vivo* and *in vitro* models have been utilized (D'Souza El-Guindy *et al.*, 2010; Plackett and Kovacs, 2008; Nagy, 2008). In cell culture, acute alcohol has been defined as the treatment of cells with varying doses of ethanol for up to 24h with ethanol, whereas chronic alcohol is less stringent with studies examining 48h up to 7 days of ethanol exposure *in vitro* (Szabo and Mandrekar, 2009; Kishore *et al.*, 2004). In rodent models, acute alcohol administration (one occurrence) is performed via intraperitoneal injection or oral gavage (Plackett and Kovacs, 2008). Both methods produce alcohol-related alterations in inflammation and immunity. Binge-drinking models consist of repeated ethanol exposure for 3–4 consecutive days either by injection or oral gavage (Callaci *et al.*, 2004; Pruett *et al.*, 2004). There are several models used to recapitulate chronic alcohol in humans including the Lieber-DeCarli Diet, the Meadows-Cook Method, and an intragastric ethanol infusion model. The Lieber-DeCarli diet is used in both mice and rats and is based on a high-fat liquid diet containing a specific amount of calories from ethanol, with alcohol-fed animals being compared to pair-fed controls (Lieber and Decarli, 1976). This method results in both liver pathology and immune system changes similar to those observed in humans. A continuous intragastric ethanol infusion model was developed by Tsukamoto and colleagues to mimic many of the features of human alcoholic liver disease including hepatic steatosis (accumulation of lipids in the liver) and elevated liver enzyme levels (Nagy, 2008).

Table 4.1. The effects of different drinking patterns on components of inflammation.

	Acute/binge alcohol	Chronic alcohol
Pro-inflammatory cytokines	↓TNF-α ↓IL-1 ↓IL-6 ↓Neutrophil chemotactants (IL-8, MIP-2, CINC) ↓G-CSF	↑TNF-α ↑IL-1 ↑IL-6
Macrophages	↓Cytokine production ↓Phagocytosis	↑Kupffer cell activation in liver ↑Alveolar macrophage activation ↑TNF-α production
Neutrophils	↓Chemotaxis ↓Superoxide production ↓Phagocytosis	↓Chemotaxis ↓Superoxide production ↓Phagocytosis
Reactive oxygen species	Decreased production by phagocytes	Increased production in liver and lung

↑, Increased relative to no alcohol controls; ↓, Decreased relative to no alcohol controls; TNF, tumour necrosis factor; IL, interleukin; MIP-2, monocyte inflammatory protein-2; CINC, cytokine induced neutrophil chemoattractant; G-CSF, granulocyte colony-stimulating factor.

The Meadows-Cook method uses continuous alcohol administration in the animals' drinking water, which mimics chronic alcohol use minus liver disease (Cook *et al.*, 2007).

Acute Alcohol Consumption and Inflammation

Suppression of inflammatory cells and mediators

Inflammation is a key feature of innate immunity and represents the body's first response to injury and pathogens (Janeway and Medzhitov, 2002). Acute alcohol exposure is associated with decreased inflammatory mediators, such as tumour necrosis factor-alpha (TNF-α), granulocyte colony-stimulating factor (G-CSF), interleukin (IL)-1 and IL-6, in addition to chemokines IL-8 and monocyte chemotactic protein (MCP-1) (Goral *et al.*, 2008; Szabo and Mandrekar, 2009) (Table 4.1). Studies have shown that acute ethanol treatment inhibits the production of pro-inflammatory cytokines in response to a variety of microbial compounds, such as lipopolysaccharide (LPS), polyinosinic–polycytidylic acid (poly I:C), peptidoglycan and unmethylated DNA. For example, ethanol suppressed pro-inflammatory cytokine production induced by these compounds by macrophages from various organ compartments. LPS-induced TNF-α (Nelson *et al.*, 1989) by alveolar macrophages was inhibited by acute ethanol exposure, as was poly I:C-induced IL-6 and IL-12 production by murine peritoneal macrophages (Pruett *et al.*, 2004). Additionally, TNF-α and IL-6 levels from mouse splenic macrophages was impaired following stimulation with peptidoglycan or unmethylated DNA (Goral *et al.*, 2008; Szabo and Mandrekar, 2009). Interestingly, the observed immune suppression by acute ethanol is not dependent on the type of alcohol as similar findings were observed after both beer and vodka ingestion in humans (Szabo and Mandrekar, 2009).

Furthermore, it was shown that acute ethanol exposure inhibited TNF-α-induced endothelial cell activation (He *et al.*, 2005), which may negatively affect the recruitment of leukocytes to the sites of inflammation. Recruitment and activation of innate immune cells at the sites of infection and injury is crucial for mounting an effective immune response. Impaired pro-inflammatory cytokine and chemokine production, as seen with acute ethanol exposure, may limit infiltration of these cells. This was demonstrated in the lung, where acute ethanol attenuated production of TNF-α by alveolar macrophages following stimulation with LPS (Kolls *et al.*, 1995). TNF-α, along with IL-1, is important for the production of chemokines that recruit neutrophils. In rodent models of acute ethanol exposure, monocyte inflammatory protein-2 (MIP-2) and cytokine-induced neutrophil chemoattractant (CINC) were inhibited resulting in decreased neutrophil infiltration egress into the lung in response to bacteria or LPS (Zhang *et al.*, 1997; Boe *et al.*, 2003). Through this negative regulation of TNF-α, ethanol may also impair interactions between lymphocytes and endothelial cells, thereby decreasing recruitment of lymphocytes to the site of inflammation. A single intraperitoneal injection of a high dose of ethanol (5 g/kg) significantly inhibited TNF-α-induced endothelial cell activation, as shown by decreases in adhesion molecule expression, chemokine production and lymphocyte adhesion (Saeed *et al.*, 2004). The proposed mechanism for this phenomenon is through the disruption of NFκB activation leading to decreased TNF-α (Saeed *et al.*, 2004). In another study, moderate ethanol consumption in human volunteers (0.8 g/kg) increased levels of IL-10, an anti-inflammatory cytokine, and impaired the ability of human monocytes to stimulate T cells (Szabo *et al.*, 2001).

Acute alcohol and Toll-like receptors

Innate immune cells, which respond to an inflammatory stimulus, recognize pathogens via pattern recognition receptors such as those found in the Toll-like receptor family (TLRs), which are specific for certain microbial components (Janeway and Medzhitov, 2002). Upon binding of their ligands, TLRs initiate complex signalling cascades and induce an immune response to the invading pathogens (Takeda *et al.*, 2003). The effects of alcohol on the activation of several TLRs have been studied including TLR2, TLR3, TLR4 and TLR9, which recognize flagellin, viral RNA, LPS and unmethylated DNA, respectively. Acute ethanol was shown to inhibit poly I:C and LPS-induced production of IL-6 and IL-12, while increasing IL-10 (Goral *et al.*, 2004; Pruett *et al.*, 2005) suggesting disruptions in TLR3 and TLR4 signalling. Additionally, acute ethanol altered TLR3-induced gene expression involved in type I interferon (IFN) amplification and may lead to suppression of inflammation (Pruett *et al.*, 2004). Activation of the TLR9 pathway in macrophages was also suppressed following stimulation with unmethylated DNA (Goral and Kovacs, 2005). Interestingly, TLR2 is not affected by treatment with acute ethanol, as evidenced by a lack of inhibition of TNF-α production following ligand binding (Oak *et al.*, 2006).

Toll-like receptor mediated signalling

As shown in Fig. 4.2, TLRs initiate inflammatory responses through intracellular signal transduction cascades, which include the activation of major pathways such as mitogen-activated protein kinases (MAPKs) and nuclear factor kappa-light-chain-enhancer of activated B cells (NFκB) (Takeda *et al.*, 2003; Kawai and Akira, 2006). Alcohol is known to inhibit activation of these pathways in inflam-

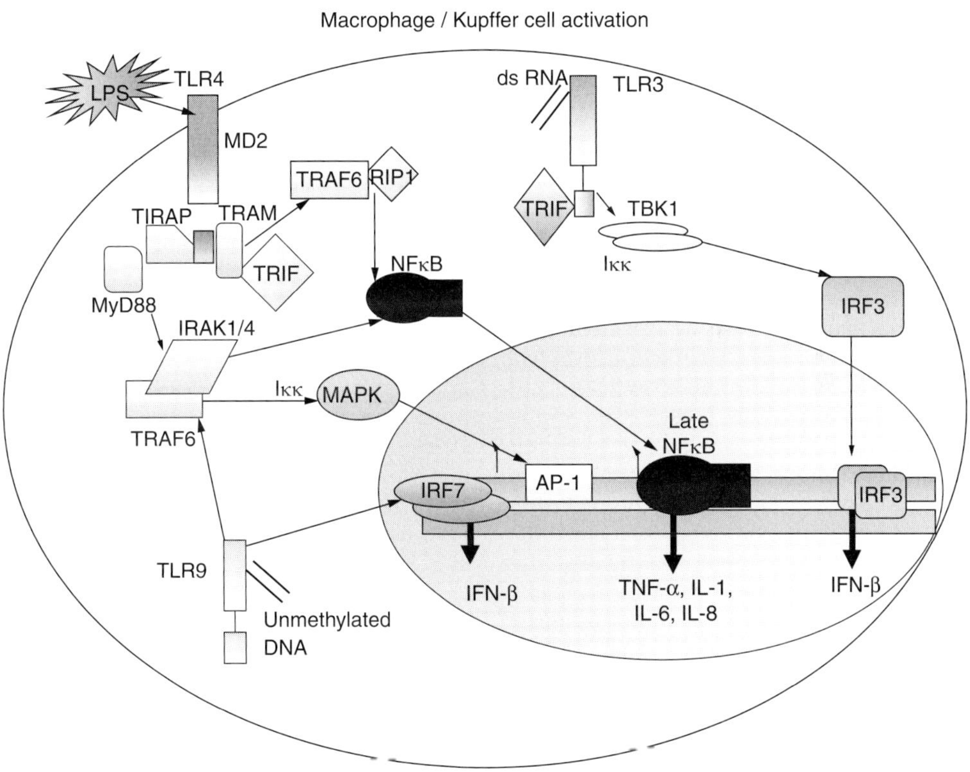

Fig. 4.2. A summary schematic of TLR signalling pathways perturbed by alcohol use in inflammation. Abbreviations: lipopolysaccharide (LPS), double-stranded RNA (ds RNA), nuclear factor kappa-light-chain-enhancer of activated B cells (NFκB), mitogen-activated protein kinases (MAPK), activator protein-1 (AP-1), Interleukin-1 receptor-associated kinase (IRAK), TNF Receptor Associated Factor-6 (TRAF6), interferon regulatory factor (IRF), interferon beta (IFN-β), inhibitor of kappa B kinase (Iκκ), TANK-binding kinase-1 (TBK-1), TIR-domain-containing adapter-inducing interferon-β (TRIF), TRIF-related adaptor molecule (TRAM), Myeloid differentiation primary response gene 88 (MYD88).

matory cells, as demonstrated in numerous reports. *In vitro*, ethanol was observed to downregulate phosphorylation of p38 (MAPK) in leukocytes and attenuated activation of NFκB in human monocytes after LPS (Arbabi *et al.*, 1999; Mandrekar *et al.*, 1999; Mandrekar *et al.*, 2007). These transcription factors were also inhibited by acute ethanol in peritoneal macrophages following activation with poly I:C (TLR3 ligand) (Pruett *et al.*, 2004). Other TLRs were affected by acute alcohol including TLR2, 4 and 9, as evidenced by diminished p38 and extracellular signal-regulated kinase (ERK1/2) phosphorylation in murine macrophages (Goral and Kovacs, 2005).

Signalling triggered by TLRs interacting with ligands is a complex process and, for TLR4, involves the formation of a receptor complex composed of CD14, MD-2 and the receptor itself (Fitzgerald *et al.*, 2004). The receptor complex then associates with intracellular signalling domains (Fig. 4.2), reminiscent of signalling within the immunological synapses in T cells formed after recognition of antigen presented in the context of MHCs present on antigen-presenting cells (Peters and Preedy, 1998; Phelan *et al.*, 2002). It has been suggested that lipid rafts comprising sphingolipids and cholesterol within the cell membrane allow for this close interaction between multiple membrane molecules (Pike, 2003; Hancock, 2006). This hypothesis implies that cell membrane proteins will freely diffuse within the plasma membrane or will form interactive assemblies through lipid rafts, depending upon activation. TLRs were shown to translocate to lipid rafts following recognition of pathogen-associated molecular patterns (PAMPs) in macrophages (Szabo *et al.*, 2007).

Early studies attempting to elucidate the mechanism by which ethanol affects inflammation and immune function examined changes in the cell membrane, and demonstrated that acute alcohol exposure increases membrane fluidity (Zambell *et al.*, 2004; Greiffenstein *et al.*, 2007). Interestingly, chronic alcohol has the opposite effect on cell membranes because it was shown to increase cholesterol content, which may lead to stiffening (Osborne *et al.*, 1994; Diebel *et al.*, 2002). These observations present an intriguing explanation for the opposing actions of acute and chronic alcohol on the inflammatory response, such that increased fluidity caused by short-term exposure to ethanol could impair the formation of signalling complexes within the lipid raft, leading to diminished activation of intracellular signalling and decreased production of inflammatory mediators. In contrast, more rigid membranes of the cells following chronic alcohol could delay the dissociation of lipid rafts, and result in prolonged signalling and increases in the production of pro-inflammatory mediators, which will be discussed later in this chapter.

Several studies have investigated the possible link between the increased membrane fluidity and the anti-inflammatory effect of acute ethanol in TLR signalling. *In vitro* exposure of acute ethanol and LPS and peptidoglycan (TLR4 andTLR2 ligands) did not disrupt lipid raft formation as measured by the distribution of lipid raft markers (Dolganiuc *et al.*, 2006). The recruitment of TLR4 to lipid rafts and the membrane distribution of CD14 were, however, affected by acute ethanol following stimulation with LPS (Dai *et al.*, 2005; Dolganiuc *et al.*, 2006). These observations were further confirmed by confocal microscopy, which showed impairment of re-organization of actin and subsequent co-localization of TLR4 and CD14 in macrophage membranes (Dai and Pruett, 2006). However, no changes in TLR2 recruitment to lipid rafts were observed (Dolganiuc *et al.*, 2006), which may be a reason for lack of changes in TLR2 signalling mentioned above. The results from these studies suggest that acute ethanol exposure inhibits the inflammatory response by modifying the formation of signalling complexes within the cell membrane after the introduction of microbial products.

Acute alcohol consumption and trauma

The immune response to trauma and injury has been described as biphasic and can result in either resolution or death. Early events result in a systemic inflammatory response (SIRS), which is mainly mediated by innate immune cells and the production of pro-inflammatory cytokines. In many patients, a compensatory anti-inflammatory response syndrome (CARS) can develop, which is associated with immune suppression and anti-inflammatory cytokine production (Bone, 1996; Murphy *et al.*, 2004). In contrast to the suppressive nature of acute ethanol exposure alone, the combination of alcohol and injury greatly exaggerates both the systemic inflammatory response and subsequent immune suppression (Bird *et al.*, 2009). In a mouse model of acute alcohol and burn injury, increased systemic and pulmonary inflammation was observed (Bird *et al.*, 2009). This enhanced inflammation was linked to increases in the expression of adhesion molecules (ICAM-1) and TLR4 signalling, because genetic deletion of either resulted in reduced levels of pro-inflammatory cytokines and pulmonary neutrophil infiltration (Bird *et al.*, 2010a,b). Alcohol exposure prior to injury results in increases in gut leakiness, as evidenced by elevated bacterial translocation (Choudhry *et al.*, 2002). Alcohol combined with injury has been shown to cause increases in gut leakiness, resulting in bacteria and pro-inflammatory mediators (i.e. cytokines and endotoxin) being carried from the gut to distal organs, primarily the lung and liver. Animal models have shown that these pro-inflammatory factors released from the gut after burn lead to neutrophil activation, endothelial cell activation and damage, and acute lung injury (Magnotti and Deitch, 2005).

In addition to burn, inflammation is greatly enhanced after other injuries in the presence of acute or binge alcohol. In fact, alcohol intoxication was shown to modulate the immediate pro-inflammatory cytokine response to haemorrhage (Phelan *et al.*, 2002). Furthermore, marked up-regulation of haemorrhage-induced tissue pro-inflammatory cytokine expression immediately post fluid resuscitation with increased neutrophil apoptosis, attenuated phagocytic activity and oxidative burst, and impaired neuromodulation of stimulated cytokine release were also observed after ethanol treatment (Molina *et al.*, 2004). These alterations in markers of host defence are associated with a marked increase in the morbidity and mortality resulting from *Klebsiella* pneumonia during the recovery period (Greiffenstein *et al.*, 2007). Improved haemodynamic homeostasis of alcohol-intoxicated haemorrhaged animals should improve organ function, prevent tissue injury and decrease susceptibility to infections and its associated morbidity. Both ethanol and gut ischaemia/reperfusion are known to impair the intestinal barrier function and increase the occurrence of sepsis following trauma (Osborne *et al.*, 1994; Diebel *et al.*, 2002), which has been suggested to be a combined effect of ethanol and ischaemia/reperfusion on epithelial function. In studies examining epithelial cells in culture, the production of TNF-α and IL-6 was elevated in the presence of ethanol, hypoxia and bacterial infection (Amin *et al.*, 2008). These data suggest that ethanol and ischaemia/reperfusion might have a synergistic effect on inflammatory cytokine production and barrier dysfunction following injury.

Chronic Alcohol Consumption and Inflammation

Hyper-state of inflammation after chronic alcohol use

Chronic alcohol abusers have increased levels of pro-inflammatory cytokines, such as TNF-α, IL-1 and IL-6 (Khoruts *et al.*, 1991; McClain *et al.*, 1993; Table 4.1). These elevated inflammatory mediators contribute to numerous illnesses with alcohol-related diseases such as alcoholic liver disease (McClain *et al.*, 1999). The augmentation of inflammation by alcohol has also been linked to neurodegeneration and tumourigenesis (Machida *et al.*, 2009, Qin *et al.*, 2008). Alcohol-mediated inflammation seems to stem from two major sources: products released from alcohol-damaged cells and leakage of gut microflora and bacterial components (Wang *et al.*, 2010). Alcohol metabolism also leads directly to the release of reactive oxygen species (ROS) and a state of hypoxia, both of which are potent inducers of inflammation (Wang *et al.*, 2010).

Alcoholic liver disease

The liver is the first major internal organ to be exposed to alcohol after the gastrointestinal tract. One of the major inflammatory diseases associated with chronic alcohol use is alcoholic liver disease (ALD). A hallmark of ALD is fibrosis, which is thought to result from hepatic injury followed by chronic inflammation. Kupffer cells, liver resident macrophages, become activated during ethanol-induced liver injury and produce high levels of inflammatory mediators, including TNF-α and ROS (Nagy, 2003; Mandrekar and Szabo, 2009; Wu and Cederbaum, 2009). These inflammatory mediators can then cause cell death and fibrosis of the liver (Nagy, 2003; Hines and Wheeler, 2004). The mechanism for Kupffer cell activation is hypothesized to be linked to increased levels of endotoxin (LPS) in the blood of alcoholics (Thurman *et al.*, 1998; Hines and Wheeler, 2004). The LPS-activated Kupffer cells can then produce TNF-α, IL-1, IL-6 and multiple chemokines, causing vascular permeability and increased infiltration of leukocytes to the liver (Nagy, 2003). Normally, bacteria and their products do not penetrate the intestinal epithelium. Excessive ethanol consumption disrupts the epithelial barrier, however, allowing increased translocation of bacteria and endotoxin from the gut lumen into the underlying tissue and the bloodstream (Rao *et al.*, 2004). Once in the circulation, these bacterial products, such as LPS, affect multiple organ systems, including the liver (Fukui *et al.*, 1991). Additionally, chronic ethanol exposure further increases the sensitivity of Kupffer cells to inflammatory stimuli, which leads to an additional production of TNF-α, as well as sensitizing hepatocytes to the damage by TNF-α and increasing susceptibility to infection (Kishore *et al.*, 2004). Increased TNF-α is accompanied by the up-regulation of p38 and ERK1/2 activity, which can be blocked by inhibitors (Kishore *et al.*, 2001, 2002; Cao *et al.*, 2002). Studies of MAP kinase involvement in synthesis of TNF-α imply a link between the activation of p38 and ERK1/2 and TNF-α mRNA stabilization. Therefore, the ethanol-induced increases in MAPK activation may contribute to the excessive sensitivity of Kupffer cells to LPS and augmented TNF-α production after chronic ethanol exposure (Nagy, 2003). The generation of ROS by NADPH oxidase was shown to be an important contributor to the increased activation of ERK1/2 in Kupffer cells after chronic ethanol and LPS exposure (Thakur *et al.*, 2006).

Bacteria are not the only pathogens affected by ethanol exposure in the liver. There are numerous studies linking chronic alcohol use with more severe viral infections of the liver, which were shown to increase the development of liver fibrosis (Regev and Jeffers, 1999). In addition, the prevalence of the hepatitis C virus is significantly higher in alcoholics than in the general population (Szabo and Mandrekar, 2009). Several studies demonstrate that alcohol alters dendritic cell function and limits the T cell response to hepatitis C virus (Dolganiuc *et al.*, 2003; Mandrekar *et al.*, 2004). Another virus, cytomegalovirus (CMV), also causes severe hepatitis in ethanol-fed mice because of a delayed induction of IL-12 and IFN-γ (Jerrells, 2002).

Because of the increased levels of LPS in ALD, it is not surprising that TLR4 signalling is important in liver inflammation after chronic alcohol exposure. In alcoholic liver disease, TLR4 signalling was shown to be crucial because the mutation of one of the components of the receptor complex CD14 resulted in protection from early alcoholic liver fat accumulation, known as steatosis (Uesugi *et al.*, 2001; Yin *et al.*, 2001). Additionally, mice genetically deficient in TLR4 did not develop liver inflammation and disease after being exposed to chronic alcohol via the Lieber-DeCarli diet (Hritz *et al.*, 2008). After binding its ligand, TLR4 signals through two different cascades, one using MyD88 and the other using another adaptor protein, TIR-domain-containing adapter-inducing IFN-β (TRIF). Both pathways result in the translocation of NFκB to the nucleus and the increased production of pro-inflammatory cytokines (Fig. 4.2). The recruitment of TRIF to the TLR4 complex also leads to the production of type I interferon. Both MyD88- and TRIF-mediated activation are important in alcoholic liver disease (Szabo *et al.*, 2011). In addition, chronic alcohol use leads to increased interleukin-1 receptor-associated kinase 1 (IRAK-1) phosphorylation, increased IκB kinase (IKK) activity, and increased NFκB nuclear translocation and DNA transactivation in human monocytes (Mandrekar and Szabo, 2009).

To combat the LPS-induced inflammation after chronic alcohol, the liver can detoxify and excrete LPS and produce increased amounts of the anti-inflammatory cytokine, IL-10. In the liver, IL-10 is mainly secreted by Kupffer cells, and has inhibitory effects on both the innate and adaptive arms of the immune system. In phagocytes, such as Kupffer cells and macrophages, IL-10 inhibits the production of pro-inflammatory cytokines, such as TNF-α, IL-1 and IL-6 (Wang *et al.*, 2010). However, chronic alcohol modulates the liver's response to inflammation by increasing sensitization of Kupffer cells as described above, impairs the liver's ability to produce anti-inflammatory cytokines (IL-10), which promotes the release of ROS and acetaldehyde, and finally hinders the ability of the liver to clear LPS (Wang *et al.*, 2010).

Failure to mount a controlled and appropriate resolution of inflammation leads to numerous chronic inflammatory diseases, such as ALD (Mandal *et al.*, 2010). Resolution is complex and involves multiple mechanisms to eliminate infiltrating leucocytes and normalizing resident cell activation. With chronic alcohol use, however, there is a failure to resolve inflammation and there is increased interest in treatments that might promote the end of the inflammatory response (Mandal *et al.*, 2010). One such anti-inflammatory molecule is adiponectin, which is an anti-inflammatory mediator produced in adipose tissue. Interestingly, the treatment of mice with large doses of adiponectin during chronic alcohol administration prevented TNF expression and liver injury in addition to reducing TNF production in culture of Kupffer cells following chronic alcohol and LPS. In liver injury, adiponectin utilizes AMP-activated protein kinase (AMPK) in hepatocytes, whereas in macrophages multiple signalling pathways are utilized including MAPK, NFκB and protein kinase A (PKA), leading to the production of IL-10 (Mandal *et al.*, 2010). Owing to high concentrations of adiponectin in the circulation and its complex structure, strategies to increase endogenous expression as well as its downstream targets, such as the IL-10/haem oxygenase-1 (HO-1) are now being undertaken (Mandal *et al.*, 2010). Little is known about IL-10 regulation and activity in the liver after chronic alcohol use, although lack of IL-10 resulted in inflammation in liver cirrhosis in alcohol abusers. Moreover, IL-10-deficient mice are more sensitive to ethanol-induced liver injury. Treating monocytes with recombinant IL-10 reduced the effects of ethanol using a HO-1-dependent mechanism. The IL-10/HO-1 pathway was shown to be involved in the suppression of Kupffer cell activation after chronic alcohol. Interestingly, ethanol does not increase the expression of HO-1; however, studies suggest that the induction of HO-1 prevents inflammation in the intestine and liver and prevents damage to hepatocytes after ethanol exposure (Mandal *et al.*, 2010).

Alcoholic lung

Chronic alcohol consumption has been linked to increases in lung infections, with bacterial pneumonia being the most common disease associated with alcohol abuse (Nelson and Kolls, 2002). Even in the late 18th century, it was noted that alcoholics had increased susceptibility to tuberculosis and pneumonia. The increased infection rate among alcoholics has been linked to impaired function of alveolar macrophages and increased reactive oxidants due to inadequate levels of glutathione in the epithelial lining fluid (Moss *et al.*, 2000). The initiation of the inflammatory response in the lung is crucial for a successful immune response to pathogens. One of the key mediators is TNF-α, which is produced by the alveolar macrophages and is important in host defence against an array of bacteria including *Streptococcus pneumoniae*, *Staphylococcus aureus*, *Legionella pneumophila*, *Klebsiella pneumoniae* and *Mycobacterium tuberculosis* (Nelson and Kolls, 2002; Szabo and Mandrekar, 2009). As discussed in detail above, acute alcohol has been demonstrated repeatedly to suppress TNF-α; however, the effect of chronic alcohol use is unclear. There is evidence showing that chronic alcohol intoxication increases the release of TNF-α through the up-regulation of the TNF-α converting enzyme activity and stabilization of TNF-α mRNA. In contrast, other studies find that chronic alcohol suppresses this mediator (Standiford and Danforth, 1997; Omidvari *et al.*, 1998). In humans, lower levels of TNF-α following LPS-stimulation of alveolar macrophages were observed from chronic alcoholic patients compared with non-alcoholics (Omidvari *et al.*, 1998; Szabo and Mandrekar, 2009). In rodent alveolar macrophages decreases of TNF-α, as well as the TNF-α -induced chemokines MIP-2 and MIP-1α, were observed after LPS stimulation in culture (Standiford and Danforth, 1997). Chronic alcohol use also affects neutrophils, resulting in hypo-responsiveness of these cells to chemotactic signals. In addition, these neutrophils are less efficient at bacterial clearance owing to impaired superoxide generation and phagocytosis (Szabo and Mandrekar, 2009).

Acute respiratory distress syndrome (ARDS) can result from increased inflammation and subsequent pulmonary dysfunction. Historically, alcohol abuse has been associated with increased incidence and severity of ARDS in critically ill patients (Moss *et al.*, 1999). Epidemiological studies conducted with patients in the intensive care unit demonstrated that alcohol abuse was a significant co-morbid variable that increased the incidence of ARDS almost threefold. Additionally, 50% of all ARDS patients had a significant history of alcohol abuse, making it a common association in this population (Esper *et al.*, 2006). Both clinical and animal model studies of chronic alcohol use demonstrate significant changes in the lungs, including epithelial and endothelial cell function, surfactant synthesis and secretion, and barrier function. Decreased glutathione in the epithelial lining fluid is also observed. Importantly, the decreased levels of glutathione observed in chronic alcoholic patients did not significantly increase even after abstaining for 1 week. Barrier function in these patients seemed to be disrupted as based on increased protein levels in the epithelial lining fluid (Boe *et al.*, 2009).

Summary and Conclusions

The effect of alcohol on inflammation and inflammatory diseases is extremely complex owing to its biphasic nature. Both acute and chronic alcohol exposure lead to immunomodulation of the innate and adaptive arms of the immune response, resulting in increased susceptibility to pathogens as well as distal organ injury. Ethanol affects multiple signalling pathways, including those involved in oxidative stress, Toll-like receptor signalling and cytokine production. Studies examining anti-inflammatory agents and compounds involved in the resolution of inflammation are of utmost importance to relieve the medical burden imposed by alcohol use and abuse.

References

Amin, P.B., Diebel, L.N. and Liberati, D.M. (2008) The synergistic effect of ethanol and shock insults on Caco-2 cytokine production and apoptosis. *Shock* 29, 631–635.

Arbabi, S., Garcia, I., Bauer, G.J. and Maier, R.V. (1999) Alcohol (ethanol) inhibits IL-8 and TNF: role of the p38 pathway. *Journal of Immunology* 162, 7441–7445.

Bird, M.D., Choudhry, M.A., Molina, P.E. and Kovacs, E.J. (2009) Alcohol and trauma: a summary of the Satellite Symposium at the 30th Annual Meeting of the Shock Society. *Alcohol* 43, 247–252.

Bird, M.D., Morgan, M.O., Ramirez, L., Yong, S. and Kovacs, E.J. (2010a) Decreased pulmonary inflammation after ethanol exposure and burn injury in intercellular adhesion molecule-1 knockout mice. *Journal of Burn Care Research* 31, 652–660.

Bird, M.D., Zahs, A., Deburghgraeve, C., Ramirez, L., Choudhry, M.A., *et al.* (2010b) Decreased pulmonary inflammation following ethanol and burn injury in mice deficient in TLR4 but not TLR2 signaling. *Alcoholism: Clinical and Experimental Research* 34, 1733–1741.

Boe, D.M., Nelson, S., Zhang, P., Quinton, L. and Bagby, G.J. (2003) Alcohol-induced suppression of lung chemokine production and the host defense response to Streptococcus pneumoniae. *Alcoholism: Clinical and Experimental Research* 27, 1838–1845.

Boe, D.M., Vandivier, R.W., Burnham, E.L. and Moss, M. (2009) Alcohol abuse and pulmonary disease. *Journal of Leukocyte Biology* 86, 1097–1104.

Bone, R.C. (1996) Sir Isaac Newton, sepsis, SIRS, and CARS. *Critical Care Medicine* 24, 1125–1128.

Callaci, J.J., Juknelis, D., Patwardhan, A., Sartori, M., Frost, N., *et al.* (2004) The effects of binge alcohol exposure on bone resorption and biomechanical and structural properties are offset by concurrent bisphosphonate treatment. *Alcoholism: Clinical and Experimental Research* 28, 182–191.

Cao, Q., Mak, K.M. and Lieber, C.S. (2002) Dilinoleoylphosphatidylcholine decreases LPS-induced TNF-alpha generation in Kupffer cells of ethanol-fed rats: respective roles of MAPKs and NF-kappaB. *Biochemical and Biophysical Research Communications* 294, 849–853.

Centers for Disease Control (2011) *Alcohol and Public Health* [Online]. Available at: http://www.cdc.gov/alcohol/ (accessed 1 April 2011).

Choudhry, M.A., Fazal, N., Goto, M., Gamelli, R.L. and Sayeed, M.M. (2002) Gut-associated lymphoid T cell suppression enhances bacterial translocation in alcohol and burn injury. *American Journal of Physiology–Gastrointestinal and Liver Physiology* 282, G937–G947.

Cook, R.T., Schlueter, A.J., Coleman, R.A., Tygrett, L., Ballas, Z.K., *et al.* (2007) Thymocytes, pre-B cells, and organ changes in a mouse model of chronic ethanol ingestion–absence of subset-specific glucocorticoid-induced immune cell loss. *Alcoholism: Clinical and Experimental Research* 31, 1746–1758.

D'souza El-Guindy, N.B., Kovacs, E.J., De Witte, P., Spies, C., Littleton, J.M., *et al.* (2010) Laboratory models available to study alcohol-induced organ damage and immune variations: choosing the appropriate model. *Alcoholism: Clinical and Experimental Research* 34, 1489–1511.

Dai, Q. and Pruett, S.B. (2006) Ethanol suppresses LPS-induced Toll-like receptor 4 clustering, reorganization of the actin cytoskeleton, and associated TNF-alpha production. *Alcoholism: Clinical and Experimental Research* 30, 1436–1444.

Dai, Q., Zhang, J. and Pruett, S.B. (2005) Ethanol alters cellular activation and CD14 partitioning in lipid rafts. *Biochemical and Biophysical Research Communications* 332, 37–42.

Diebel, L.N., Liberati, D.M., Dulchavsky, S.A., Diglio, C.A. and Brown, W.J. (2002) Ethanol impairs intestinal barrier defense by modulation of immunoglobulin A transport. *Surgery* 132, 573–581; discussion 581.

Dolganiuc, A., Kodys, K., Kopasz, A., Marshall, C., Mandrekar, P., *et al.* (2003) Additive inhibition of dendritic cell allostimulatory capacity by alcohol and hepatitis C is not restored by DC maturation and involves abnormal IL-10 and IL-2 induction. *Alcoholism: Clinical and Experimental Research* 27, 1023–1031.

Dolganiuc, A., Bakis, G., Kodys, K., Mandrekar, P. and Szabo, G. (2006) Acute ethanol treatment modulates Toll-like receptor-4 association with lipid rafts. *Alcoholism: Clinical and Experimental Research* 30, 76–85.

Driscoll, T.R., Harrison, J.A. and Steenkamp, M. (2004) Review of the role of alcohol in drowning associated with recreational aquatic activity. *Injury Prevention* 10, 107–113.

Esper, A., Burnham, E.L. and Moss, M. (2006) The effect of alcohol abuse on ARDS and multiple organ dysfunction. *Minerva Anestesiologica* 72, 375–381.

Fitzgerald, K.A., Rowe, D.C. and Golenbock, D.T. (2004) Endotoxin recognition and signal transduction by the TLR4/MD2-complex. *Microbes and Infection* 6, 1361–1367.

Fukui, H., Brauner, B., Bode, J.C. and Bode, C. (1991) Plasma endotoxin concentrations in patients with alcoholic and non-alcoholic liver disease: reevaluation with an improved chromogenic assay. *Journal of Hepatology* 12, 162–169.

Goral, J. and Kovacs, E.J. (2005) In vivo ethanol exposure down-regulates TLR2-, TLR4-, and TLR9-mediated macrophage inflammatory response by limiting p38 and ERK1/2 activation. *Journal of Immunology* 174, 456–463.

Goral, J., Choudhry, M.A. and Kovacs, E.J. (2004) Acute ethanol exposure inhibits macrophage IL-6 production: role of p38 and ERK1/2 MAPK. *Journal of Leukocyte Biology* 75, 553–559.

Goral, J., Karavitis, J. and Kovacs, E.J. (2008) Exposure-dependent effects of ethanol on the innate immune system. *Alcohol* 42, 237–247.

Greiffenstein, P., Mathis, K.W., Stouwe, C.V. and Molina, P.E. (2007) Alcohol binge before trauma/hemorrhage impairs integrity of host defense mechanisms during recovery. *Alcoholism: Clinical and Experimental Research* 31, 704–715.

Hancock, J.F. (2006) Lipid rafts: contentious only from simplistic standpoints. *Nature Reviews Molecular Cell Biology,* 7, 456–462.

Hanna, E.Z., Chou, S.P. and Grant, B.F. (1997) The relationship between drinking and heart disease morbidity in the United States: results from the National Health Interview Survey. *Alcoholism: Clinical and Experimental Research,* 21, 111–118.

He, H.T., Lellouch, A. and Marguet, D. (2005) Lipid rafts and the initiation of T cell receptor signaling. *Seminars in Immunology* 17, 23–33.

Hines, I.N. and Wheeler, M.D. (2004) Recent advances in alcoholic liver disease III. Role of the innate immune response in alcoholic hepatitis. *American Journal of Physiology – Gastrointestal and Liver Physiology* 287, G310–G314.

Hingson, R. (2004) Advances in measurement and intervention for excessive drinking. *American Joural of Preventive Medicine* 27, 261–263.

Hritz, I., Mandrekar, P., Velayudham, A., Catalano, D., Dolganiuc, A., *et al.* (2008) The critical role of toll-like receptor (TLR) 4 in alcoholic liver disease is independent of the common TLR adapter MyD88. *Hepatology* 48, 1224–1231.

Janeway, C.A., Jr and Medzhitov, R. (2002) Innate immune recognition. *Annual Reviews of Immunology* 20, 197–216.

Jerrells, T.R. (2002) Association of alcohol consumption and exaggerated immunopathologic effects in the liver induced by infectious organism. *Frontiers in Bioscience* 7, d1487.

Kawai, T. and Akira, S. (2006) TLR signaling. *Cell Death and Differentiation* 13, 816–825.

Khoruts, A., Stahnke, L., Mcclain, C.J., Logan, G. and Allen, J.I. (1991) Circulating tumor necrosis factor, interleukin-1 and interleukin-6 concentrations in chronic alcoholic patients. *Hepatology* 13, 267–276.

Kishore, R., Mcmullen, M.R. and Nagy, L.E. (2001) Stabilization of tumor necrosis factor alpha mRNA by chronic ethanol: role of A + U-rich elements and p38 mitogen-activated protein kinase signaling pathway. *Journal of Biological Chemistry* 276, 41930–41937.

Kishore, R., Hill, J.R., Mcmullen, M.R., Frenkel, J. and Nagy, L.E. (2002) ERK1/2 and Egr-1 contribute to increased TNF-alpha production in rat Kupffer cells after chronic ethanol feeding. *American Journal of Physiology– Gastrointestal and Liver Physiology* 282, G6–G15.

Kishore, R., Mcmullen, M.R., Cocuzzi, E. and Nagy, L.E. (2004) Lipopolysaccharide-mediated signal transduction: Stabilization of TNF-alpha mRNA contributes to increased lipopolysaccharide-stimulated TNF-alpha production by Kupffer cells after chronic ethanol feeding. *Comparative Hepatology* 3 Suppl 1, S31.

Kolls, J.K., Xie, J., Lei, D., Greenberg, S., Summer, W.R., *et al.* (1995) Differential effects of in vivo ethanol on LPS-induced TNF and nitric oxide production in the lung. *American Journal of Physiology* 268, L991–L998.

Lieber, C.S. and Decarli, L.M. (1976) Animal models of ethanol dependence and liver injury in rats and baboons. *Federation Proceedings* 35, 1232–1236.

Machida, K., Tsukamoto, H., Mkrtchyan, H., Duan, L., Dynnyk, A., *et al.* (2009) Toll-like receptor 4 mediates synergism between alcohol and HCV in hepatic oncogenesis involving stem cell marker Nanog. *Proceedings of the National Academy of Sciences of the United States of America* 106, 1548–1553.

Magnotti, L.J. and Deitch, E.A. (2005) Burns, bacterial translocation, gut barrier function, and failure. *Journal of Burn Care and Rehabilation* 26, 383–391.

Mandal, P., Pritchard, M.T. and Nagy, L.E. (2010) Anti-inflammatory pathways and alcoholic liver disease: role of an adiponectin/interleukin-10/heme oxygenase-1 pathway. *World Journal of Gastroenterology* 16, 1330–1336.

Mandrekar, P. and Szabo, G. (2009) Signalling pathways in alcohol-induced liver inflammation. *Journal of Hepatology* 50, 1258–1266.

Mandrekar, P., Catalano, D. and Szabo, G. (1999) Inhibition of lipopolysaccharide-mediated NFkappaB activation by ethanol in human monocytes. *International Immunology,* 11, 1781–1790.

Mandrekar, P., Catalano, D., Dolganiuc, A., Kodys, K. and Szabo, G. (2004) Inhibition of myeloid dendritic cell accessory cell function and induction of T cell anergy by alcohol correlates with decreased IL-12 production. *Journal of Immunology* 173, 3398–3407.

Mandrekar, P., Jeliazkova, V., Catalano, D. and Szabo, G. (2007) Acute alcohol exposure exerts anti-inflammatory effects by inhibiting IkappaB kinase activity and p65 phosphorylation in human monocytes. *Journal of Immunology,* 178, 7686–7693.

Mcclain, C., Hill, D., Schmidt, J. and Diehl, A.M. (1993) Cytokines and alcoholic liver disease. *Seminars in Liver Disease* 13, 170–182.

Mcclain, C.J., Barve, S., Deaciuc, I., Kugelmas, M. and Hill, D. (1999) Cytokines in alcoholic liver disease. *Seminars in Liver Disease* 19, 205–219.

Mcdonald, A.J., 3rd, Wang, N. and Camargo, C.A., Jr (2004) US emergency department visits for alcohol-related diseases and injuries between 1992 and 2000. *Archives of Internal Medicine* 164, 531–537.

Mokdad, A.H., Marks, J.S., Stroup, D.F. and Gerberding, J.L. (2004) Actual causes of death in the United States, 2000. *Journal of the American Medical Association* 291, 1238–1245.

Molina, P.E., Zambell, K.L., Norenberg, K., Eason, J., Phelan, H., *et al.* (2004) Consequences of alcohol-induced early dysregulation of responses to trauma/hemorrhage. *Alcohol* 33, 217–227.

Moss, M., Steinberg, K.P., Guidot, D.M., Duhon, G.F., Treece, P., *et al.* (1999) The effect of chronic alcohol abuse on the incidence of ARDS and the severity of the multiple organ dysfunction syndrome in adults with septic shock: an interim and multivariate analysis. *Chest* 116, 97S–98S.

Moss, M., Guidot, D.M., Wong-Lambertina, M., Ten Hoor, T., Perez, R.L., *et al.* (2000) The effects of chronic alcohol abuse on pulmonary glutathione homeostasis. *American Journal of Respiratory and Critical Care Medicine,* 161, 414–419.

Murphy, T.J., Paterson, H.M., Mannick, J.A. and Lederer, J.A. (2004) Injury, sepsis, and the regulation of Toll-like receptor responses. *Journal of Leukocyte Biology* 75, 400–407.

Nagy, L.E. (2003) Recent insights into the role of the innate immune system in the development of alcoholic liver disease. *Experimental Biology and Medicine (Maywood)* 228, 882–890.

Nagy, L.E. (ed) (2008) *Alcohol: Methods and Protocols.* Humana Press, New Jersey.

Nelson, S. and Kolls, J.K. (2002) Alcohol, host defence and society. *Nature Reviews in Immunology* 2, 205–209.

Nelson, S., Bagby, G.J., Bainton, B.G. and Summer, W.R. (1989) The effects of acute and chronic alcoholism on tumor necrosis factor and the inflammatory response. *Journal of Infectious Disease* 160, 422–429.

Oak, S., Mandrekar, P., Catalano, D., Kodys, K. and Szabo, G. (2006) TLR2- and TLR4-mediated signals determine attenuation or augmentation of inflammation by acute alcohol in monocytes. *Journal of Immunology* 176, 7628–7635.

Omidvari, K., Casey, R., Nelson, S., Olariu, R. and Shellito, J.E. (1998) Alveolar macrophage release of tumor necrosis factor-alpha in chronic alcoholics without liver disease. *Alcoholism: Clinical and Experimental Research* 22, 567–572.

Osborne, D.L., Aw, T.Y., Cepinskas, G. and Kvietys, P.R. (1994) Development of ischemia/reperfusion tolerance in the rat small intestine. An epithelium-independent event. *Journal of Clinical Investigation* 94, 1910–1918.

Peters, T.J. and Preedy, V.R. (1998) Metabolic consequences of alcohol ingestion. *Novartis Foundation Symposium* 216, 19–24; discussion 24–34.

Phelan, H., Stahls, P., Hunt, J., Bagby, G.J. and Molina, P.E. (2002) Impact of alcohol intoxication on hemodynamic, metabolic, and cytokine responses to hemorrhagic shock. *Journal of Trauma* 52, 675–682.

Pike, L.J. (2003) Lipid rafts: bringing order to chaos. *Journal of Lipid Research* 44, 655–67.

Plackett, T.P. and Kovacs, E.J. (2008) Acute models of ethanol exposure to mice. *Methods in Molecular Biology* 447, 3–9.

Pruett, S.B., Zheng, Q., Fan, R., Matthews, K. and Schwab, C. (2004) Acute exposure to ethanol affects Toll-like receptor signaling and subsequent responses: an overview of recent studies. *Alcohol* 33, 235–239.

Pruett, S.B., Fan, R., Zheng, Q. and Schwab, C. (2005) Differences in IL-10 and IL-12 production patterns and differences in the effects of acute ethanol treatment on macrophages in vivo and in vitro. *Alcohol* 37, 1–8.

Qin, L., He, J., Hanes, R.N., Pluzarev, O., Hong, J.S. and Crews, F.T. (2008) Increased systemic and brain cytokine production and neuroinflammation by endotoxin following ethanol treatment. *Journal of Neuroinflammation* 5, 10.

Rao, R.K., Seth, A. and Sheth, P. (2004) Recent advances in alcoholic liver disease I. Role of intestinal permeability and endotoxemia in alcoholic liver disease. *American Journal of Physiology–Gastrointestal and Liver Physiology* 286, G881–G884.

Regev, A. and Jeffers, L.J. (1999) Hepatitis C and alcohol. *Alcoholism: Clinical and Experimental Research* 23, 1543–1551.

Rehm, J., Gmel, G., Sempos, C.T. and Trevisan, M. (2003) Alcohol-related morbidity and mortality. *Alcohol Research and Health* 27, 39–51.

Saeed, R.W., Varma, S., Peng, T., Tracey, K.J., Sherry, B., *et al.* (2004) Ethanol blocks leukocyte recruitment and endothelial cell activation in vivo and in vitro. *Journal of Immunology* 173, 6376–6383.

Schermer, C.R. (2006) Alcohol and injury prevention. *Journal of Trauma* 60, 447–451.

Standiford, T.J. and Danforth, J.M. (1997) Ethanol feeding inhibits proinflammatory cytokine expression from murine alveolar macrophages ex vivo. *Alcoholism: Clinical and Experimental Research* 21, 1212–1217.

Szabo, G. and Mandrekar, P. (2009) A recent perspective on alcohol, immunity, and host defense. *Alcoholism: Clinical and Experimental Research* 33, 220–232.

Szabo, G., Mandrekar, P., Dolganiuc, A., Catalano, D. and Kodys, K. (2001) Reduced alloreactive T-cell activation after alcohol intake is due to impaired monocyte accessory cell function and correlates with elevated IL-10, IL-13, and decreased IFNgamma levels. *Alcoholism: Clinical and Experimental Research* 25, 1766–1772.

Szabo, G., Dolganiuc, A., Dai, Q. and Pruett, S.B. (2007) TLR4, ethanol, and lipid rafts: a new mechanism of ethanol action with implications for other receptor-mediated effects. *Journal of Immunology* 178, 1243–1249.

Szabo, G., Mandrekar, P., Petrasek, J. and Catalano, D. (2011) The unfolding web of innate immune dysregulation in alcoholic liver injury. *Alcoholism: Clinical and Experimental Research* 35,782–786.

Takeda, K., Kaisho, T. and Akira, S. (2003) Toll-like receptors. *Annual Reviews of Immunology* 21, 335–376.

Thakur, V., Pritchard, M.T., Mcmullen, M.R., Wang, Q. and Nagy, L.E. (2006) Chronic ethanol feeding increases activation of NADPH oxidase by lipopolysaccharide in rat Kupffer cells: role of increased reactive oxygen in LPS-stimulated ERK1/2 activation and TNF-alpha production. *Journal of Leukocyte Biology* 79, 1348–1356.

Thurman, R.G., Bradford, B.U., Iimuro, Y., Knecht, K.T., Arteel, G.E., *et al.* (1998) The role of gut-derived bacterial toxins and free radicals in alcohol-induced liver injury. *Journal of Gastroenterology and Hepatology* 13 Suppl, S39–S50.

US Department of Health and Human Services and US Department of Agriculture (2010) *Dietary Guidelines for Americans*, 7th edn. Government Printing Office, Washington, DC.

Uesugi, T., Froh, M., Arteel, G.E., Bradford, B.U. and Thurman, R.G. (2001) Toll-like receptor 4 is involved in the mechanism of early alcohol-induced liver injury in mice. *Hepatology* 34, 101–108.

Wang, H.J., Zakhari, S. and Jung, M.K. (2010) Alcohol, inflammation, and gut-liver-brain interactions in tissue damage and disease development. *World Journal of Gastroenterology* 16, 1304–1313.

World Health Organization (2010) *Global Strategy to Reduce the Harmful Use of Alcohol.* WHO Press, Geneva, Switzerland.

Wu, D. and Cederbaum, A.I. (2009) Oxidative stress and alcoholic liver disease. *Seminars in Liver Disease* 29, 141–154.

Yin, M., Bradford, B.U., Wheeler, M.D., Uesugi, T., Froh, M., *et al.* (2001) Reduced early alcohol-induced liver injury in CD14-deficient mice. *Journal of Immunology* 166, 4737–4742.

Zambell, K.L., Phelan, H., Vande Stouwe, C., Zhang, P., Shellito, J.E., *et al.* (2004) Acute alcohol intoxication during hemorrhagic shock: impact on host defense from infection. *Alcoholism: Clinical and Experimental Research* 28, 635–642.

Zhang, P., Nelson, S., Summer, W.R. and Spitzer, J.A. (1997) Acute ethanol intoxication suppresses the pulmonary inflammatory response in rats challenged with intrapulmonary endotoxin. *Alcoholism: Clinical and Experimental Research* 21, 773–778.

5 Vitamin D and Inflammation

T. Barker*
The Orthopedic Specialty Hospital, Murray, Utah, USA

Introduction

Vitamin D is a fat-soluble vitamin that was discovered in 1922 (McCollum *et al.*, 1922). In addition to regulating calcium and bone homeostasis, vitamin D regulates a variety of other physiological functions, including, but not limited to, the modulation of inflammatory cytokines. Inflammatory cytokines are small polypeptides or glycoproteins (≤30kDa) secreted by nearly every nucleated cell in the body. Cytokines regulate and orchestrate host defence and repair processes, and participate in and marshal intercellular signalling. Thus, inflammatory cytokines are vital to the function of the immune system. The ability of vitamin D to regulate cytokine production is the focus of this chapter.

Endogenous vitamin D concentration is influenced by a variety of factors, including dietary (i.e. oily fish, dairy, fortified foods and drinks, dietary supplements, etc.), environmental (i.e. sun exposure, latitude, season, etc.), demographic (i.e. age, body mass index, fat composition, etc.), and genetic (e.g. polymorphisms in metabolism and transport genes) factors. In plants, ergosterol is activated by irradiation and forms ergocalciferol (vitamin D_2). Ergosterol is not found in humans. In contrast, 7-dehydrocholesterol is synthesized in sebaceous glands in the skin and is secreted onto the surface of the skin in humans. Upon sun exposure, 7-dehydrocholesterol is converted to pre-vitamin D_3. Pre-vitamin D_3 is isomerized into vitamin D_3 (cholecalciferol). Cholecalciferol on the skin can diffuse to the circulation. In the circulation, a vitamin-D-binding protein transports cholecalciferol. Cholecalciferol obtained from food and supplement sources is incorporated into chylomicrons and transported by the lymphatic system into the venous circulation.

* Author, tyler.barker@imail.org

Circulating cholecalciferol is transported to the liver where it is hydroxylated by 25-hydroxylase (25-OHase), which forms the major circulating metabolite of vitamin D, 25-hydroxyvitamin D (25(OH)D; Fig. 5.1). 25(OH)D is the common metabolite used to identify vitamin D status and serves as a substrate for other hydroxylase enzymes. In the kidney, 1α-hydroxylase (1α-OHase; encoded by CYP27B1) converts 25(OH)D to 1,25-dihydroxyvitamin D (1,25(OH)D), whereas 24-hydroxylase (24-OHase; encoded by CYP24A1) converts 25(OH)D to 24,25-dihyroxyvitamin D (24,25(OH)D). High serum calcium or phosphate levels stimulate 24-OHase to produce 24,25(OH)D (Holick, 2007; Lappe, 2011). Although 24,25(OH)D is considered inactive, the circulating 24,25(OH)D-to-25(OH)D concentration ratio could be influential in determining an individual's response to supplemental vitamin D (Wagner *et al.*, 2011) and 24,25(OH)D increases hydrogen peroxide production by binding to and blocking catalase activity (Nemere *et al.*, 2006).

Low serum vitamin D, elevated parathyroid hormone, or low serum calcium or phosphate stimulate the production of 1,25(OH)D (calcitrol; Fig. 5.1), the active, hormonal form of vitamin D. This active form is pivotal in regulating serum calcium homeostasis by modulating calcium absorption in the intestines, reabsorption in the kidneys and resorption in the bone (along with phosphate). 1,25(OH)D is also instrumental in regulating inflammatory cytokines and is synthesized from extrarenal sources.

The immune actions of vitamin D were first documented when receptors for 1,25(OH)D were detected in various neoplastic cell lines (Eisman *et al.*, 1979; Manolagas *et al.*, 1980). Shortly thereafter, cancer cell studies demonstrated that the binding of 1,25(OH)D to the vitamin D receptor (VDR) induced anti-proliferative and pro-differentiation responses (Abe *et al.*, 1981; Colston *et al.*, 1981). These immune modulating properties were later extended in other immune cells (Abe *et al.*, 1983; Bhalla *et al.*, 1984). Of these immune cells, monocytes and dendritic cells express the VDR intracellularly

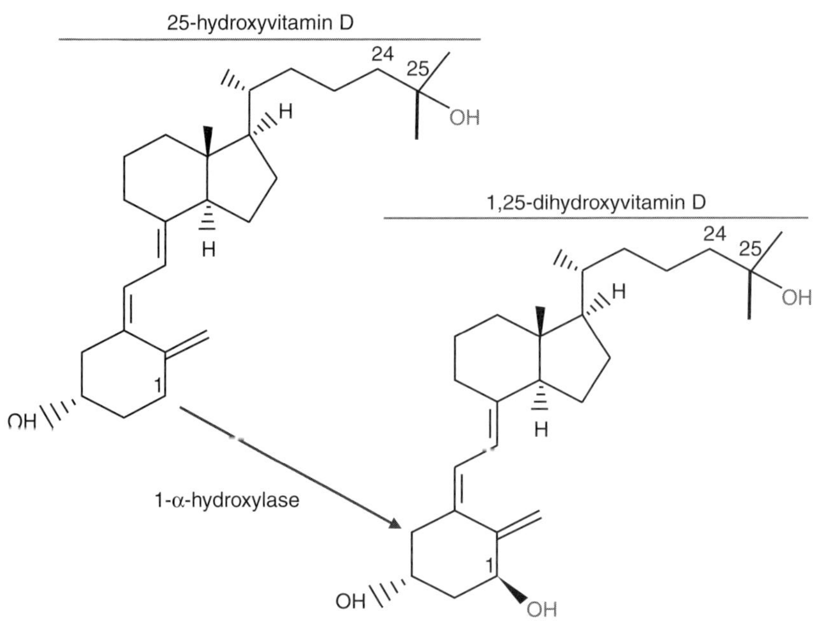

Fig. 5.1. 25-Hydroxyvitamin D (25(OH)D; top left) is a pro-hormone that serves as the major vitamin D circulating metabolite, acts as the vitamin D status measure, and is the precursor to the active hormonal form of vitamin D, 1,25-dihydroxyvitamin D (1,25(OH)D; bottom right). The enzyme 1-α-hydroxylase (encoded by CYP27B1) hydroxylates 25(OH)D at the C-1 position to form 1,25(OH)D. In addition to being found in the kidney, 1-α-hydroxylase is present in various immune cells.

(Provvedini *et al.*, 1983; Rigby *et al.*, 1987; Muller *et al.*, 1992; Penna and Adorini, 2000; Hewison *et al.*, 2003), whereas T and B lymphocytes express VDR following activation or stimulation (Bhalla *et al.*, 1983; Provvedini *et al.*, 1983; Provvedini and Manolagas, 1989; Veldman *et al.*, 2000).

Immune cells also participate in vitamin D metabolism. Peripheral blood mononuclear cells express 1α-OHase and 24-OHase (Hewison *et al.*, 2003; Fritsche *et al.*, 2003; Gottfried *et al.*, 2006; Chen *et al.*, 2007; Penna *et al.*, 2007; Sigmundsdottir *et al.*, 2007; Heine *et al.*, 2008; Correale *et al.*, 2009; Szeles *et al.*, 2009). In patients with sarcoidosis disease, circulating 1,25(OH)D concentrations were elevated. These elevations were due to an increased 1α-OHase activity (Bell *et al.*, 1979; Papapoulos *et al.*, 1979) and, importantly, in disease-associated macrophages (Barbour *et al.*, 1981; Adams *et al.*, 1983; Adams and Gacad, 1985).

Vitamin D Status or Supplementation and Inflammatory Cytokines

The influence of vitamin D status, or alterations therein, on circulating cytokines is receiving increasing attention (Table 5.1). One determinant of vitamin D status is season (Tangpricha *et al.*, 2002). Low serum 25(OH)D and interleukin (IL)-10 concentrations have been observed in newborns born during the winter as opposed to those born during the summer (Zittermann *et al.*, 2004). More recently, Khoo *et al.* (2011b) examined the seasonal variation in vitamin D status and circulating cytokines. During the summer, serum 25(OH)D and 1,25(OH)D increases occurred concurrently with tumour necrosis factor (TNF)-α, IL-1β, IL-6, interferon (IFN)-γ and IL-10 decreases (Khoo *et al.*, 2011b). The cytokine decreases occurred concomitantly with suppressed Toll-like receptor (TLR)-2 and -4 expression on monocytes, implying that the increase in vitamin D status during the summer downregulates cytokine production, possibly through the TLR-2 and TLR-4 signalling pathways (Khoo *et al.*, 2011b).

Obesity is another determinant of vitamin D status. Obesity results in hypovitaminosis D (Wortsman *et al.*, 2000) and systemic cytokine challenge (Berg and Scherer, 2005). In obese patients, those in a low vitamin D tertile (serum 25(OH)D between 35.1 and 60.2 nmol/l) were more obese (greater fat percentage, fat mass (kg) and truncal fat mass) and displayed greater circulating TNF-α and IL-6 concentrations than those in a high tertile (serum 25(OH)D between 70.6 and 112.8 nmol/l) (Bellia *et al.*, 2011). Furthermore, serum 25(OH)D inversely correlated with TNF-α and IL-6 (Bellia *et al.*, 2011). The authors suggested that inflammatory markers decrease as serum 25(OH)D concentrations increase in obese individuals (Bellia *et al.*, 2011).

Supplemental vitamin D increases serum 25(OH)D concentration, and it is suggested that 100 IU of vitamin D intake increases serum 25(OH)D concentration by ~1.0 ng/ml (Barger-Lux *et al.*, 1998). Given this knowledge, it is surprising that few studies have examined the prospective influence of supplemental vitamin D on serum 25(OH)D and circulating cytokine concentrations. In pathophysiological conditions (i.e. congestive heart failure, multiple sclerosis, osteoporosis in post-menopausal women or end-stage renal disease), vitamin D supplementation with or without calcium for various durations increased vitamin D status and IL-10, and decreased transforming growth factor-β1, IL-1β, IL-6 and IL-8, whereas TNF-α remained unchanged or decreased (Mahon *et al.*, 2003a; Inanir *et al.*, 2004; Schleithoff *et al.*, 2006; Stubbs *et al.*, 2010) (Table 5.1). Following vitamin D supplementation in post-menopausal women, serum TNF-α and IL-6 concentrations were not significantly different (Table 5.1; Gannage-Yared *et al.*, 2003). In healthy adults, and despite inconsistent cytokine results (Zittermann *et al.*, 2009; Yusupov *et al.*, 2010; Barnes *et al.*, 2011), supplemental vitamin D increased circulating 25(OH)D and decreased TNF-α, IFN-γ, IL-4, IL-8 and IL-10 (Table 5.1). Additionally, a high dose of supplemental vitamin D increased the proportion of IL-10⁺ CD4⁺ T cells and decreased the IFN-γ⁺/IL-4⁺ ratio in patients with relapsing remitting multiple sclerosis (Smolders *et al.*,

Table 5.1. Vitamin D and inflammatory cytokines.

Vitamin D intervention or determinant	Dose/duration or vitamin D status[a] demarcation	Population	Cytokine results	Reference
Season	Winter versus summer	Newborns	Low serum 25(OH)D and IL-10 in infants born during the winter	Zittermann *et al.* (2004)
Season	Seasonal variation	Healthy males	High serum 25(OH)D and low TNF-α, IL-1β, IFN-γ, IL-6 and IL-10 production during summer	Khoo *et al.* (2011)
Obesity	Serum 25(OH)D tertiles	Obese[b]	Upper tertile had lower serum TNF-α and IL-6 concentrations	Bellia *et al.* (2011)
Cholecalciferol	800 IU/day for 12 weeks – menopausal women	Healthy post-concentrations	No change in serum TNF-α or IL-6	Gannage-Yared *et al.* (2003)
Cholecalciferol	200, 400 or 600 IU/day for 22 weeks	Young and old adults	No significant influence on TNF-α, IL-6 or IL-10 serum concentrations	Barnes *et al.* (2011)
Cholecalciferol	3332 IU/day for 12 months adults	Overweight	No change in plasma IL-6 but a ↓ TNF-α concentrations	Zittermann *et al.* (2009)
Cholecalciferol	2000 IU/day for 3 months	Adults	↓ IFN-γ, IL-4, IL-8, and IL-10 but no change in IL-6 and IL-2 serum concentrations	Yusupov *et al.* (2010)
Cholecalciferol	2000 IU/day for 9 months	Congestive heart failure patients	↑ IL-10 and ameliorated the increase in TNF-α plasma concentrations	Schleithoff *et al.* (2006)
Cholecalciferol	20,000 IU/day for 12 weeks – remitting MS patients	Relapsing	↑ Proportion of IL-10$^+$ and ↓ the IFN-γ$^+$-to-IL-4$^+$ ratio expression in CD4$^+$ T cells	Smolders *et al.* (2010)
Cholecalciferol	50,000 IU once, twice and/or three times weekly for 8 weeks	End-stage renal disease	↓ Serum IL-8, IL-6 and TNF concentrations	Stubbs *et al.* (2010)
Cholecalciferol	1000 IU/day for 6 months	MS patients	No change in TNF-α, IFN-γ, or IL-2 mRNA in PBMC	Mahon *et al.* (2003)
Calcitriol	0.5 μg/day for 6 months	Post-menopausal patients with osteoporosis	↓ Serum IL-1 and TNF-α but no change in IL-6 concentrations	Inanir *et al.* (2004)
Calcitriol	0.5 μg/day for 7 days	Glucocorticoid-resistant asthma patients	↑ IL-10 in CD3$^+$CD4$^+$ T cells	Urry *et al.* (2010)

[a]Vitamin D status as reflected by serum 25(OH)D concentration. [b]Obese patients undergoing bariatric surgery. 25(OH)D, 25-hydroxyvitamin D; IL, interleukin; IFN, interferon; MS, multiple sclerosis; PBMC, peripheral blood mononuclear cells; TNF, tumour necrosis factor.

2010) (Table 5.1). Vitamin D supplementation in its active form also increased IL-10 expression in $CD3^+CD4^+$ T cells (Urry *et al.*, 2009). These data indicate that supplemental vitamin D modulates circulating concentrations and immune cell expression of different inflammatory cytokines.

Regulation of inflammatory cytokines by vitamin D

The identification of VDR in peripheral blood mononuclear cells (Bhalla *et al.*, 1983; Provvedini *et al.*, 1983) and the production of 1,25(OH)D from activated macrophages acquired from sarcoidosis patients (Adams *et al.*, 1983; Adams and Gacad, 1985; Adams *et al.*, 1985) ignited research endeavours investigating vitamin D as an immuno-modulator, especially in isolated immune cells obtained from experimental animals (Boonstra *et al.*, 2001; Froicu *et al.*, 2003; Mahon *et al.*, 2003b). These earlier results laid the foundation for future studies examining the cytokine-modulating property of 1,25(OH)D.

Reports identifying the influence of 1,25(OH)D on IL-1β production are varied. Results indicate that 1,25(OH)D inhibits, does not alter or increases IL-1β (Iho *et al.*, 1985; Bhalla *et al.*, 1986; Tsoukas *et al.*, 1989; Rigby and Waugh, 1992). Regarding TNF-α, 1,25(OH)D inhibits TNF-α production or secretion from a variety of immune cells (Sadeghi *et al.*, 2006; Almerighi *et al.*, 2009; Khoo *et al.*, 2011b; Lysandropoulos *et al.*, 2011). Furthermore, 1,25(OH)D blocks TNF-α production from peripheral blood mononuclear cells stimulated with *Candida albicans*, tuberculosis or mycobacteria, and from activated macrophages infected with mycobacteria (Martineau *et al.*, 2007; Prabhu *et al.*, 2009; Khoo *et al.*, 2011a). Although there are discrepancies that could relate to differences in immune cells and immune cell activation states, data suggest that vitamin D inhibits the production of pro-inflammatory cytokines.

IFN-γ is a T helper 1 (T_{H1})-type cytokine that possesses pro- and anti-inflammatory properties. Although the exposure of activated $CD4^+$ and $CD8^+$ T cells to 1,25(OH)D has been reported to be ineffective at altering IFN-γ production (Willheim *et al.*, 1999; Thien *et al.*, 2005), the majority of the data suggest that 1,25(OH)D (or an analogue) blocks IFN-γ production (Reichel *et al.*, 1987b; Rigby *et al.*, 1987; Staeva-Vieira and Freedman, 2002; Bartels *et al.*, 2007; Penna *et al.*, 2007; Almerighi *et al.*, 2009; Jeffery *et al.*, 2009; Baeke *et al.*, 2011; Lysandropoulos *et al.*, 2011). Consistent with an inhibitory regulation, 1,25(OH)D reduces IFN-γ production from immune cells infected with bacteria or immune cells acquired from patients with disparate diseases (e.g. Crohns disease or rheumatoid arthritis) Bartels *et al.*, 2007; Martineau *et al.*, 2007; Jeffery *et al.*, 2009; Prabhu *et al.*, 2009; Colin *et al.*, 2010). The ability of vitamin D to down-regulate IFN-γ could be dependent on VDR levels (Baeke *et al.*, 2010).

Similar to IFN-γ, IL-6 possesses pro- and anti-inflammatory properties. Conflicting reports exist regarding the influence of vitamin D on IL-6 production (Willheim *et al.*, 1999; Jiang *et al.*, 2011). The ability of vitamin D to increase IL-6 could plausibly be reliant on the presence of other inflammatory cytokines, such as IL-4 (Thien *et al.*, 2005). None the less, most data indicate that 1,25(OH)D decreases IL-6 production (Muller *et al.*, 1991; Correale *et al.*, 2009; Khoo *et al.*, 2011a; Khoo *et al.*, 2011b) and results could be immune cell and activation specific (Peelen *et al.*, 2011).

The inhibition of IL-2 expression or production by 1,25(OH)D has been consistently reported in a variety of immune cells (Rigby *et al.*, 1984, 1987; Iho *et al.*, 1985; Lemire *et al.*, 1985; Bhalla *et al.*, 1986; Willheim *et al.*, 1999; Thien *et al.*, 2005; Jeffery *et al.*, 2009). Conversely, there are contrasting results regarding the influence of vitamin D on IL-4. 1,25(OH)D does not modulate or inhibit IL-4 production (Willheim *et al.*, 1999; Staeva-Vieira and Freedman, 2002; Baeke *et al.*, 2011), whereas others found that the presence of 1,25(OH)D increases IL-4 production in peripheral blood mononuclear cells obtained from patients with rheumatoid arthritis (Colin *et al.*, 2010).

In addition to IL-4, IL-5 and IL-10 are T helper 2 (T_{H2})-type cytokines regulated by vitamin D. In peripheral blood mononuclear cells, 1,25(OH)D inhibits IL-5 production

(Lysandropoulos *et al.*, 2011). In a variety of immune cells, 1,25(OH)D (or vitamin D analogue) enhances IL-10 expression (mRNA and protein) and production (Penna and Adorini, 2000; Barrat *et al.*, 2002; Bartels *et al.*, 2007; Heine *et al.*, 2008; Almerighi *et al.*, 2009; Correale *et al.*, 2009; Jeffery *et al.*, 2009; Matilainen *et al.*, 2010a; Baeke *et al.*, 2011; Khoo *et al.*, 2011a). Importantly, IL-10 mRNA expression seems to be time-sensitive because results indicate an initial down-regulation that is followed by an up-regulation (Matilainen *et al.*, 2010a,b). Along these lines, Baeke *et al.* (2010) indicated that 1,25(OH)D suppressed short-term but not long-term IL-10 mRNA expression in active T cells, which, similar to IFN-γ, could be dependent on VDR levels.

Mechanisms of action

The majority of the biological actions mediated by 1,25(OH)D require a nuclear or cell-surface receptor. The VDR is a high-affinity receptor for steroid hormones. The nuclear VDR acts as a ligand-activated transcription factor. Upon interaction with 1,25(OH)D, VDR heterodimerizes with the retinoic X receptor (RXR) (Provvedini *et al.*, 1983; Veldman *et al.*, 2000). This 1,25(OH)D–VDR–RXR complex binds to the vitamin D response elements and regulates cytokine gene transcription (Alroy *et al.*, 1995; D'Ambrosio *et al.*, 1998; Heine *et al.*, 2008).

Numerous studies have investigated the influence of 1,25(OH)D on cytokine regulation. From these studies, the mechanisms by which vitamin D regulates IFN-γ, IL-2 and IL-10 are the best characterized. 1,25(OH)D down-regulates the activation of the IFN-γ promoter (Cippitelli and Santoni, 1998), which is mediated by the VDR–RXR complex. Likewise, IL-2 and IL-10 mRNA expression is ligand-dependently repressed by 1,25(OH)D treatment (Matilainen *et al.*, 2010b). Similar reports identifying the ligand–receptor regulatory influence on other cytokines, such as IL-12B (Gynther *et al.*, 2011), are increasing.

In addition to the VDR–RXR complex, vitamin D regulates inflammatory cytokines by modulating the expression and activity of nuclear factor (NF)κB (D'Ambrosio *et al.*, 1998; Dong *et al.*, 2003; Mahon *et al.*, 2003b). The bioactive, hormonal form of vitamin D impairs NFκB gene expression (Mahon *et al.*, 2003b). 1,25(OH)D induces IκBα (Hansdottir *et al.*, 2010), an inhibitor of NFκB activation, and impairs the nuclear translocation of p65 and subsequent binding to the p105 promoter (Geldmeyer-Hilt *et al.*, 2011). Thus, vitamin D impairs the activation of NFκB. The ability of vitamin D to inhibit NFκB is specific to 1,25(OH)D because other vitamin D metabolites (i.e. 25(OH)D and 24,25(OH)D) are reportedly ineffective at regulating NFκB (Yu *et al.*, 1995). Interestingly, the inhibitory influence of vitamin D on NFκB is challenged by inflammatory cytokines, such as TNF-α (Farmer *et al.*, 2000).

Vitamin D also regulates cytokine expression or production by modulating the nuclear factor of activated T cells (NFAT). The repression of IL-2 transcription by 1,25(OH)D is mediated by repressing NFAT activity (Alroy *et al.*, 1995; Takeuchi *et al.*, 1998). Thus, in addition to VDR–RXR and NFκB, vitamin D regulates cytokine expression by modulating NFAT.

Vitamin D also regulates cytokine production by interfering with the signalling cascade or cross-talk between cytokines. For example, TNF-α is a pro-inflammatory cytokine that induces IL-6. 1,25(OH)D inhibits the induction of IL-6 by TNF-α, which seems to be dependent upon p38 inhibition (Nonn *et al.*, 2006). 1,25(OH)D also inhibits the induction of IFN-γ induced by IL-12 (Thien *et al.*, 2005). These are important results because they identify that vitamin D indirectly regulates cytokine production by altering the association between mutually related cytokines.

The non-genomic responses elicited by vitamin D occur rapidly and are mediated by cell-surface receptors. The non-genomic events mediated by vitamin D include, but are not limited to, mitogen-activated protein kinase (MAPK), protein kinase C (PKC), cGMP, phosphoinositide metabolism and cytosolic calcium (Dusso *et al.*, 2005). For example, in human monocytes, 1,25(OH)D reduced MAPK (Sadeghi *et al.*, 2006), which, as demonstrated in peripheral blood mononuclear cells, could be linked to the upregulation of MAPK phosphatase-1 (Zhang *et al.*, 2012). Although the non-genomic influence of vitamin D on cytokine expression or production is an exciting area of research, future investigations are clearly warranted.

Reciprocal regulation of inflammatory cytokines on vitamin D metabolism

It also seems that inflammatory cytokines regulate vitamin D metabolism in immune cells. In pulmonary alveolar macrophages acquired from healthy subjects and tuberculosis patients, IL-2 and IFN-γ induce 1,25(OH)D synthesis from 25(OH)D (Koeffler *et al.*, 1985; Reichel *et al.*, 1987a). In monocytes, the increased production of 1,25(OH)D by IFN-γ is mediated by an upregulation in TLR 2/1 that induces 1α-OHase (Edfeldt *et al.*, 2010). The induction of 1α-OHase and subsequent 1,25(OH)D production induced by IFN-γ is also mediated by Janus kinase-signal transducer and activator of transcription (JAK-STAT), NFκB and p38MAPK pathways in monocytes (Stoffels *et al.*, 2006; Stoffels *et al.*, 2007). In B cells, IL-4 induces 1α-OHase (Heine *et al.*, 2008). IL-4 has, however, also been shown to induce the catabolism of 25(OH)D to 24,25(OH)D in monocytes, thereby suggesting that the regulatory influence of IL-4 on vitamin D metabolism is immune-cell specific (Edfeldt *et al.*, 2010). Nevertheless, these data indicate that inflammatory cytokines regulate vitamin D metabolism in circulating immune cells, which could influence autocrine or paracrine mechanisms in peripheral tissue.

Summary and Conclusions

Adaptive immune cells express vitamin D receptors and enzymes involved in vitamin D metabolism. This allows adaptive immune cells to convert 25(OH)D to its active, hormonal form and to regulate intracellular processes, including cytokine expression and production (Fig. 5.2). From isolated immune cells, results predominately indicate that vitamin D mediates a shift from T_{H1}- to T_{H2}-type cytokines by inhibiting the former and accentuating the production of the latter. This observation requires further investigation, however. Data also indicate that T_{H1}-type cytokines induce 1,25(OH)D, whereas the regulatory influence of T_{H2}-type cytokines on vitamin D metabolism awaits future resolution. Furthermore, the interactions between vitamin D, vitamin D metabolism and receptors, and inflammatory cytokines could exhibit different properties and responses *in vivo*. Future studies are needed to identify whether results obtained *in vitro* translate to *in vivo* conditions.

In conclusion, vitamin D is a fat-soluble vitamin that modulates inflammatory cytokines. Vitamin D regulates inflammatory cytokines at the transcriptional and translational levels, and this regulation is immune-cell and cytokine specific. Furthermore, the ability of vitamin D to modulate inflammatory cytokines is condition specific because patients with different pathophysiological or physiological characteristics display disparate responses to supplemental interventions.

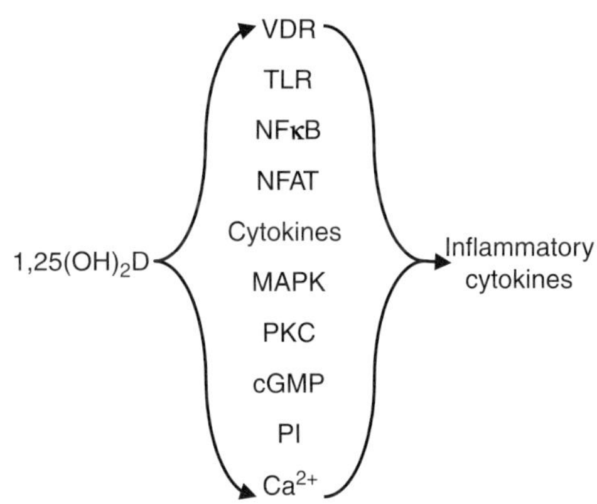

Fig. 5.2. Vitamin D targets in cytokine regulation. The active, hormonal form of vitamin D, 1,25(OH)D, regulates cytokine production by binding to the vitamin D receptor (VDR), suppressing Toll-like receptor (TLR)-mediated pathways, inhibiting NFκB nuclear presence and activation, repressing NFAT activity and interfering with signalling cascades or cross-talk between inflammatory cytokines. It is also plausible that vitamin D regulates cytokine production by modulating MAPK, PKC, cGMP, phosphoinositide (PI) metabolism and cytosolic calcium (Ca^{2+}), but confirmation of this speculation awaits future research.

Acknowledgements

The author would like to recognize the research efforts of those who have contributed to this field of study. The author thanks Vanessa T. Henriksen for critically reviewing this chapter. The author would also like to thank Dr Maret G. Traber (Oregon State University and the Linus Pauling Institute) for her mentoring and support. Work on this chapter was supported by The Deseret Foundation (Intermountain Healthcare, Salt Lake City, Utah), USANA Health Sciences, Inc. (Salt Lake City, Utah), The Orthopedic Specialty Hospital (TOSH, Murray, Utah) and Intermountain Healthcare. Special thanks to TOSH and Intermountain Healthcare for their continued support.

References

Abe, E., Miyaura, C., Sakagami, H., Takeda, M., Konno, K., *et al.* (1981) Differentiation of mouse myeloid leukemia cells induced by 1 alpha,25-dihydroxyvitamin D3. *Proceedings of the National Academy of Sciences of the United States of America* 78, 4990–4994.

Abe, E., Miyaura, C., Tanaka, H., Shiina, Y., Kuribayashi, T., *et al.* (1983) 1 alpha,25-dihydroxyvitamin D3 promotes fusion of mouse alveolar macrophages both by a direct mechanism and by a spleen cell-mediated indirect mechanism. *Proceedings of the National Academy of Sciences of the United States of America* 80, 5583–5587.

Adams, J.S. and Gacad, M.A. (1985) Characterization of 1 alpha-hydroxylation of vitamin D3 sterols by cultured alveolar macrophages from patients with sarcoidosis. *The Journal of Experimental Medicine* 161, 755–765.

Adams, J.S., Sharma, O.P., Gacad, M.A. and Singer, F.R. (1983) Metabolism of 25-hydroxyvitamin D3 by cultured pulmonary alveolar macrophages in sarcoidosis. *The Journal of Clinical Investigation* 72, 1856–1860.

Adams, J.S., Singer, F.R., Gacad, M.A., Sharma, O.P., Hayes, M.J., *et al.* (1985) Isolation and structural identification of 1,25-dihydroxyvitamin D3 produced by cultured alveolar macrophages in sarcoidosis. *Journal of Clinical Endocrinology and Metabolism* 60, 960–966.

Almerighi, C., Sinistro, A., Cavazza, A., Ciaprini, C., Rocchi, G., *et al.* (2009) 1Alpha,25-dihydroxyvitamin D3 inhibits CD40L-induced pro-inflammatory and immunomodulatory activity in human monocytes. *Cytokine* 45, 190–197.

Alroy, I., Towers, T.L. and Freedman, L.P. (1995) Transcriptional repression of the interleukin-2 gene by vitamin D3: direct inhibition of NFATp/AP-1 complex formation by a nuclear hormone receptor. *Molecular and Cellular Biochemistry* 15, 5789–5799.

Baeke, F., Korf, H., Overbergh, L., van, E.E., Verstuyf, A., *et al.* (2010) Human T lymphocytes are direct targets of 1,25-dihydroxyvitamin D3 in the immune system. *Journal of Steroid Biochemistry and Molecular Biology* 121, 221–227.

Baeke, F., Korf, H., Overbergh, L., Verstuyf, A., Thorrez, L., *et al.* (2011) The vitamin D analog, TX527, promotes a human CD4+CD25highCD127low regulatory T cell profile and induces a migratory signature specific for homing to sites of inflammation. *The Journal of Immunology* 186, 132–142.

Barbour, G.L., Coburn, J.W., Slatopolsky, E., Norman, A.W. and Horst, R.L. (1981) Hypercalcemia in an anephric patient with sarcoidosis: evidence for extrarenal generation of 1,25-dihydroxyvitamin D. *New England Journal of Medicine* 305, 440–443.

Barger-Lux, M.J., Heaney, R.P., Dowell, S., Chen, T.C. and Holick, M.F. (1998) Vitamin D and its major metabolites: serum levels after graded oral dosing in healthy men. *Osteoporosis International* 8, 222–230.

Barnes, M.S., Horigan, G., Cashman, K.D., Hill, T.R., Forsythe, L.K., *et al.* (2011) Maintenance of wintertime vitamin D status with cholecalciferol supplementation is not associated with alterations in serum cytokine concentrations among apparently healthy younger or older adults. *The Journal of Nutrition* 141, 476–481.

Barrat, F.J., Cua, D.J., Boonstra, A., Richards, D.F., Crain, C., *et al.* (2002) In vitro generation of interleukin 10-producing regulatory CD4(+) T cells is induced by immunosuppressive drugs and inhibited by T helper type 1 (Th1)- and Th2-inducing cytokines. *The Journal of Experimental Medicine* 195, 603–616.

Bartels, L.E., Jorgensen, S.P., Agnholt, J., Kelsen, J., Hvas, C.L., *et al.* (2007) 1,25-dihydroxyvitamin D3 and dexamethasone increase interleukin-10 production in CD4+ T cells from patients with Crohn's disease. *International Immunopharmacology* 7, 1755–1764.

Bell, N.H., Stern, P.H., Pantzer, E., Sinha, T.K. and DeLuca, H.F. (1979) Evidence that increased circulating 1 alpha, 25-dihydroxyvitamin D is the probable cause for abnormal calcium metabolism in sarcoidosis. *The Journal of Clinical Investigation* 64, 218–225.

Bellia, A., Garcovich, C., D'Adamo, M., Lombardo, M., Tesauro, M., *et al.* (2011) Serum 25-hydroxyvitamin D levels are inversely associated with systemic inflammation in severe obese subjects. *Internal and Emergency Medicine* DOI: 10.1007/s11739-011-0559-x.

Berg, A.H. and Scherer, P.E. (2005) Adipose tissue, inflammation, and cardiovascular disease. *Circulation Research* 96, 939–949.

Bhalla, A.K., Amento, E.P., Clemens, T.L., Holick, M.F. and Krane, S.M. (1983) Specific high-affinity receptors for 1,25-dihydroxyvitamin D3 in human peripheral blood mononuclear cells: presence in monocytes and induction in T lymphocytes following activation. *Journal of Clinical Endocrinology and Metabolism* 57, 1308–1310.

Bhalla, A.K., Amento, E.P., Serog, B. and Glimcher, L.H. (1984) 1,25-Dihydroxyvitamin D3 inhibits antigen-induced T cell activation. *The Journal of Immunology* 133, 1748–1754.

Bhalla, A.K., Amento, E.P. and Krane, S.M. (1986) Differential effects of 1,25-dihydroxyvitamin D3 on human lymphocytes and monocyte/macrophages: inhibition of interleukin-2 and augmentation of interleukin-1 production. *Cellular Immunology* 98, 311–322.

Boonstra, A., Barrat, F.J., Crain, C., Heath, V.L., Savelkoul, H.F., *et al.* (2001) 1alpha,25-Dihydroxyvitamin d3 has a direct effect on naive CD4(+) T cells to enhance the development of Th2 cells. *The Journal of Immunology* 167, 4974–4980.

Chen, S., Sims, G.P., Chen, X.X., Gu, Y.Y., Chen, S., *et al.* (2007) Modulatory effects of 1,25-dihydroxyvitamin D3 on human B cell differentiation. *The Journal of Immunology* 179, 1634–1647.

Cippitelli, M. and Santoni, A. (1998) Vitamin D3: a transcriptional modulator of the interferon-gamma gene. *European Journal of Immunology* 28, 3017–3030.

Colin, E.M., Asmawidjaja, P.S., van Hamburg, J.P., Mus, A.M., van, D.M., *et al.* (2010) 1,25-dihydroxyvitamin D3 modulates Th17 polarization and interleukin-22 expression by memory T cells from patients with early rheumatoid arthritis. *Arthritis and Rheumatism* 62, 132–142.

Colston, K., Colston, M.J. and Feldman, D. (1981) 1,25-dihydroxyvitamin D3 and malignant melanoma: the presence of receptors and inhibition of cell growth in culture. *Endocrinology* 108, 1083–1086.

Correale, J., Ysrraelit, M.C. and Gaitan, M.I. (2009) Immunomodulatory effects of Vitamin D in multiple sclerosis. *Brain* 132, 1146–1160.

D'Ambrosio, D., Cippitelli, M., Cocciolo, M.G., Mazzeo, D., Di Lucia, P., *et al.* (1998) Inhibition of IL-12 production by 1,25-dihydroxyvitamin D3. Involvement of NF-kappaB downregulation in transcriptional repression of the p40 gene. *The Journal of Clinical Investigation* 101, 252–262.

Dong, X., Craig, T., Xing, N., Bachman, L.A., Paya, C.V., *et al.* (2003) Direct transcriptional regulation of RelB by 1alpha,25-dihydroxyvitamin D3 and its analogs: physiologic and therapeutic implications for dendritic cell function. *Journal of Biological Chemistry* 278, 49378–49385.

Dusso, A.S., Brown, A.J. and Slatopolsky, E. (2005) Vitamin D. *American Journal of Physiology, Renal Physiology* 289, F8–F28.

Edfeldt, K., Liu, P.T., Chun, R., Fabri, M., Schenk, M., *et al.* (2010) T-cell cytokines differentially control human monocyte antimicrobial responses by regulating vitamin D metabolism. *Proceedings of the National Academy of Sciences of the United States of America* 107, 22593–22598.

Eisman, J.A., Martin, T.J., MacIntyre, I. and Moseley, J.M. (1979) 1,25-dihydroxyvitamin-D-receptor in breast cancer cells. *Lancet* 2, 1335–1336.

Farmer, P.K., He, X., Schmitz, M.L., Rubin, J. and Nanes, M.S. (2000) Inhibitory effect of NF-kappaB on 1,25-dihydroxyvitamin D(3) and retinoid X receptor function. *American Journal of Physiology, Endocrinology and Metabolism* 279, E213–E220.

Fritsche, J., Mondal, K., Ehrnsperger, A., Andreesen, R. and Kreutz, M. (2003) Regulation of 25-hydroxyvitamin D3-1 alpha-hydroxylase and production of 1 alpha,25-dihydroxyvitamin D3 by human dendritic cells. *Blood* 102, 3314–3316.

Froicu, M., Weaver, V., Wynn, T.A., McDowell, M.A., Welsh, J.E., *et al.* (2003) A crucial role for the vitamin D receptor in experimental inflammatory bowel diseases. *Molecular Endocrinology* 17, 2386–2392.

Gannage-Yared, M.H., Azoury, M., Mansour, I., Baddoura, R., Halaby, G., *et al.* (2003) Effects of a short-term calcium and vitamin D treatment on serum cytokines, bone markers, insulin and lipid concentrations in healthy post-menopausal women. *Journal of Endocrinological Investigations* 26, 748–753.

Geldmeyer-Hilt, K., Heine, G., Hartmann, B., Baumgrass, R., Radbruch, A., *et al.* (2011) 1,25-dihydroxyvitamin D(3) impairs NF-kappaB activation in human naive B cells. *Biochemical and Biophysical Research Communications* 407, 699–702.

Gottfried, E., Rehli, M., Hahn, J., Holler, E., Andreesen, R., *et al.* (2006) Monocyte-derived cells express CYP27A1 and convert vitamin D3 into its active metabolite. *Biochemical and Biophysical Research Communications* 349, 209–213.

Gynther, P., Toropainen, S., Matilainen, J.M., Seuter, S., Carlberg, C., *et al.* (2011) Mechanism of 1alpha,25-dihydroxyvitamin D(3)-dependent repression of interleukin-12B. *Biochimica et Biophysica Acta* 1813, 810–818.

Hansdottir, S., Monick, M.M., Lovan, N., Powers, L., Gerke, A., *et al.* (2010) Vitamin D decreases respiratory syncytial virus induction of NF-kappaB-linked chemokines and cytokines in airway epithelium while maintaining the antiviral state. *The Journal of Immunology* 184, 965–974.

Heine, G., Niesner, U., Chang, H.D., Steinmeyer, A., Zugel, U., *et al.* (2008) 1,25-dihydroxyvitamin D(3) promotes IL-10 production in human B cells. *European Journal of Immunology* 38, 2210–2218.

Hewison, M., Freeman, L., Hughes, S.V., Evans, K.N., Bland, R., *et al.* (2003) Differential regulation of vitamin D receptor and its ligand in human monocyte-derived dendritic cells. *The Journal of Immunology* 170, 5382–5390.

Holick, M.F. (2007) Vitamin D deficiency. *New England Journal of Medicine* 357, 266–281.

Iho, S., Kura, F., Sugiyama, H., Takahashi, T. and Hoshino, T. (1985) The role of monocytes in the suppression of PHA-induced proliferation and IL 2 production of human mononuclear cells by 1,25-dihydroxyvitamin D3. *Immunology Letters* 11, 331–336.

Inanir, A., Ozoran, K., Tutkak, H. and Mermerci, B. (2004) The effects of calcitriol therapy on serum interleukin-1, interleukin-6 and tumour necrosis factor-alpha concentrations in post-menopausal patients with osteoporosis. *The Journal of International Medical Research* 32, 570–582.

Jeffery, L.E., Burke, F., Mura, M., Zheng, Y., Qureshi, O.S., *et al.* (2009) 1,25-Dihydroxyvitamin D3 and IL-2 Combine to Inhibit T Cell Production of Inflammatory Cytokines and Promote Development of Regulatory T Cells Expressing CTLA-4 and FoxP3. *The Journal of Immunology* 183, 5458–5467.

Jiang, Z., Yin, X. and Jiang, Q. (2011) Natural forms of vitamin E and 13 -carboxychromanol, a long-chain vitamin E metabolite, inhibit leukotriene generation from stimulated neutrophils by blocking calcium influx and suppressing 5-lipoxygenase activity, respectively. *The Journal of Immunology* 186, 1173–1179.

Khoo, A.L., Chai, L.Y., Koenen, H.J., Kullberg, B.J., Joosten, I., *et al.* (2011a) 1,25-dihydroxyvitamin D3 modulates cytokine production induced by Candida albicans: impact of seasonal variation of immune responses. *The Journal of Infectious Diseases* 203, 122–130.

Khoo, A.L., Chai, L.Y., Koenen, H.J., Sweep, F.C., Joosten, I., *et al.* (2011b) Regulation of cytokine responses by seasonality of vitamin D status in healthy individuals. *Clinical and Experimental Immunology* 164, 72–79.

Koeffler, H.P., Reichel, H., Bishop, J.E. and Norman, A.W. (1985) gamma-Interferon stimulates production of 1,25-dihydroxyvitamin D3 by normal human macrophages. *Biochemical and Biophysical Research Communications* 127, 596–603.

Lappe, J.M. (2011) The role of vitamin D in human health: a paradigm shift. *Journal of Evidence-Based Complementary and Alternative Medicine* 16, 58–72.

Lemire, J.M., Adams, J.S., Kermani-Arab, V., Bakke, A.C., Sakai, R. *et al.* (1985) 1,25-Dihydroxyvitamin D3 suppresses human T helper/inducer lymphocyte activity in vitro. *The Journal of Immunology* 134, 3032–3035.

Lysandropoulos, A.P., Jaquiery, E., Jilek, S., Pantaleo, G., Schluep, M., *et al.* (2011) Vitamin D has a direct immunomodulatory effect on CD8+ T cells of patients with early multiple sclerosis and healthy control subjects. *Journal of Neuroimmunology* 233, 240–244.

Mahon, B.D., Gordon, S.A., Cruz, J., Cosman, F. and Cantorna, M.T. (2003a) Cytokine profile in patients with multiple sclerosis following vitamin D supplementation. *Journal of Neuroimmunology* 134, 128–132.

Mahon, B.D., Wittke, A., Weaver, V. and Cantorna, M.T. (2003b) The targets of vitamin D depend on the differentiation and activation status of CD4 positive T cells. *Journal of Cellular Biochemistry* 89, 922–932.

Manolagas, S.C., Haussler, M.R. and Deftos, L.J. (1980) 1,25-dihydroxyvitamin D3 receptors in cancer. *Lancet* 1, 828.

Martineau, A.R., Wilkinson, K.A., Newton, S.M., Floto, R.A., Norman, A.W., *et al.* (2007) IFN-gamma- and TNF-independent vitamin D-inducible human suppression of mycobacteria: the role of cathelicidin LL-37. *The Journal of Immunology* 178, 7190–7198.

Matilainen, J.M., Husso, T., Toropainen, S., Seuter, S., Turunen, M.P., *et al.* (2010a) Primary effect of 1alpha,25(OH)D on IL-10 expression in monocytes is short-term down-regulation. *Biochimica et Biophysica Acta* 1803, 1276–1286.

Matilainen, J.M., Rasanen, A., Gynther, P. and Vaisanen, S. (2010b) The genes encoding cytokines IL-2, IL-10 and IL-12B are primary 1alpha,25(OH)2D3 target genes. *Journal of Steroid Biochemistry and Molecular Biology* 121, 142–145.

McCollum, E.V., Simmonds, N. and Becker, J.E. (1922) Studies on experimental rickets. XXI. An experimental demonstration of the existence of a vitamin which promotes calcium deposition. *Journal of Biological Chemistry* 53, 293–312.

Muller, K., Diamant, M. and Bendtzen, K. (1991) Inhibition of production and function of interleukin-6 by 1,25-dihydroxyvitamin D3. *Immunology Letters* 28, 115–120.

Muller, K., Haahr, P.M., Diamant, M., Rieneck, K., Kharazmi, A. *et al.* (1992) 1,25-Dihydroxyvitamin D3 inhibits cytokine production by human blood monocytes at the post-transcriptional level. *Cytokine* 4, 506–512.

Nemere, I., Wilson, C., Jensen, W., Steinbeck, M., Rohe, B., *et al.* (2006) Mechanism of 24,25-dihydroxyvitamin D3-mediated inhibition of rapid, 1,25-dihydroxyvitamin D3-induced responses: role of reactive oxygen species. *Journal of Cellular Biochemistry* 99, 1572–1581.

Nonn, L., Peng, L., Feldman, D. and Peehl, D.M. (2006) Inhibition of p38 by vitamin D reduces interleukin-6 production in normal prostate cells via mitogen-activated protein kinase phosphatase 5: implications for prostate cancer prevention by vitamin D. *Cancer Research* 66, 4516–4524.

Papapoulos, S.E., Clemens, T.L., Fraher, L.J., Lewin, I.G., Sandler, L.M., *et al.* (1979) 1, 25-dihydroxycholecalciferol in the pathogenesis of the hypercalcaemia of sarcoidosis. *Lancet* 1, 627–630.

Peelen, E., Knippenberg, S., Muris, A.H., Thewissen, M., Smolders, J., *et al.* (2011) Effects of vitamin D on the peripheral adaptive immune system: A review. *Autoimmunity Reviews* 10, 733–743.

Penna, G. and Adorini, L. (2000) 1 Alpha,25-dihydroxyvitamin D3 inhibits differentiation, maturation, activation, and survival of dendritic cells leading to impaired alloreactive T cell activation. *Journal of Immunology* 164, 2405–2411.

Penna, G., Armuchastequi, S., Giarratana, N., Daniel, K.C., Vulcano, M., *et al.* (2007) 1 Alpha,25-dihydroxyvitamin D3 selectively modulates tolerogenic properties in myeloid but not plasmacytoid dendritic cells. *The Journal of Immunology* 178, 145–153.

Prabhu, A.S., Selvaraj, P. and Narayanan, P.R. (2009) Effect of 1,25 dihydroxyvitamin D3 on intracellular IFN-gamma and TNF-alpha positive T cell subsets in pulmonary tuberculosis. *Cytokine* 45, 105–110.

Provvedini, D.M. and Manolagas, S.C. (1989) 1 Alpha,25-dihydroxyvitamin D3 receptor distribution and effects in subpopulations of normal human T lymphocytes. *Journal of Clinical Endocrinology and Metabolism* 68, 774–779.

Provvedini, D.M., Tsoukas, C.D., Deftos, L.J. and Manolagas, S.C. (1983) 1,25-dihydroxyvitamin D3 receptors in human leukocytes. *Science* 221, 1181–1183.

Reichel, H., Koeffler, H.P., Barbers, R. and Norman, A.W. (1987a) Regulation of 1,25-dihydroxyvitamin D3 production by cultured alveolar macrophages from normal human donors and from patients with pulmonary sarcoidosis. *Journal of Clinical Endocrinology and Metabolism* 65, 1201–1209.

Reichel, H., Koeffler, H.P., Tobler, A. and Norman, A.W. (1987b) 1 alpha,25-Dihydroxyvitamin D3 inhibits gamma-interferon synthesis by normal human peripheral blood lymphocytes. *Proceedings of the National Academy of Sciences of the United States of America* 84, 3385–3389.

Rigby, W.F. and Waugh, M.G. (1992) Decreased accessory cell function and costimulatory activity by 1,25-dihydroxyvitamin D3-treated monocytes. *Arthritis and Rheumatism* 35, 110–119.

Rigby, W.F., Stacy, T. and Fanger, M.W. (1984) Inhibition of T lymphocyte mitogenesis by 1,25-dihydroxyvitamin D3 (calcitriol). *The Journal of Clinical Investigation* 74, 1451–1455.

Rigby, W.F., Denome, S. and Fanger, M.W. (1987) Regulation of lymphokine production and human T lymphocyte activation by 1,25-dihydroxyvitamin D3. Specific inhibition at the level of messenger RNA. *The Journal of Clinical Investigation* 79, 1659–1664.

Sadeghi, K., Wessner, B., Laggner, U., Ploder, M., Tamandl, D., *et al.* (2006) Vitamin D3 down-regulates monocyte TLR expression and triggers hyporesponsiveness to pathogen-associated molecular patterns. *European Journal of Immunology* 36, 361–370.

Schleithoff, S.S., Zittermann, A., Tenderich, G., Berthold, H.K., Stehle, P., *et al.* (2006) Vitamin D supplementation improves cytokine profiles in patients with congestive heart failure: a double-blind, randomized, placebo-controlled trial. *American Journal of Clinical Nutrition* 83, 754–759.

Sigmundsdottir, H., Pan, J., Debes, G.F., Alt, C., Habtezion, A., *et al.* (2007) DCs metabolize sunlight-induced vitamin D3 to 'program' T cell attraction to the epidermal chemokine CCL27. *Nature Immunology* 8, 285–293.

Smolders, J., Peelen, E., Thewissen, M., Cohen Tervaert, J.W., Menheere, P., *et al.* (2010) Safety and T cell modulating effects of high dose vitamin D3 supplementation in multiple sclerosis. *PLoS.One.* 5, e15235.

Staeva-Vieira, T.P. and Freedman, L.P. (2002) 1,25-dihydroxyvitamin D3 inhibits IFN-gamma and IL-4 levels during in vitro polarization of primary murine CD4+ T cells. *The Journal of Immunology* 168, 1181–1189.

Stoffels, K., Overbergh, L., Giulietti, A., Verlinden, L., Bouillon, R., *et al.* (2006) Immune regulation of 25-hydroxyvitamin-D3-1alpha-hydroxylase in human monocytes. *Journal of Bone and Mineral Research* 21, 37–47.

Stoffels, K., Overbergh, L., Bouillon, R. and Mathieu, C. (2007) Immune regulation of 1alpha-hydroxylase in murine peritoneal macrophages: unravelling the IFNgamma pathway. *Journal of Steroid Biochemistry and Molecular Biology* 103, 567–571.

Stubbs, J.R., Idiculla, A., Slusser, J., Menard, R. and Quarles, L.D. (2010) Cholecalciferol supplementation alters calcitriol-responsive monocyte proteins and decreases inflammatory cytokines in ESRD. *Journal of the American Society of Nephrology* 21, 353–361.

Szeles, L., Keresztes, G., Torocsik, D., Balajthy, Z., Krenacs, L., *et al.* (2009) 1,25-dihydroxyvitamin D3 is an autonomous regulator of the transcriptional changes leading to a tolerogenic dendritic cell phenotype. *The Journal of Immunology* 182, 2074–2083.

Takeuchi, A., Reddy, G.S., Kobayashi, T., Okano, T., Park, J., *et al.* (1998) Nuclear factor of activated T cells (NFAT) as a molecular target for 1alpha,25-dihydroxyvitamin D3-mediated effects. *The Journal of Immunology* 160, 209–218.

Tangpricha, V., Pearce, E.N., Chen, T.C. and Holick, M.F. (2002) Vitamin D insufficiency among free-living healthy young adults. *The American Journal of Medicine* 112, 659–662.

Thien, R., Baier, K., Pietschmann, P., Peterlik, M. and Willheim, M. (2005) Interactions of 1 alpha,25-dihydroxyvitamin D3 with IL-12 and IL-4 on cytokine expression of human T lymphocytes. *The Journal of Allergy and Clinical Immunology* 116, 683–689.

Tsoukas, C.D., Watry, D., Escobar, S.S., Provvedini, D.M., Dinarello, C.A., *et al.* (1989) Inhibition of interleukin-1 production by 1,25-dihydroxyvitamin D3. *Journal of Clinical Endocrinology and Metabolism* 69, 127–133.

Urry, Z., Xystrakis, E., Richards, D.F., McDonald, J., Sattar, Z., *et al.* (2009) Ligation of TLR9 induced on human IL-10-secreting Tregs by 1alpha,25-dihydroxyvitamin D3 abrogates regulatory function. *The Journal of Clinical Investigation* 119, 387–398.

Veldman, C.M., Cantorna, M.T. and DeLuca, H.F. (2000) Expression of 1,25-dihydroxyvitamin D(3) receptor in the immune system. *Archives of Biochemistry and Biophysics* 374, 334–338.

Wagner, D., Hanwell, H.E., Schnabl, K., Yazdanpanah, M., Kimball, S., *et al.* (2011) The ratio of serum 24,25-dihydroxyvitamin D(3) to 25-hydroxyvitamin D(3) is predictive of 25-hydroxyvitamin D(3) response to vitamin D(3) supplementation. *Journal of Steroid Biochemistry and Molecular Biology* 126, 72–77.

Willheim, M., Thien, R., Schrattbauer, K., Bajna, E., Holub, M., *et al.* (1999) Regulatory effects of 1alpha,25-dihydroxyvitamin D3 on the cytokine production of human peripheral blood lymphocytes. *Journal of Clinical Endocrinology and Metabolism* 84, 3739–3744.

Wortsman, J., Matsuoka, L.Y., Chen, T.C., Lu, Z. and Holick, M.F. (2000) Decreased bioavailability of vitamin D in obesity. *American Journal of Clinical Nutrition* 72, 690–693.

Yu, X.P., Bellido, T. and Manolagas, S.C. (1995) Down-regulation of NF-kappa B protein levels in activated human lymphocytes by 1,25-dihydroxyvitamin D3. *Proceedings of the National Academy of Sciences of the United States of America* 92, 10990–10994.

Yusupov, E., Li-Ng, M., Pollack, S., Yeh, J.K., Mikhail, M., *et al.* (2010) Vitamin D and serum cytokines in a randomized clinical trial. *International Journal of Endocrinology* 2010.

Zhang, Y., Leung, D.Y.M., Richers, B.N., Liu, Y., Remigio, L.K., *et al.* (2012) Vitamin D inhibits monocyte/macrophage proinflammatory cytokine production by targeting MAPK phosphatase-1. *The Journal of Immunology* 188, 2127–2135.

Zittermann, A., Dembinski, J. and Stehle, P. (2004) Low vitamin D status is associated with low cord blood levels of the immunosuppressive cytokine interleukin-10. *Pediatric Allergy and Immunology* 15, 242–246.

Zittermann, A., Frisch, S., Berthold, H.K., Gotting, C., Kuhn, J., *et al.* (2009) Vitamin D supplementation enhances the beneficial effects of weight loss on cardiovascular disease risk markers. *American Journal of Clinical Nutrition* 89, 1321–1327.

6 Vitamin E and Inflammation

T. Barker*
The Orthopedic Specialty Hospital, Murray, Utah, USA

Introduction

Vitamin E is a fat-soluble vitamin discovered in 1922 (Evans and Bishop, 1922). Since its discovery, it has become apparent that vitamin E possesses a variety of biological functions, including the modulation of inflammatory cytokines. The regulatory influence of vitamin E on cytokine production is the focus of this chapter. This chapter begins with an overview of vitamin E and then evidence identifying the regulatory influence of different forms of vitamin E on inflammatory cytokines, as well as the physiological mechanisms that they govern in cytokine production, is presented.

The chain-breaking antioxidant property of vitamin E prevents the propagation of free radicals in membranes and plasma lipoproteins (Traber and Atkinson, 2007). Vitamin E exists in eight different natural forms: four tocopherols (α-, β-, γ- and δ-) and four tocotrienols (α-, β-, γ- and δ-) (Fig. 6.1). Of the different vitamin E forms, α-tocopherol is the most common form in supplements and European diets, whereas γ-tocopherol is the predominant form found in the American diet (McLaughlin and Weihrauch, 1979; Lehmann *et al.*, 1986). The structural difference between the two tocopherols is that α-tocopherol is fully substituted in the chromanol ring and γ-tocopherol is unsubstituted at the C-5 position (Fig. 6.1). The chiral centers are in the 'R' configuration at the 2, 4′ and 8′ (i.e. RRR or d) positions in the naturally occurring tocopherol form. Synthetic tocopherols (called all-rac-α-tocopherol, all racemic or dl) exist in other stereoisomer forms (i.e. RSR, RRS, RSS, SRR, SSS, SRS and SSR). Tocotrienols have substituted chromanol rings and, in contrast to tocopherols, unsaturated side chains.

All forms of vitamin E are absorbed in the intestine and released into the circulation in chylomicrons. Lipoprotein lipases hydrolyse

* Author, tyler.barker@imail.org

 Nutrition and Physical Activity in Inflammatory Diseases (eds M.L. Garg and L.G. Wood)

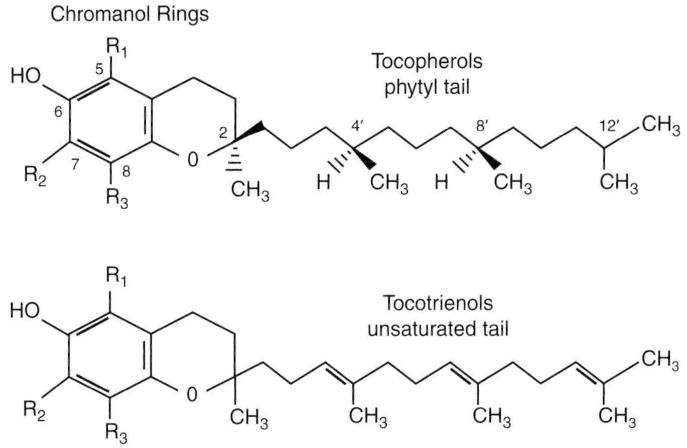

Isoforms	R_1	R_2	R_3
α	CH_3	CH_3	CH_3
β	CH_3	H	CH_3
γ	H	CH_3	CH_3
δ	H	H	CH_3

Fig. 6.1. The chemical structures of different vitamin E forms: tocopherols and tocotrienols. Tocopherols (above) have substituted chromanol rings and phytyl (saturated) side chains with three chiral centers. Tocotrienols (below) have substituted chromanol rings and unsaturated side chains. α-, β-, γ, and δ-tocopherols and tocotrienols differ in the number of methyl groups on the chromanol rings at C-5 and C-7 (isoform insert for R_1, R_2 and R_3). Regarding the side chains, the chiral centers are in the 'R' configuration at the 2, 4′ and 8′ (i.e. RRR) positions in the naturally occurring tocopherol forms (as shown above). Synthetic tocopherols exist in other stereoisomer forms (i.e. RSR, RRS, SRR, SRS and SSR; forms not shown). Figure modified from Barker and Traber (2011).

chylomicron triglycerides, resulting in fatty acid and vitamin E transfer to tissue. In the plasma and during the formation of chylomicron remnants, some of the vitamin E is transferred to high-density lipoproteins and other lipoproteins. Chylomicron remnants shuttle vitamin E to the liver (Traber, 2007). In the liver, the α-tocopherol transfer protein preferentially targets and secretes RRR-α-tocopherol into the circulation in very-low-density lipoproteins (Traber and Kayden, 1989; Traber *et al.*, 1990a; 1990b; 1992). The other forms of vitamin E are not as well recognized and are excreted in the bile (Traber, 2007). In the circulation and during lipoprotein catabolism, α-tocopherol is distributed among the various lipoproteins. Lipoproteins can be taken up by tissues and the liver, thus delivering tocopherols to peripheral tissues (Traber, 2007).

Supplemental vitamin E in different forms can differentially modulate circulating α- and γ-tocopherol concentrations. Supplemental vitamin E in the α-tocopherol form increases α-tocopherol and decreases γ-tocopherol concentrations in the circulation (Handelman *et al.*, 1985). Following equimolar supplemental doses of α- and γ-tocopherols, γ-tocopherol disappears faster (i.e. has a shorter half-life), resulting in less circulating γ-tocopherol than α-tocopherol (Leonard *et al.*, 2005). Additionally, γ-tocopherol administration increases circulating γ-tocopherol and decreases α-tocopherol concentrations (Yoshikawa *et al.*, 2005; Devaraj *et al.*, 2008). As mentioned above, the α-tocopherol transfer protein preferentially targets and secretes vitamin E in the α-tocopherol form. The discriminatory regulation by the hepatic α-tocopherol transfer protein is responsible for the contrasting circulating vitamin E metabolite responses to different forms of vitamin E intake or supplementation. The α-tocopherol transfer protein is not a likely candidate, however, for the disparate influence of contrasting vitamin E forms in cytokine regulation, which is discussed below.

Supplemental Vitamin E and Inflammatory Cytokines

The influence of supplemental vitamin E combined with other micronutrients on inflammatory cytokines has been commonly studied (Malmberg *et al.*, 2002; Vassilakopoulos *et al.*, 2002, 2003), especially in combination with vitamin C (ascorbic acid) (Petersen *et al.*, 2001; Fischer *et al.*, 2004; Mastaloudis *et al.*, 2004; Barker *et al.*, 2009a,b, 2011). There are a variety of reasons for incorporating vitamins E and C into a single supplement regimen, but one rationale is that ascorbic acid regenerates α-tocopherol (Halpner *et al.*, 1998; Bruno *et al.*, 2006) and therefore maintains vitamin E activity. Conversely, vitamin E protects against vitamin C loss during inflammatory challenge (Jiang *et al.*, 2002). Thus, the interaction between vitamins E and C is important in maintaining endogenous tocopherol and ascorbic acid concentrations during inflammatory conditions that challenge micronutrient status.

Consistent with its antioxidant property, supplemental vitamin E ameliorates inflammatory cell-derived superoxide anion release (Devaraj *et al.*, 1996; Devaraj and Jialal, 2000b). The reduction in superoxide anion release from monocytes by vitamin E has been shown to be mediated by the inhibition of protein kinase C (PKC) (Devaraj *et al.*, 1996). Regarding the cytokine-modulating property, vitamin E modulates diverse inflammatory cytokines disparately (Table 6.1). In general, vitamin E decreases interleukin (IL)-1β, tumour necrosis factor (TNF)-α, interferon (IFN)-γ, IL-8 and IL-6 and increases IL-2 and IL-4, but results are inconsistent (Table 6.1). The different mechanisms or sources of cytokine production regulated by vitamin E are discussed here.

Regulation of inflammatory cytokines by vitamin E

α-Tocopherol

Interleukin-1β is a pro-inflammatory cytokine secreted by a variety of cells, including monocytes. PKC inhibition, antioxidant enzymes (superoxide dismutase and catalase), β-tocopherol, and a cyclooxygenase (COX) inhibitor were ineffective at decreasing the release of IL-1β from activated monocytes (Devaraj and Jialal, 1999). However, α-tocopherol inhibited IL-1β release from lipopolysaccharide (LPS)-activated monocytes without affecting IL-1β mRNA (Devaraj and Jialal, 1999). Additionally, α-tocopherol decreased a major product of the 5-lipoxygenase pathway, leukotriene B_4 (LTB_4). Adding LTB_4 to α-tocopherol treated and activated monocytes reversed the inhibition of IL-1β release (Devaraj and Jialal, 1999). On the basis of the available data, it seems that α-tocopherol inhibits IL-1β release from activated monocytes without influencing IL-1β mRNA (Devaraj and Jialal, 1999), suggesting that vitamin E regulates IL-1β post-transcriptionally and possibly by inhibiting the 5-lipoxygenase pathway.

Another pro-inflammatory cytokine, TNF-α, is modulated by α-tocopherol. In smokers, but not healthy controls or diabetics, supplemental vitamin E (Table 6.1) inhibited LPS-stimulated TNF-α production in whole blood (Mol *et al.*, 1997). Following incubation with α-tocopherol, TNF-α release was inhibited and LTB_4 levels decreased (Devaraj and Jialal, 2005). The inhibition of TNF-α release was independent from PKC, the COX pathway and other antioxidants, but was reversed by LTB_4 (Devaraj and Jialal, 2005). Similar to α-tocopherol, 5-lipoxygenase inhibitors blunted TNF-α release (Devaraj and Jialal, 2005). At the mRNA level, α-tocopherol and 5-lipoxygenase inhibitors decreased TNF-α mRNA synthesis in stimulated monocytes and reduced nuclear factor (NF)κB binding activity (Devaraj and Jialal, 2005). These results indicate that α-tocopherol impairs TNF-α release from activated monocytes by inhibiting the 5-lipoxygenase pathway and reduces TNF-α synthesis by impairing NFκB binding activity. However, results were population or condition specific because patients with diverse pathophysiological or physiological conditions displayed contrasting TNF-α outcomes to vitamin E.

α-Tocopherol decreases IL-6 concentrations, an inflammatory cytokine that possess pro- and anti-inflammatory properties (Pedersen *et al.*, 2007). In patients with type 2 diabetes, plasma IL-6 concentrations were increased using α-tocopherol (Devaraj and

Table 6.1. Human supplemental vitamin E studies and inflammatory cytokine results.

Vitamin E form	Dose/duration	Population	Cytokine results	Reference
dl-α-tocopheryl acetate	800 mg/day for 30 days	Elderly	↑ PBMC IL-2 production	Meydani *et al.* (1990)
dl-α-tocopherol	400 IU/day for 48 days	Eccentric exercise in sedentary men	↓ IL-1β but no change in IL-6 or TNF-α plasma concentrations ↓ Mononuclear cell IL-6 and IL-1β production but no change TNF-α	Cannon *et al.* (1991)
d-α-tocopherol	1200 IU/day for 8 weeks	Healthy males and females	↓ IL-1β secretion from monocytes	Devaraj and Jialal (1996)
dl-α-tocopherol acetate	600 IU/day for 4 weeks	Diabetics Smokers and healthy controls	No change in whole blood TNF-α or IL-1β production ↓ Whole blood IL-1β production	Mol *et al.* (1997)
dl-α-tocopheryl acetate	50 and 100 mg/day for 24 weeks	Elderly	No change in PBMC IL-2 production but ↓ PBMC IFN-γ and ↑ IL-4 production	Pallast *et al.* (1999)
RRR-α-tocopherol	600 IU/day for 6 weeks	Normolipdemic and hypertriglyceridemic	↓ PBMC TNF-α, IL-1β and IL-8 production but no change in IL-10	van Tits *et al.* (2000)
RRR-α-tocopherol	1200 IU/day for 12 weeks	Type 2 diabetics with macro-vascular disease Type 2 diabetics without macro-vascular disease Controls	↓ Monocyte IL-1β, TNF-α and IL-6 production in all three groups	Devaraj and Jialal (2000b) Devaraj and Jialal (2000a)
RRR-α-tocopherol	400 IU/day for 60 days	End-stage renal disease patients	No change in plasma TNF-α or IL-6 concentrations	Smith *et al.* (2003)
RRR-α-tocopherol	1200 IU/day for 8 weeks	Healthy volunteers	↓ TNF-α release from activated monocytes	Devaraj and Jialal (2005)
RRR-α-tocopherol	500 mg/day for 6 weeks	Type 2 diabetics	No influence on plasma TNF-α or IL-6 concentrations	Wu *et al.* (2007)
RRR-α-tocopherol	1200 IU/day for 2 years	Coronary artery disease	↓ TNF-α release from activated monocytes	Devaraj *et al.* (2007)
RRR-α-tocopherol	800 mg/day for 6 weeks	Metabolic syndrome	↓ TNF-α whole blood production but no change in IL-1β or IL-6	Devaraj *et al.* (2008)
γ-tocopherol	800 mg/day for 6 weeks	Metabolic syndrome	No influence on whole blood TNF-α, IL-1β or IL-6 production	Devaraj *et al.* (2008)

Vitamin E nomenclature is the identified form provided in the respective publication. PBMC, peripheral blood mononuclear cells.

Jialal, 2000a). Monocytes release IL-6 under hyperglycemic conditions, which seems to be mediated through the upregulation of PKC-α and PKC-β (Jeschke *et al.*, 2002). In addition to PKC-α and PKC-β, IL-6 is regulated by p38 mitogen-activated protein kinase (MAPK) and NFκB; both of which impair IL-6 release upon inhibition (Devaraj *et al.*, 2005). Likewise, inhibiting COX-2 activation and prostaglandin E_2 (PGE_2) formation ameliorates IL-6 production (Williams and Shacter, 1997). In summary, IL-6 is regulated by PKC, p38MAPK, NFκB, COX-2 and/or PGE_2, all of which are modulated by α-tocopherol (Boscoboinik *et al.*, 1991; Tasinato *et al.*, 1995; Wu *et al.*, 1998; Venugopal *et al.*, 2002; Egger *et al.*, 2003; Devaraj and Jialal, 2005; Devaraj *et al.*, 2005).

Immune system dysfunction is a consequence of ageing, and IL-2 is routinely measured to identify immune system dysfunction in the elderly (Nagel *et al.*, 1988; Rink *et al.*, 1998). IL-2 augments T-lymphocyte proliferation in response to antigenic stimulation, including the generation of cytotoxic and suppressor T cells (Waldmann, 1989; Nakarai *et al.*, 1994). Thus, impaired IL-2 production or secretion hinders specific immune responses. Previous studies have investigated the influence of supplemental vitamin E on IL-2 in the elderly (Meydani *et al.*, 1990; Pallast *et al.*, 1999). It has been shown that, in the elderly, vitamin E supplementation increases α-tocopherol concentrations in the plasma and in peripheral blood mononuclear cells (Table 6.1; Meydani *et al.*, 1990). The increase in vitamin E occurred concomitantly with IL-2 increases and PGE_2 decreases (Meydani *et al.*, 1990). Likewise, in experimental rats, vitamin E supplementation decreased macrophage COX activity and PGE_2 production (Wu *et al.*, 1998). These are interesting results because increased COX-2 expression induces PGE_2 production (Hayek *et al.*, 1997) and could contribute to the age-associated IL-2 decrease (Walker *et al.*, 1983; Beharka *et al.*, 1997). Moreover, inhibiting COX-2 expression and PGE_2 production increases IL-2, thereby identifying a potential mechanism or source of IL-2 regulation by vitamin E. An alternative explanation of IL-2 regulation could relate to the antioxidant property of vitamin E. Specifically, lipid hydroperoxides and reactive nitrogen species regulate COX activation (Hemler and Lands, 1980; Fujimoto *et al.*, 2004). It is feasible that the peroxyl radical and reactive nitrogen scavenging properties of vitamin E (α- and γ-tocopherol forms) attenuate COX activity and increase IL-2. None the less, these results indicate that vitamin E regulates IL-2 production by modulating eicosanoid synthesis and, in theory, by scavenging reactive oxygen and nitrogen species.

On the basis of the inconsistency and variability of available data (Meydani *et al.*, 1990; Pallast *et al.*, 1999; Wu *et al.*, 2007), it is postulated that the cytokine-modulating property of vitamin E could be genetically determined. To investigate this question, Belisle *et al.* (2009) examined the interaction between vitamin E and a single nucleotide polymorphism on TNF-α production in the elderly. In elderly nursing home subjects treated with vitamin E, TNF-α production was lower in those with the A/A and A/G genotype at TNF-α -308G→A than those with the A allele treated with the placebo (Belisle *et al.*, 2009). The original results provided by Belisle *et al.* (2009) identify that the influence of supplemental vitamin E on TNF-α production is genetically determined and provide a possible explanation on why previous studies found a null effect of vitamin E on TNF-α. In a subsequent study, Belisle *et al.* (2010) investigated the influence of cytokine gene polymorphisms on respiratory tract infection and response to vitamin E in nursing home patients. In women who received supplemental vitamin E, the G/G genotype at IL-10 -819G→A was associated with a decreased incidence of lower respiratory tract infections, whereas the A/A genotype at IL-10-819G→A displayed more lower respiratory tract inflections than those who received a placebo treatment (Belisle *et al.*, 2010). These results not only suggest that the development of respiratory tract infections in nursing home patients is influenced by supplemental vitamin E, but again establish that a single nucleotide polymorphism is influential on the response to supplemental vitamin E outcomes.

γ-Tocopherol

γ-Tocopherol is another form of vitamin E that possesses antioxidant and anti-inflammatory properties. γ-Tocopherol traps reactive nitrogen species (Christen *et al.*, 1997), inhibits protein nitration and spares ascorbic acid oxidation in experimental rats during inflammatory challenge (Jiang *et al.*, 2002). Furthermore, γ-tocopherol inhibits PGE_2 production, nitrite accumulation and inducible nitric oxide synthase expression in macrophage cells challenged with LPS (Jiang *et al.*, 2000). Although evidence identifying the anti-inflammatory property of γ-tocopherol is increasing in experimental animals (Christen *et al.*, 1997; Saldeen *et al.*, 1999; Jiang *et al.*, 2000, 2001; Himmelfarb *et al.*, 2003; Jiang and Ames, 2003; Wagner *et al.*, 2007), evidence in humans is sparse (Table 6.1).

In metabolic syndrome patients, Devaraj *et al.* (2008) examined the influence of supplemental α- and γ-tocopherols alone and in combination on circulating cytokine concentrations. α-Tocopherol and combined α- and γ-tocopherol supplementation decreased plasma TNF-α concentrations, whereas γ-tocopherol supplementation alone was not influential on TNF-α (Devaraj *et al.*, 2008). Neither α- or γ-tocopherol alone or in combination modulated circulating IL-6 or IL-1β concentrations (Devaraj *et al.*, 2008). Furthermore, supplemental vitamin E enriched with γ-tocopherol increased circulating γ-tocopherol concentrations and inhibited IL-1β, TNF-α and IL-6 secretion by peripheral blood mononuclear cells *ex vivo* (Wiser *et al.*, 2008). These results imply that γ-tocopherol mixed with other tocopherols modulates inflammatory cytokine concentrations and production in metabolic syndrome and asthmatic patients.

In a model that mimics the pathology of joint disease, such as arthritis, Jiang and Ames (2003) found that γ-tocopherol inhibited the localized formation in PGE_2 and LTB_4 in experimental rats. The inhibition of PGE_2 and LTB_4 occurred concurrently with a decrease in TNF-α (Jiang and Ames, 2003). Considering the influence of PGE_2 and LTB_4 on TNF-α production, as well as other cytokines (e.g. IL-1β), it is likely that γ-tocopherol modulates cytokine production by altering eicosanoid biosynthesis and the production or accumulation of eicosanoid biosynthesis by-products (Christen *et al.*, 1997; Jiang *et al.*, 2000, 2011).

In addition to the evidence provided by Jiang and Ames (2003), several other mechanisms could be responsible for the ability of γ-tocopherol to modulate inflammatory cytokines. First, as demonstrated in peripheral blood mononuclear cells obtained from allergic asthmatic patients, γ-tocopherol modestly inhibited LPS-induced IκBα degradation and jun terminal kinase (JNK) phosphorylation (Wiser *et al.*, 2008). Second, γ-tocopherol impaired ionophore-triggered extracellular-signal regulated kinases (ERK) 1/2 phosphorylation (Jiang *et al.*, 2011). Finally, γ-tocopherol could impair cytokine production by trapping reactive nitrogen species. Overall, γ-tocopherol impairs cytokine production by: (i) perturbing IκBα degradation and inhibiting NFκB activation; (ii) abrogating JNK activation; (iii) inhibiting 5-lipoxygenase and COX-2 activation; (iv) impairing ERK phosphorylation; and (v) scavenging reactive nitrogen species.

Additional cell-signalling mechanisms regulated by vitamin E

There are additional cell-signalling pathways regulated by vitamin E that alter cytokine expression that require mentioning. As identified above, vitamin E regulates NFκB activation (Fox *et al.*, 1997). NFκB is a redox sensitive transcription factor and is a major mediator in the upregulation of inflammatory cytokines. Peroxisome proliferator-activated receptors (PPAR) are a family of transcription factors that interfere with the inflammatory signalling cascade mediated by NFκB and are upregulated by α- and γ-tocopherols (Reiter *et al.*, 2007). Vitamin E can also interfere with NFκB activation by inhibiting Akt phosphorylation, possibly by altering phosphatidylinositol 3-kinase (PI3K) activity (Kempna *et al.*, 2004). The phosphatase type 2A increase mediated by vitamin E also decreases ERK 1/2 and p38 MAPK phosphorylation and NFκB binding (Egger *et al.*, 2003). Considering the sensitivity of NFκB to reactive oxygen and nitrogen species, it is also likely that antioxidant properties of vitamin E alter NFκB activity and modulate cytokine expression.

In addition, α-tocopherol inhibits PKCα activity (Boscoboinik *et al.*, 1991; Tasinato *et al.*, 1995; Cachia *et al.*, 1998; Venugopal *et al.*, 2002). The inhibition in PKC activity is mediated by an increase in protein phosphatase type 2A activity induced by α-tocopherol (Ricciarelli *et al.*, 1998). Although PKC inhibition blocks IL-1β production in LPS-stimulated monocytes and macrophages (Grisanti *et al.*, 2011), results are inconsistent regarding the inhibition of PKC activity regulated by vitamin E (Devaraj and Jialal, 1999).

Vitamin E also alters the inflammatory signalling cascade between reciprocally regulated cytokines. For example, IL-6 is transcriptionally regulated by NFκB (among others, e.g. serum-responsive element and activating protein-1; Dendorfer *et al.*, 1994; Sanceau *et al.*, 1995), and TNF-α induces IL-6 (Van Damme *et al.*, 1987). Provocatively, vitamin E or its derivate impairs TNF-α-induced activation of NFκB (Suzuki and Packer, 1993a,b), implying that vitamin E indirectly impairs the induction of one cytokine by altering the signalling and transcriptional events induced by another cytokine.

Summary and Conclusions

In summary, vitamin E regulates inflammatory cytokine production by altering eicosanoid synthesis, cell-signalling pathways, transcription-factor activation, and the scavenging of reactive oxygen and nitrogen species. It is noteworthy that different vitamin E forms induce different signalling pathways that modulate the production of disparate cytokines. Emerging evidence indicates that the cytokine-modulating capacity of vitamin E could be dependent on a single nucleotide polymorphism. Additionally, vitamin E modifies the association between reciprocally regulated cytokines, suggesting that vitamin E impairs the induction of one cytokine by altering the events mediated by another cytokine (Fig. 6.2).

In conclusion, vitamin E is a fat-soluble vitamin that governs cytokine modulations at the transcriptional and translational levels. Importantly, this regulation is immune cell and

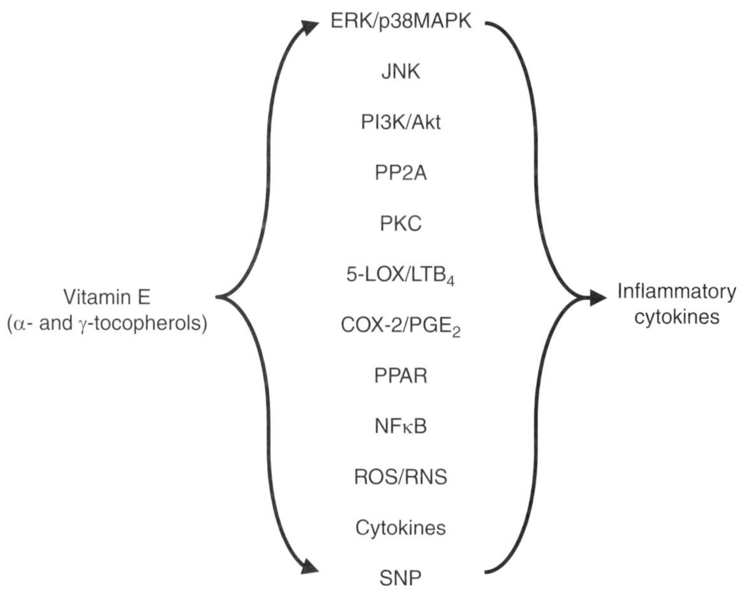

Fig. 6.2. Targets of cytokine regulation by vitamin E. Vitamin E (α- and γ-tocopherols) regulates inflammatory cytokine production by altering cell signalling pathways (ERK/p38MAPK, PI3K, PKC, PP2A), transcriptional-factor activation (PPAR, NFκB), eicosanoid biosynthesis (5-LOX/LTB_4, COX-2/PGE_2), and the scavenging of reactive oxygen (ROS) and nitrogen species (RNS). Additionally, vitamin E modifies the association between reciprocally regulated cytokines, suggesting that vitamin E could impair the induction of one cytokine by altering the preceding signalling events mediated by another cytokine. Emerging evidence also indicates that the cytokine-modulating capacity of vitamin E is dependent on single nucleotide polymorphism (SNP).

cytokine specific. Furthermore, the ability of vitamin E to mediate deviations in inflammatory cytokine production is apparently condition specific, as patients with different pathophysiological or physiological characteristics display disparate responses to supplemental interventions. Finally, an exciting and emerging research field identifies that the influence of vitamin E on cytokine regulation is genetically determined.

Acknowledgements

The author would like to recognize the research efforts of those who have contributed to this field of study. The author thanks Vanessa T. Henriksen for critically reviewing this chapter. The author would also like to thank Dr Maret G. Traber (Oregon State University and the Linus Pauling Institute) for her mentoring and support. Work on this chapter was supported by The Deseret Foundation (Intermountain Healthcare, Salt Lake City, Utah), USANA Health Sciences, Inc. (Salt Lake City, Utah), The Orthopedic Specialty Hospital (TOSH, Murray, Utah) and Intermountain Healthcare. Special thanks to TOSH and Intermountain Healthcare for their continued support.

References

Barker, T. and Traber, M.G. (2011) Does vitamin E and C supplementation improve the recovery from anterior cruciate ligament surgery. *Journal of Evidence-Based Complementary and Alternative Medicine* 16, 114–128.

Barker, T., Leonard, S.W., Hansen, J., Trawick, R.H., Ingram, R., *et al.* (2009a) Vitamin E and C supplementation does not ameliorate muscle dysfunction following anterior cruciate ligament surgery. *Free Radical Biology and Medicine* 47, 1611–1618.

Barker, T., Leonard, S.W., Trawick, R.H., Martins, T.B., Kjeldsberg, C.R., *et al.* (2009b) Modulation of inflammation by vitamin E and C supplementation prior to anterior cruciate ligament surgery. *Free Radical Biology and Medicine* 46, 599–606.

Barker, T., Martins, T.B., Hill, H.R., Kjeldsberg, C.R., Trawick, R.H., *et al.* (2011) Vitamins E and C modulate the association between reciprocally regulated cytokines after an anterior cruciate ligament injury and surgery. *American Journal of Physical Medicine and Rehabilitation* 90, 638–647.

Beharka, A.A., Wu, D., Han, S.N. and Meydani, S.N. (1997) Macrophage prostaglandin production contributes to the age-associated decrease in T cell function which is reversed by the dietary antioxidant vitamin E. *Mechanisms of Ageing and Development* 93, 59–77.

Belisle, S.E., Leka, L.S., Delgado-Lista, J., Jacques, P.F., Ordovas, J.M., *et al.* (2009) Polymorphisms at cytokine genes may determine the effect of vitamin E on cytokine production in the elderly. *The Journal of Nutrition* 139, 1855–1860.

Belisle, S.E., Hamer, D.H., Leka, L.S., Dallal, G.E., Delgado-Lista, J., *et al.* (2010) IL-2 and IL-10 gene polymorphisms are associated with respiratory tract infection and may modulate the effect of vitamin E on lower respiratory tract infections in elderly nursing home residents. *American Journal of Clinical Nutrition* 92, 106–114.

Boscoboinik, D., Szewczyk, A., Hensey, C. and Azzi, A. (1991) Inhibition of cell proliferation by alpha-tocopherol. Role of protein kinase C. *Journal of Biological Chemistry* 266, 6188–6194.

Bruno, R.S., Leonard, S.W., Atkinson, J., Montine, T.J., Ramakrishnan, R., *et al.* (2006) Faster plasma vitamin E disappearance in smokers is normalized by vitamin C supplementation. *Free Radical Biology and Medicine* 40, 689–697.

Cachia, O., Benna, J.E., Pedruzzi, E., Descomps, B., Gougerot-Pocidalo, M.A., *et al.* (1998) alpha-tocopherol inhibits the respiratory burst in human monocytes. Attenuation of p47(phox) membrane translocation and phosphorylation. *Journal of Biological Chemistry* 273, 32801–32805.

Cannon, J.G., Meydani, S.N., Fielding, R.A., Fiatarone, M.A., Meydani, M., *et al.* (1991). Acute phase response in exercise. II. Associations between vitamin E, cytokines, and muscle proteolysis. *American Journal of Physiology* 260, R1235–R1240.

Christen, S., Woodall, A.A., Shigenaga, M.K., Southwell-Keely, P.T., Duncan, M.W., *et al.* (1997) gamma-tocopherol traps mutagenic electrophiles such as NO(X) and complements alpha-tocopherol:

physiological implications. *Proceedings of the National Academy of Sciences of the United States of America* 94, 3217–3222.
Dendorfer, U., Oettgen, P. and Libermann, T.A. (1994) Multiple regulatory elements in the interleukin-6 gene mediate induction by prostaglandins, cyclic AMP, and lipopolysaccharide. *Molecular and Cellular Biology* 14, 4443–4454.
Devaraj, S. and Jialal, I. (1999) Alpha-tocopherol decreases interleukin-1 beta release from activated human monocytes by inhibition of 5-lipoxygenase. *Arteriosclerosis, Thrombosis, and Vascular Biology* 19, 1125–1133.
Devaraj, S. and Jialal, I. (2000a) Alpha tocopherol supplementation decreases serum C-reactive protein and monocyte interleukin-6 levels in normal volunteers and type 2 diabetic patients. *Free Radical Biology and Medicine* 29, 790–792.
Devaraj, S. and Jialal, I. (2000b) Low-density lipoprotein postsecretory modification, monocyte function, and circulating adhesion molecules in type 2 diabetic patients with and without macrovascular complications: the effect of {alpha}-tocopherol supplementation. *Circulation* 102, 191–196.
Devaraj, S. and Jialal, I. (2005) Alpha-tocopherol decreases tumor necrosis factor-alpha mRNA and protein from activated human monocytes by inhibition of 5-lipoxygenase. *Free Radical Biology and Medicine* 38, 1212–1220.
Devaraj, S., Li, D. and Jialal, I. (1996) The effects of alpha tocopherol supplementation on monocyte function. Decreased lipid oxidation, interleukin 1beta secretion, and monocyte adhesion to endothelium. *The Journal of Clinical Investigation* 98, 756–763.
Devaraj, S., Venugopal, S.K., Singh, U. and Jialal, I. (2005) Hyperglycemia induces monocytic release of interleukin-6 via induction of protein kinase c-{alpha} and -{beta}. *Diabetes* 54, 85–91.
Devaraj, S., Tang, R., Adams-Huet, B., Harris, A., Seenivasan, T., *et al.* (2007) Effect of high-dose α-tocopherol supplementation on biomarkers of oxidative stress and inflammation and carotid atherosclerosis in patients with coronary artery disease. *American Journal of Clinical Nutrition* 86, 1392–1398.
Devaraj, S., Leonard, S., Traber, M.G. and Jialal, I. (2008) Gamma-tocopherol supplementation alone and in combination with alpha-tocopherol alters biomarkers of oxidative stress and inflammation in subjects with metabolic syndrome. *Free Radical Biology and Medicine* 44, 1203–1208.
Egger, T., Schuligoi, R., Wintersperger, A., Amann, R., Malle, E., *et al.* (2003) Vitamin E (alpha-tocopherol) attenuates cyclo-oxygenase 2 transcription and synthesis in immortalized murine BV-2 microglia. *Biochemical Journal* 370, 459–467.
Evans, H.M. and Bishop, K.S. (1922) On the existence of a hitherto unrecognized dietary factor essential for reproduction. *Science* 56, 650–651.
Fischer, C.P., Hiscock, N.J., Penkowa, M., Basu, S., Vessby, B., *et al.* (2004) Supplementation with vitamins C and E inhibits the release of interleukin-6 from contracting human skeletal muscle. *The Journal of Physiology (London)* 558, 633–645.
Fox, E.S., Brower, J.S., Bellezzo, J.M. and Leingang, K.A. (1997) N-acetylcysteine and alpha-tocopherol reverse the inflammatory response in activated rat Kupffer cells. *The Journal of Immunology* 158, 5418–5423.
Fujimoto, Y., Uno, E. and Sakuma, S. (2004) Effects of reactive oxygen and nitrogen species on cyclooxygenase-1 and -2 activities. *Prostaglandins, Leukotrienes, and Essential Fatty Acids* 71, 335–340.
Grisanti, L.A., Woster, A.P., Dahlman, J., Sauter, E.R., Combs, C.K., *et al.* (2011) {alpha}1-Adrenergic receptors positively regulate Toll-like receptor cytokine production from human monocytes and macrophages. *The Journal of Pharmacology and Experimental Therapeutics* 338, 648–657.
Halpner, A.D., Handelman, G.J., Harris, J.M., Belmont, C.A. and Blumberg, J.B. (1998) Protection of vitamin C of loss of vitamin E in cultured rat hepatocytes. *Archives of Biochemistry and Biophysics* 359, 305–309.
Handelman, G.J., Machlin, L.J., Fitch, K., Weiter, J.J. and Dratz, E.A. (1985) Oral alpha-tocopherol supplements decrease plasma gamma-tocopherol levels in humans. *The Journal of Nutrition* 115, 807–813.
Hayek, M.G., Mura, C., Wu, D., Beharka, A.A., Han, S.N., *et al.* (1997) Enhanced expression of inducible cyclooxygenase with age in murine macrophages. *The Journal of Immunology* 159, 2445–2451.
Hemler, M.E. and Lands, W.E. (1980) Evidence for a peroxide-initiated free radical mechanism of prostaglandin biosynthesis. *Journal of Biological Chemistry* 255, 6253–6261.
Himmelfarb, J., Kane, J., McMonagle, E., Zaltas, E., Bobzin, S., *et al.* (2003) Alpha and gamma tocopherol metabolism in healthy subjects and patients with end-stage renal disease. *Kidney International* 64, 978–991.
Jeschke, M.G., Barrow, R.E., Suzuki, F., Rai, J., Benjamin, D., *et al.* (2002) IGF-I/IGFBP-3 equilibrates ratios of pro- to anti-inflammatory cytokines, which are predictors for organ function in severely burned pediatric patients. *Molecular Medicine* 8, 238–246.

Jiang, Q. and Ames, B.N. (2003) Gamma-tocopherol, but not alpha-tocopherol, decreases proinflammatory eicosanoids and inflammation damage in rats. *The Journal of the Federation of American Societies for Experimental Biology* 17, 816–822.

Jiang, Q., Elson-Schwab, I., Courtemanche, C. and Ames, B.N. (2000) gamma-tocopherol and its major metabolite, in contrast to alpha-tocopherol, inhibit cyclooxygenase activity in macrophages and epithelial cells. *Proceedings of the National Academy of Sciences of the United States of America* 97, 11494–11499.

Jiang, Q., Christen, S., Shigenaga, M.K. and Ames, B.N. (2001) gamma-tocopherol, the major form of vitamin E in the US diet, deserves more attention. *American Journal of Clinical Nutrition* 74, 714–722.

Jiang, Q., Lykkesfeldt, J., Shigenaga, M.K., Shigeno, E.T., Christen, S., *et al.* (2002) Gamma-tocopherol supplementation inhibits protein nitration and ascorbate oxidation in rats with inflammation. *Free Radical Biology and Medicine* 33, 1534–1542.

Jiang, Z., Yin, X. and Jiang, Q. (2011) Natural forms of vitamin E and 13′-carboxychromanol, a long-chain vitamin E metabolite, inhibit leukotriene generation from stimulated neutrophils by blocking calcium influx and suppressing 5-lipoxygenase activity, respectively. *The Journal of Immunology* 186, 1173–1179.

Kempna, P., Reiter, E., Arock, M., Azzi, A. and Zingg, J.M. (2004) Inhibition of HMC-1 mast cell proliferation by vitamin E: involvement of the protein kinase B pathway. *Journal of Biological Chemistry* 279, 50700–50709.

Lehmann, J., Martin, H.L., Lashley, E.L., Marshall, M.W. and Judd, J.T. (1986) Vitamin E in foods from high and low linoleic acid diets. *Journal of the American Dietetic Association* 86, 1208–1216.

Leonard, S.W., Paterson, E., Atkinson, J.K., Ramakrishnan, R., Cross, C.E., *et al.* (2005) Studies in humans using deuterium-labeled alpha- and gamma-tocopherols demonstrate faster plasma gamma-tocopherol disappearance and greater gamma-metabolite production. *Free Radical Biology and Medicine* 38, 857–866.

Malmberg, K.J., Lenkei, R., Petersson, M., Ohlum, T., Ichihara, F., *et al.* (2002) A short-term dietary supplementation of high doses of vitamin E increases T helper 1 cytokine production in patients with advanced colorectal cancer. *Clinical Cancer Research* 8, 1772–1778.

Mastaloudis, A., Morrow, J.D., Hopkins, D.W., Devaraj, S. and Traber, M.G. (2004) Antioxidant supplementation prevents exercise-induced lipid peroxidation, but not inflammation, in ultramarathon runners. *Free Radical Biology and Medicine* 36, 1329–1341.

McLaughlin, P.J. and Weihrauch, J.L. (1979) Vitamin E content of foods. *Journal of the American Dietetic Association* 75, 647–665.

Meydani, S.N., Barklund, M.P., Liu, S., Meydani, M., Miller, R.A., *et al.* (1990) Vitamin E supplementation enhances cell-mediated immunity in healthy elderly subjects. *American Journal of Clinical Nutrition* 52, 557–563.

Mol, M.J., de Rijke, Y.B., Demacker, P.N. and Stalenhoef, A.F. (1997) Plasma levels of lipid and cholesterol oxidation products and cytokines in diabetes mellitus and cigarette smoking: effects of vitamin E treatment. *Atherosclerosis* 129, 169–176.

Nagel, J.E., Chopra, R.K., Chrest, F.J., McCoy, M.T., Schneider, E.L., *et al.* (1988) Decreased proliferation, interleukin 2 synthesis, and interleukin 2 receptor expression are accompanied by decreased mRNA expression in phytohemagglutinin-stimulated cells from elderly donors. *The Journal of Clinical Investigation* 81, 1096–1102.

Nakarai, T., Robertson, M.J., Streuli, M., Wu, Z., Ciardelli, T.L., *et al.* (1994) Interleukin 2 receptor gamma chain expression on resting and activated lymphoid cells. *The Journal of Experimental Medicine* 180, 241–251.

Pallast, E.G., Schouten, E.G., de Waart, F.G., Fonk, H.C., Doekes, G., *et al.* (1999) Effect of 50- and 100-mg vitamin E supplements on cellular immune function in noninstitutionalized elderly persons. *American Journal of Clinical Nutrition* 69, 1273–1281.

Pedersen, B.K., Akerstrom, T.C., Nielsen, A.R. and Fischer, C.P. (2007) Role of myokines in exercise and metabolism. *Journal of Applied Physiology* 103, 1093–1098.

Petersen, E.W., Ostrowski, K., Ibfelt, T., Richelle, M., Offord, E., Halkjar-Kristensen, J. and Pedersen, B.K. (2001) Effect of vitamin supplementation on cytokine response and on muscle damage after strenuous exercise. *American Journal of Physiology. Cell Physiology* 280, C1570–C1575.

Reiter, E., Jiang, Q. and Christen, S. (2007) Anti-inflammatory properties of alpha- and gamma-tocopherol. *Molecular Aspects Medicine* 28, 668–691.

Ricciarelli, R., Tasinato, A., Clement, S., Ozer, N.K., Boscoboinik, D., *et al.* (1998) alpha-Tocopherol specifically inactivates cellular protein kinase C alpha by changing its phosphorylation state. *Biochemical Journal* 334, 243–249.

Rink, L., Cakman, I. and Kirchner, H. (1998) Altered cytokine production in the elderly. *Mechanisms of Ageing and Development* 102, 199–209.

Saldeen, T., Li, D. and Mehta, J.L. (1999) Differential effects of alpha- and gamma-tocopherol on low-density lipoprotein oxidation, superoxide activity, platelet aggregation and arterial thrombogenesis. *Journal of American College of Cardiology* 34, 1208–1215.

Smith, K.S., Lee, C.L., Ridlington, J.W., Leonard, S.W., Devaraj, S., *et al.* (2003) Vitamin E supplementation increases circulating vitamin E metabolites tenfold in end-stage renal disease patients. *Lipids* 38, 813–819.

Sanceau, J., Kaisho, T., Hirano, T. and Wietzerbin, J. (1995) Triggering of the human interleukin-6 gene by interferon-gamma and tumor necrosis factor-alpha in monocytic cells involves cooperation between interferon regulatory factor-1, NF kappa B, and Sp1 transcription factors. *Journal of Biological Chemistry* 270, 27920–27931.

Suzuki, Y.J. and Packer, L. (1993a) Inhibition of NF-kappa B activation by vitamin E derivatives. *Biochemical and Biophysical Research Communications* 193, 277–283.

Suzuki, Y.J. and Packer, L. (1993b) Inhibition of NF-kappa B DNA binding activity by alpha-tocopheryl succinate. *Biochemistry and Molecular Biology International* 31, 693–700.

Tasinato, A., Boscoboinik, D., Bartoli, G.M., Maroni, P. and Azzi, A. (1995) d-alpha-tocopherol inhibition of vascular smooth muscle cell proliferation occurs at physiological concentrations, correlates with protein kinase C inhibition, and is independent of its antioxidant properties. *Proceedings of the National Academy of Sciences of the United States of America* 92, 12190–12194.

Traber, M.G. (2007) Vitamin E regulatory mechanisms. *Annual Review of Nutrition* 27, 347–362.

Traber, M.G. and Atkinson, J. (2007) Vitamin E, antioxidant and nothing more. *Free Radical Biology and Medicine* 43, 4–15.

Traber, M.G. and Kayden, H.J. (1989) Preferential incorporation of alpha-tocopherol vs gamma-tocopherol in human lipoproteins. *American Journal of Clinical Nutrition* 49, 517–526.

Traber, M.G., Rudel, L.L., Burton, G.W., Hughes, L., Ingold, K.U., *et al.* (1990a) Nascent VLDL from liver perfusions of cynomolgus monkeys are preferentially enriched in RRR- compared with SRR-alpha-tocopherol: studies using deuterated tocopherols. *Journal of Lipid Research* 31, 687–694.

Traber, M.G., Sokol, R.J., Burton, G.W., Ingold, K.U., Papas, A.M., *et al.* (1990b) Impaired ability of patients with familial isolated vitamin E deficiency to incorporate alpha-tocopherol into lipoproteins secreted by the liver. *The Journal of Clinical Investigation* 85, 397–407.

Traber, M.G., Burton, G.W., Hughes, L., Ingold, K.U., Hidaka, H., *et al.* (1992) Discrimination between forms of vitamin E by humans with and without genetic abnormalities of lipoprotein metabolism. *Journal of Lipid Research* 33, 1171–1182.

Van Damme, J., Opdenakker, G., Simpson, R.J., Rubira, M.R., Cayphas, S., *et al.* (1987) Identification of the human 26-kD protein, interferon beta 2 (IFN-beta 2), as a B cell hybridoma/plasmacytoma growth factor induced by interleukin 1 and tumor necrosis factor. *The Journal of Experimental Medicine* 165, 914–919.

van Tits, L.J., Demacker, P.N., de Graaf, J., Hak-Lemmers, H.L. and Stalenhoef, A.F. (2000) α-Tocopherol supplementation decreases production of superoxide and cytokines by leukocytes ex vivo in both normolipidemic and hypertriglyceridemic individuals. *American Journal of Clinical Nutrition* 71, 458–464.

Vassilakopoulos, T., Katsaounou, P., Karatza, M.H., Kollintza, A., Zakynthinos, S., *et al.* (2002) Strenuous Resistive Breathing Induces Plasma Cytokines: Role of Antioxidants and Monocytes. *American Journal of Respiratory and Critical Care Medicine* 166, 1572–1578.

Vassilakopoulos, T., Karatza, M.H., Katsaounou, P., Kollintza, A., Zakynthinos, S., *et al.* (2003) Antioxidants attenuate the plasma cytokine response to exercise in humans. *Journal of Applied Physiology* 94, 1025–1032.

Venugopal, S.K., Devaraj, S., Yang, T. and Jialal, I. (2002) Alpha-tocopherol decreases superoxide anion release in human monocytes under hyperglycemic conditions via inhibition of protein kinase C-alpha. *Diabetes* 51, 3049–3054.

Wagner, J.G., Jiang, Q., Harkema, J.R., Illek, B., Patel, D.D., *et al.* (2007) Ozone enhancement of lower airway allergic inflammation is prevented by gamma-tocopherol. *Free Radical Biology and Medicine* 43, 1176–1188.

Waldmann, T.A. (1989) The multi-subunit interleukin-2 receptor. *Annual Review of Biochemistry* 58, 875–911.

Walker, C., Kristensen, F., Bettens, F. and deWeck, A.L. (1983) Lymphokine regulation of activated (G1) lymphocytes. I. Prostaglandin E2-induced inhibition of interleukin 2 production. *The Journal of Immunology* 130, 1770–1773.

Williams, J.A. and Shacter, E. (1997) Regulation of macrophage cytokine production by prostaglandin E2. Distinct roles of cyclooxygenase-1 and -2. *Journal of Biological Chemistry* 272, 25693–25699.

Wiser, J., Alexis, N.E., Jiang, Q., Wu, W., Robinette, C., *et al.* (2008) In vivo gamma-tocopherol supplementation decreases systemic oxidative stress and cytokine responses of human monocytes in normal and asthmatic subjects. *Free Radical Biology and Medicine* 45, 40–49.

Wu, D., Mura, C., Beharka, A.A., Han, S.N., Paulson, K.E., *et al.* (1998) Age-associated increase in PGE2 synthesis and COX activity in murine macrophages is reversed by vitamin E. *American Journal of Physiology. Cell Physiology* 275, C661–C668.

Wu, J.H., Ward, N.C., Indrawan, A.P., Almeida, C.A., Hodgson, J.M., *et al.* (2007) Effects of alpha-tocopherol and mixed tocopherol supplementation on markers of oxidative stress and inflammation in type 2 diabetes. *Clinical Chemistry* 53, 511–519.

Yoshikawa, S., Morinobu, T., Hamamura, K., Hirahara, F., Iwamoto, T., *et al.* (2005) The effect of gamma-tocopherol administration on alpha-tocopherol levels and metabolism in humans. *European Journal of Clinical Nutrition* 59, 900–905.

7 Vitamin C, B-Complex Vitamins and Inflammation

A. Oliveira* **and C. Lopes**
Department of Clinical Epidemiology, Public Health Institute, University of Porto, Portugal

Introduction

Inflammation is believed to play a major role in the pathogenesis of atherosclerosis (Ross, 1999; Libby *et al.*, 2002; Hansson *et al.*, 2006). Prospective studies and primary prevention trials have systematically associated high-sensitivity C-reactive protein (hs-CRP), an acute-phase protein widely considered to be a marker of systemic inflammation, to cardiovascular risk (Ridker, 2007; Nakou *et al.*, 2008; Devaraj *et al.*, 2009; Kaptoge *et al.*, 2010). Elevated hs-CRP levels have been also associated with the severity of coronary plaques and carotid intima-media thickness (Sitzer *et al.*, 2002) and with the components of the metabolic syndrome (Esposito and Giugliano, 2004).

Traditionally, many researchers have regarded lipids as the central mediators of atherosclerosis. This belief is supported by the 'oxidation hypothesis' (i.e. the atherosclerotic process mainly consists of the accumulation of lipids within the artery wall and of the oxidation of native low-density lipoprotein (LDL) molecules that once oxidized are preferentially taken up in the artery wall) (Williams and Tabas, 1998; Jessup *et al.*, 2004). The oxidation hypothesis, by itself, supports an important role of diet and other lifestyles in atherogenesis, because LDL can be oxidized by smoking, for example, and oxidation can be prevented by dietary antioxidants, such as vitamins and polyphenols (effects that will be discussed later in this chapter).

During the past decades, a plausible model linking lipids and inflammation to atherogenesis has re-emerged. The realization that inflammation might play an important

* Corresponding author, acmatos@med.up.pt

role in the pathogenesis of atherosclerosis suggests new opportunities for its prevention and treatment. Possible pharmacological and non-pharmacological approaches could be used to reduce the inflammatory state. Indeed, healthy diets have been suggested for their potential to reduce the pro-inflammatory milieu, by acting through mechanisms such as improving the production of adiponectin (a hormone produced by adipocytes with anti-inflammatory properties) and reducing the production of pro-inflammatory molecules, such as C-reactive protein (CRP) by the liver (Giugliano *et al.*, 2006). These mechanisms will improve insulin sensitivity and endothelial function at the vascular level and, in the long run, reduce an individual's predisposition to metabolic syndrome, type 2 diabetes and coronary heart disease (Fig. 7.1).

Via multiple biological pathways, involving serum total or LDL-cholesterol, blood pressure, insulin sensitivity, oxidative stress and endothelial dysfunction (Hu and Willett, 2002), inflammation might be a potential pathway by which diet, and particularly water-soluble vitamins, fibre and low fruit and vegetable intake, can modulate coronary risk (Fig. 7.2).

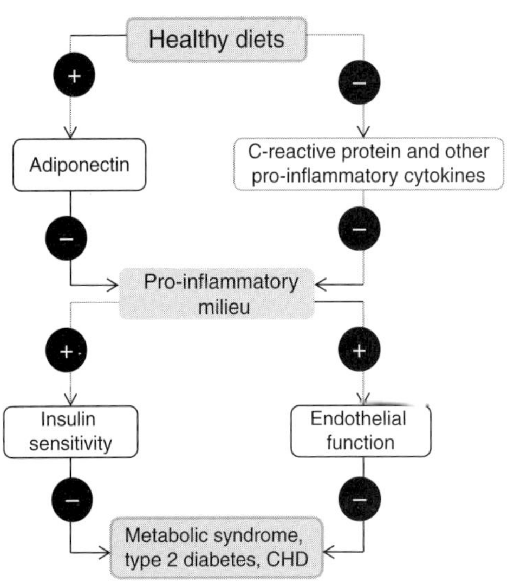

Fig. 7.1. Contribution of healthy diets to a lower generation of a pro-inflammatory milieu and its relationship with a decreased incidence of metabolic syndrome, type 2 diabetes and coronary heart disease (CHD). From Giugliano *et al.*, 2006, with permission from Elsevier Ltd.

Inflammation can be defined as the elevation of various pro-inflammatory cytokines (e.g. interleukin-1, tumour necrosis factor-alpha (TNF-α)), adhesion molecules (e.g. intercellular adhesion molecule-1, selectins), stimuli with proinflammatory hepatic effects (e.g. interleukin-6 (IL-6)) or the products of hepatic stimulation, such as serum amyloid A and CRP. The Centre for Disease Control and the American Heart Association Consensus Panel (Pearson *et al.*, 2003) note that CRP values >10 mg/l represent acute infection or inflammatory disease and should not be used in the evaluation of cardiovascular disease risk. Accordingly, mainly sub-clinical inflammation will be the focus of this chapter, because it probably represents the main pathway by which diet could exert its effects.

Water-soluble Vitamins and Inflammation

Scientific research in the past several years has demonstrated a beneficial effect of various nutrients, such as fatty acids (monounsaturated and polyunsaturated n-3), fibre and antioxidant vitamins (C, E and β-carotene), owing to their antioxidant and anti-inflammatory properties (Hu and Willett, 2002; Parikh *et al.*, 2005; Giugliano *et al.*, 2006). In this chapter we will present evidence focused on the effects of vitamin C and B-complex vitamins on inflammation.

Throughout the literature, water-soluble vitamins have been related to inflammatory markers, including those studies that have assessed plasma or serum levels of vitamins (Friso *et al.*, 2001; Folsom *et al.*, 2003; Ford *et al.*, 2003; van Herpen-Broekmans *et al.*, 2004; Wannamethee *et al.*, 2006; Aasheim *et al.*, 2008; Shen *et al.*, 2010) or vitamin supplement use (Bruunsgaard *et al.*, 2003; Mangoni *et al.*, 2003; Vermeulen *et al.*, 2003; Block *et al.*, 2004; Ullegaddi *et al.*, 2004; Durga *et al.*, 2005; Dusitanond *et al.*, 2005; Klerk *et al.*, 2005; Bo *et al.*, 2007; Rizzo *et al.*, 2008; Block *et al.*, 2009), as well as those that have measured dietary vitamin intake (Folsom *et al.*, 2003; Wannamethee *et al.*, 2006; Oliveira *et al.*, 2009). Whereas observational studies hold inverse and independent associations between water-soluble

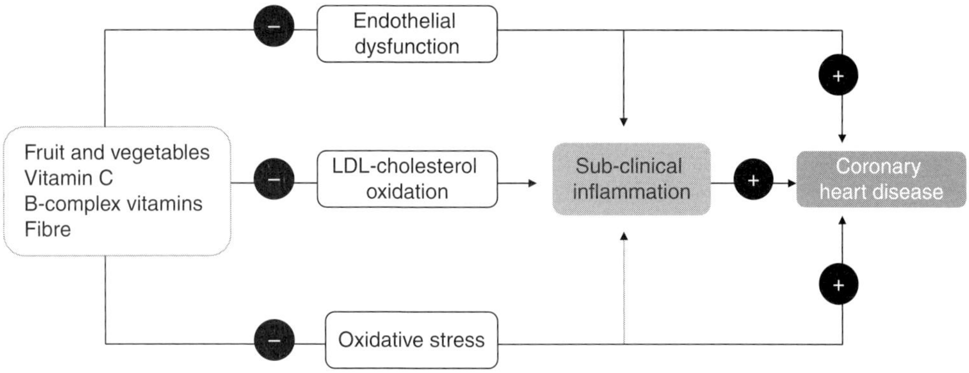

Fig. 7.2. Mechanisms through which 'healthy' diets may lead to a reduced risk of coronary heart disease, including a potential role of sub-clinical inflammation. LDL, low-density lipoprotein. Adapted from Giugliano *et al.*, 2006, with permission from Elsevier Ltd.

vitamins and inflammation, supplementation studies report inconsistent results regarding the ability of these vitamins to reduce systemic and vascular inflammation *in vivo*.

Vitamin C

Vitamin C (ascorbic acid or ascorbate) is an essential water-soluble nutrient, mainly present in fruit and vegetables. Vitamin C primarily exerts its effect on host defence mechanisms and immune homeostasis by acting as a potent antioxidant (Kelley and Bendich, 1996). Although its antioxidant effects, with respect to both reactive oxygen and nitrogen species, are relatively well established, vitamin C effects on inflammatory markers have not been extensively examined. Observational studies have shown protective effects of vitamin C over some inflammatory mediators (Ford *et al.*, 2003; van Herpen-Broekmans *et al.*, 2004; Wannamethee *et al.*, 2006; Aasheim *et al.*, 2008; Oliveira *et al.*, 2009) and controlled trials have reported no effects (Bruunsgaard *et al.*, 2003) or slightly protective effects for high-risk individuals (Block *et al.*, 2004; Rizzo *et al.*, 2008). According to some authors (Aguirre and May, 2008), the latter results might be due to the fact that 'antioxidant therapies are applied too little and too late'. In fact, these trials might not have targeted the right group (mainly secondary prevention in advanced atherosclerotic disease has been studied), or might not have used adequate amounts of vitamin supplements (vitamin C given orally, even at high doses, does not seem to achieve sustained serum levels that might be required for an effective anti-inflammatory activity) (Talaulikar and Manyonda, 2011).

Observational epidemiological evidence

In a cross-sectional analysis of the third National Health and Nutrition Examination Survey data (USA), the authors reported that CRP concentrations were inversely and significantly associated with serum concentrations of vitamin C, among other nutrients (Ford *et al.*, 2003). The authors suggested that the inflammatory process, through the production of reactive oxygen species, may deplete stores of antioxidants, and help to explain this inverse association. Wannamethee *et al.* (2006) also reported a significant inverse association between both dietary and plasma vitamin C and markers of inflammation in a cross-sectional study of 3258 men aged 60–79 years who had no history of cardiovascular disease or diabetes (the study sample was drawn from general practices in 24 British towns). The authors found that plasma vitamin C had a stronger inverse association with hs-CRP than dietary vitamin C. It was pointed out that the strength of the association between vitamin C and inflammatory markers may well have been underestimated because measurements of vitamin C (particularly dietary vitamin C) are imprecise, contributing to the differences found between plasma and dietary vitamin C results. Although plasma/serum levels of vitamin C might not be the best indicator of vitamin C status because excess is excreted in the urine, of all the vitamins, vitamin C exhibits possibly the strongest and most significant correlation between intake and biochemical indices, so that its intake can be predicted with moderate precision (Nelson, 1991).

Another study measuring dietary vitamin C intake in the general population of Porto, Portugal suggested that the probability of changing hs-CRP category (low to average risk or average to high risk) was inversely associated with the increase in vitamin C intake in men (Oliveira *et al.*, 2009). In another study in the general population of the Netherlands, the authors found that serum vitamin C was inversely related to hs-CRP (van Herpen-Broekmans *et al.*, 2004). Aasheim *et al.* (2008) also reported that vitamin C serum concentrations were moderately inversely associated with elevated hs-CRP concentrations, comparing 110 obese Norwegian patients seeking weight-loss treatment and 58 healthy controls. These studies suggest a possible protective effect of vitamin C through an influence on the inflammatory process.

Experimental evidence

The Antioxidant Supplementation in Atherosclerosis Prevention (ASAP) study was a randomized controlled trial conducted among 45–69-year-old men with mild hypercholesterolemia and no overt signs of inflammation. It was designed to test whether supplementation twice a day with either 91 mg of α-tocopherol, 250 mg of slow-release ascorbic acid or a combination of α-tocopherol and vitamin C retarded the progression of common carotid atherosclerosis. To elucidate the underlying mechanisms, Bruunsgaard *et al.* (2003) investigated the effects of the vitamin supplements on inflammatory markers *in vivo*, and found that long-term combined supplementation with α-tocopherol and vitamin C, in reasonable doses, had no detectable systemic anti-inflammatory effects in this population. One possible limitation could be the dosages used in the study that might be too low to induce an anti-inflammatory effect, even in combination.

Another non-randomized, controlled trial evaluated the combined effect of vitamin C (1000 UI/day) and E (1000 mg/day) supplementation for 4 weeks on the plasma cytokine levels of 13 Italian volunteers, who were older men (mean age: 67 years; age range: 65–73 years) with impaired fasting glucose (Rizzo *et al.*, 2008). A combined administration of vitamin E and C was found to decrease plasma levels of TNF-α and 8-isoprostane, a marker of oxidative stress. In another study, Block *et al.* (2004) found a significant reduction in hs-CRP as a result of 2 months treatment with 500 mg/day of vitamin C among both active and passive smokers. In a subsequent study, a placebo-controlled parallel-design study examined the separate effects of 1000 mg/day of vitamin C and 800 IU/day of vitamin E versus placebo for 2 months in healthy non-smokers (Block *et al.*, 2009). Vitamin E supplementation had no significant effects. For vitamin C, no treatment effect was seen when all participants were analysed; but among participants at elevated cardiovascular risk (hs-CRP≥1.0 mg/l), vitamin C significantly reduced the median hs-CRP concentrations by 25.3% versus placebo (median reduction in the vitamin C group, 0.25 mg/l, 16.7%).

Vitamin C has been related to other inflammatory mediators, such as resistin – a hormone produced by fat cells (adipokine). Growing evidence has suggested that this protein, highly expressed in monocytes and macrophages in humans, might have an involvement in the inflammatory process, being induced by increased cytokine levels, and by directly stimulating the further production of pro-inflammatory cytokines, thus leading to inflammation amplification (Reilly *et al.*, 2005; Silswal *et al.*, 2005). The efficacy of vitamin C treatment in reducing serum resistin levels was evaluated in a randomized study, which involved administering 2 g of ascorbic acid orally for 2 weeks (n = 40; experimental group) or no supplementation (n = 40; control group) (Bo *et al.*, 2007). Authors observed that short-term vitamin C supplementation significantly reduced resistin levels, independently of changes in other inflammatory or metabolic variables (including hs-CRP), with each unit increase of vitamin C corresponding to a decrease of about 0.10 units of resistin levels, $p<0.001$. This suggests a specific direct effect of antioxidant substances on resistin expression from monocytes/macrophages. Additionally, levels of two oxidative stress markers were significantly different between groups: nitrotyrosine, which is associated with cell damage and inflammation, was decreased in the intervention group, whereas glutathione (an endogenous antioxidant) was increased.

Further research is needed to better understand the anti-inflammatory effects of oral vitamin C supplementation. The supplementation dose of greater than about 500 mg might stay in the gut and cause osmotic diarrhoea and other gastrointestinal upset (Talaulikar and Manyonda, 2011).

Biological plausibility

Strong biological plausibility supports potential anti-inflammatory effects of vitamin C. In general, ascorbate is believed to modify the early steps of atherosclerosis (Aguirre and May, 2008). It acts in three major vascular cell types: endothelial cells, vascular smooth muscle cells and macrophages. It helps to prevent endothelial dysfunction, stimulates type IV collagen synthesis and enhances cell proliferation. Ascorbate also inhibits differentiation, recruitment and proliferation of vascular smooth muscle in areas of vascular damage, decreases oxidative stress related to macrophage activation and enhances several aspects of macrophage function (Aguirre and May, 2008). In some studies, it was also described that vitamin C decreases uptake and degradation of oxidized LDL (Aguirre and May, 2008).

Vitamin C could also have a direct effect on cytokine production. Hartel *et al.* (2004) found in healthy adult volunteers that vitamin C, in a dose-dependent manner, inhibited lipopolysaccharide-induced IL-6 and TNF-α production, as well as IL-2 production after stimulation *in vitro*. These authors suggest several potential mechanisms underlying the immunomodulating effect of vitamin C, including both oxidative and non-oxidative processes. Oxidative damage leads to an inappropriate activation of the transcription factor, nuclear factor-kappa B (NFκB) and, subsequently, to an overexpression of inflammatory proteins. Because most activation pathways of NFκB are reliant on reactive oxygen species, vitamin C may protect against deregulation of the immune-inflammatory response by its antioxidant properties (Bowie and O'Neill, 2000). Vitamin C could also inhibit not only the initial expression of pro-inflammatory cytokines but also their autocrine stimulation pathways via NFκB (Bowie and O'Neill, 2000; Carcamo *et al.*, 2002b). Vitamin C can also act by inhibiting granulocyte–macrophage-colony-stimulating factor, IL-3- and IL-5-induced signal transduction pathways (Carcamo *et al.*, 2002a). Moreover, it has been demonstrated that vitamin C could inhibit T cell apoptosis signalling pathways (Campbell *et al.*, 1999) and FAS-induced apoptotic death in human monocytes (Perez-Cruz *et al.*, 2003).

Although all these potential mechanisms may be enrolled in immunomodulation by vitamin C, the role of vitamin C in the complex cytokine network has not been yet completely defined and further studies are needed to elucidate these mechanisms.

B-complex vitamins

Folate and the 'homocysteine hypothesis'

B-complex vitamins, such as folate (also called folic acid or vitamin B9), have been suggested to have potential beneficial effects on surrogate end points such as endothelial function in patients at high cardiovascular risk (Chambers *et al.*, 2000; Mangoni *et al.*, 2005). Folic acid treatment is safe, nontoxic and believed to be cost effective, and could be easily incorporated into a global food fortification strategy, in combination with other vitamins and micronutrients (Jacques *et al.*, 1999; Tice *et al.*, 2001). Grain fortification with folic acid was predicted to decrease coronary heart disease events by 8% in women and 13% in men, with a comparable reduction in cardiovascular mortality (Tice *et al.*, 2001). Current evidence does not support the use of folic acid as an anti-inflammatory agent, however. Studies are limited to small trials on different study populations, using folic acid often in combination with other vitamins and for different treatment periods (Das, 2003; Mangoni, 2006).

Nevertheless, a strong biological plausibility favours the potential effectiveness of a folic-acid-based treatment strategy on the pro-inflammatory state associated with atherosclerosis. At least two mechanisms might explain it: (i) enhancing endothelial nitric oxide (eNO) production; and (ii) lowering of homocysteine concentrations, as discussed below.

The ability of folate to increase eNO synthesis seems to be independent of its capacity to lower plasma homocysteine levels. On the basis of a literature review conducted by Das (2003), it was described that folate enhances eNO synthesis showing anti-inflammatory actions by stimulating endogenous tetrahydrobiopterin [H(4)B] regeneration. This cofactor necessary for eNO synthesis inhibits intracellular superoxide generation and thus enhances the half-life of eNO. H(4)B in turn enhances eNO generation and increases arginine transport into cells. Additionally, folic acid increases the concentration of omega-3 polyunsaturated fatty acids (PUFAs), which also enhance eNO synthesis. Other dietary components and hormones are involved in eNO synthesis. Vitamin C increases eNO synthesis by increasing intracellular H(4)B and its stabilization. Insulin stimulates H(4)B synthesis and PUFA metabolism suppresses the production of the pro-inflammatory cytokine TNF-α and superoxide anion, and enhances eNO generation (Das, 2003). It remains to be determined whether a combination of folic acid, vitamins B12, B6 and C, H(4)B, L-arginine and omega-3 fatty acids, in appropriate amounts, might form a novel approach in the prevention and management of cardiovascular end points.

Vitamins such as B6, B12 and folic acid are also implicated in homocysteine metabolism. The relationship between elevated blood levels of homocysteine and low levels of related factors such as vitamins B6, B12 and folate and its impact on atherosclerotic process have been studied since the 1970s (McCully, 1969; Wald *et al.*, 2002; Humphrey *et al.*, 2008). Homocysteine concentrations are an independent risk factor for cardiovascular disease and B-complex vitamins, particularly folic acid, are important cofactors in homocysteine metabolism. Therefore, it has been suggested that supplementation with these vitamins might decrease cardiovascular risk and reduce morbidity and mortality associated with stroke and coronary heart disease. This principle forms the basis of the 'homocysteine hypothesis' (Clarke and Armitage, 2000). Nowadays, controversies over the homocysteine hypothesis still exist and the benefits of B-vitamin supplementation in the prevention of cardiovascular diseases are still under discussion. Results from clinical trials have been inconsistent, with large-scale trials suggesting that folic acid and B-vitamin supplements might not provide the assumed protection (Ntaios *et al.*, 2008, 2009; Antoniades *et al.*, 2009). Furthermore, these findings raise questions about whether the combination of folic acid and B-vitamins might actually be harmful. In addition, homocysteine has several potentially deleterious vascular actions. Most known forms of damage or injury are due to homocysteine-mediated oxidative stress (owing to its auto-oxidative potential, thereby increasing the production of reactive oxygen species), but are also due to impaired endothelial function, stimulation of mitogenesis and induction of thrombosis (Haynes, 2002).

B-complex vitamins, however, also have a series of *in vitro* effects indicating a direct anti-atherogenic action and the results of some studies, especially for vitamin B6, suggest an inverse relationship with cardiovascular risk, at least in part, independent of homocysteinemia (Friso *et al.*, 2001; Shen *et al.*, 2010), as presented in the next section.

Vitamin B6

The utilization of B-complex vitamins in the presence of underlying inflammatory processes has been described as a possible mechanism to explain the decreased vitamin B6 levels in certain pathological conditions. Pyridoxal 59-phosphate (PLP), the active form of vitamin B6, has been inversely associated with inflammation in patients with rheumatoid arthritis (Roubenoff *et al.*, 1995; Chiang *et al.*, 2003) and inflammatory bowel disease (Saibeni *et al.*, 2003) and lower concentrations of this coenzyme have been reported to be an independent risk factor for cardiovascular diseases (Robinson *et al.*, 1998; Friso *et al.*, 2004). Although the causal factor remains to be clarified, inflammation has been suggested as facilitating the redistribution of PLP from circulation to tissues with high demand. Because vitamin B6 is involved in nucleic acid synthesis, and consequently in mRNA and protein synthesis, the production of cytokines and inflammatory mediators during the inflammatory response might increase the use of PLP (Friso *et al.*, 2001).

PLP participates in a wide range of reactions, including homocysteine metabolism; because plasma PLP is an important determinant of total plasma homocysteine, the relationship between low PLP and certain diseases has been frequently explained by an abnormal homocysteine metabolism. None the less, Friso and colleagues (2001), in participants from the population-based Framingham Heart Study cohort, suggested a new potential pathophysiological link between the active form of vitamin B6 and coronary heart disease: independent of plasma homocysteine, low circulating PLP is associated with increased levels of hs-CRP (Friso *et al.*, 2001). Despite the lack of a pathophysiological explanation for the association between PLP and markers of acute-phase status, the authors suggested that PLP might be acting as a coenzyme for the inflammation-related functions, e.g. the production of cytokines and other polypeptide mediators during the inflammatory response might require an increased utilization of this coenzyme. Furthermore, this model is consistent with the observation that vitamin B6 deficiency is associated with an impairment in differentiation and maturation of monocyte-derived macrophages and T lymphocytes, inflammatory cells whose activation leads to the release of several enzymes and cytokines (Rall and Meydani, 1993). Vitamin B6 deficiency was also reported to change the regulation of IL-2 production (Meydani *et al.*, 1991).

Folsom *et al.* (2003) attempted to reproduce these findings, but they did not find either a significant association between PLP and serum CRP in healthy middle-aged adults or B-vitamin status (evaluated by dietary and serum levels of vitamin B6, B12 and folic acid) to be strongly correlated with circulating markers of inflammation, endothelial dysfunction or thrombogenesis. Similarly, Friso *et al.* (2001) reported no significant differences in folic acid concentrations in subjects with normal or elevated hs-CRP levels. More recently, Shen *et al.* (2010) evaluated the cross-sectional association of vitamin B6 status with markers of inflammation and oxidative stress in Porto Rican adults living in the USA, and found that there was a strong inverse relationship between plasma PLP concentration and plasma hs-CRP levels. This negative association persisted after plasma homocysteine was controlled for.

Further studies are needed to clarify whether decreases of inflammatory levels associated with PLP play a role in the cascade of metabolic events related to certain diseases. If confirmed, this could help to explain the complex mechanisms by which this metabolite acts as a risk factor for cardiovascular diseases.

Experimental evidence

A few experimental studies have investigated the effects of supplementation with B-complex vitamins, mainly folic acid with or without other B-vitamins, on concentrations of inflammatory markers. Dusitanond *et al.* (2005) conducted a randomized controlled trial on 285 patients from the VITAmins TO Prevent Stroke study. Patients were randomized to daily combined treatment with folic acid (2 mg), vitamin B6 (25 mg) and vitamin B12 (0.5 mg) versus placebo for 6 months. Apart from a significant reduction in plasma homocysteine concentrations among the supplementation group, the two randomized treatment groups did not differ in hs-CRP and IL-6 levels at 6 months. Mangoni *et al.* (2003) evaluated the effects of 4-week folic acid supplementation (5 mg/day) versus placebo on hs-CRP, white blood cells, fibrinogen and homocysteine concentrations of 24 healthy chronic cigarette smokers (Mangoni *et al.*, 2003). A significant reduction in homocysteine and fibrinogen was observed, but concentrations of hs-CRP and white blood cells did not change. Klerk *et al.* (2005), in a randomized placebo controlled trial among 276 older adults, investigated the effect of folic acid supplementation (0.8 mg/day) for 1 year on markers of endothelial function, fibrinolysis and inflammation. Despite a 24% reduction in plasma homocysteine concentration in the folic acid group compared with the placebo group, there was no clear change in any of the haemostasis markers, nor CRP.

Vermeulen *et al.* (2003) performed a placebo-controlled 2-year trial among 158 healthy siblings of patients with premature atherosclerotic disease to determine the effect of daily folic acid (5 mg) plus vitamin B6 (250 mg) treatment as compared with placebo (n = 80) on markers of endothelial function and inflammation. Vitamin treatment significantly lowered homocysteine concentrations, but again no significant changes in hs-CRP, soluble vascular cell adhesion molecule-1 and E-selectin levels were observed. Durga *et al.* (2005) in a double-blind, randomized, placebo-controlled trial among 530 men and post-menopausal women assessed the effects of a 1-year treatment with folic acid (0.8 mg/day) versus placebo on serum concentrations of hs-CRP and soluble intercellular adhesion molecule-1. Despite a significant reduction in plasma homocysteine concentrations, folic acid treatment did not induce any significant changes in blood concentrations of these inflammatory markers. Ullegaddi *et al.* (2004) assigned 24 patients within 12 h of symptom onset from an acute ischemic stroke to receive daily oral supplements with combined folic acid (5 mg), vitamin B2 (5 mg), vitamin B6 (50 mg) and vitamin B12 (0.4 mg) compared with placebo (n = 24), and investigated the effect of 2-week treatment on CRP and homocysteine levels. Vitamin supplementation suppressed the expected increase in CRP post-stroke, suggesting some anti-inflammatory activity, but did not affect plasma homocysteine concentrations, probably owing to the relatively short treatment period.

The heterogeneity found across studies mainly regarding population sets (subjects with different cardiovascular risk profiles were included), treatment periods (from 2 weeks to 2 years) and concurrent use of different drug treatments might explain some of the results. A possible solution would pass through the design of studies in homogeneous populations with similar cardiovascular risk and drug treatment.

Fruit and vegetables

Fruit and vegetables are major dietary sources of antioxidant vitamins, in particular vitamin C. Several studies have related fruit and vegetable consumption to decreased inflammatory marker levels (Sanchez-Moreno *et al.*, 2003, 2004; Freese *et al.*, 2004; Gao *et al.*, 2004; Watzl *et al.*, 2005; Esmaillzadeh *et al.*, 2006; Kelley *et al.*, 2006; Riso *et al.*, 2006; Wannamethee *et al.*, 2006; Oliveira *et al.*, 2009). Most studies were randomized trials with very specific exposures such as a tomato-based drink (Riso *et al.*, 2006), high-pressurized orange juice (Sanchez-Moreno *et al.*, 2003), carotenoid-rich vegetables and fruit (Watzl *et al.*, 2005), sweet cherries (Kelley *et al.*, 2006), berries and apple (Freese *et al.*, 2004), and the vegetable soup 'gazpacho' (Sanchez-Moreno *et al.*, 2004). Most found decreased inflammatory levels with the intake of these food items; however one failed to show a reduction in hs-CRP after several weeks of intervention (Freese *et al.*, 2004).

From the few observational studies conducted, an inverse association between fruit and vegetable intake and inflammatory markers have been reported (Gao *et al.*, 2004; Esmaillzadeh *et al.*, 2006; Wannamethee *et al.*, 2006; Oliveira *et al.*, 2009), some of them only among the elderly (Gao *et al.*, 2004; Wannamethee *et al.*, 2006). A study conducted among Portuguese adults concluded that for each 100 g increase in fruit and vegetable intake, there was 30% less probability of changing hs-CRP category (low to moderate risk, or moderate to high risk) (Oliveira *et al.*, 2009). Overall, the effects were weaker in overweight men and women. Further research is needed on the separate effects of fruit and vegetables, by sex, body mass index categories and in a broader age spectrum.

Fruit and vegetables are the main dietary sources of vitamin C, but also contain a great variety of bioactive compounds with antioxidant properties, such as polyphenols, which are able to act at different levels of the inflammatory cascade that lead to plaque formation (Maron, 2004). These components all together are believed to contribute to the anti-inflammatory effects of fruit and vegetables. Indeed, a study by Brighenti *et al.* (2005) conducted in 243 non-diabetic subjects concluded that dietary total antioxidant capacity, rather than single antioxidant compounds, are inversely and independently correlated with plasma concentrations of hs-CRP. Also, in a crossover intervention, 33 healthy adults received high versus low total antioxidant capacity diets for 2 weeks that did not differ in the intake of macronutrients, dietary fibre, alcohol or daily servings of fruit and vegetables (Valtuena *et al.*, 2008). Plasma hs-CRP concentrations decreased following the high total antioxidant capacity diet compared with the low counterpart.

The anti-inflammatory properties of certain vitamins and other bioactive compounds with antioxidant capacity have been attributed to their ability to modulate the NFκB DNA-binding activity (Carcamo *et al.*, 2002a; Choi *et al.*, 2004). This activation is primarily promoted by oxidative stress and leads to the cytokine-induced expression of CAM molecules in the vascular endothelium and to the TNF-α- and IL-6-induced production of CRP by the liver.

Limitations across Studies

When reviewing the literature relating to water-soluble vitamins and inflammation, some conceptual and methodological limitations should be considered. Diet has been traditionally studied through the effects of single nutrients and/or foods on health outcomes. Although this type of analysis has been quite valuable and has led to many important nutritional findings, it has important limitations (Willett, 1998; Hu, 2002; Schulze and Hoffmann, 2006). The first one is related to the simple fact that people do not eat isolated nutrients or foods, but rather meals with complex combinations of nutrients that are likely to be interactive or synergistic. Therefore, the high level of inter-correlation among nutrients makes it difficult to examine their separate effects (as is the case for water-soluble vitamins, examined in this chapter). Moreover, the effect of a single nutrient, such as vitamins, may be too small to be detected. When a large number of nutrients or foods are being studied together, statistically significant associations might also be found simply by chance. In addition, the single nutrient analysis could potentially be confounded by the effect of an overall eating behaviour (Willett, 1998; Hu, 2002; Schulze and Hoffmann, 2006). For all these reasons, measuring diet is a demanding and challenging task. Measurements of vitamins (particularly dietary vitamin sources) are somewhat imprecise so the strengths of associations with inflammatory and haemostatic markers may well have been underestimated.

Summary and Conclusions

Several epidemiological studies have related water-soluble vitamins to markers of systemic inflammation, largely sustained by multiple plausible biological mechanisms. Although observational studies hold inverse and independent associations, most randomized clinical trials show inconsistent results regarding the ability of water-soluble vitamins to reduce systemic and vascular inflammation *in vivo*. Studies have focused on different measures of vitamin status: dietary vitamin intake (scarce evidence), plasma or serum levels, or vitamin supplement use, which could contribute to the heterogeneity in the data. Additionally, the different dosages used in each experiment, the different treatment periods, the use of vitamins alone or in combination with others, and the different population sets with various degrees of cardiovascular risk do not help to find comparable and consistent results.

Vitamin C (ascorbic acid) has been the water-soluble vitamin most consistently associated with the inflammatory process, probably owing to its well-recognized antioxidant effects. Ascorbate is believed to modify the early steps of atherosclerosis, acting in three major vascular cell types: endothelial cells (helping to prevent endothelial dysfunction), vascular smooth muscle cells (inhibiting proliferation of vascular smooth muscle in areas of vascular damage) and macrophages (decreasing oxidative stress related to macrophage activation).

Basic research data also support the hypothesis that folic acid might represent an effective therapeutic option to reduce the inflammatory response in atherosclerosis either by lowering homocysteine concentrations, a pro-inflammatory and pro-atherosclerotic factor, and/or by directly interacting with endothelial nitric oxide production to reduce the generation of reactive oxygen species. Despite this promising approach, current evidence does not support the use of folic acid as an anti-inflammatory agent. Further research should disentangle the effect of water-soluble vitamins in the inflammatory process. Greater homogeneity in study populations may be necessary to enhance the interpretation of data from future research.

References

Aasheim, E.T., Hofso, D., Hjelmesaeth, J., Birkeland, K.I. and Bohmer, T. (2008) Vitamin status in morbidly obese patients: a cross-sectional study. *The American Journal of Clinical Nutrition* 87, 362–369.

Aguirre, R. and May, J.M. (2008) Inflammation in the vascular bed: importance of vitamin C. *Pharmacology and Therapeutics* 119, 96–103.

Antoniades, C., Antonopoulos, A.S., Tousoulis, D., Marinou, K. and Stefanadis, C. (2009) Homocysteine and coronary atherosclerosis: from folate fortification to the recent clinical trials. *European Heart Journal,* 30 6–15.

Block, G., Jensen, C., Dietrich, M., Norkus, E.P., Hudes, M., *et al.* (2004) Plasma C-reactive protein concentrations in active and passive smokers: influence of antioxidant supplementation. *Journal of the American College of Nutrition,* 23, 141–147.

Block, G., Jensen, C.D., Dalvi, T.B., Norkus, E.P., Hudes, M., *et al.* (2009) Vitamin C treatment reduces elevated C-reactive protein. *Free Radical Biology and Medicine* 46, 70–77.

Bo, S., Ciccone, G., Durazzo, M., Gambino, R., Massarenti, P., *et al.* (2007) Efficacy of antioxidant treatment in reducing resistin serum levels: a randomized study. *PLoS clinical trials* 2, e17.

Bowie, A.G. and O'Neill, L.A. (2000) Vitamin C inhibits NF-kappa B activation by TNF via the activation of p38 mitogen-activated protein kinase. *Journal of Immunology* 165, 7180–7188.

Brighenti, F., Valtuena, S., Pellegrini, N., Ardigo, D., Del Rio, D., *et al.* (2005) Total antioxidant capacity of the diet is inversely and independently related to plasma concentration of high-sensitivity C-reactive protein in adult Italian subjects. *The British Journal of Nutrition* 93, 619–625.

Bruunsgaard, H., Poulsen, H.E., Pedersen, B.K., Nyyssonen, K., Kaikkonen, J., *et al.* (2003) Long-term combined supplementations with alpha-tocopherol and vitamin C have no detectable anti-inflammatory effects in healthy men. *The Journal of Nutrition* 133, 1170–1173.

Campbell, J.D., Cole, M., Bunditrutavorn, B. and Vella, A.T. (1999) Ascorbic acid is a potent inhibitor of various forms of T cell apoptosis. *Cellular Immunology* 194, 1–5.

Carcamo, J.M., Borquez-Ojeda, O. and Golde, D.W. (2002a)Vitamin C inhibits granulocyte macrophage-colony-stimulating factor-induced signaling pathways. *Blood* 99, 3205–3212.

Carcamo, J.M., Pedraza, A., Borquez-Ojeda, O. and Golde, D.W. (2002b) Vitamin C suppresses TNF alpha-induced NF kappa B activation by inhibiting I kappa B alpha phosphorylation. *Biochemistry* 41, 12995–13002.

Chambers, J.C., Ueland, P.M., Obeid, O.A., Wrigley, J., Refsum, H., *et al.* (2000) Improved vascular endothelial function after oral B vitamins: An effect mediated through reduced concentrations of free plasma homocysteine. *Circulation* 102, 2479–2483.

Chiang, E.P., Bagley, P.J., Selhub, J., Nadeau, M. and Roubenoff, R. (2003) Abnormal vitamin B(6) status is associated with severity of symptoms in patients with rheumatoid arthritis. *The American Journal of Medicine* 114, 283–287.

Choi, J.S., Choi, Y.J., Park, S.H., Kang, J.S. and Kang, Y.H. (2004) Flavones mitigate tumor necrosis factor-alpha-induced adhesion molecule upregulation in cultured human endothelial cells: role of nuclear factor-kappa B. *The Journal of Nutrition* 134, 1013–1019.

Clarke, R. and Armitage, J. (2000) Vitamin supplements and cardiovascular risk: review of the randomized trials of homocysteine-lowering vitamin supplements. *Seminars in Thrombosis and Hemostasis* 26, 341–348.

Das, U.N. (2003) Folic acid says NO to vascular diseases. *Nutrition* 19, 686–692.

Devaraj, S., Singh, U. and Jialal, I. (2009) The evolving role of C-reactive protein in atherothrombosis. *Clinical Chemistry* 55, 229–238.

Durga, J., Van Tits, L.J., Schouten, E.G., Kok, F.J. and Verhoef, P. (2005) Effect of lowering of homocysteine levels on inflammatory markers: a randomized controlled trial. *Archives of Internal Medicine* 165, 1388–1394.

Dusitanond, P., Eikelboom, J.W., Hankey, G.J., Thom, J., Gilmore, G., *et al.* (2005) Homocysteine-lowering treatment with folic acid, cobalamin, and pyridoxine does not reduce blood markers of inflammation, endothelial dysfunction, or hypercoagulability in patients with previous transient ischemic attack or stroke: a randomized substudy of the VITATOPS trial. *Stroke; a Journal of Cerebral Circulation* 36, 144–146.

Esmaillzadeh, A., Kimiagar, M., Mehrabi, Y., Azadbakht, L., Hu, F.B., *et al.* (2006) Fruit and vegetable intakes, C-reactive protein, and the metabolic syndrome. *The American Journal of Clinical Nutrition* 84, 1489–1497.

Esposito, K. and Giugliano, D. (2004) The metabolic syndrome and inflammation: association or causation? *Nutrition, Metabolism, and Cardiovascular Diseases* 14, 228–232.

Folsom, A.R., Desvarieux, M., Nieto, F.J., Boland, L.L., Ballantyne, C.M., *et al.* (2003) B vitamin status and inflammatory markers. *Atherosclerosis* 169, 169–174.

Ford, E.S., Liu, S., Mannino, D.M., Giles, W.H. and Smith, S.J. (2003) C-reactive protein concentration and concentrations of blood vitamins, carotenoids, and selenium among United States adults. *European Journal of Clinical Nutrition* 57, 1157–1163.

Freese, R., Vaarala, O., Turpeinen, A.M. and Mutanen, M. (2004) No difference in platelet activation or inflammation markers after diets rich or poor in vegetables, berries and apple in healthy subjects. *European Journal of Nutrition* 43, 175–182.

Friso, S., Jacques, P.F., Wilson, P.W., Rosenberg, I.H. and Selhub, J. (2001) Low circulating vitamin B(6) is associated with elevation of the inflammation marker C-reactive protein independently of plasma homocysteine levels. *Circulation* 103, 2788–2791.

Friso, S., Girelli, D., Martinelli, N., Olivieri, O., Lotto, V., *et al.* (2004) Low plasma vitamin B-6 concentrations and modulation of coronary artery disease risk. *The American Journal of Clinical Nutrition* 79, 992–998.

Gao, X., Bermudez, O.I. and Tucker, K.L. (2004) Plasma C-reactive protein and homocysteine concentrations are related to frequent fruit and vegetable intake in Hispanic and non-Hispanic white elders. *The Journal of Nutrition* 134, 913–918.

Giugliano, D., Ceriello, A. and Esposito, K. (2006) The effects of diet on inflammation: emphasis on the metabolic syndrome. *Journal of the American College of Cardiology* 48, 677–685.

Hansson, G.K., Robertson, A.K. and Soderberg-Naucler, C. (2006) Inflammation and atherosclerosis. *Annual Review of Pathology* 1, 297–329.

Hartel, C., Strunk, T., Bucsky, P. and Schultz, C. (2004) Effects of vitamin C on intracytoplasmic cytokine production in human whole blood monocytes and lymphocytes. *Cytokine* 27, 101–106.

Haynes, W.G. (2002) Hyperhomocysteinemia, vascular function and atherosclerosis: effects of vitamins. *Cardiovascular Drugs and Therapy* 16, 391–399.

Hu, F.B. (2002) Dietary pattern analysis: a new direction in nutritional epidemiology. *Current Opinion in Lipidology* 13, 3–9.

Hu, F.B. and Willett, W.C. (2002) Optimal diets for prevention of coronary heart disease. *JAMA : the Journal of the American Medical Association* 288, 2569–2578.

Humphrey, L.L., Fu, R., Rogers, K., Freeman, M. and Helfand, M. (2008) Homocysteine level and coronary heart disease incidence: a systematic review and meta-analysis. *Mayo Clinic Proceedings. Mayo Clinic* 83, 1203–1212.

Jacques, P.F., Selhub, J., Bostom, A.G., Wilson, P.W. and Rosenberg, I.H. (1999) The effect of folic acid fortification on plasma folate and total homocysteine concentrations. *The New England Journal of Medicine* 340, 1449–1454.

Jessup, W., Kritharides, L. and Stocker, R. (2004) Lipid oxidation in atherogenesis: an overview. *Biochemical Society Transactions* 32, 134–138.

Kaptoge, S., Di Angelantonio, E., Lowe, G., Pepys, M.B., Thompson, S.G., *et al.* (2010) C-reactive protein concentration and risk of coronary heart disease, stroke, and mortality: an individual participant meta-analysis. *Lancet* 375, 132–140.

Kelley, D.S. and Bendich, A. (1996) Essential nutrients and immunologic functions. *The American Journal of Clinical Nutrition* 63, 994S–996S.

Kelley, D.S., Rasooly, R., Jacob, R.A., Kader, A.A. and Mackey, B.E. (2006) Consumption of Bing sweet cherries lowers circulating concentrations of inflammation markers in healthy men and women. *The Journal of Nutrition* 136, 981–986.

Klerk, M., Durga, J., Schouten, E.G., Kluft, C., Kok, F.J., *et al.* (2005) No effect of folic acid supplementation in the course of 1 year on haemostasis markers and C-reactive protein in older adults. *Thrombosis and Haemostasis* 94, 96–100.

Libby, P., Ridker, P.M. and Maseri, A. (2002) Inflammation and atherosclerosis. *Circulation* 105, 1135–1143.

Mangoni, A.A. (2006) Folic acid, inflammation, and atherosclerosis: false hopes or the need for better trials? *Clinica Chimica Acta; International Journal of Clinical Chemistry* 367, 11–19.

Mangoni, A.A., Arya, R., Ford, E., Asonganyi, B., Sherwood, R.A., *et al.* (2003) Effects of folic acid supplementation on inflammatory and thrombogenic markers in chronic smokers. A randomised controlled trial. *Thrombosis Research* 110, 13–17.

Mangoni, A.A., Sherwood, R.A., Asonganyi, B., Swift, C.G., Thomas, S., *et al.* (2005) Short-term oral folic acid supplementation enhances endothelial function in patients with type 2 diabetes. *American Journal of Hypertension* 18, 220–226.

Maron, D.J. (2004) Flavonoids for reduction of atherosclerotic risk. *Current Atherosclerosis Reports* 6, 73–78.

McCully, K.S. (1969) Vascular pathology of homocysteinemia: implications for the pathogenesis of arteriosclerosis. *The American Journal of Pathology* 56, 111–128.

Meydani, S.N., Ribaya-Mercado, J.D., Russell, R.M., Sahyoun, N., Morrow, F.D., *et al.* (1991) Vitamin B-6 deficiency impairs interleukin 2 production and lymphocyte proliferation in elderly adults. *The American Journal of Clinical Nutrition* 53, 1275–1280.

Nakou, E.S., Liberopoulos, E.N., Milionis, H.J. and Elisaf, M.S. (2008) The role of C-reactive protein in atherosclerotic cardiovascular disease: an overview. *Current Vascular Pharmacology* 6, 258–270.

Nelson, M. (1991) The validation of dietary assessments. In: Margetts, M.B. and Nelson, M. (eds) *Design Concepts in Nutritional Epidemiology*. Oxford Medical Publication, New York, pp. 241–272.

Ntaios, G., Savopoulos, C., Grekas, D. and Hatzitolios, A. (2009) The controversial role of B-vitamins in cardiovascular risk: An update. *Archives of Cardiovascular Diseases* 102, 847–854.

Ntaios, G.C., Savopoulos, C.G., Chatzinikolaou, A.C., Kaiafa, G.D. and Hatzitolios, A. (2008) Vitamins and stroke: the homocysteine hypothesis still in doubt. *The Neurologist* 14, 2–4.

Oliveira, A., Rodriguez-Artalejo, F. and Lopes, C. (2009) The association of fruits, vegetables, antioxidant vitamins and fibre intake with high-sensitivity C-reactive protein: sex and body mass index interactions. *European Journal of Clinical Nutrition* 63, 1345–1352.

Parikh, P., Mcdaniel, M.C., Ashen, M.D., Miller, J.I., Sorrentino, M., *et al.* (2005) Diets and cardiovascular disease: an evidence-based assessment. *Journal of the American College of Cardiology* 45, 1379–1387.

Pearson, T.A., Mensah, G.A., Alexander, R.W., Anderson, J.L., Cannon, R.O., 3rd, *et al.* (2003) Markers of inflammation and cardiovascular disease: application to clinical and public health practice: A statement for healthcare professionals from the Centers for Disease Control and Prevention and the American Heart Association. *Circulation* 107, 499–511.

Perez-Cruz, I., Carcamo, J.M. and Golde, D.W. (2003). Vitamin C inhibits FAS-induced apoptosis in monocytes and U937 cells. *Blood* 102, 336–343.

Rall, L.C. and Meydani, S.N. (1993) Vitamin B6 and immune competence. *Nutrition Reviews* 51, 217–225.

Reilly, M.P., Lehrke, M., Wolfe, M.L., Rohatgi, A., Lazar, M.A., *et al.* (2005) Resistin is an inflammatory marker of atherosclerosis in humans. *Circulation* 111, 932–939.

Ridker, P.M. (2007) Inflammatory biomarkers and risks of myocardial infarction, stroke, diabetes, and total mortality: implications for longevity. *Nutrition Reviews* 65, S253–S259.

Riso, P., Visioli, F., Grande, S., Guarnieri, S., Gardana, C., *et al.* (2006) Effect of a tomato-based drink on markers of inflammation, immunomodulation, and oxidative stress. *Journal of Agricultural and Food Chemistry* 54, 2563–2566.

Rizzo, M.R., Abbatecola, A.M., Barbieri, M., Vietri, M.T., Cioffi, M., *et al.* (2008) Evidence for anti-inflammatory effects of combined administration of vitamin E and C in older persons with impaired fasting glucose: impact on insulin action. *Journal of the American College of Nutrition* 27, 505–511.

Robinson, K., Arheart, K., Refsum, H., Brattstrom, L., Boers, G., *et al.* (1998) Low circulating folate and vitamin B6 concentrations: risk factors for stroke, peripheral vascular disease, and coronary artery disease. European COMAC Group. *Circulation* 97, 437–443.

Ross, R. (1999) Atherosclerosis-an inflammatory disease. *The New England Journal of Medicine* 340, 115–126.

Roubenoff, R., Roubenoff, R.A., Selhub, J., Nadeau, M.R., Cannon, J.G., *et al.* (1995) Abnormal vitamin B6 status in rheumatoid cachexia. Association with spontaneous tumor necrosis factor alpha production and markers of inflammation. *Arthritis and Rheumatism* 38, 105–109.

Saibeni, S., Cattaneo, M., Vecchi, M., Zighetti, M.L., Lecchi, A., *et al.* (2003) Low vitamin B(6) plasma levels, a risk factor for thrombosis, in inflammatory bowel disease: role of inflammation and correlation with acute phase reactants. *The American Journal of Gastroenterology* 98, 112–117.

Sanchez-Moreno, C., Cano, M.P., De Ancos, B., Plaza, L., Olmedilla, B., *et al.* (2003) High-pressurized orange juice consumption affects plasma vitamin C, antioxidative status and inflammatory markers in healthy humans. *The Journal of Nutrition* 133, 2204–2209.

Sanchez-Moreno, C., Cano, M.P., De Ancos, B., Plaza, L., Olmedilla, B., *et al.* (2004) Consumption of high-pressurized vegetable soup increases plasma vitamin C and decreases oxidative stress and inflammatory biomarkers in healthy humans. *The Journal of Nutrition* 134, 3021–3025.

Schulze, M.B. and Hoffmann, K. (2006) Methodological approaches to study dietary patterns in relation to risk of coronary heart disease and stroke. *The British Journal of Nutrition* 95, 860–869.

Shen, J., Lai, C.Q., Mattei, J., Ordovas, J.M. and Tucker, K.L. (2010) Association of vitamin B-6 status with inflammation, oxidative stress, and chronic inflammatory conditions: the Boston Puerto Rican Health Study. *The American Journal of Clinical Nutrition* 91, 337–342.

Silswal, N., Singh, A.K., Aruna, B., Mukhopadhyay, S., Ghosh, S., *et al.* (2005) Human resistin stimulates the pro-inflammatory cytokines TNF-alpha and IL-12 in macrophages by NF-kappaB-dependent pathway. *Biochemical and Biophysical Research Communications* 334, 1092–1101.

Sitzer, M., Markus, H.S., Mendall, M.A., Liehr, R., Knorr, U., *et al.* (2002) C-reactive protein and carotid intimal medial thickness in a community population. *Journal of Cardiovascular Risk* 9, 97–103.

Talaulikar, V.S. and Manyonda, I.T. (2011) Vitamin C as an antioxidant supplement in women's health: a myth in need of urgent burial. *European Journal of Obstetrics, Gynecology, and Reproductive Biology,* 157, 10–13.

Tice, J.A., Ross, E., Coxson, P.G., Rosenberg, I., Weinstein, M.C., *et al.* (2001) Cost-effectiveness of vitamin therapy to lower plasma homocysteine levels for the prevention of coronary heart disease: effect of grain fortification and beyond. *JAMA : the Journal of the American Medical Association* 286, 936–943.

Ullegaddi, R., Powers, H.J. and Gariballa, S.E. (2004) B-group vitamin supplementation mitigates oxidative damage after acute ischaemic stroke. *Clinical science (London)* 107, 477–484.

Valtuena, S., Pellegrini, N., Franzini, L., Bianchi, M.A., Ardigo, D., *et al.* (2008) Food selection based on total antioxidant capacity can modify antioxidant intake, systemic inflammation, and liver function without altering markers of oxidative stress. *The American Journal of Clinical Nutrition* 87, 1290–1297.

Van Herpen-Broekmans, W.M., Klopping-Ketelaars, I.A., Bots, M.L., Kluft, C., Princen, H., *et al.* (2004) Serum carotenoids and vitamins in relation to markers of endothelial function and inflammation. *European Journal of Epidemiology* 19, 915–921.

Vermeulen, E.G., Rauwerda, J.A., Van Den Berg, M., De Jong, S.C., Schalkwijk, C., *et al.* (2003) Homocysteine-lowering treatment with folic acid plus vitamin B6 lowers urinary albumin excretion but not plasma markers of endothelial function or C-reactive protein: further analysis of secondary endpoints of a randomized clinical trial. *European Journal of Clinical Investigation* 33, 209–215.

Wald, D.S., Law, M. and Morris, J.K. (2002) Homocysteine and cardiovascular disease: evidence on causality from a meta-analysis. *Bristish Medical Journal* 325, 1202.

Wannamethee, S.G., Lowe, G.D., Rumley, A., Bruckdorfer, K.R. and Whincup, P.H. (2006) Associations of vitamin C status, fruit and vegetable intakes, and markers of inflammation and hemostasis. *The American Journal of Clinical Nutrition* 83, 567–574.

Watzl, B., Kulling, S.E., Moseneder, J., Barth, S.W. and Bub, A. (2005) A 4-wk intervention with high intake of carotenoid-rich vegetables and fruit reduces plasma C-reactive protein in healthy, nonsmoking men. *The American Journal of Clinical Nutrition* 82, 1052–1058.

Willett, W.C. (1998) *Nutritional Epidemiology.* Oxford University Press, New York.

Williams, K.J. and Tabas, I. (1998) The response-to-retention hypothesis of atherogenesis reinforced. *Current Opinion in Lipidology* 9, 471–474.

8 Phytonutrients and Inflammation

D. Heber*
UCLA Center for Human Nutrition, Los Angeles, California, USA

Introduction

International epidemiological studies suggest, but do not prove, that consistently higher intakes of fruits, vegetables, whole grains and plant proteins are associated with a markedly reduced risk of cancer, heart disease and chronic diseases of ageing (World Cancer Research Fund, 1997). Recent studies of hunter–gatherer populations in the outback of Australia have revealed that these individuals ate more than 800 different varieties of plant based foods (Cordain *et al.*, 2000) but, when they moved into urban areas and begin eating so-called 'street foods', they began to develop nutritional deficiencies and common chronic diseases of ageing (Lee, 1996).

Epidemiological and anthropological observations can, however, only provide evidence of association and not prove causality.

* Author, dheber@mednet.ucla.edu

Both experimental and clinical intervention studies of phytonutrients in modifying inflammation have been conducted to examine the hypothesis that increased intake of phytonutrients can modify inflammation. Ageing is associated with an increased risk of chronic disease and a decline in adaptive immune function (Mahbub *et al.*, 2011). Inflammation can occur, however, as the result of abdominal obesity combined with a reduced intake of fruits and vegetables (Temple, 2000). The changes in immune function with ageing have been called both 'inflammaging' and immunosenescence (Willett, 1994). Dietary studies are therefore complex and can be confounded by uncontrolled variables. It is not clear whether the inflammation seen with ageing is due to the ageing process itself or is secondary to obesity and reduced intake of phytonutrients with anti-inflammatory properties. It is clear, however, that many phytonutrients have anti-inflammatory activity and may help support immune function during ageing based on evidence from studies in cell culture, with animal models and a limited number of studies in humans.

Antioxidant and Anti-inflammatory Actions of Phytonutrients

Mechanisms of antioxidant effects

Fruits, vegetables and grains contain thousands of phytonutrients. Many of these are either absorbed into the body from the gastrointestinal tract or further metabolized by commensal bacteria to absorbable phytonutrients. Phytonutrients are commonly called antioxidants, on the basis of their ability to trap singlet oxygen.

Oxidant stress and radical oxygen species

The production of radical oxygen species endogenously, as a result of normal oxidative metabolic reactions and by external forces, can damage biological structures and molecules including lipids, protein and DNA in a chain reaction. Ageing increases endogenous oxygen radical production from the mitochondria and can be associated with a decreased enzymatic component of oxidant defence. Increased physical activity generates free radicals as a result of increased oxygen consumption during exercise. Ultraviolet radiation, infection, trauma and pollutants are all potential stimulants of oxidant stress and inflammation. Environmental pollutants are sources for free radicals including nitrogen dioxide, ozone, cigarette smoke, radiation, halogenated hydrocarbons, heavy metals and certain pesticides.

The antioxidant network

There is evidence that antioxidants can help prevent this damage under certain circumstances. There are robust and multiple defence mechanisms against this outcome within all living organisms including both enzymatic and chemical components that prevent radical formation, remove radicals before damage can occur, repair oxidative damage, eliminate damaged molecules and prevent mutations (Blot *et al.*, 1993).

Cells contain a number of antioxidants that have various roles in protecting against free radical reactions. The major water-soluble antioxidant metabolites are glutathione (GSH) and vitamin C, which reside primarily in the cytoplasm and mitochondria. Many water-soluble enzymes also catalyse these reactions. Glutathione peroxidase catalyses the reaction between GSH and hydrogen peroxide to form water and oxidized glutathione, which is stable. Vitamin E and the carotenoids are the principal lipid-soluble antioxidants. Vitamin E is the major lipid-soluble antioxidant in cell membranes that can break the chain of lipid peroxidation (Gordon, 1996). Vitamin E is recycled by a reaction with vitamin C: vitamin C quenches free radicals in aqueous systems but also regenerates cellular vitamin E, which helps to control lipid peroxidation. Beta carotene also traps free radicals in concert with vitamin E.

Polyphenols occur widely in plants and flavonoids occur in all plant foods. This broad class of compounds includes flavonols, flavones, isoflavones, flavonones, flavanol and anthocyanins. Polyphenols comprise the most frequent and highest dose of phytonutrients ingested daily. They are an important component of the antioxidant network but there is a need for much more research on their mechanisms of action.

Studies investigating the antioxidant properties of phytosterols can be misleading for several reasons. First, the cells of the body maintain exquisite antioxidant balance through the molecular induction of antioxidant defence enzymes. It is difficult to show the impact of dietary antioxidant administration on cells in the body owing to these endogenous defences. In addition, *in vitro* cell assays can be misleading. For example, vitamin C can become a pro-oxidant *in vitro* and produce hydrogen peroxide in adequate amounts to kill cells (Doll and Peto, 1981). In human plasma there are also large amounts of uric acid that also acts as an antioxidant. It is therefore difficult to show changes in plasma antioxidant activity with intake of antioxidant phytonutrients. There are many inconsistencies in the scientific literature in this respect. Finally, the oxygen radical absorbing capacity (ORAC) of various fruits and vegetables is a property of foods in a test tube, but does not consider the bioavailability, metabolism and pharmacokinetics of phytonutrients ingested within a matrix of a fruit, vegetable or grain.

Phytonutrient functions beyond antioxidation

There are complementary and overlapping mechanisms of phytonutrient action, including modulation of detoxification enzymes, stimulation of the immune system, reduction of platelet aggregation, modulation of cholesterol synthesis and hormone metabolism, reduction of blood pressure, and antibacterial and antiviral effects. Phytonutrients also often interact with the host to stimulate, suppress or modulate enzyme activities important in DNA repair, detoxification and cell metabolism. Phytonutrients interact with nuclear receptors and impact cellular signalling involved in cell proliferation and apoptosis. They can also act as oxygen radical scavengers to reduce proliferation and protect DNA from damage (Lampe, 1999). Phytonutrients, unlike drugs, have multiple mechanisms of action that complicate their study in traditional reductionist study designs. Furthermore, it is common for phytonutrients to interact in additive, synergistic or antagonistic ways (Clement *et al.*, 2001).

Although many of the cellular and molecular effects of phytonutrients have been examined primarily in animal and cell-culture models, experimental dietary studies in humans have also shown the capacity of vegetables and fruits and their constituents to modulate some potential disease-preventive mechanisms (Adams *et al.*, 2006).

Mechanisms of anti-inflammatory effects

Components of the cell-signalling network, especially those that converge on the ubiquitous eukaryotic redox-sensitive transcription factor, nuclear factor-kappa B (NFκB), have been implicated in the pathogenesis of many inflammation-associated disorders. A wide variety of phytonutrients can alter or correct undesirable cellular functions caused by abnormal pro-inflammatory signal transmissions, mediated by NFκB. The modulation of cellular signalling involved in chronic inflammatory responses, induced by anti-inflammatory phytonutrients, has been studied extensively using cancer cell models and animals bearing tumours. Induction of phase-2 detoxifying or antioxidant genes represents an important cellular defence in response to oxidative and electrophilic insults. Nuclear transcription factor erythroid 2p45 (NF-E2)-related factor 2 (Nrf2) plays a crucial role in regulating phase-2 detoxifying/antioxidant gene induction. Many antioxidant phytonutrients have been found to activate this particular redox-sensitive transcription factor, thereby potentiating the cellular antioxidant or detoxification capacity. Figures 8.1 and 8.2 show the various subcellular signalling systems involved in inflammation that may be affected by phytonutrients.

Key Dietary Phytonutrients

Flavonoids

Flavonoids and their polymers form a large class of food constituents and are a subclass of polyphenols (Fig. 8.3) that are further divided

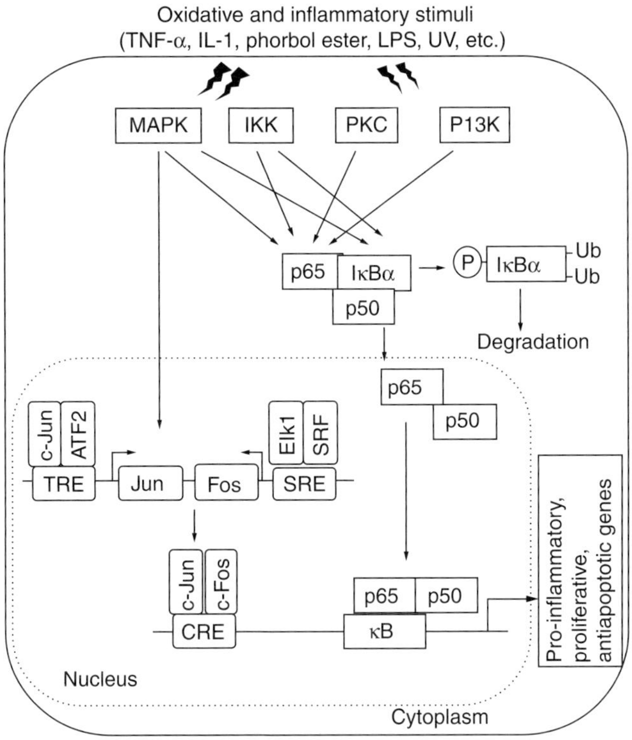

Fig. 8.1. The NFκB and AP-1 mediated signalling pathway. Exposure of cells to oxidative and pro-inflammatory stimuli causes activation of a series of upstream kinases such as MAPKs, IKK, PKC and PI3K, which then activate NFκB by phosphorylation-mediated degradation of IκBα. Activated upstream kinases may also phosphorylate p65, the active subunit of NFκB. Free activated NFκB, in the form of the p65–p50 heterodimer, translocates to the nucleus, where it binds to κB sequences located in the promoter of a target gene. Alternatively, MAPKs can activate the AP-1 components, c-Jun and c-Fos, leading to the binding of AP-1 (c-Jun–c-Fos heterodimer) to the cyclic AMP response element (CRE) sequences of the target gene promoter. (From Surh *et al.*, 2005, with permission from the American Society of Nutrition.)

into subclasses on the basis of their chemical structure. More than 60 years ago, extracts of foods presumably containing flavonoids were shown to have beneficial biological properties (Epstein, 2001). Although these early results were not corroborated, modulation of many biological systems by flavonoids, tannins and other phytonutrients has been demonstrated by many investigators (Berg and Daniel, 1988). These polyphenolic compounds represent one of the most prevalent classes of compounds in vegetables, nuts, fruits and beverages such as coffee, tea and red wine (Middleton and Kandaswami, 1993). However, what may be more important than the total flavonoid content of a food is the content of flavonoid and tannin subclasses. For example, soy and soy-based foods are unique sources of isoflavones, whereas tea is rich in catechins, and each seems to confer unique health-related biological properties.

The average total intake of flavonoids in the USA has been estimated to be 1 g/day (Hollman and Katan, 1997; Kuhnau, 1976), but recent studies have indicated that the intake varies widely (Scalbert and Williamson, 2000). More than 8000 compounds with a flavonoid structure have been identified. The classes of flavonoids include flavones, flavonols, flavanones, flavanols, anthocyanins and isoflavones (Fig. 8.3). The flavonoid natural products exert a wide range of biochemical and pharmacological properties, with one of the most investigated effects

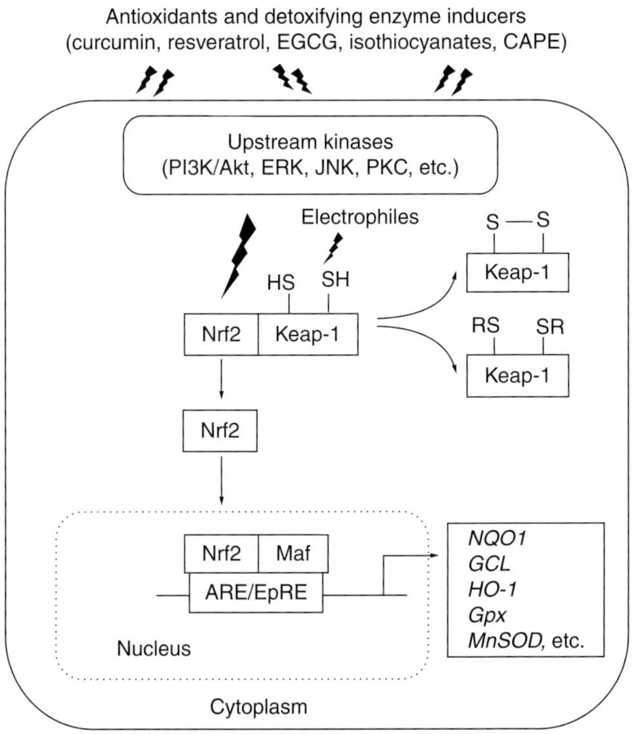

Fig. 8.2. Activation of Nrf2 signalling and induction of phase II detoxifying and antioxidant genes. The transcription factor Nrf2 is kept sequestered in the cytoplasm as an inactive complex with its cytosolic repressor Keap-1. Chemopreventive phytochemicals activate diverse upstream kinases, which in turn stimulate dissociation of Nrf2 from Keap-1. Alternatively, electrophiles generated endogenously or from chemopreventive phytochemicals can facilitate dissociation of Nrf2 from Keap-1 by either oxidation (forming disulfide bonds –S–S–) or covalent modification (RS) of cysteine thiols of Keap-1. Once released from Keap-1 repression, Nrf2 translocates to the nucleus, forms a heterodimer with small Maf protein, and binds to the ARE/EpRE sequences located in the promoter region of genes encoding antioxidant and detoxifying enzymes. (From Surh *et al.*, 2005, with permission from the American Society of Nutrition.)

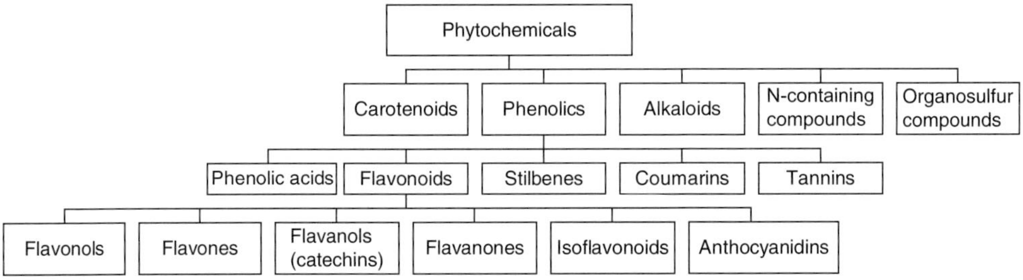

Fig. 8.3. Classes of phytochemicals.

being their cancer preventive activities. The cancer protective effects of flavonoids have been attributed to a wide variety of mechanisms, including free-radical scavenging, modifying enzymes that activate or detoxify carcinogens, and inhibiting the induction of the transcription factor activator protein-1 (AP-1) activity by tumour promoters (Canivenc-Lavier *et al.*, 1996; Beecher, 2003). Flavonoids also have inhibitory effects on the activities of many enzymes, including β-glucuronidase (Kim *et al.*, 1994), lipoxygenase (Laughton *et al.*, 1991; Schewe *et al.*, 2002), cyclooxygenase (Raso *et al.*, 2001), inducible nitric oxide synthase (Raso *et al.*, 2001), monooxygenase (Siess *et al.*, 1995), thyroid peroxidase (Doerge and Chang, 2002) and xanthine oxidase (Sheu *et al.*, 1998).

Anthocyanins

The anthocyanins are very widespread in more than 25 families of plant foods, and provide red, blue and purple colours to berries, cherries, grapes, rhubarb and plums. They are of great nutritional interest because of the marked daily intake of 180–215 mg/day in the USA, with more consumed during summer months (Hertog *et al.*, 1993a). Similar to most other flavanoids, anthocyanins occur naturally in fruits and vegetables as glycosides. The de-glycosylated or aglycone forms of anthocyanins are known as anthocyanidins.

These bioactive compounds have several effects on human health. The natural electron deficiency of anthocyanins makes these compounds particularly reactive as free-radical scavengers, as well as acting indirectly through antioxidant actions that protect DNA from damage. Other activities include the regulation of enzymes important in metabolizing xenobiotics and carcinogens, and the modulation of nuclear receptors, gene expression and sub-cellular signalling pathways of proliferation, angiogenesis and apoptosis (Zafra-Stone *et al.*, 2007).

Green tea polyphenols

Tea is one of the most popular beverages in the world. The beneficial effects of green tea are attributed to the polyphenolic compounds present in green tea, particularly the catechins, which make up 30% of the dry weight of green tea leaves (Graham, 1992). These catechins are present in higher quantities in green tea than in black or oolong tea, because of differences in the processing of tea leaves after harvest. For green tea, fresh tea leaves from the plant *Camellia sinensis* are steamed and dried to inactivate the polyphenol oxidase enzyme, a process that essentially maintains the polyphenols in their monomeric forms. Black tea, on the other hand, is produced by extended fermentation of tea leaves, which results in the polymeric compounds thearubigins and theaflavins.

Green tea and its constituent catechins are best known for their antioxidant properties, which have led to their evaluation in a number of diseases associated with reactive oxygen species, such as cancer, cardiovascular and neurodegenerative diseases. The consumption of tea has been associated with a decreased risk of developing cancer of the ovary (Zhang *et al.*, 2002), oral cavity (Hsu *et al.*, 2002), colon (Su and Arab, 2002) and stomach (Setiawan *et al.*, 2001). This beneficial health effect has been attributed to the catechins in tea, with their strong antioxidant and anti-angiogenic activity as well as their potential to inhibit cell proliferation and modulate carcinogen metabolism (Demeule *et al.*, 2002; Kazi *et al.*, 2002).

Green tea has also shown to be hypocholesterolemic (Yang and Koo, 2000) and to prevent the development of atherosclerotic plaques (Chyu *et al.*, 2004). Among age-associated pathologies and neurodegenerative diseases, green tea has been shown to afford significant protection against Parkinson's disease, Alzheimer's disease and ischaemic damage (Mandel and Youdin, 2004). Green tea has also shown anti-diabetic effects in animal models of insulin resistance (Wu *et al.*, 2004) and has been shown to promote energy expenditure (Dulloo *et al.*, 1999).

Soy isoflavones

Soy protein is the highest quality protein found in the plant kingdom, and it is eaten by two thirds of the world's population. Interest in soy proteins and cancer prevention arose from the observation that naturally occurring phytonutrients within soy protein – the isoflavones genistein and daidzein – were able to inhibit the growth of both oestrogen-receptor positive and negative breast cancer cells *in vitro* (Peterson and Barnes, 1996). In addition, studies of populations eating soy protein indicate that they have a lower incidence of breast cancer and other common cancers compared with populations such as the US population where soy foods are rarely eaten. These studies provide only supportive evidence for a positive role of soy foods, because the diets of the populations eating more soy protein are also richer in fruits, vegetables and whole cereals and grains in comparison with the US diet.

Genistein and daidzein are phytoestrogens that antagonize the actions of estradiol in the breast and the uterus but demonstrate oestrogen-like beneficial activities in the bone, on serum lipids and in the brain. These observations are explained by the existence of two oestrogen receptors called alpha and beta. Soy isoflavones bind with very low affinity (1/50,000 to 1/100,000 the affinity of oestradiol) to the alpha-oestradiol receptor, but bind equally well to the beta-oestradiol receptor (Clarkson *et al.*, 2001).

Soy protein isoflavones have been shown to influence not only sex hormone metabolism and biological activity but also intracellular enzymes, protein synthesis, growth factor action, malignant cell proliferation, differentiation and angiogenesis, providing strong evidence that these substances might have a protective role in cancer (Kim *et al.*, 2002).

Soy food intake has also been shown to have beneficial effects on cardiovascular disease, although data directly linking soy food intake to clinical outcomes of cardiovascular disease have been sparse. A recent study among the participants of the Shanghai Women's Health Study, a population-based prospective cohort study of approximately 75,000 Chinese women, documented a dose–response relationship between soy food intake and risk of coronary heart disease, providing direct evidence that soy food consumption may reduce the risk of coronary heart disease in women.

Glucosinolates and allyl sulfides

Cruciferous vegetable consumption has been associated with a reduced risk of cancer of the lung, stomach, colon and rectum. The health benefit of cruciferous vegetables such as broccoli, Brussels sprouts, cabbage and bok choy have been attributed to their high concentration of glucosinolates, which are found in significant amounts in these vegetables. These compounds are normally chemically conjugated to sugar residues and are stable. When the plant cell is crushed or chewed, however, myrosinase enzymes are activated and break these stabilized chemical structures to yield volatile and highly reactive compounds such as isothiocyanate. The body normally detoxifies itself in two steps so that it can get rid of these compounds. Phase I enzymes add an electron to the compound and Phase II enzymes catalyse a reaction that links a sugar or sulfate residue on the activated toxin so that it becomes water soluble and is excreted in the urine. Isothiocyanates act as anticarcinogens by inducing Phase II conjugating enzymes, in particular glutathione S-tranferases (GSTs), which metabolize isothiocyanates (Finley, 2003).

Many studies have reported the beneficial effects on health of consuming garlic. Garlic has a high concentration of sulfur-containing compounds. The thiosulfinates, including allicin, seem to be the active substances in garlic. Allicin is formed when alliin, a sulfur-containing amino acid, comes into contact with the enzyme alliinase when raw garlic is chopped, crushed or chewed. The antimicrobial, hypolipidemic, antioxidant, and antithrombotic effects that have been attributed to garlic are thought to be related to allicin and other breakdown products.

Many randomized clinical trials have studied the effects of garlic on lipid levels. Results from two meta-analyses (Warshafsky *et al.*, 1993; Silagy and Neil, 1994) of garlic's effect on total cholesterol show a significant reduction in total cholesterol levels (9–12%) compared with placebo. More recently, additional trials have been published, with conflicting results (Saradeth *et al.*, 1994; Neil *et al.*, 1996; Berthold *et al.*, 1998; Isaacsohn *et al.*, 1998). However, a meta-analysis published in 2000 (Stevinson *et al.*, 2000) that included these trials concluded that garlic is superior to placebo in reducing total cholesterol levels, but that the extent of the effect is modest (4–6%). A recent review of ten trials assessing the effect of garlic on thrombotic risk showed modest but significant decreases in platelet aggregation with garlic compared with placebo (Ackermann, 2001).

The sulfur compounds inhibit cell proliferation of cancer cells, modulate cell-cycle activity and interfere with hormone action in cancer cells (Hirsch *et al.*, 2000; Munday and Munday, 2001; Nakagawa *et al.*, 2001; Pinto and Rivlin, 2001). Allicin is the major ingredient in crushed garlic and has been shown to inhibit the proliferation of human mammary, endometrial and colon cancer cells (Hirsch *et al.*, 2000).

Carotenoids

Carotenoids comprise a class of natural fat-soluble pigments that are found in many red, deep green and orange/yellow coloured fruits and vegetables. Their major biochemical functions are determined by the extended system of conjugated double bonds, which is also responsible for their colour (Britton, 1995). The orange/yellow colour of many fruits and vegetables can be seen when the carotenoid-containing chromoplasts are usually devoid of chlorophyll, but considerable amounts are also present in green parts of the plants where chlorophyll masks the carotenoids. The most prominent carotenes are β-carotene, α-carotene and lycopene; zeaxanthin and lutein, α-and β-cryptoxanthin, canthaxanthin and astaxanthin are structurally different carotenoids that exist to a lesser extent in foods.

Tomatoes and tomato products, including ketchup, tomato juice, salsa and pasta sauce, are the richest sources of lycopene in the American diet, accounting for more than three quarters of the total lycopene intake of Americans (Minorsky, 2002). Several studies have linked the consumption of tomatoes and tomato products with a decreased risk of cancer and cardiovascular disease. The health benefits of lycopene have been attributed to its antioxidant properties, although other mechanisms of lycopene action are possible, including the modulation of intercellular communication, hormonal and immune system changes, and alterations of metabolic pathways (Rao and Agarwal, 2000). In breast cancer cells, lycopene can interfere with insulin-like growth factor 1–stimulated tumour cell proliferation (Karas *et al*, 2000).

The relationship between lycopene intake and prostate cancer risk has been reported and supported by studies linking low plasma levels of lycopene with increased risk (Giovannucci *et al.*, 1995, 2002; Gann *et al*, 1999). Lycopene administration may reduce proliferation and increase apoptosis in human prostate tissue where lycopene is the predominant carotenoid (Kucuk *et al.*, 1999).

Lutein and zeaxanthin are xanthophyll carotenoids found particularly in dark-green leafy vegetables. They are widely distributed in tissues and are the principal carotenoids in the eye lens and macular region of the retina. Epidemiologic studies indicating an inverse relationship between xanthophyll intake or status and both cataract and age-related macular degeneration (ARMD) suggest these compounds can play a protective role in the eye.

ARMD is a major cause of irreversible blindness among the elderly in the Western world, affecting about 20% of the population above the age of 65 (Khachik *et al*, 2002). Lutein and zeaxanthin are the pigments responsible for the coloration of the macula lutea ('yellow spot') of the retina, which is the area of maximal visual acuity. Lutein and zeaxanthin are essential for maintaining the proper anatomy and function of the retina. Epidemiological data support the concept that the macular pigments have a protective role. According to the Eye Disease Case-Control Study, subjects with the highest quintile of carotenoid intake had a 43% reduced risk of ARMD compared with subjects in the lowest quintile (Seddon *et al.*, 1994) and lower levels of lutein and zeaxanthin have been reported in the retina from donors suffering from ARMD (Bone *et al.*, 2001).There is also some evidence from a small intervention study that visual function is improved in patients suffering from atrophic AMD when lutein alone or lutein together with other nutrients is supplemented (Richer *et al.*, 2004). Supplementation studies have shown that subjects who are able to modify their diet through increased intake of spinach and corn can experience significant increases in plasma levels of lutein and macular pigment density within 4 weeks

(Hammond *et al.*, 1997). Some observational studies have also shown these xanthophylls may help reduce the risk of certain types of cancer, particularly those of the breast and lung. Emerging studies also suggest a potential contribution of lutein and zeaxanthin to the prevention of heart disease and stroke.

Phytonutrients and Human Health

Phytonutrients in the prevention of cancer

There is evidence which associates increased intake of fruit and vegetable with a reduced risk of cancers of the lung, colon, breast, cervix, oesophagus, oral cavity, stomach, bladder, pancreas and ovary (Block *et al.*, 1992). Many of these cancers have been associated with chronic inflammation. In order for a tumour to grow, it must grow its own blood supply through angiogenesis, which results from the secretion by endothelial cells of vascular endothelial growth factor (VEGF). Chronic inflammation contributes to cancer not only as a consequence of a direct effect of pro-inflammatory mediators on cellular signalling but also by creating a state of oxidative stress. The transformed cells are often surrounded by innate immune cells, inflammatory macrophages, fibroblasts and endothelial cells, which release a distinct set of pro-inflammatory mediators and hence exacerbate the generation of reactive oxygen species (Coussens and Werb, 2002). This can create a vicious loop between oxidative stress and inflammation, which in turn favours tumourigenesis. Carcinogenesis provides a multistep process that can be explored to elucidate the anti-inflammatory effects of phytonutrients.

Phytonutrients found in fruits and vegetables can affect the above processes by several mechanisms. Free-radical damage, which induces oxidative stress, can cause DNA damage that in turn can lead to base mutation, DNA cross-linking, and chromosomal breakage and rearrangement. This damage may be limited by dietary antioxidants in fruits and vegetables through the modulation of detoxification enzymes, scavenging of oxidative agents, stimulation of the immune system, hormone metabolism, and regulation of gene expression in cell proliferation and apoptosis (Dragsted *et al.*, 1993; Pool-Zobel *et al.*, 1998; Singh *et al.*, 2002).

Phytonutrients in the prevention of cardiovascular disease

There is a large body of observational (epidemiological, case-control, or prospective and retrospective cohort) evidence on the relationship between inflammation and the risk for cardiovascular disease. Oxidized low-density lipoprotein (LDL) has been proposed as an atherogenic factor in heart disease, promoting cholesterol ester accumulation and stimulation of phagocytosis by macrophages with subsequent foam cell formation (Berliner *et al.*, 1997; Witzum and Berliner, 1998). Dietary antioxidants from fruits and vegetables become incorporated into LDL, becoming oxidized themselves, thus preventing oxidation of polyunsaturated fatty acids on phospholipids. Phytonutrients have other effects indirectly related to inflammation including reducing platelet aggregation, modulation of cholesterol synthesis and absorption and reducing blood pressure (Sanchez-Moreno *et al.*, 2000). C-reactive protein, an inflammatory marker, may be a stronger predictor of cardiovascular disease than LDL cholesterol (Ridker *et al.*, 2002) and the anti-inflammatory activity of phytonutrients may play an important role in heart health.

Studies have shown an inverse correlation between death from myocardial infarction and vitamin E intake (Stephens *et al.*, 1996), an inverse correlation between vitamin C and carotid wall thickness (Kritchevsky *et al.*, 1995), and an inverse correlation between carotenoids and myocardial infarction (Street *et al.*, 1994). Vitamin C deficiency may be associated with an increased risk of myocardial infarction (Nyyssonen *et al.*, 1997), whereas dietary intake of flavonoids (30 mg/day) is correlated with 50% reduction in cardiovascular disease mortality when compared with an intake of 19 mg/day (Hertog *et al.*, 1993b).

Plant-rich diets and weight management

Abdominal obesity has been shown to be associated with systemic inflammation. To date, there is no evidence that increasing fruits and vegetables without making other changes in the diet will impact body fat or body weight (Tohill *et al.*, 2004). Ongoing research is, however, investigating the impact of specific dietary patterns and physical activity on energetics and obesity. The contribution of specific macronutrients to satiety, especially the impact of increased dietary protein intake together high volume/ low calorific density fruits and vegetables, might provide an additional key to controlling energy intake. Fruits and vegetables are high in water and fibre, and are 10–20-fold less calorie dense than grains. Although promoting satiety and decreasing energy intake, plant foods also provide a rich supply of micronutrients, a wealth of phytonutrients, increased amounts of dietary fibre compared with refined grains and a balance of omega-3 and omega-6 fatty acids. Evidence suggests that increasing these foods while decreasing total energy intake is an effective strategy for weight management (Rolls *et al.*, 2005). Although obesity is often considered synonymous with overnutrition, the dietary patterns of overweight and obese individuals might be more accurately depicted as overnutrition of calories but undernutrition of many essential vitamins, minerals and phytonutrients. The increased incidence of obesity has been associated with an increased incidence of heart disease, breast cancer, prostate cancer and colon cancer in comparison with populations eating a dietary pattern consisting of less meat and more fruits, vegetables, cereals and whole grains (Willett, 1994, 1995; Temple, 2000).

Several studies have sought to characterize dietary patterns and relate these patterns to body weight and other nutritional parameters. A prospective study of 737 non-overweight women in the Framingham Offspring/Spouse cohort examined the relationship between dietary patterns and the development of overweight over a 12-year period. Participants were grouped into one of five dietary patterns at baseline: (i) a heart-healthy pattern (low fat, nutritionally varied); (ii) light eating pattern (lower calories, but proportionately more fat and fewer micronutrients); (iii) wine and moderate eating pattern; (iv) high fat pattern; and (v) empty calorie pattern (rich in sweets and fat, and low in fruits and vegetables). Women in the heart-healthy cluster consumed more servings of vegetables and fruits than women in each of the other four clusters. During the 12-year period, 214 cases of overweight developed in this cohort. Compared with women in the heart-healthy group, women in the empty calorie group were at a significantly higher risk for becoming overweight (Quatromoni *et al.*, 2002).

In another analysis of dietary patterns among 179 older rural adults, those in the high-nutrient-dense cluster (higher intake of dark green/yellow vegetables, citrus/melons/ berries, and other fruits and vegetables) had lower energy intakes and lower waist circumferences than those in the low-nutrient-dense cluster (higher intake of breads, sweets, desserts, processed meats, eggs, fats and oil). Those with a low-nutrient-dense pattern were twice as likely to be obese (Ledikewe *et al.*, 2004). Similar observations were reported utilizing data from the Canadian Community Health Survey from 2000–2001. The frequency of eating fruits and vegetables was positively related to being physically active and not being overweight (Perez, 2002).

In a controlled clinical trial, families with obese parents and non-obese children were randomized into either a comprehensive behavioural weight management programme that featured encouragement to increase fruit and vegetable consumption or to decrease intake of high-fat, high-sugar foods. During a 1-year period, parents in the increased fruit and vegetable group showed significantly greater decreases in percentage of being overweight than in the group attempting to reduce fat and sugar (Epstein, 2001).

Summary and Conclusions

Phytonutrients from different plants can interact to inhibit inflammation (e.g. soy isoflavones and green tea catechins). It has also been proposed that the additive and synergistic effects of phytonutrients in fruits and vegetables are responsible for their antioxidant and anticancer activities, and that the benefit of plant-based diets is attributed in part to the complex mixture of phytonutrients present in whole foods (Eberhardt *et al.*, 2000; Dhu *et al.*, 2002; Sun *et al.*, 2002). Clearly, no single antioxidant can replace the natural combination of thousands of phytonutrients that exist in whole foods. Given the history of diverse intake of plant foods by humans, it is sensible to encourage a diverse intake. The exact amounts of fruits and vegetables needed each day to minimize the risks of chronic diseases of ageing resulting from inflammation are not known and will require a great deal of additional research. The benefits of fruits and vegetables on the dietary pattern and the evidence of benefit suggest, however, that it is not premature to advise an increased intake of a variety of colourful fruits and vegetables.

Humans and a few primate species have trichromatic colour vision so that they are able to distinguish red from green (Dominy and Lucas, 2001). All other mammals have dichromatic vision and cannot distinguish between the two colours. One hypothesis for the evolution of this visual ability was that it provided an advantage by enabling primates to distinguish red fruits from the green background of forest leaves. Today colours are still used to promote food choices and contrasting colours have been shown to be one of the key factors in food selection (Drewnowski, 1996). Many individuals eat only two to three servings per day of fruits and vegetables without regard to the phytonutrient contents of the foods being eaten. Certain phytonutrients give fruits and vegetables their colours and also indicate their unique physiological roles. All of the colored phytonutrients that absorb light in the visible spectrum have antioxidant properties (Kahkonen *et al.*, 1999). In artificial membrane systems, it is possible to show synergistic interactions of lutein and lycopene in antioxidant capacity and there are well-known antioxidant interactions of vitamin C and vitamin E based on their solubilities in hydrophilic and hydrophobic compartments of cells (Sander *et al.*, 2004).

Current dietary recommendations from the National Cancer Institute in the USA emphasize increasing the daily consumption of fruits and vegetables from diverse sources such as citrus fruits, cruciferous vegetables, and green and yellow vegetables (Steinmetz and Potter, 1996). A method for selecting fruits and vegetables on the basis of colours keyed to the content of phytonutrients is a way of translating the science of phytonutrient nutrition into dietary guidelines for the public (Heber and Bowerman, 2001). It can also help consumers change dietary patterns to include more fruits and vegetables by including one serving from each of the seven colour groups each day (Table 8.1).

Although the colour method may be superior to the current system of simply encouraging increased fruit and vegetable intakes, it does not account for actual phytonutrient delivery to the consumer. Today, there is no labelling law that requires fruit and vegetable

Table 8.1. Colour code groups of fruits and vegetables.

Colour	Phytochemical	Fruits and vegetables
Red	Lycopene	Tomatoes and tomato products (soups, juice, pasta sauce), watermelon, pink grapefruit
Red/purple	Anthocyanins and polyphenols	Berries, grapes, red wine
Orange	α- and β-Carotene	Carrots, mangoes, pumpkin
Orange/yellow	β-Cryptoxanthin and flavonoids	Cantaloupe, peaches, oranges, papaya
Yellow/green	Lutein and zeaxanthin	Spinach, avocado, honeydew, kiwi, Romaine lettuce
Green	Glucosinolates and indoles	Broccoli, cabbage, cauliflower kale, Brussels sprouts
White/green	Allyl sulfides	Leeks, onion, garlic, chives

manufacturers to list the phytonutrients in their products. Furthermore, fruits and vegetables are developed and grown more for the need to transport them over long distances and extend their shelf life rather than for their flavour or nutritional content. Research in this area needs to continue on the more than 25,000 phytonutrients provided by fruits and vegetables. These important phytonutrients are widely distributed among different plant species, but the delivery of phytonutrients and their effects on biomarkers relevant to health promotion and disease prevention need to be documented.

References

Ackermann, R.T., Mulrow, C.D., Ramirez, G., Gardner, C.D., Morbidoni, L., *et al.* (2001) Garlic shows promise for improving some cardiovascular risk factors. *Archives of Internal Medicine* 161, 813–824.

Adams, L.S., Seeram, N.P., Hardy, M.L., Carpenter, C., Heber, D. (2006) Analysis of the interactions of botanical extract combinations against the viability of prostate cancer cell lines. *Evidence Based Complementary and Alternative Medicine* 3, 117–124.

Beecher, G.R. (2003) Overview of dietary flavonoids: nomenclature, occurrence and intake. *Journal of Nutrition* 133, 3248S–3254S.

Berg, P.A. and Daniel, P.T. (1988) Effects of flavonoid compounds on the immune system. In: *Plant Flavonoids in Biology and Medicine II: Biochemical, Cellular, and Medicinal Properties.* Alan R. Liss, Inc., New York.

Berliner, J., Leitinger, N., Watson, A., Huber, J., Fogelman, A., *et al.* (1997). Oxidized lipids in atherogenesis: formation, destruction and action. *Journal of Thrombosis and Haemostasis* 78, 195–199.

Berthold, H.K., Sudhop, T., and von Bergmann, K. (1998) Effect of a garlic oil preparation on serum lipoproteins and cholesterol metabolism: a randomized controlled trial. *Journal of the American Medical Association* 279, 1900–1902.

Block, G., Patterson, B. and Subar, A. (1992) Fruit, vegetables, and cancer prevention: a review of the epidemiological evidence. *Nutrition and Cancer* 18, 1–29.

Blot, W.J., Li, J.Y., Taylor, P.R., Guo, W., Dawsey, S., *et al.* (1993). Nutrition intervention trials in Linxian, China: supplementation with specific vitamin/mineral combinations, cancer incidence, and disease-specific mortality in the general population. *Journal of the National Cancer Institute* 85, 1483–1492.

Bone, R.A., Landrum, J.T., Mayne, S.T., Gomez, C.M., Tibor, S.E., *et al.* (2001) Macular pigment in donor eyes with and without AMD: a case-control study. *Investigative Ophthalmology and Visual Sciences* 42, pp. 235–240.

Britton, G. (1995) Structure and properties of carotenoids in relation to function. *FASEB Journal* 9, 1551–1558.

Canivenc-Lavier, M.C., Vernevaut, M.F., Totis, M., Siess, M.H., Magdalou, J., *et. al.* (1996) Comparative effects of flavonoids and model inducers on drug-metabolizing enzymes in rat liver. *Toxicology* 114, 19–27.

Chu, Y.F., Sun, J., Wu, X., Liu, R.H. (2002). Antioxidant and antiproliferative activities of vegetables. *Journal of. Agriculture and Food Chemistry.* 50, pp. 6910–6916.

Chyu, K.Y., Babbidge, S.M., Zhao, X., Dandillaya, R., Rietveld, A.G. (2004) Differential effects of green tea-derived catechin on developing versus established atherosclerosis in apolipoprotein E-null mice. *Circulation* 109, 2448–2253.

Clarkson, T.B., Anthony, M.S. and Morgan, T.M. (2001) Inhibition of postmenopausal atherosclerosis progression: a comparison of the effects of conjugated equine estrogens and soy phytoestrogens. *Journal of Clinical Endocrinology and Metabolism* 86, 41–47.

Clement, M.V., Ramalingam, J., Long, L.H., Halliwell, B. (2001). The in vitro cytotoxicity of ascorbate depends on the culture medium used to perform the assay and involves hydrogen peroxide. *Antioxidants and Redox Signaling* 3, 157–163.

Cordain, L., Miller, J.B., Eaton, S.B., Mann, N., Holt, S.H., *et al.* (2000) Plant-animal subsistence ratios and macronutrient energy estimations in worldwide hunter-gatherer diets. *American Journal of Clinical Nutrition* 71, 682–692.

Coussens, L.M. and Werb, Z. (2002). Inflammation and cancer. *Nature* 420, 860-867.

Demeule, M., Michaud-Levesque, J., Annabi, B., Gingras, D., Boivin, D., *et al.* (2002) Green tea catechins as novel antitumor and antiangiogenic compounds. *Current Medicinal Chemistry - Anti-Cancer Agents* 2, 441–463.

Doerge, D.R. and Chang, H.C. (2002) Inactivation of thyroid peroxidase by soy isoflavones, in vitro and in vivo. *Journal of Chromatography B - Analytical Technologies in the Biomedical and Life Sciences.* 777, 269–279.

Doll, R. and Peto, R. (1981) The causes of cancer: quantitative estimates of avoidable risks of cancer in the United States today. *Journal of the National Cancer Institute.* 66, 1191–1308.

Dominy, N.J. and Lucas, P.W. (2001) Ecological importance of trichromatic vision to primates. *Nature* 410, 363–366.

Dragsted, L.O., Strube, M., Larson, J.C. (1993) Cancer-protective factors in fruits and vegetables: biochemical and biological background. *Pharmacology and Toxicology* 72, 116–135.

Drewnowski, A. (1996) From asparagus to zucchini: mapping cognitive space for vegetable names. *Journal of the American College of Nutrition* 15, 147–153.

Dulloo, A.G., Duret, C., Rohrer, D., Girardier, L., Mensi, N., *et al.* (1999) Efficacy of a green tea extract rich in catechin polyphenols and caffeine in increasing 24-h energy expenditure and fat oxidation in humans. *American Journal of Clinical Nutrition* 70, 1040–1045.

Eberhardt, M.V., Lee, C.Y. and Liu, R.H. (2000) Dietary modification of human macular pigment density. *Nature* 405, 903–904.

Epstein, L.H. (2001) Increasing fruit and vegetable intake and decreasing fat and sugar intake in families at risk for childhood obesity. *Obesity Research* 9, 171–178.

Finley, J.W. (2003) The antioxidant responsive element (ARE) may explain the protective effects of cruciferous vegetables on cancer. *Nutrition Reviews* 61, 250–254.

Gann, P.H., Ma, J., Giovannucci, E., Willett, W., Sacks, F.M., *et al.* (1999) Lower Prostate Cancer Risk in Men with Elevated Plasma Lycopene Levels: Results of a Prospective Analysis. *Cancer Research* 59, 1225–1230.

Giovannucci, E., Ascherio, A., Rimm, E.B., Stampfer, M.J., Colditz, G.A., *et al.* (1995) Intake of carotenoids and retinol in relation to risk of prostate cancer. *Journal of the National Cancer Institute* 87, 1767–1776.

Giovannucci, E., Rimm, E.B., Liu, Y., Stampfer, M.J. and Willett, W.C. (2002) A prospective study of tomato products, lycopene, and prostate cancer risk. *Journal of the National Cancer Institute* 94, 391–398.

Gordon, M.H. (1996) Dietary antioxidants in disease prevention. *Natural Product Reports* 13, 265–273.

Graham, H.N. (1992) Green tea composition, consumption, and polyphenol chemistry. *Preventive Medicine* 21, 334–350.

Hammond, B.R., Johnson, E.J., Russell, R.M., Krinsky, N.I., Yeum, K.J., *et al.* (1997) Dietary modification of human macular pigment density. *Investigative Ophthalmology and Visual Sciences* 38, 1795–1801.

Heber, D. and Bowerman, S. (2001) *What Color is Your Diet?* Harper Collins/Regan, New York.

Hertog, M.G.L., Hollman, P.C., Katan, M.B. and Kromhout, D. (1993a) Intake of potentially anticarcinogenic flavonoids and their determinants in adults in The Netherlands. *Nutrition and Cancer* 20, 21–29.

Hertog, E.J., Feskens, E.J., Hollman, P.C., Katan, M.B. and Kromhout, D. (1993b) Dietary antioxidant flavonoids and risk of coronary heart disease: the Zutphen Elderly Study. *The Lancet* 342, 1007–1011.

Hirsch, K., Danilenko, M., Giat, J., Miron, T., Rabinkov, A., *et al.* (2000) Effect of purified allicin, the major ingredient of freshly crushed garlic, on cancer cell proliferation. *Nutrition and Cancer* 38, 245–254.

Hollman, P.C. and Katan, M.B. (1997) Absorption, metabolism and health effects of dietary flavonoids in man. *Biomedical Pharmacotherapy* 51, 305–310.

Hsu, S.D., Singh, B.B., Lewis, J.B., Borke, J.L., Dickinson, D.P., *et al.* (2002) Chemoprevention of oral cancer by green tea. *General Dentistry* 50, 140–146.

Isaacsohn, J.L., Moser, M., Stein, E.A., Dudley, K., Davey, J.A., *et al.* (1998) Garlic powder and plasma lipids and lipoproteins: a multicenter, randomized, placebo-controlled trial. *Archives of Internal Medicine* 158, 1189–1194.

Kähkönen, M., Hopia, A., Vuorela, H., Rauha, J.P., Pihlaja, K., *et al.* (1999) Antioxidant Activity of Plant Extracts Containing Phenolic Compounds. *Journal of Agriculture and Food Chemistry* 47, 3954–3962.

Karas, M., Amir, H., Fishman, D., Danilenko, M., Segal, S., *et al.* (2000) Lycopene interferes with cell cycle progression and insulin-like growth factor I signaling in mammary cancer cells. *Nutrition and Cancer* 36, 101–111.

Kazi, A., Smith, D.M., Daniel, K., Zhong, S., Gupta, P., *et al.* (2002) Potential molecular targets of tea polyphenols in human tumor cells: significance in cancer prevention. *In Vivo* 16, 397–403.

Khachik, F., deMoura, F.F., Zhao, D.Y., Aebischer, C.P. and Bernstein, P.S. (2002) Transformations of selected carotenoids in plasma, liver, and ocular tissues of humans and in nonprimate animal models. *Investigative Ophthalmology and Visual Sciences* 43, 3383–3392.

Kim, D.H., Kim, H.S., Imamura, L. and Kobashi, K. (1994) Kinetic studies on a sulfotransferase from Klebsiella K-36, a rat intestinal bacterium. *Biological and Pharmaceutical Bulletin* 17, 543–545.

Kim, M.H., Gutierrez, A.M. and Goldfarb, R.H. (2002). Different mechanisms of soy isoflavones in cell cycle regulation and inhibition of invasion. *Anticancer Research* 22, 3811–3817.

Kritchevsky, S.B., Shimakawa, T., Tell, G.S., Dennis, B., Carpenter, M., *et al.* (1995). Dietary antioxidants and carotid artery wall thickness. The ARIC Study. Atherosclerosis Risk in Communities Study. *Circulation* 92, 2142–2150.

Kucuk, O., Sakr, W., Sarkar, F., Djuric, Z. and Li, Y.W. (1999) Lycopene supplementation in men with prostate cancer (Pca) reduced grade and volume of preneoplasia (PIN) and tumor, decreases serum prostate specific antigen (PSA) and modulates biomarkers of growth and differentiation. International Carotenoid Meeting; Cairns, Australia (abstract).

Kuhnau, J. (1976) A class of semi-essential food components: their role in human nutrition. *World Review of Nutrition and Dietetics* 24, 117–191.

Lampe, J.W. (1999). Health effects of vegetables and fruit: assessing mechanisms of action in human experimental studies. *American Journal of Clinical Nutrition* 70(3 Suppl), 475S–490S.

Laughton, M.J., Evans, P.J., Moroney, M.A., Hoult, J.R. and Halliwell, B. (1991) Inhibition of mammalian 5-lipoxygenase and cyclo-oxygenase by flavonoids and phenolic dietary additives. Relationship to antioxidant activity and to iron ion-reducing ability. *Biochemical Pharmacology* 42, 1673–1681.

Ledikewe, J.H., Smiciklas-Wright, H., Mitchell, D.C., Miller, C.K., Jensen, G.L. (2004) Dietary patterns of rural older adults are associated with weight and nutritional status. *Journal of the American Geriatric Society* 52, 589–595.

Lee, A. (1996) The transition of Australian aboriginal diet and nutritional health. *World Review of Nutrition and Dietetics* 79, 1–52.

Mahbub, S., Brubaker, A.L. and Kovacs, E.J. (2011) Aging of the Innate Immune System: An Update. *Current Immunology Reviews* 7, 104–115.

Mandel, S. and Youdim, M.B. (2004) Catechin polyphenols: neurodegeneration and neuroprotection in neurodegenerative diseases. *Free Radical Biology and Medicine* 37, 304–317.

Middleton, E., Jr and Kandaswami, C. (1993) The impact of of plant flavonoids on mammalian biology: implications for immunity, inflammation and cancer. In *The Flavonoids. Advances in Research since 1986.* Chapman & Hall, London.

Minorsky, P.V. (2002) Lycopene and human health. *Plant Physiolology* 130, 1077–1078.

Munday, R. and Munday, C.M. (2001) Relative activities of organosulfur compounds derived from onions and garlic in increasing tissue activities of quinone reductase and glutathione transferase in rat tissues. *Nutrition and Cancer* 40, 205–210.

Nakagawa, H., Tsuta, K., Kiuchi, K., Senzaki, H., Tanaka, K., *et al.* (2001) Growth inhibitory effects of diallyl disulfide on human breast cancer cell lines. *Carcinogenesis* 22, 891–897.

Neil, H.A., Silagy, C.A., Lancaster, T., Hodgeman, J., Vos, K., *et al.* (1996) Garlic powder in the treatment of moderate hyperlipidaemia: a controlled trial and meta-analysis. *Journal of the Royal College of Physicians London* 30, 329–334.

Nyyssönen, K., Parviainen, M.T., Salonen, R., Tuomilehto, J. and Salonen, J.T. (1997) Vitamin C deficiency and risk of myocardial infarction: prospective population study of men from eastern Finland. *British Medical Journal* 314, 634–638.

Perez, C.E. (2002) Fruit and vegetable consumption. *Health Reports* 13, 23–31.

Peterson, G. and Barnes, S. (1996) Genistein inhibits both estrogen and growth factor-stimulated proliferation of human breast cancer cells. *Cell Growth and Differentiation* 7, 1345–1351.

Pinto, J.T. and Rivlin, R.S. (2001) Antiproliferative effects of allium derivatives from garlic. *Journal of Nutrition* 131, 1058S–1060S.

Pool-Zobel, B.L., Bub, A., Liegibel, U.M., Treptow-van Lishaut, S. and Rechkemmer, G. (1998). Mechanisms by which vegetable consumption reduces genetic damage in humans. *Cancer Epidemiolology, Biomarkers and Prevention* 7, 891–899.

Quatromoni, P.A., Copenhafer, D.L., D'Agostino, R.B., Millen, B.E. (2002) Dietary patterns predict the development of overweight in women: The Framingham Nutrition Studies. *Journal of the American Dietetic Association* 102, 1240–1246.

Rao, A.V.R., and Agarwal, S.J. (2000) Role of antioxidant lycopene in cancer and heart disease. *Journal of the American College of Nutrition* 19, 563–569.

Raso, G.M., Meli, R., Di Carlo, G., Pacilio, M. and Di Carlo, R. (2001) Inhibition of inducible nitric oxide synthase and cyclooxygenase-2 expression by flavonoids in macrophage J774A.1. *Life Sciences* 68, 921–931.

Richer, S., Stiles, W., Statkute, L., Pulido, J., Frankowski, J., *et al.* (2004) Double-masked, placebo-controlled, randomized trial of lutein and antioxidant supplementation in the intervention of atrophic age-related macular degeneration: the Veterans LAST study (Lutein Antioxidant Supplementation Trial). *Optometry* 75, 216–230.

Ridker, P.M., Rifai, N., Rose, L., Buring, J.E. and Cook, N.R. (2002). Comparison of C-reactive protein and low-density lipoprotein cholesterol levels in the prediction of first cardiovascular events. *New England Journal of Medicine* 347, 1557–1565.

Rolls, B., Drewnowski, A. and Ledikewe, J. (2005) Changing the energy density of the diet as a strategy for weight management *Journal of the American Dietetic Association* 105, 98–103.

Sanchez-Moreno, C., Jimenez-Escrig, A. and Saura-Calixto, F. (2000) Study of low-density lipoprotein oxidizability indexes to measure the antioxidant activity of dietary polyphenols. *Nutrition Research* 20, 941–953.

Sander, C., Chang, H., Hamm, F., Elsner, P. and Thiele, J.J. (2004) Role of oxidative stress and the antioxidant network in cutaneous carcinogenesis. *International Journal of Dermatology* 43, 326–335.

Saradeth, T., Seidl, S. and Resch, K.L. (1994) Does garlic alter the lipid pattern in normal volunteers? *Phytomedicine* 1, 183–185.

Scalbert, A. and Williamson, G. (2000). Dietary intake and bioavailability of polyphenols. *Journal of Nutrition* 130(8S Suppl), 2073S–2085S.

Schewe, T., Kuhn, H. and Sies, H. J. (2002). Flavonoids of cocoa inhibit recombinant human 5-lipoxygenase. *Nutrition* 132, 1825–1829.

Seddon, J.M., Ajani, U.A., Sperduto, R.D., Hiller, R., Blair, N., *et al.* (1994) Dietary carotenoids, vitamins A, C, and E, and advanced age-related macular degeneration. Eye Disease Case-Control Study Group. *Journal of the American Medical Association* 272, 1413–1420.

Setiawan, V.W., Zhang, Z.F., Yu, G.P., Lu, Q.Y., Li, Y.L., *et al.* (2001) Protective effect of green tea on the risks of chronic gastritis and stomach cancer. *International Journal of Cancer* 92, 600–604.

Sheu, S.Y., Lai, C.H. and Chiang, H.C. (1998) Inhibition of xanthine oxidase by purpurogallin and silymarin group. *Anticancer Research* 18, 263–267.

Shih, H., Pickwell, G.V. and Quattrochi, L.C. (2000) Differential effects of flavonoid compounds on tumor promoter-induced activation of the human CYP1A2 enhancer. *Archives of Biochemistry and Biophysics* 373, 287–294.

Siess, M.H., Leclerc, J., Canivenc-Lavier, M.C., Rat, P. and Suschetet, M. (1995) Heterogenous effects of natural flavonoids on monooxygenase activities in human and rat liver microsomes. *Toxicology and Applied Pharmacology* 130, 73–78.

Silagy, C. and Neil, A. (1994) Garlic as a lipid lowering agent–a meta-analysis. *Journal of the Royal College of Physicians London* 28, 39–45.

Singh, R.P., Dhanalakshmi, S. and Agarwal, R. (2002). Phytochemicals as cell cycle modulators–a less toxic approach in halting human cancers. *Cell Cycle* 1, 156–161.

Steinmetz, K.A. and Potter, J.D. (1996) Vegetables, fruit, and cancer prevention: a review. *Journal of the American Dietetic Association* 96, 1027–1039.

Stephens, N.G., Parsons, A., Schofield, P.M., Kelly, F., Cheeseman, K., *et al.* (1996). Randomised controlled trial of vitamin E in patients with coronary disease: Cambridge Heart Antioxidant Study (CHAOS). *The Lancet* 347, 781–786.

Stevinson, C., Pittler, M.H. and Ernst, E. (2000) Garlic for treating hypercholesterolemia. A meta-analysis of randomized clinical trials. *Annals of Internal Medicine* 133, 420–429.

Street, D.A., Comstock, G.W. and Salkeld, R.M. (1994). Serum antioxidants and myocardial infarction. Are low levels of carotenoids and alpha-tocopherol risk factors for myocardial infarction? *Circulation* 90, 1154–1161.

Su, L.J. and Arab, L. (2002) Tea consumption and the reduced risk of colon cancer – results from a national prospective cohort study. *Public Health Nutrition* 5, 419–425.

Sun, J., Chu, Y.F., Wu, X., Liu, R.H. (2002) Antioxidant and antiproliferative activities of common fruits. *Journal of Agriculture and Food Chemistry* 50, 7449–7454.

Surh, Y.J., Kundu, J.K., Na, H.K. and Lee, J.S. (2005) Redox-sensitive transcription factors as prime targets for chemoprevention with anti-inflammatory and antioxidative phytochemicals. *Journal of Nutrition* 135, 2993S–3001S.

Temple, N.J. (2000) Antioxidants and disease: more questions than answers. *Nutrition Research* 20, 449–459.

Tohill, B.C., Seymour, J., Serdula, M., Kettel-Khan, L. and Rolls, B.J. (2004) What epidemiologic studies tell us about the relationship between fruit and vegetable consumption and body weight. *Nutrition Reviews* 62, 365–372.

United States Department of Agriculture, Agricultural Research Service (1998) *Food and Nutrient Intakes by Individuals in the United States, by Sex and Age, 1994–1996. Nationwide Food Surveys Report No. 96-2.* USDA, Washington, DC.
Warshafsky, S., Kamer, R.S. and Sivak, S.L. (1993) Effect of garlic on total serum cholesterol. A meta-analysis. *Annals of Internal Medicine* 119, 599–695.
Watson, R.R. and Leonard, T.K. (1986) Selenium and vitamins A, E, and C: nutrients with cancer prevention properties. *Journal of the American Dietetic Association* 86, 505–510.
Willett, W.C. (1994) Diet and health: what should we eat? *Science* 264, 532–537.
Willett, W.C. (1995) Diet, nutrition and avoidable cancer. *Environmental Health Perspectives* 103(Suppl.8), 165–170.
Witzum, J.L. and Berliner, J.A. (1998). Oxidized phospholipids and isoprostanes in atherosclerosis. *Current Opinions in Lipidology* 9, 441–448.
World Cancer Research Fund & American Institute for Cancer Research (1997) *Food, Nutrition, and the Prevention of Cancer: A Global Perspective.* American Institute for Cancer Research Washington, DC.
Wu, L.Y., Juan, C.C., Hwang, L.S., Hsu, Y.P., Ho, P.H., *et al.* (2004) Green tea supplementation ameliorates insulin resistance and increases glucose transporter IV content in a fructose-fed rat model. *European Journal of Nutrition* 43, 116–124.
Yang, T.T. and Koo, M.W. (2000) Chinese green tea lowers cholesterol level through an increase in fecal lipid excretion. *Life Sciences* 66, 411–423.
Zafra-Stone, S., Yasmin, T., Bagchi, M., Chatterjee, A., Vinson, J.A., *et al.* (2007) Berry anthocyanins as novel antioxidants in human health and disease prevention. *Molecular Nutrition and Food Research* 51, 675–683.
Zhang, M., Binns, C.W. and Lee, A.H. (2002) Tea consumption and ovarian cancer risk: a case-control study in China. *Cancer Epidemiology and Biomarkers Review* 11, 713–718.

9 Trace Elements and Inflammation

S. Samman,*,[1] H.T. O'Connor,[2] K.S. Bell-Anderson[1] and M. Foster[1]

[1]*Discipline of Nutrition & Metabolism, School of Molecular Bioscience, University of Sydney, Australia;* [2]*Discipline of Exercise & Sport Science, Faculty of Health Sciences, University of Sydney, Australia*

Introduction

Inflammation is an integral part of the innate immune system's response to trauma or infection. The acute inflammatory response is initiated upon detection of inducers, such as microbial infections, oxygen radicals and tissue damage, by sensors such as Toll-like receptors (TLRs) and other pattern recognition receptors. A rapid increase in blood flow and capillary permeability at the site of insult facilitates entry of leucocytes and chemical mediators into tissue, resulting in the cardinal signs of inflammation: pain, redness, swelling and heat. The purpose of inflammation is to protect the host from the spread of infection or tissue damage, whereupon the inflammatory response is resolved and homeostasis is restored. In typical cases, the inflammatory response is localised to the site where the

* Corresponding author, samir.samman@sydney.edu.au

inflammatory inducer is present; however, an increasing number of inflammatory conditions have been described where the initiating trigger is not well defined and inflammation appears to be chronic (Medzhitov, 2010; Nathan and Ding, 2010). Chronic inflammation is characterized by elevated production of cytokines, tissue macrophage infiltration and sustained activation of inflammatory signalling pathways (Hotamisligil, 2006).

Activation of the immune system is an energy-demanding process that requires mechanisms for redistribution of nutrients away from metabolic tissues to fuel proliferation of immune cells and the production of mediators of inflammation. Inflammation is often associated with increased oxidative stress owing to the production of reactive oxygen species (ROS), which draws on available antioxidants such as vitamins C and E, and triggers cellular antioxidative responses (Foster and Samman, 2010). Activity of antioxidative enzymes requires the presence of inorganic nutrients such as manganese, copper, zinc, iron and selenium at active sites or as structural components. This suggests that, in chronic inflammation, utilization and requirement of some vitamins and minerals are increased. The presence of low-grade systemic inflammation in chronic diseases such as obesity, type 2 diabetes mellitus (DM) and atherosclerosis, has highlighted the role for nutrition in the management of cardiometabolic symptoms in concert with a reduction in inflammation. Despite extensive investigations in this area, the specific cellular mechanisms that are involved in the initiation of chronic inflammation are unclear. Processes of inflammation, including cytokine signalling, seem to be influenced by nutrient status. The aim of this chapter is to evaluate the literature on the roles of iron and zinc in inflammation, and their interactions with chronic disease.

Inflammation and Nutrient Status

Optimal immune function is dependent on the availability and balance of nearly all macronutrients and micronutrients. Data from observational studies demonstrate positive associations between the consumption of Western diets and the pro-inflammatory state. High intakes of saturated and *trans* fatty acids, and high glycaemic index carbohydrate have been linked to elevated concentrations of C-reactive protein (CRP) (Kontogianni *et al.*, 2006). The Western diet is also typically high in n-6 relative to n-3 polyunsaturated fatty acids (PUFAs). N-6 arachidonic acid and n-3 eicosapentaenoic acid are essential for the production of inflammatory-modulating eicosanoids. N-6-derived eicosanoids are powerful inflammatory agents compared with those derived from n-3 fatty acids. The impact of increasing n-3 fatty acids (marine oils) by diet or supplementation on inflammatory markers is the subject of intense research. It is likely that the effects of n-3 PUFAs *in vivo* are complex and influenced by disease state, genetic predisposition and the presence of micronutrients such as zinc and iron that impact on fatty acid desaturase activity and the synthesis of prostaglandins (Cunnane, 1982; Cunnane and McAdoo, 1987; Eder and Kirchgessner, 1996).

Nutrient deficiencies, such as protein-energy malnutrition, are a major cause of immunodeficiency because of the high requirements for amino acids and energy for immune cell proliferation and synthesis of protein mediators. Under-nutrition impairs immune function and increases susceptibility to disease but insights into the mechanisms of action are complicated by the fact that stimulation of the immune system can also impair nutritional status. Mounting an immune response requires energy and amino acids, but also demands micronutrients (Cunningham-Rundles *et al.*, 2005). The generation of energy itself requires vitamin B coenzymes, such as thiamine, riboflavin and niacin. Minerals such as iron and copper are essential at active sites of proteins involved in oxidative phosphorylation and the generation of ATP.

It is well documented that circulating levels of many micronutrients decrease rapidly owing to inflammation (Thurnham *et al.*, 2005). The mechanisms by which this occurs are not clear, but probably involve the utilization of micronutrients for immune activities. Micronutrients such as zinc and iron may influence inflammatory signalling pathways at different levels and in a variety of ways, including via the modulation of cytokine production. Reduced serum concentrations of zinc and iron might be part of the physiological defence mechanism to limit supply of biologically available micronutrients to invading pathogens. In infection, serum vitamin A concentrations decline rapidly but are able to recover without vitamin A supplementation when the infection is resolved. This supports the notion that the coordinated response to inflammation includes the redistribution of micronutrients to tissues or cellular compartments. In contrast, the redistribution of micronutrients in non-resolving inflammation may contribute to the pathogenesis of a range of chronic conditions, including obesity, atherosclerosis and DM. It is known, for example, that impaired zinc and iron utilization in chronic disorders compromises the many functions of these nutrients and further exacerbates the processes of disease.

Iron

Iron metabolism and homeostasis

Most living organisms require iron. The majority of body iron in humans is located in erythrocytes in association with haemoglobin, and the remainder is distributed in myoglobin, a range of enzymes, is stored in the liver, or appears in the plasma. The essentiality of iron relates to its ability to bind oxygen for transport to tissues and for short-term storage in muscle. The presence of iron in mitochondrial enzymes, e.g. dehydrogenase or cytochrome, facilitates the flow of electrons that is needed for the production of metabolic energy. Other iron-containing enzymes are involved in numerous metabolic pathways including protein and DNA metabolism and collagen synthesis (MacPhail, 2007; Samman, 2007a).

Unlike many other trace minerals where nutrient balance is maintained by excretion of excess, body iron is strictly conserved. Relatively small amounts of iron are excreted through the gastrointestinal tract, skin and kidneys. The regulation of iron balance includes the recycling of senescent erythrocytes, which ensures that adequate levels of iron are available for optimal function while preventing toxicity. Significant losses of iron occur when salvage mechanisms are bypassed, primarily by direct loss of intact red blood cells, e.g. through menstrual blood losses or in people with gastrointestinal infections or ulcers. Iron is stored as ferritin or haemosiderin with the principal sites of storage being the liver, bone marrow and spleen. Dietary haem iron, from animal sources, is soluble in the intestine and is absorbed intact by haem carrier protein (HCP1) (MacPhail, 2007; Samman, 2007a). Because the iron is shielded by haem, its absorption is not affected significantly by the composition of the background diet, and its bioavailability is considered relatively high. In contrast, non-haem iron, from fruit and vegetables, is absorbed with poorer efficiency by a divalent metal transporter (DTM1), which requires iron to be in the ferrous state.

Iron homeostasis is achieved by mechanisms that either conserve iron or facilitate its absorption depending on body iron requirements. The absorption and flux of iron through the duodenal enterocytes and macrophages of the reticulo-endothelial system (RES) involves a group of similar receptors, proteins and functions (Wessling-Resnick, 2010). DMT1 requires ferroreductase activity to reduce Fe(III) to Fe(II) to facilitate absorption (Gunshin *et al.*, 1997), and duodenal cytochrome B probably fulfils this function (McKie *et al.*, 2001). Basolateral iron transport across the intestinal mucosa is then achieved by ferroportin. Absorbed iron is ultimately bound to transferrin and delivered to peripheral tissues. Macrophages export iron in a similar manner to duodenal enterocytes, i.e. they also depend on ferroportin (Wessling-Resnick, 2010). The expression and action of ferroportin are regulated primarily by hepcidin (Knutson *et al.*, 2003).

The role of hepcidin in the regulation of iron

Hepcidin is a 25-amino acid peptide that is synthesised by hepatocytes, macrophages, neutrophils and adipocytes (Bekri *et al.*, 2006; Kemna *et al.*, 2008; Wessling-Resnick, 2010). When first isolated from plasma, hepcidin was named 'liver-expressed antimicrobial peptide' (LEAP-1) (Krause *et al.*, 2000). It was also isolated from human urine and called 'hepcidin' to acknowledge its hepatic origin and *in vitro* bactericidal effect (Park *et al.*, 2001).

Hepcidin binds to ferroportin, resulting in its internalization and degradation. The binding of hepcidin to ferroportin prevents export of iron across the intestinal mucosa and from macrophages that contain phagocytosed iron from senescent red blood cells (Nemeth *et al.*, 2004). The role of hepcidin seems to be post-transcriptional down-regulation of ferroportin, but because the discovery of hepcidin is still relatively recent, an understanding of its actions and control mechanisms is still evolving (Wessling-Resnick, 2010). The circulating hepcidin concentration seems to be regulated by body iron status and physiological demands. Synthesis is reduced by hypoxia and iron deficiency and conversely increased by iron loading (Nicolas *et al.*, 2002). Infection and inflammation increase hepcidin synthesis, and this discovery has enhanced our understanding of the association between iron and innate immunity (Ganz, 2003; Wessling-Resnick, 2010).

Iron status, infection and inflammation

It is well established that serum iron concentrations decrease markedly in response to systemic inflammation or infection (Cartwright *et al.*, 1946). Studies in patients with infectious diseases, such as tuberculosis, have demonstrated that supplementation with iron increases mycobacterial growth (Kochan, 1973; Lounis *et al.*, 2001) and is associated with increased morbidity and mortality (Murray *et al.*, 1978). The deleterious impact of iron supplementation in parasitic disease such as malaria is well documented (Prentice, 2008). Patients with hereditary haemochromatosis and those with thalassemia treated with frequent blood transfusions are known to have increased susceptibility to infection (Ozkalay *et al.*, 2006; Doherty, 2007). Iron status therefore appears to influence the progression of infectious disease with iron deficiency conferring resistance (Moalem *et al.*, 2004). It has been hypothesized that from an evolutionary perspective, iron deficiency is an adaptive, protective response especially prevalent in areas where there is a high burden of infectious disease (Denic and Agarwal, 2007).

As with infection, most inflammatory conditions are influenced by iron status and generally are associated with increased iron stores (Wessling-Resnick, 2010). Iron loading is associated with atherosclerosis (Yuan, 1999), neurodegeneration (Graham *et al.*, 2000) and chronic liver disease (Wallace and Subramaniam, 2009). More recently, increased inflammation and iron stores have been correlated with established risk factors of DM, obesity and the metabolic syndrome (Vari *et al.*, 2007; Rajpathak *et al.*, 2009). In contrast, iron deficiency improves inflammation and clinically is known as the anaemia of chronic disease, more recently described as the anaemia of inflammation (AI): the latter idiom reflects a greater understanding of the underlying pathophysiology of iron deficiency. AI is usually a mild anaemia, which is associated clinically with most infections, rheumatoid or autoimmune disorders (Ganz and Nemeth, 2009), malignancy (Maccio *et al.*, 2005) and multiple myeloma (Ludwig *et al.*, 2004).

Several biochemical mechanisms seem to contribute to the development of AI. Limitation in the iron supply for erythropoiesis is considered to be a major factor, along with increased destruction of erythrocytes and cytokine-mediated suppression of erythrocyte production and maturation (Ganz and Nemeth, 2009). Evidence that supports the importance of limited iron supply in the development of AI includes the increased incorporation of zinc protoporphyrin into protoporphyrin IX during the synthesis of haem (Hastka *et al.*, 1993). This indicates that insufficient iron reaches the sites of haem synthesis in the developing erythrocytes resulting in a greater incorporation of zinc. Histological support for this mechanism also comes from reduced iron-specific staining of nucleated erythrocyte precursors (sideroblasts) (Cartwright, 1966). Studies using damaged, iron-radiolabelled hepatocytes show that inflammation or infection results in the delayed appearance of radiolabelled iron in the circulation and accumulation of iron in the reticuloendothelial system (Noyes *et al.*, 1960). Although it has been known for some time that AI resulted in the sequestration of iron in macrophages and subsequent development of hypoferraemia, until the discovery of hepcidin, the underpinning mechanisms involved were unknown.

Hepcidin and inflammation

A number of studies show that hepcidin is elevated by inflammation, with interleukin (IL)-6 purported to be a key mediator, but other cytokines may also contribute. The regulation of hepcidin synthesis is predominantly transcriptional with the STAT3 pathway transducing the effect of IL-6 via the canonical STAT3 binding site in the proximal hepcidin promoter (Wrighting and Andrews, 2006; Pietrangelo *et al.*, 2007; Verga Falzacappa *et al.*, 2007). Supporting the important impact of IL-6, diseases associated with IL-6 excess including Castleman's syndrome, multiple myeloma and juvenile chronic arthritis are all associated with elevated hepcidin and AI (Nemeth and Ganz, 2009). In the case of Castleman's syndrome, treatment with anti-IL-6 receptor antibody decreases hepcidin concentrations and corrects the anaemia (Kawabata *et al.*, 2007). Other mediators of hepcidin include bone morphogenic proteins (BMP), which are putative stimulators of hepcidin synthesis (Wang *et al.*, 2005). Synthesis of another regulatory protein, hemojuvelin, which acts as a co-receptor for BMP, seems to be augmented by inflammation. Mutations resulting in the loss of hemojuvelin lead to low rates of transcription of hepcidin and iron overload (Papanikolaou *et al.*, 2004). Finally, ferroportin expression itself is reduced by inflammation (Yang *et al.*, 2002). Although hepcidin is probably the most important regulator of ferroportin, other mechanisms impacting production and trafficking of ferroportin secondary to inflammation are potentially independent of hepcidin (Ganz and Nemeth, 2009).

Diagnosis of the anaemia of inflammation

AI is characterized by low serum iron, low iron binding (e.g. low transferrin) and inadequate erythropoiesis despite adequate iron stores in bone marrow (Roy, 2010). Serum ferritin levels are normal or high, unlike the clinical profile in iron deficiency where serum ferritin is below the reference range. Elevated ferritin concentrations are likely to be the result of macrophage iron loading and inflammation-stimulated ferritin synthesis (Roy, 2010). Erythrocytes can be microcytic and hypochromic, especially in children who have higher iron requirements for growth or if AI has been of long duration. The abnormal erythrocyte morphology is thought to be the result of progressive depletion of iron stores (Ganz and Nemeth, 2009).

Because ferritin is increased by inflammation, it has been used in conjunction with serum transferrin receptor to determine the serum transferrin receptor/log serum ferritin ratio. Serum transferrin receptor is produced when erythroid precursors have produced sufficient haemoglobin to shed the receptor. As iron availability to the erythron decreases or as erythroid capacity increases, serum transferrin in the plasma increases (Roy, 2010). Despite the iron restriction in AI, serum transferrin receptor is not elevated but remains in the normal range owing to down-regulation by pro-inflammatory cytokines (Skikne, 2008). The serum transferrin to log serum ferritin ratio has been suggested as a marker that discriminates between iron-deficiency anaemia and AI, whereby a ratio of >1.5 is consistent with iron deficiency and <0.8 is consistent with AI (Brugnara, 2003).

Iron, inflammation and obesity

A link between obesity and iron deficiency was first made more than 40 years ago (Seltzer and Mayer, 1963). Initially this association was dismissed and largely attributed to poor diet, increased blood volume and body surface area in the obese (Pinhas-Hamiel *et al.*, 2003). It was not until 2007 with the publication of a study by Yanoff *et al.* (2007) reporting significant associations between obesity, CRP and iron deficiency that there was renewed interest in the area of iron status in the obese. More recently a number of studies have reported an association between obesity and iron deficiency or 'hypoferremia' in adults (Ausk and Ioannou, 2008; Menzie *et al.*, 2008) and children (Aeberli *et al.*, 2009). This is supported further by data from the National Health and Examination Survey (NHANES III) showing that overweight children in the USA were twice as likely to be iron deficient compared with normal weight children (Nead *et al.*, 2004). A recent systematic review also reported a tendency for lower transferrin saturation and higher ferritin concentrations in obese populations (Fig. 9.1), consistent with the inflammatory hepcidin hypothesis (Cheng *et al.*, 2011).

Because obesity is known to be a state of chronic low-grade inflammation, a mechanistic link between inflammation in obesity and hypoferremia is plausible. In obese populations, higher circulating hepcidin concentrations have been reported (Aeberli *et al.*, 2009; Tussing-Humphreys *et al.*, 2010). The underpinning mechanisms that lead to higher hepcidin levels in obesity are yet to be elucidated but the elevation of IL-6 is well documented in obesity (Shoelson *et al.*, 2007) and this cytokine is known to stimulate hepcidin expression through signalling and activation of STAT-3, which binds to the promoter region of the hepcidin gene (HAMP) inducing mRNA transcription (De Domenico *et al.*, 2008). One *in vitro* study involving leptin, which is markedly increased in obesity, suggests that leptin may stimulate hepcidin expression also through the STAT-3 pathway (Chung *et al.*, 2007). Recent studies have demonstrated hepcidin expression in adipose tissue, which may contribute further to elevated hepcidin concentrations in the obese (Bekri *et al.*, 2006), though studies comparing expression of hepcidin mRNA in hepatic and adipose tissue in obese participants have yielded conflicting results (Bekri *et al.*, 2006; Tussing-Humphreys *et al.*, 2010).

At present, there are insufficient studies in the obese that compare iron and inflammatory markers with hepcidin simultaneously to provide detailed evidence about the abnormalities of iron metabolism. Studies that employ appropriate control groups and

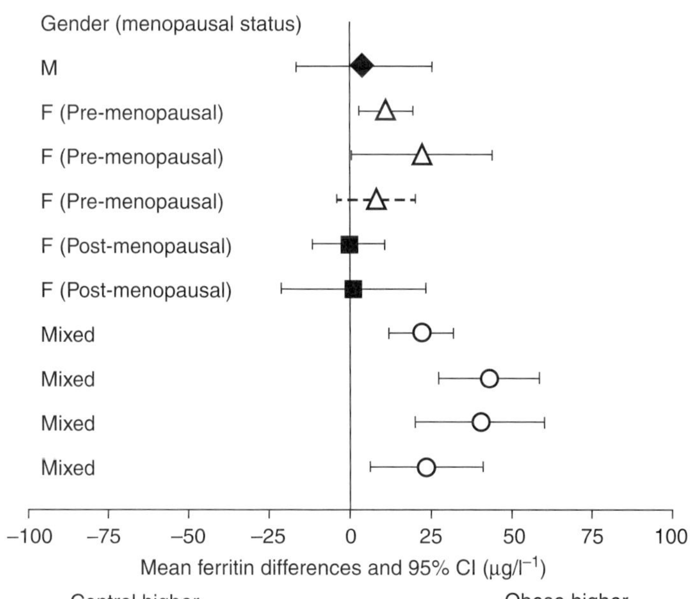

Fig. 9.1. The relationship between obesity and hypoferraemia in adults. Forest plot summarizing mean serum ferritin differences between obese (body-mass index >30 kg/m^2) and non-obese groups (body-mass index <30 kg/m^2). Figure modified from Cheng *et al.*, 2011 (*Obesity Reviews*, John Wiley & Sons Ltd).

measure hepcidin and other biomarkers of iron status are warranted. Clinically, iron deficiency may add further to the burden of obesity and complicate weight management. Iron deficiency has been associated with fatigue, depression and reduced exercise capacity and this may impact negatively on the efficacy of behavioural weight management programmes aimed at increasing physical activity and improving motivation and psychological well-being (Brownlie *et al.*, 2002; Vahdat Shariatpanaahi *et al.*, 2007). Restricted energy diets used for weight management may be low in iron, particularly for women during reproductive years where requirements are higher (O'Connor *et al.*, 2011). Treatment of iron deficiency including improved dietary iron intake and/or iron supplementation might not be efficacious in obesity, because obesity related inflammation may alter iron absorption and circulation, a situation similar to AI (Shoelson *et al.*, 2007; Roy, 2010). Unfortunately, the independent effect of iron deficiency on weight management and the treatment of hypoferraemia in obesity are yet to be adequately evaluated.

Zinc

Zinc metabolism and homeostasis

Zinc was established as an essential trace element following the reporting of zinc deficiency in humans (Prasad *et al.*, 1961). Similar to iron, dietary zinc is subject to complex interactions in the gastrointestinal tract that promote or interfere with its bioavailability (Samman, 2011). The adult human body contains 1.5–2.5 g of zinc, which is distributed in all tissues but mostly in fat-free mass such as bone and muscle. The content and distribution of total body zinc is maintained through powerful retention and recycling mechanisms. At the cellular level, an intricate arrangement of cellular homeostatic mechanisms has evolved to regulate the intracellular zinc content and its distribution within the mammalian cell. Although much is yet unknown, the maintenance of cellular zinc homeostasis is believed to involve complex interactions between zinc sensors, such as metal responsive element-binding transcription factor-1 (MTF-1), and cell-signalling machinery; the transcriptional and/or post-translational regulation of two recently discovered classes of zinc transporters, the ZnT (SLC30) and Zip (SLC39) transporter families; the trafficking of zinc through the cell by metallothionein (MT); and the synthesis and/or degradation of proteins that bind zinc with high affinity.

Zinc is involved in a number of metabolic processes including protein and nucleic acid synthesis, and is essential for the synthesis and action of insulin. It is the most common catalytic metal ion in the cytoplasm of cells. Carbonic anhydrase was the first discovered zinc metalloenzyme; other enzymes include carboxypeptidase, alkaline phosphatase, DNA/RNA polymerase and superoxide dismutase. As a component of metalloenzymes, zinc participates in the reaction at the active site or provides structural integrity to the enzyme. Genes such as those involved in the regulation of the redox state, fatty acid metabolism, signal transduction and platelet activation, have been recognized as potential candidates for regulation by zinc: some genes are positively affected, others negatively, whereas some are affected only by extremes of zinc status. Zinc-containing proteins in the human genome, known as 'zinc fingers', are able to interact with DNA and act as transcriptional mediators. Zinc serves as a structural component that allows for the coordinate binding of amino acids, mainly cysteine and histidine residues, in the protein chain to form a finger-like structure (Samman 2007b,c). Zinc finger proteins with redox switch capabilities have also been identified, wherein the thiol groups of zinc-coordinating cysteines can be reversibly modified by oxidation and reduction reactions with concomitant release and binding of zinc (Foster and Samman, 2010).

The involvement of zinc in the immune system is well recognized (Kruse-Jarres, 1989), with an initial consequence of zinc deficiency being an impairment of immunological functions (Prasad, 2008). Intracellular zinc concentrations have been shown to influence the induction of inflammatory cytokines that regulate acute inflammation and that are also known to generate ROS (Foster and Samman, 2010); inflammatory and oxidative-stress-related pathways seem to intersect in numerous ways with both, for example, influencing NFκB and nitric oxide (NO) signalling. Sustained expression of pro-inflammatory cytokines and impaired signalling in inflammation and oxidative stress contribute to the pathology of a range of chronic disorders, including cardiovascular disease (CVD) and DM. Perturbations of zinc homeostasis are also associated with these disorders, suggesting an interrelationship between zinc, inflammation and oxidative stress (Foster and Samman, 2010).

Zinc and acute inflammation

Zinc may affect the generation of cytokines by influencing the normal development and function of immune cells. For example, zinc deficiency decreases the activity of serum thymulin, which is required for the maturation of T-helper cells (Prasad, 2007); even a mild deficiency of zinc has been shown to lead to an imbalance of T-helper 1 (Th1) and T-helper 2 (Th2) functions, decrease the recruitment of T-naive cells (Beck *et al.*, 1997) and reduce natural-killer (NK) cell lytic activity (Tapazoglou *et al.*, 1985).

A number of *in vitro* studies have measured cytokine production in response to zinc depletion or supplementation in stimulated and unstimulated cells. Human-derived promyelocytic leukaemia (HL-60) and human vascular endothelial cells cultured in zinc-deficient media demonstrated significantly higher generation of tumour necrosis factor (TNF)-α and IL-1β cytokines than cells cultured under physiological zinc concentrations (Prasad *et al.*, 2010). The effect of zinc deficiency on cytokine levels was not apparent in unstimulated cells; before phorbol myristate acetate (PMA) or lipopolysaccharide (LPS) stimulation, both groups of cells produced only trace amounts of TNF-α and IL-1β regardless of the zinc concentration of the media and despite negative changes in oxidative stress markers in the zinc-deficient cells (Prasad *et al.*, 2010). Similarly, in peripheral blood mononuclear cells isolated from healthy adults and treated with 3 or 30 μM zinc, no difference was observed in the protein levels of TNF-α, IL-1β, IL-6, IL-12 and interferon (IFN)-γ; however, an increase in all cytokines was seen with ≥100 μM zinc (Chang *et al.*, 2006), which may indicate that high extracellular zinc levels act as an inflammatory trigger in primary mononuclear cells.

In human intervention studies measuring the effects of zinc on plasma cytokine levels or cytokine production in primary human blood cells (Table 9.1), supplementation with ≥45 mg zinc/day is reported to decrease pro-inflammatory cytokine mRNA and protein synthesis in stimulated mononuclear cells (Prasad *et al.*, 2004, 2007; Bao *et al.*, 2008). Conversely, increased cytokine levels have been shown in stimulated mononuclear cells isolated from populations supplemented with ≤20 mg zinc/day (Aydemir *et al.*, 2006; Kahmann *et al.*, 2008; Sandstead *et al.*, 2008), suggesting a dose effect of zinc. Measurements of plasma cytokine levels in response to zinc supplementation support a difference in effect depending on zinc dose; plasma concentrations of IL-6 have been shown to decrease with zinc supplementation of 45 mg/day (Bao *et al.*, 2010b) but to increase with 10 mg zinc/day (Mariani *et al.*, 2008; Mocchegiani *et al.*, 2008). The significance of these changes is unclear but the ability of zinc supplementation to influence cytokine levels in humans is consistently reported.

Zinc, C-reactive protein and NFκB

In mediating the acute inflammatory response, the endocrine actions of cytokines enhance the ability of the innate immune system to eradicate infection; these changes include an increase in the expression of NFκB-sensitive genes, and an increase in the plasma concentrations of acute phase proteins, including CRP. A number of studies have investigated the relationship between zinc and CRP concentrations in humans (Table 9.2). In observational studies, there seems to be an inverse association between CRP and serum zinc concentrations in geriatric (Craig *et al.*, 1990) and surgical patients (Oakes *et al.*, 2008).

Table 9.1. Effects of zinc supplementation in humans on plasma cytokine concentrations or *ex vivo* cytokine release in isolated blood cells.

Study (author, year)	Description of participants	Study design/*ex vivo* cell culture conditions	Zn dose (mg/day)	Outcome
Aydemir *et al.*, 2006	Healthy adults; M; 19–31 years	Controlled before and after trial, 10 days; isolated cells stimulated with LPS for 2 h (monocytes/granulocytes) or by antigen presentation for 2 days (T lymphocytes)	15	Greater release of TNF-α, IL-1β, IFN-γ in stimulated cells (monocytes, granulocytes, and T lymphocytes, respectively) derived from Zn supplemented subjects compared with placebo group
Bao *et al.*, 2008	Adults with sickle cell disease; n = 36, M and F; 18–47 years	RCT, parallel, 13 weeks; PBMC stimulated with LPS or PHA-P for 24 h	75	Decrease in LPS-induced TNF-α and IL-1β mRNA and protein concentrations and increase in PHA-P induced IL-2 mRNA levels in Zn compared with placebo group
Bao *et al.*, 2010b	Healthy older adults; n = 40, M and F; 56–83 years	RCT, parallel, 26 weeks	45	Decrease in plasma IL-6 concentrations in Zn supplement group
Kahmann *et al.*, 2008	Healthy older adults; n = 19, M and F; 65–82 years	Uncontrolled before and after trial, 48 days; PBMC stimulated with LPS for 72 h	10	Zn supplementation resulted in lower basal IL-6, higher induced IL-6, TNF-α and IFN-γ levels
Mariani *et al.*, 2008	Healthy older adults; n = 39, M and F; 60–83 years	Uncontrolled before and after trial, 48 days	10	Increase in plasma IL-6 concentrations with Zn
Mocchegiani *et al.*, 2008	Healthy older adults; n = 110, M and F; 65–85 years	Uncontrolled before and after trial, 48 days	10	No change in TNF-α but increase in plasma IL-6 concentrations with Zn
Prasad *et al.*, 2004	Healthy adults; n = 20, M and F; 19–50 years	RCT, parallel, 8 weeks; isolated PBMC stimulated with LPS for 24 h	45	Zn reduced levels of LPS-induced TNF-α and IL-1β mRNA
Prasad *et al.*, 2007	Healthy older adults; n = 50, M and F; 55–87 years	RCT, parallel, 52 weeks; whole blood stimulated for 4 h and isolated PBMC for 24 h with LPS	45	No change in percentage of whole blood cells positive for IL-1β or TNF-α in Zn supplement group; decrease in *ex vivo* generation of TNF-α in PBMC from Zn supplement group
Raqib *et al.*, 2004	Children with *Shigella*-infection, n = 56; M & F; age 1–5 years	RCT, parallel, 2 weeks; isolated PBMC stimulated with PHA for 72 h	20	No significant effects of Zn on PHA-induced cytokine release
Sandstead *et al.*, 2008	Children; n = 54, M & F; 6–7 years	RCT, parallel, 10 weeks; isolated mononuclear cells stimulated with PHA-P for 48 h	20	Greater release of IL-2 & IFN-γ in stimulated cells derived from Zn supplemented compared with control subjects

Abbreviations: F, female; IFN, interferon; IL, interleukin; LPS, lipopolysaccharide; M, male; PBMC, peripheral blood mononuclear cells; PHA, phytohaemagglutinin; RCT, randomized controlled trial; TNF, tumour necrosis factor.

Table 9.2. Studies investigating the relationship between zinc and C-reactive protein.

Study (author, year)	Description of participants	Study design	Outcome
Bao *et al.*, 2010b	Healthy elderly adults, n = 40	RCT, parallel, 26 weeks, 45 mg Zn/day	Decrease in plasma CRP with Zn supplementation
Brown *et al.*, 1993	Children (Peruvian), n = 153, 11–19 months	Cross-sectional	Trend for lower serum Zn in children with elevated CRP
Craig *et al.*, 1990	Acutely ill geriatric patients n = 238, long stay geriatric patients n = 50, controls n = 71	Case-control	CRP levels were higher and inversely correlated with serum Zn in acutely ill geriatric patients
Kelishadi *et al.*, 2010	Obese children, n = 60, 6–10 years	RCT, crossover, 16 weeks (8 + 8 weeks with 4-week washout period), 20 mg Zn/day	Decrease in plasma CRP with Zn supplementation
Kuvibidila and Vuvu, 2009	Non-pregnant women (Congalese): n = 77 (lactating), n = 30 (non-lactating)	Cross-sectional	Zn concentration was lower in lactating than in non-lactating women; CRP levels were within reference range and not different between groups
Oakes *et al.*, 2008	11 elective knee athroplasty patients	Cohort; time course (pre-operatively and at 12, 24, 48, 72, 168 h post-operatively)	Post-operative increase in CRP levels and decrease in plasma Zn concentrations
Raqib *et al.*, 2004	Children with *Shigella* infection, n = 56, 1–5 years	RCT, parallel, 2 weeks, 20 mg Zn/day	No effect of Zn on serum CRP concentrations
Rashidi *et al.*, 2009	Adults undergoing haemodialysis, n = 55	RCT, parallel, 6 weeks, 50 mg Zn/day	CRP levels were above the reference range; trend for CRP to decrease with Zn supplementation

Abbreviations: CRP, C-reactive protein; RCT, randomized controlled trial.

Zinc supplementation trials have shown a decrease in CRP levels in healthy adults (Bao *et al.*, 2010b), patients undergoing haemodialysis (Rashidi *et al.*, 2009) and in obese children (Kelishadi *et al.*, 2010). In contrast, no significant effects of zinc supplementation on serum CRP levels were observed in *Shigella*-infected children (Raqib *et al.*, 2004); however, the period of supplementation (2 weeks) may have been insufficient to demonstrate a response. Overall, the balance of evidence suggests an inverse relationship between zinc and CRP levels in humans.

The effects of zinc on NFκB activity seem to depend on the health and/or zinc status of the host. Diet-induced zinc deficiency in a murine model of polymicrobial sepsis enhanced NFκB binding activity in vital organs and the expression of a range of NFκB targeted genes known to increase systemic inflammation. Short-term zinc repletion before the onset of sepsis significantly reduced these effects (Bao *et al.*, 2010a). In humans, NFκB activation and the mRNA levels of the NFκB-regulated IL-2 cytokine and IL-2Rα receptor were decreased in the peripheral blood mononuclear cells of elderly subjects with plasma zinc levels below the reference range. These effects were corrected with zinc supplementation (Prasad *et al.*, 2006).

Atherosclerosis

An altered distribution of zinc among its principal plasma proteins has been observed in atherosclerosis (Malavolta *et al.*, 2007) and the ease with which labile zinc is transported into endothelial cells (Rowe and Bobilya, 2000) suggests that the vascular endothelium may be particularly affected by perturbations in zinc homeostasis and metabolism (Beattie and Kwun, 2004). Zinc has also been linked to several cardiovascular risk factors including plasma lipoprotein concentrations, haemostasis and antioxidant status (Hughes and Samman, 2006; Foster *et al.*, 2010).

Zinc deficiency has been suggested to exacerbate the detrimental effects of specific fatty acids, such as linoleic acid, and inflammatory cytokines, such as TNF-α, on vascular endothelial functions. Endothelial cells rendered zinc deficient demonstrated considerably higher levels of apoptotic cell death and caspase-3 activity than control cells when stimulated with linoleic acid and TNF-α. This effect was blocked by concurrent administration of zinc to the culture medium (Meerarani *et al.*, 2000). Conversely, increases in intracellular free zinc levels resulted in a rise in oxidative-stress-related apoptosis of endothelial cells (Wiseman *et al.*, 2007), highlighting that a change in the cellular zinc concentration in either direction could promote cell death in the endothelium.

Cellular zinc deficiency has been shown to upregulate NFκB activity in endothelial cells (Hennig *et al.*, 1999) and high levels of NFκB have been found to be present in the smooth muscle cells of the atherosclerotic lesion (Bourcier *et al.*, 1997). NFκB is a component of the adhesion molecule upregulation process; is involved in the promotion of smooth muscle cell proliferation (de Martin *et al.*, 2000); and mediates signal transduction by TLR. Each of these functions plays an important role in the initiation of the innate immune response and is implicated in atherogenesis (Pasterkamp *et al.*, 2004).

The release of NO by the endothelium plays a role in vascular homeostasis. One way in which the relationship between NO and zinc may promote atherogenesis relates to Nrf2 expression in vascular cells, which is a key factor in the cellular protection against oxidative stress and inflammation. A release of intracellular zinc from proteins containing zinc–sulfur complexes, stimulated by inducible NOS-derived NO, has been shown to be a crucial component of an Nrf2-dependent signalling pathway that activates the glutathione redox cycle in endothelial cells, ultimately protecting against oxidative damage (Cortese-Krott *et al.*, 2009).

The anti-inflammatory and antioxidant potential of zinc is supported by a recent zinc supplementation study. In a trial in healthy elderly subjects, supplementation with 45 mg Zn/day for 6 months was associated with an increase in antioxidant power and a decrease in plasma concentrations of CRP, IL-6, macrophage chemo-attractant protein 1 (MCP-1), vascular endothelial cell adhesion molecule 1 (VCAM-1) and oxidative stress markers. Taken together with the potential high-density-lipoprotein-raising effect of zinc (Foster *et al.*, 2010), these data indicate that zinc may exert an atheroprotective effect under some conditions (Bao *et al.*, 2010b).

Diabetes

Both type 1 and type 2 diabetes mellitus (DM) exhibit an impaired immune function as part of their pathogenesis that ultimately results in a decreased functional β-cell mass; whereas type 1 DM is primarily an autoimmune disorder that leads to rapid β-cell destruction, the failure of β cells in type 2 DM occurs over a prolonged period and involves the chronic activation of the innate immune system (Donath *et al.*, 2003). The sustained or aberrant expression in DM of a number of immune mediators, including NFκB, IL-1β and IL-6, suggests a potential interaction between the impaired immunity and the perturbed cellular zinc homeostasis associated with the disease.

Zinc has the ability to regulate both negatively and positively the signalling pathways of TLR and the IL-1 receptor, which may reflect its ability to induce or inhibit NFκB activation. Increased concentrations of IL-1β have been observed in the pancreatic islet in humans with type 2 DM (Maedler *et al.*, 2002), and human islets have been shown to respond to metabolic stress *in vitro* by increasing IL-6 release (Ehses *et al.*, 2007). A prospective examination of the effects of IL-1β, IL-6 and TNF-α on the development of type 2 DM found that participants with detectable levels of IL-1β and elevated levels of IL-6 in plasma had a threefold increased risk of developing DM compared with the reference group (Spranger *et al.*, 2003). Both IL-1β and IL-6 are pleiotropic and are known to exert both beneficial and detrimental effects on a variety of cell types, including the pancreatic β cells, depending on the cytokine concentration and the duration of exposure. Higher doses and longer exposure times impair glucose-stimulated insulin secretion and, at least in the case of IL-1β, increase β-cell apoptosis (Donath *et al.*, 2010).

The destruction of β cells can be mediated by autoreactive T-lymphocytes such as $CD4^+$ and $CD8^+$ cells; cytokines have been shown to induce the expression of the Fas (CD95, APO-1) receptor in the β cell, thereby sensitizing it to T-lymphocyte-mediated destruction (Donath *et al.*, 2003). The involvement of T cells in β-cell failure, and inflammation more broadly, further implicates perturbations in zinc homeostasis in the pathogenesis of DM. Zinc deficiency is well known to disrupt the development and function of T cells by causing, for instance, a reduction in thymic involution (Wellinghausen *et al.*, 1997) and a decrease in the $CD4^+$ to $CD8^+$ cell ratio (Prasad, 2008), both effects that have been shown to be corrected by zinc supplementation. High zinc doses also produce adverse consequences, including the inhibition of T cell functions and aberrant expression of cytokines (Ibs and Rink, 2003), and a paradoxical decrease in Cu-Zn superoxide dismutase activity (Abdallah and Samman, 1993; Samman 1993).

Summary and Conclusions

Deficiencies of iron and zinc are prevalent globally, and supplements of these nutrients are widely available, thus making the extremes of iron and zinc status achievable within the same population. Inflammation augments iron metabolism significantly through the action of hepcidin. Enhanced understanding of the action of hepcidin and inflammatory-driven regulation of iron status is important for improved diagnosis and treatment of anaemia under conditions of infectious or chronic disease. Similarly, deficiency and overload of zinc can influence markers of inflammation. High zinc doses produce adverse consequences similar to those observed in zinc-deficient conditions, such as the inhibition of T-cell functions and aberrant expression of cytokines. Further investigation of the molecular mechanisms that underpin the transport, sensing and distribution of zinc and iron are necessary to explain their effects in humans.

Recognition of the public health importance of zinc and iron continues to expand, as does knowledge of the multitude of biological pathways affected by these nutrients and their interaction with inflammation. Impaired homeostasis, chronic inflammation and increased levels of oxidative stress feature prominently in a number of disorders, including obesity, atherosclerosis and DM; the interplay of zinc and iron with these variables warrants further examination.

References

Abdallah, S.M. and Samman, S. (1993) The effect of increasing dietary zinc on the activity of superoxide dismutase and zinc concentration in erythrocytes of healthy female subjects. *European Journal of Clinical Nutrition* 47, 327–332.

Aeberli, I., Hurrell, R.F. and Zimmermann, M.B. (2009) Overweight children have higher circulating hepcidin concentrations and lower iron status but have dietary iron intakes and bioavailability comparable with normal weight children. *International Journal of Obesity* 33, 1111–1117.

Ausk, K.J. and Ioannou, G.N. (2008) Is obesity associated with anemia of chronic disease? A population-based study. *Obesity* 16, 2356–2361.

Aydemir, T.B., Blanchard, R.K. and Cousins, R.J. (2006) Zinc supplementation of young men alters metallothionein, zinc transporter, and cytokine gene expression in leukocyte populations. *Proceedings of the National Academy of Sciences USA* 103, 1699–1704.

Bao, B., Prasad, A.S., Beck, F.W.J., Snell, D., Suneja, A., *et al.* (2008) Zinc supplementation decreases oxidative stress, incidence of infection, and generation of inflammatory cytokines in sickle cell disease patients. *Translational Research* 152, 67–80.

Bao, S., Liu, M.J., Lee, B., Besecker, B., Lai, J.P., *et al.* (2010a) Zinc modulates the innate immune response in vivo to polymicrobial sepsis through regulation of NF-κB. *American Journal of Physiology* 298, L744–L754.

Bao, B., Prasad, A.S., Beck, F.W.J., Fitzgerald, J.T., Snell, D., *et al.* (2010b) Zinc decreases C-reactive protein, lipid peroxidation, and inflammatory cytokines in elderly subjects: a potential implication of zinc as an atheroprotective agent. *American Journal of Clinical Nutrition* 91, 1634–1641.

Beattie, J.H. and Kwun, I.S. (2004) Is zinc deficiency a risk factor for atherosclerosis? *British Journal of Nutrition* 91, 177–181.

Beck, F.W.J., Prasad, A.S., Kaplan, J., Fitzgerald, J.T. and Brewer, G.J. (1997) Changes in cytokine production and T cell subpopulations in experimentally induced zinc-deficient humans. *American Journal of Physiology* 272, E1002–E1007.

Bekri, S., Gual, P., Anty, R., Luciani, N., Dahman, M., *et al.* (2006) Increased adipose tissue expression of hepcidin in severe obesity is independent from Diabetes and NASH. *Gastroenterology* 131, 788–796.

Bourcier, T., Sukhova, G. and Libby, P. (1997) The nuclear factor kB signaling pathway participates in dysregulation of vascular smooth muscle cells in vitro and in human atherosclerosis. *Journal of Biological Chemistry* 272, 15817–15824.

Brown, K.H., Lanata, C.F., Yuen, M.L., Peerson, J.M., Butron, B., *et al.* (1993) Potential magnitude of the misclassification of a population's trace element status due to infection: Example from a survey of young Peruvian children. *American Journal of Clinical Nutrition* 58, 549–554.

Brownlie, T., 4th, Utermohlen, V., Hinton, P.S. and Haas, J.D. (2002) Marginal iron deficiency without anemia impairs aerobic adaptation among previously untrained women. *American Journal of Clinical Nutrition* 75, 734–742.

Brugnara, C. (2003) Iron deficiency and erythropoiesis: New diagnostic approaches. *Clinical Chemistry* 49, 1573–1578.

Cartwright, G.E. (1966) The anemia of chronic disorders. *Seminars in Hematology* 3, 351–375.

Cartwright, G.E., Lauritsen, M.A., Jones, P.J., Merrill, I.M. and Wintrobe, M.M. (1946) The anemia of infection. I. Hypoferremia, hypercupremia, and alterations in porphyrin metabolism in patients. *Journal of Clinical Investigation* 25, 65–80.

Chang, K.L., Hung, T.C., Hsieh, B.S., Chen, Y.H., Chen, T.F., *et al.* (2006) Zinc at pharmacologic concentrations affects cytokine expression and induces apoptosis of human peripheral blood mononuclear cells. *Nutrition* 22, 465–474.

Cheng, H.L., Bryant, C., Cook, R., O'Connor, H., Rooney, K., *et al.* (2011) The relationship between obesity and hypoferraemia in adults: a systematic review. *Obesity Reviews* doi: 10.1111/j.1467-789X.2011.00938.x.

Chung, B., Matak, P., McKie, A.T. and Sharp, P. (2007) Leptin increases the expression of the iron regulatory hormone hepcidin in HuH7 human hepatoma cells. *Journal of Nutrition* 137, 2366–2370.

Cortese-Krott, M.M., Suschek, C.V., Wetzel, W., Kröncke, K.D. and Kolb-Bachofen, V. (2009) Nitric oxide-mediated protection of endothelial cells from hydrogen peroxide is mediated by intracellular zinc and glutathione. *American Journal of Physiology* 296, C811–C820.

Craig, G.M., Evans, S.J. and Brayshaw, B.J. (1990) An inverse relationship between serum zinc and C-reactive protein levels in acutely ill elderly hospital patients. *Postgraduate Medical Journal* 66, 1025–1028.

Cunnane, S.C. (1982) Differential regulation of essential fatty acid metabolism to the prostaglandins: Possible basis for the interaction of zinc and copper in biological systems. *Progress in Lipid Research* 21, 73–90.

Cunnane, S.C. and McAdoo, K.R. (1987) Iron intake influences essential fatty acid and lipid composition of rat plasma and erythrocytes. *Journal of Nutrition* 117, 1514–1519.

Cunningham-Rundles, S., McNeeley, D.F. and Moon, A. (2005) Mechanisms of nutrient modulation of the immune response. *Journal of Allergy & Clinical Immunology* 115, 1119–1128.

De Domenico, I., McVey Ward, D. and Kaplan, J. (2008) Regulation of iron acquisition and storage: consequences for iron-linked disorders. *Nature Reviews Molecular Cell Biology* 9, 72–81.

de Martin, R., Hoeth, M., Hofer-Warbinek, R. and Schmid, J.A. (2000) The transcription factor NF-κB and the regulation of vascular cell function. *Arteriosclerosis, Thrombosis, and Vascular Biology* 20, E83–E88.

Denic, S. and Agarwal, M.M. (2007) Nutritional iron deficiency: An evolutionary perspective. *Nutrition* 23, 603–614.

Doherty, C.P. (2007) Host-pathogen interactions: The role of iron. *Journal of Nutrition* 137, 1341–1344.

Donath, M.Y., Størling, J., Maedler, K. and Mandrup-Poulsen, T. (2003) Inflammatory mediators and islet beta-cell failure: A link between type 1 and type 2 diabetes. *Journal of Molecular Medicine* 81, 455–470.

Donath, M.Y., Böni-Schnetzler, M., Ellingsgaard, H., Halban, P.A. and Ehses, J.A. (2010) Cytokine production by islets in health and diabetes: Cellular origin, regulation and function. *Trends in Endocrinology and Metabolism* 21, 261–267.

Eder, K. and Kirchgessner, M. (1996) Zinc deficiency and the desaturation of linoleic acid in rats force-fed fat-free diets. *Biological Trace Element Research* 54, 173–183.

Ehses, J.A., Perren, A., Eppler, E., Ribaux, P., Pospisilik, J.A., *et al.* (2007) Increased number of islet-associated macrophages in type 2 diabetes. *Diabetes* 56, 2356–2370.

Foster, M. and Samman, S. (2010) Zinc and redox signaling: Perturbations associated with cardiovascular disease and diabetes mellitus. *Antioxidants & Redox Signaling* 13, 1549–1573.

Foster, M.J., Petocz, P. and Samman, S. (2010) The effect of zinc supplementation on plasma lipoprotein cholesterol in humans: A meta-analysis of controlled trials. *Atherosclerosis* 210, 344–352.

Ganz, T. (2003) Hepcidin, a key regulator of iron metabolism and mediator of anemia of inflammation. *Blood* 102, 783–788.

Ganz, T. and Nemeth, E. (2009) Iron sequestration and anemia of inflammation. *Seminars in Hematology* 46, 387–393.

Graham, J.M., Paley, M.N.J., Grünewald, R.A., Hoggard, N. and Griffiths, P.D. (2000) Brain iron deposition in Parkinson's disease imaged using the PRIME magnetic resonance sequence. *Brain* 123, 2423–2431.

Gunshin, H., Mackenzie, B., Berger, U.V., Gunshin, Y., Romero, M.F., *et al.* (1997) Cloning and characterization of a mammalian proton-coupled metal-ion transporter. *Nature* 388, 482–488.

Hastka, J., Lasserre, J.J., Schwarzbeck, A., Strauch, M. and Hehlmann, R. (1993) Zinc protoporphyrin in anemia of chronic disorders. *Blood* 81, 1200–1204.

Hennig, B., Meerarani, P., Toborek, M. and McClain, C.J. (1999) Antioxidant-like properties of zinc in activated endothelial cells. *Journal of the American College of Nutrition* 18, 152–158.

Hotamisligil, G.S. (2006) Inflammation and metabolic disorders. *Nature* 444, 860–867.

Hughes, S. and Samman, S. (2006) The effect of zinc supplementation in humans on plasma lipids, antioxidant status and thrombogenesis. *Journal of the American College of Nutrition* 25, 285–291.

Ibs, K.H. and Rink, L. (2003) Zinc-altered immune function. *Journal of Nutrition* 133, 1452S–1456S.

Kahmann, L., Uciechowski, P., Warmuth, S., Plümäkers, B., Gressner, A.M., *et al.* (2008) Zinc supplementation in the elderly reduces spontaneous inflammatory cytokine release and restores T cell functions. *Rejuvenation Research* 11, 227–237.

Kawabata, H., Tomosugi, N., Kanda, J., Tanaka, Y., Yoshizaki, K., *et al.* (2007) Anti-interleukin 6 receptor antibody tocilizumab reduces the level of serum hepcidin in patients with multicentric Castleman's disease. *Haematologica* 92, 857–858.

Kelishadi, R., Hashemipour, M., Adeli, K., Tavakoli, N., Movahedian-Attar, A., *et al.* (2010) Effect of zinc supplementation on markers of insulin resistance, oxidative stress, and inflammation among prepubescent children with metabolic syndrome. *Metabolic Syndrome and Related Disorders* 8, 505–510.

Kemna, E.H.J.M., Tjalsma, H., Willems, H.L. and Swinkels, D.W. (2008) Hepcidin: From discovery to differential diagnosis. *Haematologica* 93, 90–97.

Knutson, M.D., Vafa, M.R., Haile, D.J. and Wessling-Resnick, M. (2003) Iron loading and erythrophagocytosis increase ferroportin 1 (FPN1) expression in J774 macrophages. *Blood* 102, 4191–4197.

Kochan, I. (1973) The role of iron in bacterial infections, with special consideration of host-tubercule bacillus interaction. *Current Topics Microbiology and Immunology* 60, 1–30.

Kontogianni, M.D., Zampelas, A. and Tsigos, C. (2006) Nutrition and inflammatory load. *Annals of the New York Academy of Science* 1083, 214–238.

Krause, A., Neitz, S., Mägert, H.-J., Schulz, A., Forssmann, W.-G., *et al.* (2000) LEAP-1, a novel highly disulfide-bonded human peptide, exhibits antimicrobial activity. *FEBS Letters* 480, 147–150.

Kruse-Jarres, J.D. (1989) The significance of zinc for humoral and cellular immunity. *Journal of Trace Elements and Electrolytes in Health and Disease* 3, 1–8.

Kuvibidila, S. and Vuvu, M. (2009) Unusual low plasma levels of zinc in non-pregnant Congolese women. *British Journal of Nutrition* 101, 1783–1786.

Lounis, N., Truffot-Pernot, C., Grosset, J., Gordeuk, V.R. and Boelaert, J.R. (2001) Iron and Mycobacterium tuberculosis infection. *Journal of Clinical Virology* 20, 123–126.

Ludwig, H., Pohl, G. and Osterborg, A. (2004) Anemia in multiple myeloma. *Clinical Advances in Hematology and Oncology* 2, 233–241.

Maccio, A., Madeddu, C., Massa, D., Mudu, M.C., Lusso, M.R., *et al.* (2005) Hemoglobin levels correlate with interleukin-6 levels in patients with advanced untreated epithelial ovarian cancer: Role of inflammation in cancer-related anemia. *Blood* 106, 362–367.

MacPhail, P. (2007) Iron. In: Mann, J.I. and Truswell, A.S. (eds) *Essentials of Human Nutrition*, 3rd edn. Oxford University Press, Oxford, UK, pp. 125–137.

Maedler, K., Sergeev, P., Ris, F., Oberholzer, J., Joller-Jemelka, H.I., *et al.* (2002) Glucose-induced beta cell production of IL1-beta contributes to glucotoxicity in human pancreatic islets. *Journal of Clinical Investigation* 110, 851–860.

Malavolta, M., Piacenza, F., Costarelli, L., Giacconi, R., Muti, E., *et al.* (2007) Combining UHR-SEC-HPLC-ICP-MS with flow cytometry to quantify metallothioneins and to study zinc homeostasis in human PBMC. *Journal of Analytical Atomic Spectrometry* 22, 1193–1198.

Mariani, E., Cattini, L., Neri, S., Malavolta, M., Mocchegiani, E., *et al.* (2008) Simultaneous evaluation of circulating chemokine and cytokine profiles in elderly subjects by multiplex technology: Relationship with zinc status. *Biogerontology* 7, 449–459.

McKie, A.T., Barrow, D., Latunde-Dada, G.O., Rolfs, A., Sager, G., *et al.* (2001) An iron-regulated ferric reductase associated with the absorption of dietary iron. *Science* 291, 1755–1759.

Medzhitov, R. (2010) Inflammation 2010: New adventures of an old flame. *Cell* 140, 771–776.

Meerarani, P., Ramadass, P., Toborek, M., Bauer, H.C., Bauer, H., and Hennig, B. (2000) Zinc protects against apoptosis of endothelial cells induced by linoleic acid and tumor necrosis factor alpha. *American Journal of Clinical Nutrition* 71, 81–87.

Menzie, C.M., Yanoff, L.B., Denkinger, B.I., McHugh, T., Sebring, N.G., Calis, K.A. and Yanovski, J.A. (2008) Obesity-related hypoferremia is not explained by differences in reported intake of heme and nonheme iron or intake of dietary factors that can affect iron absorption. *Journal of the American Dietetic Association* 108, 145–148.

Moalem, S., Weinberg, E.D. and Percy, M.E. (2004) Hemochromatosis and the enigma of misplaced iron: implications for infectious disease and survival. *BioMetals* 17, 135–139.

Mocchegiani, E., Giacconi, R., Costarelli, L., Muti, E., Cipriano, C., *et al.* (2008) Zinc deficiency and IL-6–174G/C polymorphism in old people from different European countries: Effect of zinc supplementation. ZINCAGE study. *Experimental Gerontology* 43, 433–444.

Murray, M.J., Murray, A.B., Murray, M.B. and Murray, C.J. (1978) The adverse effect of iron repletion on the course of certain infections. *British Medical Journal* 2, 1113–1115.

Nathan, C. and Ding, A. (2010) Nonresolving inflammation. *Cell* 140, 871–882.

Nead, K.G., Halterman, J.S., Kaczorowski, J.M., Auinger, P. and Weitzman, M. (2004) Overweight children and adolescents: a risk group for iron deficiency. *Pediatrics* 114, 104–108.

Nemeth, E. and Ganz, T. (2009) The role of hepcidin in iron metabolism. *Acta Haematologica* 122, 78–86.

Nemeth, E., Tuttle, M.S., Powelson, J., Vaughn, M.B., Donovan, A., *et al.* (2004) Hepcidin regulates cellular iron efflux by binding to ferroportin and inducing its internalization. *Science* 306, 2090–2093.

Nicolas, G., Chauvet, C., Viatte, L., Danan, J.L., Bigard, X., *et al.* (2002) The gene encoding the iron regulatory peptide hepcidin is regulated by anemia, hypoxia, and inflammation. *Journal of Clinical Investigation* 110, 1037–1044.
Noyes, W.D., Bothwell, T.H. and Finch, C.A. (1960) The role of the reticulo-endothelial cell in iron metabolism. *British Journal of Haematology* 6, 43–55.
Oakes, E.J.C., Lyon, T.D.B., Duncan, A., Gray, A., Talwar, D., *et al.* (2008) Acute inflammatory response does not affect erythrocyte concentrations of copper, zinc and selenium. *Clinical Nutrition* 27, 115–120.
O'Connor, H., Munas, Z., Griffin, H., Rooney, K., Cheng, H.L., *et al.* (2011) Nutritional adequacy of energy restricted diets for young obese women. *Asia Pacific Journal of Clinical Nutrition* 20, 206–211.
Ozkalay, N., Anil, M., Agus, N., Helvaci, M. and Sirti, S. (2006) Community-acquired meningitis and sepsis caused by Chryseobacterium meningosepticum in a patient diagnosed with Thalassemia Major. *Journal of Clinical Microbiology* 44, 3037–3039.
Papanikolaou, G., Samuels, M.E., Ludwig, E.H., MacDonald, M.L.E., Franchini, P.L., *et al.* (2004) Mutations in HFE2 cause iron overload in chromosome 1q-linked juvenile hemochromatosis. *Nature Genetics* 36, 77–82.
Park, C.H., Valore, E.V., Waring, A.J. and Ganz, T. (2001) Hepcidin, a urinary antimicrobial peptide synthesized in the liver. *Journal of Biological Chemistry* 276, 7806–7810.
Pasterkamp, G., van Keulen, J.K. and de Kleijn, D.P.V. (2004) Role of Toll-like receptor 4 in the initiation and progression of atherosclerotic disease. *European Journal of Clinical Investigation* 34, 328–334.
Pietrangelo, A., Dierssen, U., Valli, L., Garuti, C., Rump, A., *et al.* (2007) STAT3 is required for IL-6-gp130-dependent activation of hepcidin in vivo. *Gastroenterology* 132, 294–300.
Pinhas-Hamiel, O., Newfield, R.S., Koren, I., Agmon, A., Lilos, P., *et al.* (2003) Greater prevalence of iron deficiency in overweight and obese children and adolescents. *International Journal of Obesity and Related Metabolic Disorders* 27, 416–418.
Prasad, A.S. (2007) Zinc: mechanisms of host defense. *Journal of Nutrition* 137, 1345–1349.
Prasad, A.S. (2008) Zinc in human health: Effect of zinc on immune cells. *Molecular Medicine* 14, 353–357.
Prasad, A.S., Halsted, J.A. and Nadami, M. (1961) Syndrome of iron deficiency anaemia, hepatosplenomegaly, hypogonadism, dwarfism and geophagia. *American Journal of Medicine* 31, 532–546.
Prasad, A.S., Bao, B., Beck, F.W.J., Kucuk, O. and Sarkar, F.H. (2004) Antioxidant effect of zinc in humans. *Free Radical Biology & Medicine* 37, 1182–1190.
Prasad, A.S., Bao, B., Beck, F.W.J. and Sarkar, F.H. (2006) Correction of interleukin-2 gene expression by in vitro zinc addition to mononuclear cells from zinc deficient human subjects: A specific test for zinc deficiency in humans. *Translational Research* 148, 325–333.
Prasad, A.S., Beck, F.W.J., Bao, B., Fitzgerald, J.T., Snell, D.C., *et al.* (2007) Zinc supplementation decreases incidence of infections in the elderly: Effect of zinc on generation of cytokines and oxidative stress. *American Journal of Clinical Nutrition* 85, 837–844.
Prasad, A.S., Bao, B., Beck, F.W.J. and Sarkar, F.H. (2010) Zinc-suppressed inflammatory cytokines by induction of A20-mediated inhibition of nuclear factor-κB. *Nutrition* 27, 816–823.
Prentice, A.M. (2008) Iron metabolism, malaria, and other infections: What is all the fuss about? *Journal of Nutrition* 138, 2537–2541.
Rajpathak, S.N., Crandall, J.P., Wylie-Rosett, J., Kabat, G.C., Rohan, T.E. and Hu, F.B. (2009) The role of iron in type 2 diabetes in humans. *Biochimica et Biophysica Acta* 1790, 671–681.
Raqib, R., Roy, S.K., Rahman, M.J., Azim, T., Ameer, S.S., *et al.* (2004) Effect of zinc supplementation on immune and inflammatory responses in pediatric patients with shigellosis. *American Journal of Clinical Nutrition* 79, 444–450.
Rashidi, A.A., Salehi, M., Piroozmand, A. and Sagheb, M.M. (2009) Effects of zinc supplementation on serum zinc and C reactive protein concentrations in hemodialysis patients. *Journal of Renal Nutrition* 19, 475–478.
Rowe, D.J. and Bobilya, D.J. (2000) Albumin facilitates zinc acquisition by endothelial cells. *Proceedings of the Society for Experimental Biology & Medicine* 224, 178–186.
Roy, C.N. (2010) Anemia of inflammation. *Hematology* 2010, 276–280.
Samman, S. (1993) Dietary versus cellular zinc: the antioxidant paradox. *Free Radicals in Biology & Medicine* 14, 95–96.
Samman, S. (2007a) Iron. *Nutrition & Dietetics* 64, S126–S130.
Samman, S. (2007b) Zinc. *Nutrition & Dietetics* 64, S131–S134.

Samman, S. (2007c) Zinc and copper. In: Mann, J.I. and Truswell, A.S. (eds) *Essentials of Human Nutrition*, 3rd edn. Oxford University Press, Oxford, UK, pp 138–144.

Samman, S. (2011) Challenges and opportunities in the assessment of zinc status. *Nutrition & Dietetics* 68, 95–96.

Sandstead, H.H., Prasad, A.S., Penland, J.G., Beck, F.W.J., Kaplan, J., *et al.* (2008) Zinc deficiency in Mexican American children: influence of zinc and other micronutrients on T cells, cytokines, and antiinflammatory plasma proteins. *American Journal of Clinical Nutrition* 88, 1067–1073.

Seltzer, C.C. and Mayer, J. (1963) Serum iron and iron-binding capacity in adolescents. II. Comparison of obese and nonobese subjects. *American Journal of Clinical Nutrition* 13, 354–361.

Shoelson, S.E., Herrero, L. and Naaz, A. (2007) Obesity, inflammation, and insulin resistance. *Gastroenterology* 132, 2169–2180.

Skikne, B.S. (2008) Serum transferrin receptor. *American Journal of Hematology* 83, 872–875.

Spranger, J., Kroke, A., Möhlig, M., Hoffman, K., Bergmann, M.M., *et al.* (2003) Inflammatory cytokines and the risk to develop type 2 diabetes: Results of the prospective population-based European Prospective Investigation into Cancer and Nutrition (EPIC)-Potsdam Study. *Diabetes* 52, 812–817.

Tapazoglou, E., Prasad, A.S., Hill, G., Brewer, G.J. and Kaplan, J. (1985) Decreased natural killer cell activity in zinc deficient subjects with sickle cell disease. *Journal of Laboratory & Clinical Medicine* 105, 19–22.

Thurnham, D.I., Mburu, A.S., Mwaniki, D.L. and De Wagt, A. (2005) Micronutrients in childhood and the influence of subclinical inflammation. *Proceedings of the Nutrition Society* 64, 502–509.

Tussing-Humphreys, L.M., Nemeth, E., Fantuzzi, G., Freels, S., Guzman, G., *et al.* (2010) Elevated systemic hepcidin and iron depletion in obese premenopausal females. *Obesity* 18, 1449–1456.

Vahdat Shariatpanaahi, M., Vahdat Shariatpanaahi, Z., Moshtaaghi, M., Shahbaazi, S.H. and Abadi, A. (2007) The relationship between depression and serum ferritin level. *European Journal of Clinical Nutrition* 61, 532–535.

Vari, I.S., Balkau, B., Kettaneh, A., André, P., Tichet, J., *et al.* (2007) Ferritin and transferrin are associated with metabolic syndrome abnormalities and their change over time in a general population. *Diabetes Care* 30, 1795–1801.

Verga Falzacappa, M.V., Vujic Spasic, M., Kessler, R., Stolte, J., Hentze, M.W., *et al.* (2007) STAT3 mediates hepatic hepcidin expression and its inflammatory stimulation. *Blood* 109, 353–358.

Wallace, D.F. and Subramaniam, V.N. (2009) Co-factors in liver disease: The role of HFE-related hereditary hemochromatosis and iron. *Biochimica et Biophysica Acta* 1790, 663–670.

Wang, R.-H., Li, C., Xu, X., Zheng, Y., Xiao, C., *et al.* (2005) A role of SMAD4 in iron metabolism through the positive regulation of hepcidin expression. *Cell Metabolism* 2, 399–409.

Wellinghausen, N., Kirchner, H. and Rink, L. (1997) The immunobiology of zinc. *Immunology Today* 18, 519–521.

Wessling-Resnick, M. (2010) Iron homeostasis and the inflammatory response. *Annual Reviews of Nutrition* 30, 105–122.

Wiseman, D.A., Wells, S.M., Hubbard, M., Welker, J.E. and Black, S.M. (2007) Alterations in zinc homeostasis underlie endothelial cell death induced by oxidative stress from acute exposure to hydrogen peroxide. *American Journal of Physiology* 292, L165–L177.

Wrighting, D.M. and Andrews, N.C. (2006) Interleukin-6 induces hepcidin expression through STAT3. *Blood* 108, 3204–3209.

Yang, F., Liu, X.-B., Quinones, M., Melby, P.C., Ghio, A., *et al.* (2002) Regulation of reticuloendothelial iron transporter MTP1 (Slc11a3) by Inflammation. *Journal of Biological Chemistry* 277, 39786–39791.

Yanoff, L.B., Menzie, C.M., Denkinger, B., Sebring, N.G., McHugh, T., *et al.* (2007) Inflammation and iron deficiency in the hypoferremia of obesity. *International Journal of Obesity* 31, 1412–1419.

Yuan, X.M. (1999) Apoptotic macrophage-derived foam cells of human atheromas are rich in iron and ferritin, suggesting iron-catalysed reactions to be involved in apoptosis. *Free Radical Research* 30, 221–231.

10 Resistance Exercise and Inflammation

G. Paulsen*,[1] and J.M. Peake[2,3,4]

[1]Norwegian School of Sport Sciences, Oslo, Norway; [2]School of Human Movement Studies and [3]Centre for Military and Veterans' Health, The University of Queensland, Brisbane, Australia; [4]Centre of Excellence for Applied Sport Science Research, Queensland Academy of Sport, Brisbane, Australia

Introduction

Intensive exercise can acutely alter trafficking and redistribution of immune cells, and also affects immune cell activity and the levels of circulating humoral factors (e.g. cytokines). Thus, exercise may initiate transient mild systemic inflammation. The immune response to exercise is generally modified by the exercise load, and immunity might even be compromised if the load is intense and long lasting. Accordingly, athletes engaging in strenuous, prolonged exercise activities (>90 min) may be more prone to developing infection and illness in the hours after exercise, as explained by the 'open window' hypothesis (Pedersen *et al.*, 1996). On the contrary, regular exercise training at moderate to high intensity can, over time, strengthen our immune system (see Chapter 11; Walsh *et al.*, 2011a,b).

The inflammatory response to traditional resistance exercise training, principally weight lifting, has received little attention. It seems, however, that the inflammatory response to a bout of resistance exercise resembles that of aerobic endurance exercise in many respects (see Chapter 11, and extensive reviews by others: Shephard *et al.*, 1991; Gabriel and Kindermann,

* Corresponding author, goran.paulsen@nih.no

1997; Nieman, 1997; Pedersen and Hoffman-Goetz, 2000; Walsh *et al.*, 2011a,b). This is not surprising because the acute physiological responses to endurance and resistance exercise are overlapping. Both exercise modes stimulate the cardiovascular system, as indicated by increased cardiac output and blood flow, especially to the lungs and working muscles. Both exercise modes may also induce haemoconcentration, resulting from movement of fluid from the circulation into the working muscle, and increased sweating and respiration (gross loss of fluid; Collins *et al.*, 1989). Together with the 'pumping' effect of dynamic muscle contractions, the increased extracellular fluid pressure will stimulate lymph flow and increased emptying of lymph into the circulation (Olszewski *et al.*, 1977). Additionally, both exercise modes will stimulate the sympathetic nervous as well as the endocrine system, leading to increased blood levels of adrenaline, noradrenaline, growth hormone and cortisol (Gabriel and Kindermann, 1997; Kraemer and Ratamess, 2005). All of these physiological changes to exercise can influence inflammatory and immunological responses. Both the cardiopulmonary stress and the hormone response will typically be greater, however, during intensive aerobic endurance exercise than during traditional resistance exercise (Hurley *et al.*, 1984; Collins *et al.*, 1991; Nieman *et al.*, 1995; Risøy *et al.*, 2003; Kraemer and Ratamess, 2005).

When considering resistance training as a form of exercise, it is important to recognize the great variety of resistance exercise programmes. Generally, by applying heavy loads, few repetitions (<5) and long rest intervals (3–5 min), the changes in cardiac output and hormone responses will be small or moderate (Kraemer and Ratamess, 2005; Crewther *et al.*, 2006). By contrast, circuit exercise training, including moderate loads, many repetitions (e.g. 20–30) and short rest intervals (e.g. 10–30 s), is intermediate to endurance exercise (e.g. running and cycling). The selection of resistance exercises in a given session will also influence the physiological response. Exercises for smaller muscle groups (e.g. the arms and calves) will induce significantly less cardiovascular stress than multiple-joint exercises for the legs, chest and back (e.g. squats, deadlifts, bench press and rowing exercises). Thus, depending on the programme design, inflammatory responses to resistance exercise can vary considerably.

The most noticeable difference between traditional aerobic endurance and high-force resistance exercises is the level of muscle motor unit recruitment and force generation. Effective resistance exercise depends on large/full muscle activation, typically achieved by lifting heavy loads (McDonagh and Davies, 1984; Folland and Williams, 2007). Consequently, the energy required during resistance exercise must be provided by the anaerobic energy system (Tesch *et al.*, 1986). The increased utilization of aerobic energy transfer during resistance exercise is primarily driven by the need to restore cellular homeostasis during the rest intervals (the periods between sets), e.g. replenishment of creatine phosphate and restoring the ion-concentration equilibrium across the myofibre membranes (Glaister, 2005; Allen *et al.*, 2008). The large force-generation and anaerobic metabolic stress are the major stimuli for muscle growth (Wernbom *et al.*, 2007, 2008; Spiering *et al.*, 2008). During exercise, however, these stress factors rapidly induce fatigue and even damage in the working muscles, which can require prolonged recovery periods (>1 day). Eccentric exercise (lengthening muscle actions under load) typically involves large force production and commonly results in muscle damage, which makes this type of exercise a popular model for research purposes (Stauber *et al.*, 1989; Evans and Cannon, 1991; Peake *et al.*, 2005a). We should, nevertheless, keep in mind that the degree of muscle damage induced by unaccustomed eccentric exercise is typically much greater than that seen after a bout of traditional resistance (and endurance) exercise. For example, the recovery time from eccentric exercise is often several days or weeks (Clarkson and Hubal, 2002), compared with 1–3 days after traditional resistance exercise (Raastad and Hallen, 2000; Ahtiainen *et al.*, 2003, 2004; Raastad *et al.*, 2003; Judge and Burke, 2010). Thus, the results from studies examining unaccustomed eccentric exercise may have limited application in this context, but are still considered important to understanding some of the mechanisms behind any altered immunological responsiveness to resistance exercise.

Leucocytosis Induced by Resistance Exercise

As soon as we start to exercise at a high intensity (e.g. >70% of maximal capacity), the concentration of freely circulating blood leucocytes rises (Fig. 10.1). This is especially true for natural killer (NK) cells and neutrophils (also known as 'neutrophilic granulocytes'; Gabriel and Kindermann, 1997; Pedersen and Hoffman-Goetz, 2000). The most important mechanism behind this acute leucocytosis seems to be increased cardiac output.[1] Increased blood pressure and flow velocity flushes out leucocytes trapped in low-pressure blood vessels in the upper part of the lungs. These effects are mediated in part by increased blood concentrations of catecholamines such as adrenaline and noradrenaline during exercise (Shephard, 2001; Walsh *et al.*, 2011b). Adrenaline and noradrenaline increase blood pressure and bind to adrenoreceptors on the surface of leucocytes. In turn, they reduce the adherence of the leucocytes to the endothelium in the spleen, liver and perhaps bone marrow, by lowering the number of adhesion molecules. In addition, the combined action of muscle contractions, increased blood flow through the lymph tissue and amplified sympathetic activity mobilizes lymphocytes in lymphatic tissue in the spleen, lymph nodes and gastrointestinal tract (Pedersen and Hoffman-Goetz, 2000; Shephard, 2001, 2003; Kruger *et al.*, 2008). Positive correlations between the mobilization of NK cells and the noradrenaline response to resistance exercise have been reported (Stock *et al.*, 1995; Ramel *et al.*, 2003). These events are probably quite similar during resistance and aerobic endurance modes of exercise, although less marked with resistance exercise (Gabriel *et al.*, 1994; Nieman *et al.*, 1995; Brenner *et al.*, 1999; Natale *et al.*, 2003).

Resistance exercise with short rest intervals (e.g. 1 min), a relatively high number of repetitions (e.g. 10) and the use of large muscle groups (e.g. squats) can induce high blood lactate concentration and a marked hormonal response, including increased levels of adrenaline/noradrenaline, growth hormone and cortisol (Hakkinen and Pakarinen, 1993;

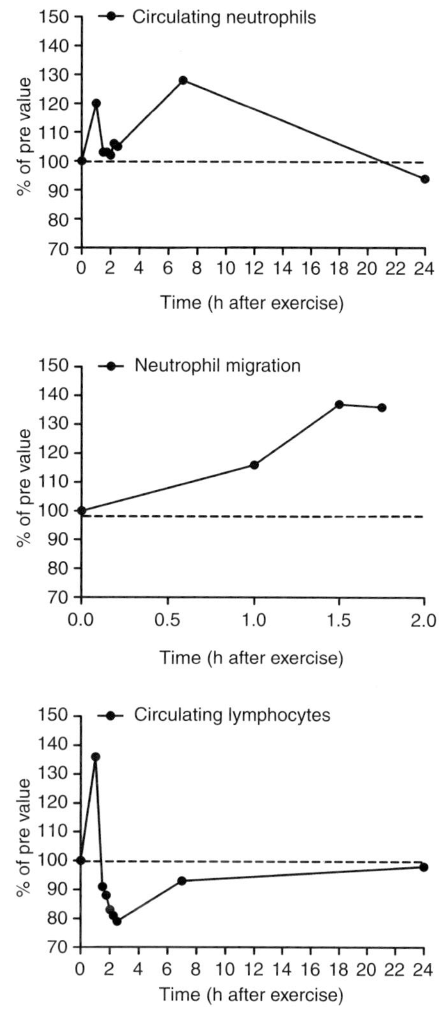

Fig. 10.1. Systemic inflammatory responses to a bout of resistance exercise: One-legged leg press (5 × 3 RM) and knee-extensions (5 × 6 RM); (a) and (c) show counts of freely circulating neutrophils and lymphocytes (including NK cells), whereas (b) displays the migration of neutrophils stimulated by the chemotactic effect of plasma (for methodological details, see Grimstad and Benestad, 1982). The assay measures the chemotactic gradient in the plasma, which increased 1.5 h after exercise and indicates that there was an increased release of chemoattractive substances (e.g. chemokines) to the circulation during and/or after exercise, possibly from the exercised muscles. All values are relative to baseline. Data are from eight resistance-trained males (figures redrawn from data published by Risøy *et al.*, 2003).

Stock *et al.*, 1995; Kraemer *et al.*, 1996, 1998, 1990, 1987; Ahtiainen *et al.*, 2004; Fragala *et al.*, 2011). Miles *et al.* (2003) observed an association between lactate levels and the increased numbers of circulating B and T lymphocytes after squat exercise in women. Lactate itself does probably not mediate these immune responses directly. Instead, other factors that are sensitive to exercise intensity such as growth hormone (Kraemer and Ratamess, 2005) appear to mobilize neutrophils and monocytes following exercise (Kappel *et al.*, 1993; Risøy *et al.*, 2003; Paulsen *et al.*, 2005).

In general, the amplitude of the leucocytosis immediately after resistance exercise seems more dependent on the anaerobic intensity than on the training level (strength) and absolute workload (Miles *et al.*, 2003). For example, Kruger *et al.* (2011) observed acute leucocytosis (~25% increase of total leucocyte counts) after a session of whole body resistance exercise at 75% of 1 repetition maximum (RM), but not at 60% of 1 RM (with equal number of repetitions; three sets per exercise). Mayhew *et al.* (2005) reported significantly greater lymphocytosis and monocytosis immediately after leg press exercise (10 × 10 reps) with 1 min rest intervals compared with the same bout but with 3 min rest intervals (equal total work). Of note, the increased blood concentration of neutrophils (neutrophilia) 1.5 h after exercise was not affected by the rest periods; and Kruger *et al.* (2011) observed neutrophilia 3 h after both 75% and 60% of 1 RM exercise intensity. This implies that different factors might regulate the acute versus delayed leucocytosis after resistance exercise training.

Delayed Leucocytosis

Both endurance and resistance exercise seem to stimulate a biphasic change in the number of circulating leucocytes (Fig. 10.1). As described, the neutrophils, lymphocytes and monocytes increase during exercise, but fall towards baseline within approximately 30 min after exercise. Then a second, delayed rise in the neutrophil count starts as the number of lymphocytes decreases below baseline. The following neutrophilia and lymphopenia may last for several hours, but cell counts are typically normalized within 24 h. The delayed neutrophilia can be observed together with a delayed monocytosis (Gabriel and Kindermann, 1997; Malm *et al.*, 1999; Paulsen *et al.*, 2005).

In order to distinguish effects of resistance exercise from aerobic endurance exercise, muscle damage is generally greater following resistance exercise, at least if we exclude very long-duration endurance competitions, such as the marathon and triathlons. Exercise-induced muscle damage is primarily caused by large mechanical forces and strain (lengthening of the working muscles; Proske and Morgan, 2001). However, metabolic stress from anaerobic energy transfer and ischaemia–reperfusion-cycles may also play a role (Uchiyama *et al.*, 2006; Tee *et al.*, 2007). Damage to extracellular structures, the sarcolemma and intracellular structures may induce the synthesis of complement components and their derivatives, lipid mediators (e.g. prostaglandins) and cytokines (e.g. interleukin (IL)-1β, IL-6 and IL-8). These inflammatory mediators have chemoattractive effects, meaning that they will recruit immune cells into the damaged tissue (Evans and Cannon, 1991; MacIntyre *et al.*, 1995; Peake *et al.*, 2005a). As these inflammatory mediators diffuse into the circulation, they may also mobilize marginated leucocytes and accelerate the release of granulocytes from bone marrow (Opdenakker *et al.*, 1998). Thus, exercise-induced muscle damage per se might cause a leucocytosis. Muscle damage, however, probably does not alter the number of circulating leucocytes during exercise, as reflected by the time lag between damage and generation of these mediators. Seemingly, the delayed response to muscle-damaging exercise may be more pronounced than the acute leucocytosis, and largely reflects increased numbers of neutrophilic granulocytes and, to some extent, a monocytosis (Pizza *et al.*, 1996; Paulsen *et al.*, 2005). In contrast, in the hours after resistance exercise, the lymphocyte numbers are often below pre-exercise values (Gabriel and Kindermann, 1997; Malm *et al.*, 1999; Paulsen *et al.*, 2005), but this event is probably less related to muscle damage.

Delayed leucocytosis can occur in response to cortisol, because cortisol is known to mobilize both bone marrow-stored and marginated neutrophils, increase their half-life in the circulation and decrease their exit from the blood (Nakagawa *et al.*, 1998). Some (Ramel *et al.*, 2003) but not all authors (Kraemer *et al.*, 1996; Risøy *et al.*, 2003) have reported an association between the leucocytosis and cortisol following resistance exercise. These findings point to a chemoattractive substance in the circulation as a plausible mechanism for the delayed leucocytosis. In favour of this assumption, Risøy *et al.* (2003) measured chemotactic activity in plasma after heavy resistance exercise and observed an increase between 5 min and 5 h after exercise that was (moderately) correlated to the delayed neutrophilia (5 h after exercise; Fig. 10.1). The neutrophilia was accompanied by increased numbers of band neutrophils, which indicates augmented release of 'young' neutrophils from the bone marrow. Paulsen *et al.* (2005) have also reported an increase in chemotactic activity in plasma 1 h after unaccustomed eccentric exercise, which was followed by a strong delayed leucocytosis (primarily neutrophilia; about 100% increase over baseline). The technique used by Risøy *et al.* (2003) and Paulsen *et al.* (2005) is based on the migration of neutrophils *in vitro* (in migration chambers), and gives a measure of chemotactic activity of unidentified factors in plasma (Grimstad and Benestad, 1982). It is unlikely that a single substance is solely responsible for this chemotactic activity because we would expect a number of potential substances to play a role in integrated synergy (e.g. cytokines/chemokines and complement products).

If the delayed leucocytosis after resistance exercise is truly related to muscle damage, there should be a relationship between markers of muscle damage and leucocytosis. Indeed, the leucocytosis after eccentric exercise follows the same 'repeated-bout' pattern as muscle function, blood creatine kinase activity and muscle soreness (Pizza *et al.*, 1996, 2001; McHugh, 2003).[2] Pizza *et al.* (1996) reported a lower number and reduced activation (CD11b and CD64 expression) of circulating neutrophils and monocytes after a second (repeated) bout compared with an initial unaccustomed bout of eccentric exercise. This has not been verified, however, after repeated bouts of traditional resistance exercise (Risøy *et al.*, 2003; McFarlin *et al.*, 2005; Hulmi *et al.*, 2010). Furthermore, the limited evidence available indicates that the leucocytosis after resistance exercise is similar between untrained and trained subjects (Ramel *et al.*, 2004). By contrast, classical muscle damage markers are higher in untrained than in trained subjects after eccentric exercise (Newton *et al.*, 2008). Only moderate correlations between markers of muscle damage and leucocytosis have been reported (Kayashima *et al.*, 1995; Nieman *et al.*, 2005; Paulsen *et al.*, 2005). Similarly, the leucocytosis that develops after heart attacks (myocardial necrosis) or trauma does not seem to correlate with the extent of damage in a linear, dose–response manner (Latini *et al.*, 1994; Rainer *et al.*, 1999). Thus, the amplitude of the delayed leucocytosis after exercise is not a good marker for muscle damage. One plausible explanation for this is that the delayed leucocytosis is induced by several factors, some related to muscle damage and others not (e.g. systematic stress of the exercise (Saxton *et al.*, 2003) and the hormone responses). An interesting finding, however, is a positive correlation between reduced muscle function (a reliable marker of muscle damage; Warren *et al.*, 1999) and the relative increase in circulating band ('young') neutrophils (differential counts on blood smears) after unaccustomed eccentric exercise with the elbow flexors (Paulsen, Bøyum, Benestad and Raastad, unpublished observations). Muscle damage may therefore be more closely related to the mobilization of young leucocytes from the bone marrow following unaccustomed eccentric exercise compared with other forms of exercise.

In summary, traditional resistance exercise induces an immediate increase in the number of freely circulating leucocytes, which is most likely primarily due to increased cardiac blood flow and catecholamine secretion. After exercise the leucocyte numbers decline towards baseline, but neutrophil counts will typically increase again in a delayed leucocytosis, while lymphocyte counts drop below baseline. Normalization of cell counts is expected within 24h. Resistance exercise sessions that involve classic multi-joint exercises, such as the squat and deadlift, 8–12 repetitions, short rest intervals (about 1min) and multiple sets per exercise (e.g. 3 sets), are expected to induce significant leucocytosis (and delayed lymphopenia). Muscle damage, induced by high-mechanical loading of the exercised muscles, might play a part in the delayed leucocytosis. Leucocytosis is not, however, a reliable marker for muscle damage.

Cytokines

Exercise evokes an acute-phase response that, to a certain extent, is similar to what can be seen during sepsis (Evans and Cannon, 1991; Shephard, 2001). Elevated levels of cytokines are a conspicuous finding during the acute-phase response, and cytokines are plausible candidates to mobilize leucocytes during and after exercise. Blood concentrations of pro-inflammatory cytokines, such as IL-1, IL-3, IL-6, IL-8, colony-stimulating factors (CSFs) and tumour necrosis factor (TNF)-α, are associated with leucocytosis during infection/ sepsis (Opdenakker *et al.*, 1998; Rankin, 2004). A large number of cytokines and chemokines increase in the circulation during and after exercise, including both pro- and anti-inflammatory cytokines/chemokines (Moldoveanu *et al.*, 2001; Shephard, 2002; Suzuki *et al.*, 2003). IL-6 and granulocyte (G)-CSF have been found to correlate positively with delayed neutrophilia after strenuous endurance exercise (Yamada *et al.*, 2002; Suzuki *et al.*, 2003). Paulsen *et al.* (2005) also reported a moderate relationship between G-CSF and delayed neutrophilia after eccentric exercise. Compared with strenuous endurance exercise, a moderate, but longer-lasting (hours to days) elevation of circulating cytokines (especially IL-6) seems to characterize the response to unaccustomed eccentric exercise (Smith *et al.*, 2000; MacIntyre *et al.*, 2001; Moldoveanu *et al.*, 2001; Shephard, 2002; Suzuki *et al.*, 2002; Peake *et al.*, 2005a). The cytokine response to traditional resistance exercise varies considerably among studies, but is generally milder than that following strenuous endurance exercise (Brenner *et al.*, 1999; Risøy *et al.*, 2003; Nieman *et al.*, 2004; Buford *et al.*, 2009; Izquierdo *et al.*, 2009; Kawada *et al.*, 2010; Kruger *et al.*, 2011). To illustrate this variability, Buford *et al.* (2009) found no increase in IL-1β, IL-6, IL-8 and TNF-α after traditional resistance exercise (squat, leg press, knee-extension; 3 × 10 reps at 80% of 1RM, 3min rest periods), whereas Nieman *et al.* (2004) found a 4–6-fold increase in IL-6, IL-8 and IL-10 after a large volume, whole-body workout (a total of 40 sets). Some of the variations between studies are likely to be explained by the workout session (load/intensity, volume, rest-intervals, etc.), sampling time points and training status of the subjects. Different observations might also be related to the cytokine assays applied (e.g. different sensitivity and detection levels).

Izquierdo *et al.* (2009) observed a stronger response of IL-6 and IL-10 after a bout of leg press (5 × 10RM) conducted after a 7-week training period, compared with a similar bout conducted before the training period. On the other hand, IL-1β increased relatively more after the first compared with the second bout, whereas the IL-1 receptor antagonist, IL-1ra, showed the opposite response. Thus, this suggests that a period of resistance exercise training alters the acute cytokine response to a bout of resistance exercise in favour of anti-inflammatory over pro-inflammatory cytokines. This assumption is supported by studies on repeated bouts of eccentric exercise (Hirose *et al.*, 2004; Smith *et al.*, 2007).

The cytokine response to exercise has primarily been linked to metabolism and muscle damage. IL-6 is secreted by the working muscles during exercise, and the secretion rate is strongly related to muscle glycogen depletion (Pedersen and Febbraio, 2008). The notion that cytokines are linked to the extent of exercise-induced muscle damage, as suggested after extreme long-distance running and eccentric exercise (MacIntyre *et al.*, 2001; Nieman *et al.*, 2004) is less certain (Pedersen and Hoffman-Goetz 2000; Moldoveanu 2001; Peake *et al.*, 2005b, 2006). If there is a genuine link between muscle damage and the cytokine response, one would expect a reduced cytokine response after a repeated bout of exercise, as for other muscle damage markers (e.g. muscle function and creatine kinase; McHugh, 2003). Studies have reported, however, an equally strong cytokine response in the circulation (e.g. IL-6 and G-CSF) after the second, repeated bout compared with the initial bout of unaccustomed eccentric exercise (Hirose *et al.*, 2004; Willoughby *et al.*, 2003). Hence, these findings do not intuitively fit well with the concept that circulating (pro-inflammatory) cytokines are directly related to muscle damage and the inflammatory response after eccentric exercise (or resistance exercise). In summary, the inflammatory cytokine response to resistance exercise is not exclusively due to muscle damage. Therefore, both metabolic and hormonal responses (e.g. adrenalin, cortisol and growth hormone) are plausible candidates to drive the cytokine response to resistance exercise.

Myokines: cytokines produced by skeletal muscles

The cytokine levels in plasma are determined by their production and elimination rates. Cytokines are regularly cleared from the circulation by splanchnic organs and the kidneys (to the urine), whereas the sources of production are more difficult to ascertain (Moldoveanu *et al.*, 2001; Suzuki *et al.*, 2002). Potential sources include leucocytes accumulated at sites of inflammation (owing to tissue damage or infection), circulating leucocytes, splanchnic tissue, skeletal muscle and adipose tissue (Moldoveanu *et al.*, 2001; Suzuki *et al.*, 2002; Rankin, 2004; Zaldivar *et al.*, 2006; Pedersen and Febbraio, 2008; Carlson *et al.*, 2011). In addition to myocytes and satellite cells, skeletal muscle contains epithelial cells and tissue-resident fibroblasts, mast cells, dendritic cells and leucocytes (primarily macrophages, but also T cells) that can produce significant amounts of cytokines (Curfs *et al.*, 1997; Scott *et al.*, 2004; Gosain and Gamelli, 2005). Myoblasts have the potential to produce a variety of cytokines (De Rossi *et al.*, 2000) or so-called 'myokines' (Pedersen *et al.*, 2007). IL-1β, IL-6, IL-8, IL-10 and TNF-α mRNA expression has been reported to increase in exercised muscles during the first hours after a bout of resistance exercise (Dennis *et al.*, 2004; Nieman *et al.*, 2004; Przybyla *et al.*, 2006; Louis *et al.*, 2007; Trenerry *et al.*, 2007; Deldicque *et al.*, 2008; Buford *et al.*, 2009). Increased protein expression of IL-6 has been found 3 h after maximal isokinetic (concentric/eccentric) exercise (Trenerry *et al.*, 2011) and both IL-6 and IL-8 have been observed as elevated after endurance exercise (Pedersen 2011). Histological signs of increased IL-1β and monocyte chemoattractant protein-1 (MCP-1) have been found after eccentric exercise (Cannon *et al.*, 1989; Fielding *et al.*, 1993; Hubal *et al.*, 2008). IL-1β protein has been located in the extracellular matrix and around capillaries, as well as inside the myofibres (Cannon *et al.*, 1989; Malm *et al.*, 2000), whereas MCP-1 protein has been observed in the proximity of macrophages and satellite cells (Hubal *et al.*, 2008). Thus, the protein levels of these cytokines and chemokines are not necessarily up-regulated by the myofibres themselves, but rather by other tissue-resident (stromal) cells and the accumulation of blood-borne leucocytes. The development of a local inflammatory reaction caused by exercise-induced muscle damage would intuitively be an important source of cytokine production (Hawke and Garry 2001; Charge and Rudnicki 2004; Tidball 2005). The expression of some cytokines/myokines in muscle may therefore require a significant degree of muscle damage, like that inflicted by unaccustomed eccentric exercise. Nevertheless, it is uncertain whether this is a realistic scenario after bouts of traditional resistance exercise, especially conducted on a regular basis. Indeed, increased levels of circulating MCP-1 and IL-1β have been reported after eccentric exercise (more than twofold above pre-exercise levels; Cannon *et al.*, 1991; Paulsen *et al.*, 2005). In contrast, circulating MCP-1 has been found to decrease slightly after whole-body, circuit-type resistance exercise (70–75% of 1 RM; Fatouros *et al.*, 2010).

In response to a period of resistance exercise training, the expression of TNF-α in resting skeletal muscle decreases in elderly individuals (or rather normalizes compared with young individuals; Greiwe *et al.*, 2001). TNF-α is associated with inflammatory reactions and muscle wasting (Reid and Li, 2001;

Frangogiannis *et al.*, 2002), which means that resistance exercise training may have a local anti-inflammatory effect and stimulate protein synthesis in aged skeletal muscle. In young, healthy individuals the baseline mRNA expression of IL-7 (but not IL-6) increased after a period of resistance exercise training (Haugen *et al.*, 2010). IL-7 is believed to affect myogenesis and migration of satellite cells, and may be involved in the muscular adaptation processes during resistance exercise training.

In summary, intensive resistance exercise seems to induce mild systemic inflammation that might encompass mild elevation of circulating cytokines. There appears to be a balance between pro- and anti-inflammatory cytokines, and anti-inflammatory cytokines such as IL-10 may dominate after repeated bouts of exercise (a training period). The sources of cytokine production are unclear, but certain cytokines may be produced by the exercised muscle (myokines). At present, it seems that only IL-6 is produced in sufficient quantities in skeletal muscle for release into the circulation following exercise. IL-6 release from skeletal muscle has, however, only been demonstrated after endurance exercise (Pedersen and Febbraio, 2008; Pedersen, 2011). Although evidence exists that resistance exercise increases the gene expression of several cytokines in skeletal muscle, there is currently scant evidence for cytokine protein expression changes in skeletal muscle following bouts of traditional resistance exercise. More research is required to examine the stimuli for the increased cytokine/myokine production (muscle damage versus metabolic stress), the time course of changes in cytokine/myokine expression, interactions between cytokines and the role of cytokine receptors in skeletal muscle following resistance exercise.

Activation of Mobilized Leucocytes

In response to an infection, cytokines activate circulating leucocytes. This occurs in the blood during sepsis and mainly in the inflamed tissues during other infectious episodes. The leucocytes become 'primed' and activated on their way to the site on infection. They are therefore ready to enter the infection site and attack microbes (Pyne, 1994; Dallegri and Ottonello, 1997; Opdenakker *et al.*, 1998). A similar response occurs in response to aseptic tissue damage, such as myocardial infarction (necrosis; Meisel *et al.*, 1998; Frangogiannis, 2008). Changes in the expression of adhesion molecules on the surface of primed leucocytes allow these leucocytes to adhere more effectively to endothelial cells, and thereby enter the inflamed tissue (Schmid-Schonbein, 2006). In comparison with endurance exercise (see Chapter 11), little is known about the effects of traditional resistance exercise on leucocyte chemotaxis, phagocytosis and oxidative burst activity.

Expression of adhesion molecules on the cell surface is essential for leucocyte trafficking and redistribution (Shephard, 2002, 2003; Rankin, 2004); such molecules represent 'addresses', whereas cytokines and chemokines represent 'go signals'. During aerobic exercise, the expression of adhesion molecules (e.g. CD11a, CD11b and CD18, and CD54 and CD62L) on leucocytes has been reported to increase, decrease or remain unchanged (Gabriel and Kindermann, 1998; van Eeden *et al.*, 1999; Peake *et al.*, 2004). By contrast, an increased density of adhesion molecules seems to be a more consistent finding after eccentric exercise (Pizza *et al.*, 1996; Malm *et al.*, 1999; Akimoto *et al.*, 2002; Saxton *et al.*, 2003; Simpson *et al.*, 2006). Pizza *et al.* (1996) observed increased expression of CD11b on neutrophils and monocytes after a bout of unaccustomed eccentric exercise, but an attenuated response after a repeated bout (3 weeks later). The authors speculated that the higher expression of CD11b after the first compared with the second bout was related to more severe muscle damage after the first bout, and that the damaged tissue attracted blood leucocytes. CD11b is essential for tissue infiltration of neutrophils, because CD11b antibody blocking significantly reduces the activation level and tissue accumulation of neutrophils in damaged muscles of rabbits (Brickson *et al.*, 2003; Toumi *et al.*, 2006). In humans, mutations in genes coding for adhesion molecules, such as the CD11b/CD18 integrin, increase the risk of serious infection because leucocytes fail to enter microbe-invaded tissue (Mazzone and Ricevuti, 1995).

Miles *et al.* (1998) have conducted the only study to date on the expression of adhesion molecules on leucocytes after traditional resistance exercise. They reported increased expression of CD62L (L-selectin) on circulating neutrophils (i.e. increased CD62L density) and a decreased expression of CD62L on lymphocytes after 6 × 10 repetitions of squat exercise (75% of 1 RM). As stated above, one would expect increased expression of adhesion molecules on leucocytes if the exercise-induced muscle damage is so severe that an inflammatory reaction is required. Leucocytes that leave the circulation are expected to shed CD62L, but Petridou *et al.* (2007) could not detect any changes in serum concentration of CD62L or ICAM-1, VCAM-1, E-selectin and P-selectin after 3 × 10–12 repetitions at 70–75% of 1 RM (10 exercises).

In summary, the activation level of circulating leucocytes after resistance exercise is not well characterized, but it seems that adhesion molecules are increased on innate immune cells (neutrophils and monocytes) in response to the exercise-induced muscle damage.

Infiltration of Leucocytes in the Exercised Muscles

Muscle damage attracts blood leucocytes. This has been clearly shown in animal models where the damage has been caused by contusion, toxins and local freezing (Jarvinen, 1975; Best and Hunter, 2000; Jarvinen *et al.*, 2005). Leucocytes also accumulate in the muscle tissue after unaccustomed eccentric exercise, which has been demonstrated in both animal and human models (Jones *et al.*, 1986; Armstrong *et al.*, 1991; Paulsen *et al.*, 2010a,b).

Paulsen *et al.* (2010b) observed that radiolabelled circulating leucocytes – mainly neutrophils – accumulated in the elbow flexors after 70 maximal eccentric actions, which is consistent with earlier studies (Fig. 10.2; MacIntyre *et al.*, 1996, 2000; Paulsen *et al.*, 2010a). The radiolabelled leucocytes that were traced non-invasively by a gamma camera

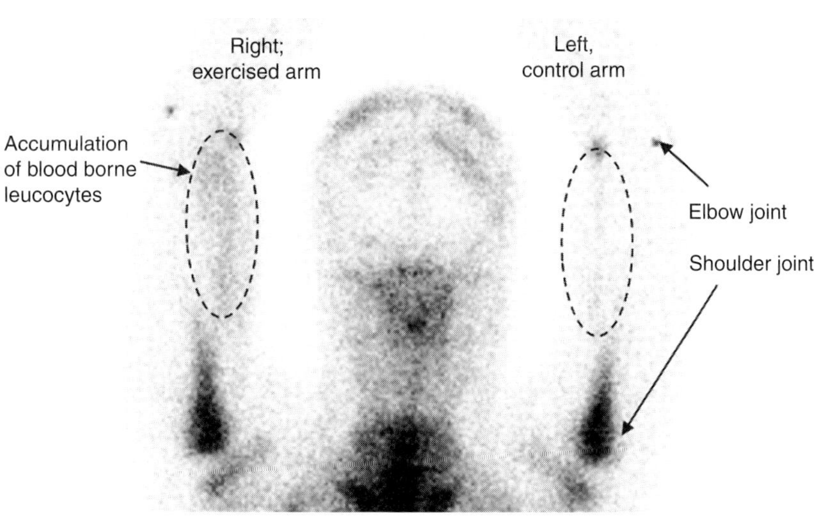

Fig. 10.2. Scintigraphic image of the arms of a subject obtained 6 h after eccentric exercise with the right elbow flexors (70 repetitions). The subject lies supine with the arms above his head. The darker areas indicate higher radioactivity from radiolabelled (technetium-99m) leucocytes (primarily neutrophils). The elbow flexors of the exercised arm display increased radioactivity that reflects accumulation of blood borne leucocytes. Note that large quantities of blood borne leucocytes are normally located in the bone marrow (e.g. caput humeri).

did not indicate extravasation and migration of leucocytes into the muscle tissue. The accumulation of radioactivity may have been on the blood side of the endothelium. Biopsies confirmed, however, that leucocytes accumulated in the extracellular space, between the myofibres. Histology analysis indicated that these leucocytes were mainly monocytes and/or macrophages, and not neutrophils. Thus, this could mean that neutrophils are primarily captured in the microvessels during and shortly after exercise (Paulsen *et al.*, 2010a,b).

Other human studies have concluded that eccentric exercise does not lead to significant inflammation in the exercised muscle tissue (Friden *et al.*, 1984; Malm *et al.*, 2000, 2004; Feasson *et al.*, 2010). A likely explanation for this discrepancy is that blood leucocyte infiltration in muscle depends on the extent of muscle damage, which in turn seems to be dictated by the exercise protocol (e.g. maximal versus submaximal eccentric actions) and the training status of research participants. Paulsen *et al.* (2010b) found a large accumulation of macrophages in approximately one third of subjects who performed unaccustomed, maximal-effort, eccentric exercise using the elbow flexors. A large reduction in muscle function (about 50%), very slow recovery (≥3 weeks) and necrosis were associated with a strong inflammatory response. Hence, it seems that some subjects are more prone than others to exercise-induced muscle damage (Chen, 2006; Hubal *et al.*, 2007).

Invasion of neutrophils, monocytes/macrophages and lymphocytes (T cells) has been reported in muscle after eccentric exercise (Round *et al.*, 1987; Fielding *et al.*, 1993). The infiltration of neutrophils and lymphocytes is, however, an inconsistent observation, whereas the infiltration of monocytes/macrophages is well documented after muscle-damaging exercise (Fig. 10.3; Stupka *et al.*, 2001; Beaton *et al.*, 2002; Peterson *et al.*, 2003; Crameri *et al.*, 2007; Mahoney *et al.*, 2008; Paulsen *et al.*, 2010b). Nevertheless, due to technical challenges in identifying the different leucocyte types, further work is needed to clarify cellular infiltration of muscle following exercise (Malm 2001, Schneider and Tiidus, 2007).

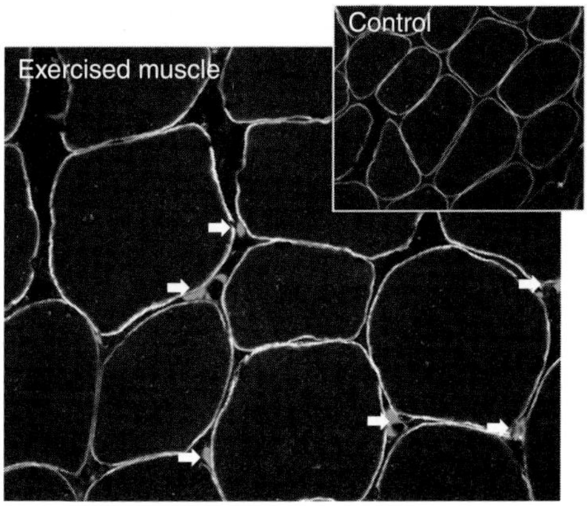

Fig. 10.3. Staining of CD68-positive cells, primarily macrophages, on a cross-section of a muscle biopsied 4 days after eccentric exercise (see arrows). The myofibre membrane is visualized by dystrophin staining. Note that macrophages are clearly present between the myofibres in the sample from the exercised muscle, whereas there are few signs of macrophages in the control sample.

Presently, it is unclear whether bouts of traditional resistance exercise, conducted on a regular basis, cause significant muscle damage and a local inflammatory response. Raastad *et al.* (2003) traced radiolabelled leucocytes in resistance-trained men after high-load leg press (5 × 3RM) and knee-extension (5 × 6RM) exercises. These investigators found at most ~30% more radiolabelled leucocytes in the exercised muscle 24h after the exercise. Unfortunately, biopsies were not collected in this study, but the accumulation of radioactivity was small compared with eccentric exercise (≥100%; MacIntyre *et al.*, 1996; Paulsen *et al.*, 2010). Thus, it is likely that most of the radiolabelled leucocytes accumulated in the microvessels and not in extravascular spaces in the exercised muscle tissue (as discussed above).

In the study by Przybyla *et al.* (2006), previously untrained subjects completed a bout of resistance exercise (4 sets at 80% of 1RM in 3 leg exercises). The number of macrophages ($CD68^+$ cells) in the exercised muscle tissue did not change significantly after exercise (72h). Others have also reported no consistent increases in the number of leucocytes in the muscle tissue after bouts of traditional resistance exercise (Staron *et al.*, 1992; Bourgeois *et al.*, 1999). On the basis of the limited evidence available, blood leucocytes only seem to infiltrate skeletal muscles in significant numbers after unaccustomed, maximal eccentric exercise (Paulsen *et al.*, 2010b) and possibly long-distance running (Hikida *et al.*, 1983). Przybyla *et al.* (2006) did, however, observe a change in the type of macrophages resident in the tissue. Specifically, there was an increase in the number of macrophages that expressed CD11b (pro-inflammatory macrophages) and CD163 (anti-inflammatory macrophages). Hence, although blood leucocytes do not infiltrate the exercised muscles (in detectable amounts) after a bout of traditional resistance exercise, the activation of tissue-resident macrophages, fibroblasts and endothelial cells may be a fundamental mechanism behind adaptation to exercise training. These cells produce an array of growth factors, such as hepatocyte growth factor (HGF), fibroblast growth factors (FGFs) and insulin-like growth factor-1 (IGF-1) and IL-6. These growth factors are important for satellite cell activation and proliferation, as well as hypertrophy of myofibres (Vandenburgh, 1987; Hawke and Garry, 2001; Spiering *et al.*, 2008; Koh and Pizza, 2009). In support of this assumption, DiPasquale *et al.* (2007) have shown that macrophages are important for skeletal muscle hypertrophy in mice.

In summary, there seems to be an important link between inflammatory cells/immune cells and myofibres during muscle damage. The importance of immune cells in the adaptation processes occurring during traditional resistance exercise training is plausible and intriguing, but not well explored in humans.

Immunosuppressive Effects of Resistance Exercise

Very strenuous endurance exercise and training periods have been associated with increased risk of upper respiratory illness (URI; Walsh *et al.*, 2011b). The increased risk of URI can be explained by a transient immunosuppressive effect of strenuous endurance exercise. The underlying mechanisms behind this effect are, however, not entirely clear (Walsh *et al.*, 2011b). Unfortunately, no research to date has investigated whether resistance exercise per se is associated with increased risk of viral or bacterial infections or other diseases. There also do not seem to be any case reports in the scientific literature.

The 'immunosuppressive' effects of strenuous exercise include a transient decreased number of circulating lymphocytes ('lymphopenia') and reduced immune cell activity, as well as decreased salivary immunoglobulin A secretion rate after exercise. Models that try to explain the immunosuppressive effects of strenuous exercise point to IL-6 and cortisol as the main culprits (Gleeson, 2007), but changes in IL-6 and cortisol are generally smaller following resistance exercise compared with endurance exercise (Nieman *et al.*, 1995; Suzuki *et al.*, 2002; Risøy *et al.*, 2003). Therefore, the immunosuppressive effects of traditional resistance exercise could be expected to be rather mild or non-existent.

Reduced salivary immunoglobulin A secretion rate seems to be the prevalent risk factor for URI after heavy endurance competition or training (Walsh *et al.*, 2011b). The effect of resistance exercise on salivary immunoglobulin A secretion rate is, however, unclear: Nieman *et al.* (2004) found a decrease, Neves Sda *et al.* (2009) found an increase, whereas others have found no changes (McDowell *et al.*, 1993; Kawada *et al.*, 2010). The decrease in salivary immunoglobulin A secretion in the study by Nieman *et al.* (2004) might reflect the large workload and long duration of resistance exercise.

Lymphopenia has, as stated above (Fig. 10.1), been reported after resistance exercise (Koch *et al.*, 2001; Risøy *et al.*, 2003; Nieman *et al.*, 2004; Carlson *et al.*, 2008; Hulmi *et al.*, 2010). After endurance exercise, cortisol probably accounts for much of this phenomenon; cortisol facilitates the egress of blood lymphocytes into lymphatic tissue and may cause apoptosis (Pedersen and Hoffman-Goetz, 2000). The lymphopenia may occur without increased cortisol levels, however (Nieman *et al.*, 1995; Risøy *et al.*, 2003; Carlson *et al.*, 2008). Low to moderate volume resistance exercise might not cause detectable lymphopenia at all (Flynn *et al.*, 1999; Neves Sda *et al.*, 2009; Hulmi *et al.*, 2010). Kruger *et al.* (2011) demonstrated that exercising at 75% of 1 RM, but not at 60% of 1 RM, induced lymphopenia. These investigators found that cortisol increased only after exercising at 75% of 1 RM, and this occurred simultaneously with lymphocyte apoptosis. *In vitro* experiments indicated that the apoptosis was initiated by glucocorticoid-receptor-dependent pathways (Kruger *et al.*, 2011). None the less, the relationship between leucocyte concentrations in the blood and the body's immune reactivity and resistance to infections is far from clear.

Nieman *et al.* (1995) observed reduced NK cell (cytotoxic) activity in men after squat exercise to exhaustion (close to 10 × 10 repetitions at 65% of 1 RM), whereas Flynn *et al.* (1999) found no decrease in elderly women (80% of 1 RM; 3 sets of 8 exercises). Moreover, Flynn *et al.* (1999) detected no change in lymphocyte proliferation. In contrast, Dohi *et al.* (2001) observed impaired lymphocyte proliferation immediately after resistance exercise in young women (6 sets of 10 RM squat exercise). This response was most evident in the strongest of the recruited subjects, which suggests that absolute work might regulate changes in lymphocyte proliferation. Miles *et al.* (2003) found impaired lymphocyte proliferation immediately after a bout of resistance exercise. This impairment was more pronounced after 3 months, but not 6 months, of training. Potteiger *et al.* (2001) observed decreased lymphocyte proliferation 3 h after resistance exercise in untrained, but not in trained, subjects.

A decreased ratio between CD4- and CD8-positive T cells (helper T cells and cytotoxic T cells) may indicate immunosuppression (Verde *et al.*, 1992). Decreased CD4/CD8 has been observed immediately after resistance exercise, but the values were normalized within 2 h (Stock *et al.*, 1995; Flynn *et al.*, 1999; Ramel *et al.*, 2003). Others have found no change in CD4/CD8 (Simonson and Jackson, 2004). The CD4/CD8 ratio seems to be stable during periods of resistance exercise training (Simonson, 2001).

Although a single session of resistance exercise is not significantly immunosuppressive, it is still plausible that high-frequency training periods (e.g. exercising every day) can induce a state of overtraining and immunosuppression. In the study by Risøy *et al.* (2003) a more pronounced and longer lasting lymphopenia was observed after 2 weeks of overreaching (including 14 sessions of resistance exercise). In line with this, NK cell activity in blood decreases during overreaching (i.e. doubling the usual training frequency, 6 sessions in 1 week; Kawada *et al.*, 2010).

In summary, traditional resistance exercise may possibly induce an immunosuppressive state shortly after exercise, because lymphopenia and reduced lymphocyte proliferation in response to mitogens have been reported. However, these changes vary between studies, most likely as a result of variation in exercise protocols. Moreover, it is unclear whether these immunological findings genuinely increase the likelihood of infection/disease, such as URI. Nevertheless, the possibility should be considered very carefully when applying overreaching protocols, which could lead to overtraining.

The immune response and the putative immunosuppressive effects of exercise may be altered by certain nutritional regimes and supplements (Nieman, 2008; Walsh *et al.*, 2011a). Unlike endurance exercise, very few studies have reported the effects of nutritional interventions on inflammatory and immune responses to resistance exercise. A number of studies have shown that the intake of carbohydrates during long-lasting endurance exercise can reduce inflammatory responses, but does not seem to attenuate exercise-induced immune dysfunction (Walsh *et al.*, 2011a). Similar effects are observed with resistance exercise. Carbohydrate supplementation reduces lymphocytosis, neutrophilia and monocytosis, and also attenuates the decrease in circulating concentrations of IL-2 and IL-5 after resistance exercise (Koch *et al.*, 2001; Chan *et al.*, 2003; Nieman *et al.*, 2004; Carlson *et al.*, 2008). Food supplementation with cysteine has been found to restore the attenuation of NK cell activity after high-intensity, high-frequency resistance exercise (Kawada *et al.*, 2010), whereas no effects (on cell counts) were found with whey protein supplementation (Hulmi *et al.*, 2010). More research is warranted to examine whether nutritional interventions alter immune responses to resistance exercise and whether such alterations influence resistance to infection.

Immunoenhancing Effects of Resistance Exercise

Providing exercise is not too strenuous and long lasting, it can actually enhance the immune system because of the transient redistribution of leucocytes during and after exercise (Edwards *et al.*, 2007b). Endurance exercise training seems to have positive effects on the immune system, because people who exercise regularly report lower incidence and severity of URI (Nieman *et al.*, 2011; Walsh *et al.*, 2011b; Wang *et al.*, 2011). Compared with endurance exercise training, little is known about the immunostimulatory effects of resistance exercise training. McFarlin *et al.* (2004, 2005, 2006) have shown improved NK cell function and reduced expression of toll-like receptor 4 on circulating leucocytes in elderly women following several months of resistance exercise training. Others, however, have found no changes in immunological variables following periods of resistance exercise training, or differences between trained and untrained subjects (Flynn *et al.*, 1999; Simonson, 2001; Hulmi *et al.*, 2010). Thus, the typical robust adaptations to resistance exercise training (i.e. increased muscle mass and strength) contrast with small or no changes in the immune system, at least within the bloodstream.

Unaccustomed eccentric exercise performed before vaccination has been reported to function as an adjuvant when the vaccine is injected in the exercised muscle (Edwards *et al.*, 2007a, 2010). Thus, the inflammatory response that is initiated by the exercise seems to enhance the immune response to the antigens of the vaccine (antibody and cell-mediated responses). The effects seem to be gender specific, however, and are not a consistent finding (Campbell *et al.*, 2010). Whether traditional resistance exercise also enhances immune responses to vaccination is unknown.

In summary, the potential immunoenhancing effects of resistance exercise training are largely unknown. It seems reasonable, however, to suggest that resistance exercise training can have similar effects as endurance exercise training. The manner in which resistance exercise affects immune cells residing in the muscle tissue might have implications for improved efficacy of vaccines that are delivered intramuscularly.

Summary and Conclusions

A bout of traditional resistance exercise typically induces a biphasic blood leucocytosis, similar to that seen after endurance exercise. An acute increase occurs during the exercise, which encompasses neutrophils, monocytes and lymphocytes, and a delayed increase occurs after exercise involving neutrophils and monocytes concomitant with a decrease below baseline of lymphocytes. The transient lymphopenia after endurance training, together with reduced activity and proliferation capability of blood lymphocytes, can possibly be viewed as a state of immunosuppression that might increase the risk of infection. Thus, there may be an 'open window' (for some hours) after exercise for microbes to invade our bodies, primarily through the upper respiratory tract. Immunosuppression is more likely to occur following intensive, large-volume resistance exercise and periods with high training frequency (overreaching/overtraining). However, taking into account the redundancy and overcapacity of the immune system in healthy subjects, it seems from an immunological point of view reasonable to conclude that resistance exercise is generally safe (Simonson 2001; Koch *et al.*, 2010). This seems also true for the elderly (>60 years; Haaland *et al.*, 2008). Regular resistance exercise training seems to have minimal effects on resting immune function. Nevertheless, on the basis of the knowledge that regular endurance exercise reduces the incidence and severity of URI (Nieman *et al.*, 2011; Walsh *et al.*, 2011b), it seems reasonable to hypothesise that regular traditional resistance training (e.g. following ACSM recommendations (2009) over months and years) has similar immunostimulatory effects. The biological significance of the acute, transient exercise-induced inflammatory response to resistance exercise is not clear. It is tempting to speculate that the increased number of circulating leucocytes, activation of the leucocytes by cytokines and egress of leucocytes into the exercised muscles could represent a part of the physiological adaptation to muscular stress. Moreover, the production of cytokines/myokines by the myofibres and stromal cells normally resident in the muscle tissue (e.g. macrophages) might prove to be important in the process of muscle hypertrophy that results from resistance exercise training. Unfortunately, few studies have investigated these possibilities in trained subjects performing traditional bouts of resistance exercise. Thus, more research is needed to elucidate interactions between the immune system and adaptation to regular strength exercise training in humans.

Acknowledgements

Professor emeritus M.D. Haakon B. Benestad is acknowledged for his valuable assistance in the preparation of the manuscript for this chapter.

Notes

[1] Leucocytosis can be defined as white blood cell count of >10 000 mm^{-3} (Opdenakker *et al.*, 1998). This means that the leucocyte cell counts after exercise often are within the wide range of reference values. We will, nevertheless, herein use the term leucocytosis to indicate an increase above baseline.

[2] The repeated-bout effect refers to the adaptation to a single bout of muscle-damaging exercise that protects the exercised muscles from damage during a repeated bout of the same type of exercise. Less delayed onset muscle soreness, lower blood levels of creatine kinase and a faster recovery of muscle function are classical signs of the repeated-bout effect (McHugh, 2003).

References

American College of Sports Medicine Position Stand (2009) Progression models in resistance training for healthy adults. *Medicine and Science in Sports and Exercise* 41, 687–708.

Ahtiainen, J.P., Pakarinen, A., Kraemer, W.J. and Hakkinen, K. (2003) Acute hormonal and neuromuscular responses and recovery to forced vs maximum repetitions multiple resistance exercises. *International Journal of Sports Medicine* 24, 410–418.

Ahtiainen, J.P., Pakarinen, A., Kraemer, W.J. and Hakkinen, K. (2004) Acute hormonal responses to heavy resistance exercise in strength athletes versus nonathletes. *Canadian Journal of Applied Physiology* 29, 527–543.

Akimoto, T., Furudate, M., Saitoh, M., Sugiura, K., Waku, T., Akama, T., *et al.* (2002) Increased plasma concentrations of intercellular adhesion molecule-1 after strenuous exercise associated with muscle damage. *European Journal of Applied Physiology* 86, 185–190.

Allen, D.G., Lamb, G.D. and Westerblad, H. (2008) Skeletal muscle fatigue, cellular mechanisms. *Physiological Reviews* 88, 287–332.

Armstrong, R.B., Warren, G.L. and Warren, J.A. (1991) Mechanisms of exercise-induced muscle fibre injury. *Sports Medicine* 12, 184–207.

Beaton, L.J., Tarnopolsky, M.A. and Phillips, S.M. (2002) Contraction-induced muscle damage in humans following calcium channel blocker administration. *Journal of Physiology* 544, 849–859.

Best, T.M. and Hunter, K.D. (2000) Muscle injury and repair. *Physical Medicine and Rehabilitation Clinics of North America* 11, 251–266.

Bourgeois, J., MacDougall, D., MacDonald, J. and Tarnopolsky, M. (1999) Naproxen does not alter indices of muscle damage in resistance-exercise trained men. *Medicine and Science in Sports and Exercise* 31, 4–9.

Brenner, I.K., Natale, V.M., Vasiliou, P., Moldoveanu, A.I., Shek, P.N., *et al.* (1999) Impact of three different types of exercise on components of the inflammatory response. *European Journal of Applied Physiology and Occupational Physiology* 80, 452–460.

Brickson, S., Ji, L.L., Schell, K., Olabisi, R., St Pierre, S.B., *et al.* (2003) M1/70 attenuates blood-borne neutrophil oxidants, activation, and myofiber damage following stretch injury. *Journal of Applied Physiology* 95, 969–976.

Buford, T.W., Cooke, M.B. and Willoughby, D.S. (2009) Resistance exercise-induced changes of inflammatory gene expression within human skeletal muscle. *European Journal of Applied Physiology* 107, 463–471.

Campbell, J.P., Edwards, K.M., Ring, C., Drayson, M.T., Bosch, J.A., *et al.* (2010) The effects of vaccine timing on the efficacy of an acute eccentric exercise intervention on the immune response to an influenza vaccine in young adults. *Brain, Behavior and Immunity* 24, 236–242.

Cannon, J.G., Fielding, R.A., Fiatarone, M.A., Orencole, S.F., Dinarello, C.A., *et al.* (1989) Increased interleukin 1 beta in human skeletal muscle after exercise. *American Journal of Physiology* 257, R451–R455.

Cannon, J.G., Meydani, S.N., Fielding, R.A., Fiatarone, M.A., Meydani, M., *et al.* (1991) Acute phase response in exercise. II. Associations between vitamin E, cytokines, and muscle proteolysis. *American Journal of Physiology* 260, R1235–R1240.

Carlson, L.A., Headley, S., Debruin, J., Tuckow, A.T., Koch, A.J., *et al.* (2008) Carbohydrate supplementation and immune responses after acute exhaustive resistance exercise. *International Journal of Sports Nutrition and Exercise Metabolism* 18, 247–259.

Carlson, L.A., Tighe, S.W., Kenefick, R.W., Dragon, J., Westcott, N.W., *et al.* (2011) Changes in transcriptional output of human peripheral blood mononuclear cells following resistance exercise. *European Journal of Applied Physiology* 111, 2919–29.

Chan, M.A., Koch, A.J., Benedict, S.H. and Potteiger, J.A. (2003) Influence of carbohydrate ingestion on cytokine responses following acute resistance exercise. *International Journal of Sports Nutrition and Exercise Metabolism* 13, 454–465.

Charge, S.B. and Rudnicki, M.A. (2004) Cellular and molecular regulation of muscle regeneration. *Physiological Reviews* 84, 209–238.

Chen, T.C. (2006) Variability in muscle damage after eccentric exercise and the repeated bout effect. *Research Quarterly for Exercise and Sport* 77, 362–371.

Clarkson, P.M. and Hubal, M.J. (2002) Exercise-induced muscle damage in humans. *American Journal of Physical Medicine and Rehabilitation* 81, S52–S69.

Collins, M.A., Cureton, K.J., Hill, D.W. and Ray, C.A. (1989) Relation of plasma volume change to intensity of weight lifting. *Medicine and Science in Sports and Exercise* 21, 178–185.

Collins, M.A., Cureton, K.J., Hill, D.W. and Ray, C.A. (1991) Relationship of heart rate to oxygen uptake during weight lifting exercise. *Medicine and Science in Sports and Exercise* 23, 636–640.

Crameri, R.M., Aagaard, P., Qvortrup, K., Langberg, H., Olesen, J., *et al.* (2007) Myofibre damage in human skeletal muscle, effects of electrical stimulation versus voluntary contraction. *Journal of Physiology* 583, 365–380.

Crewther, B., Keogh, J., Cronin, J. and Cook, C. (2006) Possible stimuli for strength and power adaptation, acute hormonal responses. *Sports Medicine* 36, 215–238.

Curfs, J.H., Meis, J.F. and Hoogkamp-Korstanje, J.A. (1997) A primer on cytokines, sources, receptors, effects, and inducers. *Clinical Microbiology Review* 10, 742–780.

Dallegri, F. and Ottonello, L. (1997) Tissue injury in neutrophilic inflammation. *Inflammation Research* 46, 382–391.

De Rossi, M., Bernasconi, P., Baggi, F., De Waal, M.R. and Mantegazza, R. (2000) Cytokines and chemokines are both expressed by human myoblasts, possible relevance for the immune pathogenesis of muscle inflammation. *International Immunology* 12, 1329–1335.

Deldicque, L., Atherton, P., Patel, R., Theisen, D., Nielens, H., *et al.* (2008) Effects of resistance exercise with and without creatine supplementation on gene expression and cell signaling in human skeletal muscle. *Journal of Applied Physiology* 104, 371–378.

Dennis, R.A., Trappe, T.A., Simpson, P., Carroll, C., Huang, B.E., *et al.* (2004) Interleukin-1 polymorphisms are associated with the inflammatory response in human muscle to acute resistance exercise. *Journal of Physiology* 560, 617–626.

DiPasquale, D.M., Cheng, M., Billich, W., Huang, S.A., van Rooijen, N., *et al.* (2007) Urokinase-type plasminogen activator and macrophages are required for skeletal muscle hypertrophy in mice. *American Journal of Physiology Cell Physiology* 293, C1278–C1285.

Dohi, K., Mastro, A.M., Miles, M.P., Bush, J.A., Grove, D.S., *et al.* (2001) Lymphocyte proliferation in response to acute heavy resistance exercise in women, influence of muscle strength and total work. *European Journal of Applied Physiology* 85, 367–373.

Edwards, K.M., Burns, V.E., Allen, L.M., McPhee, J.S., Bosch, J.A., *et al.* (2007a) Eccentric exercise as an adjuvant to influenza vaccination in humans. *Brain, Behavior and Immunity* 21, 209–217.

Edwards, K.M., Burns, V.E., Carroll, D., Drayson, M. and Ring, C. (2007b) The acute stress-induced immunoenhancement hypothesis. *Exercise and Sport Science Review* 35, 150–155.

Edwards, K.M., Campbell, J.P., Ring, C., Drayson, M.T., Bosch, J.A., *et al.* (2010) Exercise intensity does not influence the efficacy of eccentric exercise as a behavioural adjuvant to vaccination. *Brain, Behavior and Immunity* 24, 623–630.

Evans, W.J. and Cannon, J.G. (1991) The metabolic effects of exercise-induced muscle damage. *Exercise and Sport Science Review* 19, 99–125.

Fatouros, I., Chatzinikolaou, A., Paltoglou, G., Petridou, A., Avloniti, A., *et al.* (2010) Acute resistance exercise results in catecholaminergic rather than hypothalamic-pituitary-adrenal axis stimulation during exercise in young men. *Stress* 13, 461–468.

Feasson, L., Stockholm, D., Freyssenet, D., Richard, I., Duguez, S., *et al.* (2002) Molecular adaptations of neuromuscular disease-associated proteins in response to eccentric exercise in human skeletal muscle. *Journal of Physiology* 543, 297–306.

Fielding, R.A., Manfredi, T.J., Ding, W., Fiatarone, M.A., Evans, W.J., *et al.* (1993) Acute phase response in exercise. III. Neutrophil and IL-1 beta accumulation in skeletal muscle. *American Journal of Physiology* 265, R166–R172.

Flynn, M.G., Fahlman, M., Braun, W.A., Lambert, C.P., Bouillon, L.E., *et al.* (1999) Effects of resistance training on selected indexes of immune function in elderly women. *Journal of Applied Physiology* 86, 1905–1913.

Folland, J.P. and Williams, A.G. (2007) The adaptations to strength training : morphological and neurological contributions to increased strength. *Sports Medicine* 37, 145–168.

Fragala, M.S., Kraemer, W.J., Mastro, A.M., Denegar, C.R., Volek, J.S., *et al.* (2011) Leukocyte beta2-adrenergic receptor expression in response to resistance exercise. *Medicine and Science in Sports and Exercise* 43, 1422–1432.

Frangogiannis, N.G. (2008) The immune system and cardiac repair. *Pharmacology Research* 58, 88–111.

Frangogiannis, N.G., Smith, C.W. and Entman, M.L. (2002) The inflammatory response in myocardial infarction. *Cardiovascular Research* 53, 31–47.

Friden, J., Kjorell, U. and Thornell, L.E. (1984) Delayed muscle soreness and cytoskeletal alterations, an immunocytological study in man. *International Journal of Sports Medicine* 5, 15–18.

Gabriel, H. and Kindermann, W. (1997) The acute immune response to exercise, what does it mean? *International Journal of Sports Medicine* 18 Suppl 1, S28–S45.

Gabriel. H.H. and Kindermann, W. (1998) Adhesion molecules during immune response to exercise. *Canadian Journal of Physiology and Pharmacology* 76, 512–523.

Gabriel, H., Urhausen, A., Brechtel, L., Muller, H.J. and Kindermann, W. (1994) Alterations of regular and mature monocytes are distinct, and dependent of intensity and duration of exercise. *European Journal of Applied Physiology and Occupational Physiology* 69, 179–181.

Glaister, M. (2005) Multiple sprint work: physiological responses, mechanisms of fatigue and the influence of aerobic fitness. *Sports Medicine* 35, 757–777.

Gleeson, M. (2007) Immune function in sport and exercise. *Journal of Applied Physiology* 103, 693–699.

Gosain, A. and Gamelli, R.L. (2005) A primer in cytokines. *Journal of Burn Care and Rehabilitation* 26, 7–12.

Greiwe, J.S., Cheng, B., Rubin, D.C., Yarasheski, K.E. and Semenkovich, C.F. (2001) Resistance exercise decreases skeletal muscle tumor necrosis factor alpha in frail elderly humans. *FASEB Journal* 15, 475–482.

Grimstad, I.A. and Benestad, H.B. (1982) A new assay for leukocyte chemotaxis using cell retrieval, electronic particle counting and flow cytometry. *Journal of Immunological Methods* 49, 215–233.

Haaland, D.A., Sabljic, T.F., Baribeau, D.A., Mukovozov, I.M. and Hart, L.E. (2008) Is regular exercise a friend or foe of the aging immune system? A systematic review. *Clinical Journal of Sports Medicine* 18, 539–548.

Hakkinen, K. and Pakarinen, A. (1993) Acute hormonal responses to two different fatiguing heavy-resistance protocols in male athletes. *Journal of Applied Physiology* 74, 882–887.

Haugen, F., Norheim, F., Lian, H., Wensaas, A.J., Dueland, S., *et al.* (2010) IL-7 is expressed and secreted by human skeletal muscle cells. *American Journal of Physiology Cell Physiology* 298, C807–C816.

Hawke, T.J. and Garry, D.J. (2001) Myogenic satellite cells, physiology to molecular biology. *Journal of Applied Physiology* 91, 534–551.

Hikida, R.S., Staron, R.S., Hagerman, F.C., Sherman, W.M. and Costill, D.L. (1983) Muscle fiber necrosis associated with human marathon runners. *Journal of Neurological Science* 59, 185–203.

Hirose, L., Nosaka, K., Newton, M., Laveder, A., Kano, M., *et al.* (2004) Changes in inflammatory mediators following eccentric exercise of the elbow flexors. *Exercise Immunology Review* 10, 75–90.

Hubal, M.J., Rubinstein, S.R. and Clarkson, P.M. (2007) Mechanisms of variability in strength loss after muscle-lengthening actions. *Medicine and Science in Sports and Exercise* 39, 461–468.

Hubal, M.J., Chen, T.C., Thompson, P.D. and Clarkson, P.M. (2008) Inflammatory gene changes associated with the repeated-bout effect. *American Journal of Physiology Regulatory, Integrative and Comparative Physiology* 294, R1628–R1637.

Hulmi, J.J., Myllymaki, T., Tenhumaki, M., Mutanen, N., Puurtinen, R., *et al.* (2010) Effects of resistance exercise and protein ingestion on blood leukocytes and platelets in young and older men. European *Journal of Applied Physiology* 109, 343–353.

Hurley, B.F., Seals, D.R., Ehsani, A.A., Cartier, L.J., Dalsky, G.P., *et al.* (1984) Effects of high-intensity strength training on cardiovascular function. *Medicine and Science in Sports and Exercise* 16, 483–488.

Izquierdo, M., Ibanez, J., Calbet, J.A., Navarro-Amezqueta, I., Gonzalez-Izal, M., *et al.* (2009) Cytokine and hormone responses to resistance training. *European Journal of Applied Physiology* 107, 397–409.

Jarvinen, M. (1975) Healing of a crush injury in rat striated muscle. 2. A histological study of the effect of early mobilization and immobilization on the repair processes. *Acta Pathologica et Microbiologica Scandinavica [A]* 83, 269–282.

Jarvinen, T.A., Jarvinen, T.L., Kaariainen, M., Kalimo, H. and Jarvinen, M. (2005) Muscle injuries, biology and treatment. *American Journal of Sports Medicine* 33, 745–764.

Jones, D.A., Newham, D.J., Round, J.M. and Tolfree, S.E. (1986) Experimental human muscle damage, morphological changes in relation to other indices of damage. *Journal of Physiology* 375, 435–448.

Judge, L.W. and Burke, J.R. (2010) The effect of recovery time on strength performance following a high-intensity bench press workout in males and females. *International Journal of Sports Physiology and Performance* 5, 184–196.

Kappel, M., Hansen, M.B., Diamant, M., Jorgensen, J.O., Gyhrs, A., *et al.* (1993) Effects of an acute bolus growth hormone infusion on the human immune system. *Hormone and Metabolic Research* 25, 579–585.

Kawada, S., Kobayashi, K., Ohtani, M. and Fukusaki, C. (2010) Cystine and theanine supplementation restores high-intensity resistance exercise-induced attenuation of natural killer cell activity in well-trained men. *Journal of Strength and Conditioning Research* 24, 846–851.

Kayashima, S., Ohno, H., Fujioka, T., Taniguchi, N. and Nagata, N. (1995) Leucocytosis as a marker of organ damage induced by chronic strenuous physical exercise. *European Journal of Applied Physiology and Occupational Physiology* 70, 413–420.

Koch, A.J. (2010) Immune response to resistance exercise. *American Journal of Lifestyle Medicine* 4, 244–252.

Koch, A.J., Potteiger, J.A., Chan, M.A., Benedict, S.H. and Frey, B.B. (2001) Minimal influence of carbohydrate ingestion on the immune response following acute resistance exercise. *International Journal of Sports Nutrition and Exercise Metabolism* 11, 149–161.

Koh, T.J. and Pizza, F.X. (2009) Do inflammatory cells influence skeletal muscle hypertrophy? *Frontiers in Bioscience (Elite Ed)* 1, 60–71.

Kraemer, W.J. and Ratamess, N.A. (2005) Hormonal responses and adaptations to resistance exercise and training. *Sports Medicine* 35, 339–361.

Kraemer, W.J., Noble, B.J., Clark, M.J. and Culver, B.W. (1987) Physiologic responses to heavy-resistance exercise with very short rest periods. *International Journal of Sports Medicine* 8, 247–252.

Kraemer, W.J., Marchitelli, L., Gordon, S.E., Harman, E., Dziados, J.E., *et al.* (1990) Hormonal and growth factor responses to heavy resistance exercise protocols. *Journal of Applied Physiology* 69, 1442–1450.

Kraemer, W.J., Clemson, A., Triplett, N.T., Bush, J.A., Newton, R.U., *et al.* (1996) The effects of plasma cortisol elevation on total and differential leukocyte counts in response to heavy-resistance exercise. *European Journal of Applied Physiology and Occupational Physiology* 73, 93–97.

Kraemer, W.J., Hakkinen, K., Newton, R.U., McCormick, M., Nindl, B.C., *et al.* (1998) Acute hormonal responses to heavy resistance exercise in younger and older men. *European Journal of Applied Physiology and Occupational Physiology* 77, 206–211.

Kruger, K., Lechtermann, A., Fobker, M., Volker, K. and Mooren, F.C. (2008) Exercise-induced redistribution of T lymphocytes is regulated by adrenergic mechanisms. *Brain, Behavior and Immunity* 22, 324–338.

Kruger, K., Agnischock, S., Lechtermann, A., Tiwari, S., Mishra, M., *et al.* (2011) Intensive resistance exercise induces lymphocyte apoptosis via cortisol and glucocorticoid-receptor dependent pathways. *Journal of Applied Physiology* 111, 1226–1232.

Latini, R., Bianchi, M., Correale, E., Dinarello, C.A., Fantuzzi, G., *et al.* (1994) Cytokines in acute myocardial infarction, selective increase in circulating tumor necrosis factor, its soluble receptor, and interleukin-1 receptor antagonist. *Journal of Cardiovascular Pharmacology* 23, 1–6.

Louis, E., Raue, U., Yang, Y., Jemiolo, B. and Trappe, S. (2007) Time course of proteolytic, cytokine, and myostatin gene expression after acute exercise in human skeletal muscle. *Journal of Applied Physiology* 103, 1744–1751.

MacIntyre, D.L., Reid, W.D., and McKenzie, D.C. (1995) Delayed muscle soreness. The inflammatory response to muscle injury and its clinical implications. *Sports Medicine* 20, 24–40.

MacIntyre, D.L., Reid, W.D., Lyster, D.M., Szasz, I.J. and McKenzie, D.C. (1996) Presence of WBC, decreased strength, and delayed soreness in muscle after eccentric exercise. *Journal of Applied Physiology* 80, 1006–1013.

MacIntyre, D.L., Reid, W.D., Lyster, D.M. and McKenzie, D.C. (2000) Different effects of strenuous eccentric exercise on the accumulation of neutrophils in muscle in women and men. *European Journal of Applied Physiology* 81, 47–53.

MacIntyre, D.L., Sorichter, S., Mair, J., Berg, A. and McKenzie, D.C. (2001) Markers of inflammation and myofibrillar proteins following eccentric exercise in humans. *European Journal of Applied Physiology* 84, 180–186.

Mahoney, D.J., Safdar, A., Parise, G., Melov, S., Fu, M., *et al.* (2008) Gene expression profiling in human skeletal muscle during recovery from eccentric exercise. *American Journal of Physiology Regulatory, Integrative and Comparative Physiology* 294, 1901–10.

Malm, C. (2001) Exercise-induced muscle damage and inflammation, fact or fiction? *Acta Physioligica Scandinavica* 171, 233–239.

Malm, C., Lenkei, R. and Sjodin, B. (1999) Effects of eccentric exercise on the immune system in men. *Journal of Applied Physiology* 86, 461–468.

Malm, C., Nyberg, P., Engstrom, M., Sjodin, B., Lenkei, R., *et al.* (2000) Immunological changes in human skeletal muscle and blood after eccentric exercise and multiple biopsies. *Journal of Physiology* 529, 243–262.

Malm, C., Sjodin, T.L., Sjoberg, B., Lenkei, R., Renstrom, P., *et al.* (2004) Leukocytes, cytokines, growth factors and hormones in human skeletal muscle and blood after uphill or downhill running. *Journal of Physiology* 556, 983–1000.

Mayhew, D.L., Thyfault, J.P. and Koch, A.J. (2005) Rest-interval length affects leukocyte levels during heavy resistance exercise. *Journal of Strength and Conditioning Research* 19, 16–22.

Mazzone, A. and Ricevuti, G. (1995) Leukocyte CD11/CD18 integrins, biological and clinical relevance. *Haematologica* 80, 161–175.

McDonagh, M.J. and Davies, C.T. (1984) Adaptive response of mammalian skeletal muscle to exercise with high loads. *European Journal of Applied Physiology and Occupational Physiology* 52, 139–155.

McDowell, S.L., Weir, J.P., Eckerson, J.M., Wagner, L.L., Housh, T.J., *et al.* (1993) A preliminary investigation of the effect of weight training on salivary immunoglobulin A. *Research Quarterly for Exercise and Sport* 64, 348–351.

McFarlin, B.K., Flynn, M.G., Campbell, W.W., Stewart, L.K. and Timmerman, K.L. (2004) TLR4 is lower in resistance-trained older women and related to inflammatory cytokines. *Medicine and Science in Sports and Exercise* 36, 1876–1883.

McFarlin, B.K., Flynn, M.G., Phillips, M.D., Stewart, L.K. and Timmerman, K.L. (2005) Chronic resistance exercise training improves natural killer cell activity in older women. *Journal of Gerontology A Biological Science and Medical Science* 60, 1315–1318.

McFarlin, B.K., Flynn, M.G., Campbell, W.W., Craig, B.A., Robinson, J.P., *et al.* (2006) Physical activity status, but not age, influences inflammatory biomarkers and toll-like receptor 4. *Journal of Gerontology A Biological Science and Medical Science* 61, 388–393.

McHugh, M.P. (2003) Recent advances in the understanding of the repeated bout effect, the protective effect against muscle damage from a single bout of eccentric exercise. *Scandinavian Journal of Medicine and Science in Sports* 13, 88–97.

Meisel, S.R., Shapiro, H., Radnay, J., Neuman, Y., Khaskia, A.R., *et al.* (1998) Increased expression of neutrophil and monocyte adhesion molecules LFA-1 and Mac-1 and their ligand ICAM-1 and VLA-4 throughout the acute phase of myocardial infarction, possible implications for leukocyte aggregation and microvascular plugging. *Journal of the American College of Cardiology* 31, 120–125.

Miles, M.P., Leach, S.K., Kraemer, W.J., Dohi, K., Bush, J.A., *et al.* (1998) Leukocyte adhesion molecule expression during intense resistance exercise. *Journal of Applied Physiology* 84, 1604–1609.

Miles, M.P., Kraemer, W.J., Nindl, B.C., Grove, D.S., Leach, S.K., *et al.* (2003) Strength, workload, anaerobic intensity and the immune response to resistance exercise in women. *Acta Physiologica Scandinavica* 178, 155–163.

Moldoveanu, A.I., Shephard, R.J. and Shek, P.N. (2001) The cytokine response to physical activity and training. *Sports Medicine* 31, 115–144.

Nakagawa, M., Terashima, T., D'yachkova, Y., Bondy, G.P., Hogg, J.C., *et al.* (1998) Glucocorticoid-induced granulocytosis, contribution of marrow release and demargination of intravascular granulocytes. *Circulation* 98, 2307–2313.

Natale, V.M., Brenner, I.K., Moldoveanu, A.I., Vasiliou, P., Shek, P., *et al.* (2003) Effects of three different types of exercise on blood leukocyte count during and following exercise. *Sao Paulo Medical Journal* 121, 9–14.

Neves Sda, C. Jr., Lima, R.M., Simoes, H.G., Marques, M.C., Reis, V.M., *et al.* (2009) Resistance exercise sessions do not provoke acute immunosuppression in older women. *Journal of Strength and Conditioning Research* 23, 259–265.

Newton, M.J., Morgan, G.T., Sacco, P., Chapman, D.W. and Nosaka, K. (2008) Comparison of responses to strenuous eccentric exercise of the elbow flexors between resistance-trained and untrained men. *Journal of Strength and Conditioning Research* 22, 597–607.

Nieman, D.C. (1997) Immune response to heavy exertion. *Journal of Applied Physiology* 82, 1385–1394.

Nieman, D.C. (2008) Immunonutrition support for athletes. *Nutrition Review* 66, 310–320.

Nieman, D.C., Henson, D.A., Sampson, C.S., Herring, J.L., Suttles, J., *et al.* (1995) The acute immune response to exhaustive resistance exercise. *International Journal of Sports Medicine* 16, 322–328.

Nieman, D.C., Davis, J.M., Brown, V.A., Henson, D.A., Dumke, C.L., *et al.* (2004) Influence of carbohydrate ingestion on immune changes after 2h of intensive resistance training. *Journal of Applied Physiology* 96, 1292–1298.

Nieman, D.C., Dumke, C.L., Henson, D.A., McAnulty, S.R., Gross, S.J., *et al.* (2005) Muscle damage is linked to cytokine changes following a 160-km race. *Brain, Behavior and Immunity* 19, 398–403.

Nieman, D.C., Henson, D.A., Austin, M.D. and Sha, W. (2011) Upper respiratory tract infection is reduced in physically fit and active adults. *British Journal of Sports Medicine* 45, 987–982.

Olszewski, W., Engeset, A., Jaeger, P.M., Sokolowski, J. and Theodorsen, L. (1977) Flow and composition of leg lymph in normal men during venous stasis, muscular activity and local hyperthermia. *Acta Physiologica Scandinavica* 99, 149–155.

Opdenakker, G., Fibbe, W.E. and van Damme, J. (1998) The molecular basis of leukocytosis. *Immunology Today* 19, 182–189.

Paulsen, G., Benestad, H.B., Strom-Gundersen, I., Morkrid, L., Lappegard, K.T., *et al.* (2005) Delayed leukocytosis and cytokine response to high-force eccentric exercise. *Medicine and Science in Sports and Exercise* 37, 1877–1883.

Paulsen, G., Crameri, R., Benestad, H.B., Fjeld, J.G., Morkrid, L., *et al.* (2010a) Time course of leukocyte accumulation in human muscle after eccentric exercise. *Medicine and Science in Sports and Exercise* 42, 75–85.

Paulsen, G., Egner, I.M., Drange, M., Langberg, H., Benestad, H.B., *et al.* (2010b) A COX-2 inhibitor reduces muscle soreness, but does not influence recovery and adaptation after eccentric exercise. *Scandinavian Journal of Medicine and Science in Sports* 20, e195–e207.

Peake, J., Wilson, G., Hordern, M., Suzuki, K., Yamaya, K., *et al.* (2004) Changes in neutrophil surface receptor expression, degranulation, and respiratory burst activity after moderate- and high-intensity exercise. *Journal of Applied Physiology* 97, 612–618.

Peake, J., Nosaka, K. and Suzuki, K. (2005a) Characterization of inflammatory responses to eccentric exercise in humans. *Exercise Immunology Review* 11, 64–85.

Peake, J.M., Suzuki, K., Hordern, M., Wilson, G., Nosaka, K., *et al.* (2005b) Plasma cytokine changes in relation to exercise intensity and muscle damage. *European Journal of Applied Physiology* 95, 514–521.

Peake, J.M., Nosaka, K., Muthalib, M. and Suzuki, K. (2006) Systemic inflammatory responses to maximal versus submaximal lengthening contractions of the elbow flexors. *Exercise Immunology Review* 12, 72–85.

Pedersen, B.K. (2011) Muscles and their myokines. *Journal of Experimental Biology* 214, 337–346.

Pedersen, B.K. and Febbraio, M.A. (2008) Muscle as an endocrine organ, focus on muscle-derived interleukin-6. *Physiological Reviews* 88, 1379–1406.

Pedersen, B.K. and Hoffman-Goetz, L. (2000) Exercise and the immune system, regulation, integration, and adaptation. *Physiological Reviews* 80, 1055–1081.

Pedersen, B.K., Rohde, T. and Zacho, M. (1996) Immunity in athletes. *Journal of Sports Medicine and Physical Fitness* 36, 236–245.

Pedersen, B.K., Akerstrom, T.C., Nielsen, A.R. and Fischer, C.P. (2007) Role of myokines in exercise and metabolism. *Journal of Applied Physiology* 103, 1093–1098.

Peterson, J.M., Trappe, T.A., Mylona, E., White, F., Lambert, C.P., *et al.* (2003) Ibuprofen and acetaminophen, effect on muscle inflammation after eccentric exercise. *Medicine and Science in Sports and Exercise* 35, 892–896.

Petridou, A., Chatzinikolaou, A., Fatouros, I., Mastorakos, G., Mitrakou, A., *et al.* (2007) Resistance exercise does not affect the serum concentrations of cell adhesion molecules. *British Journal of Sports Medicine* 41, 76–79.

Pizza, F.X., Davis, B.H., Henrickson, S.D., Mitchell, J.B., Pace, J.F., *et al.* (1996) Adaptation to eccentric exercise, effect on CD64 and CD11b/CD18 expression. *Journal of Applied Physiology* 80, 47–55.

Pizza, F.X., Baylies, H. and Mitchell, J.B. (2001) Adaptation to eccentric exercise, neutrophils and E-selectin during early recovery. *Canadian Journal of Applied Physiology* 26, 245–253.

Potteiger, J.A., Chan, M.A., Haff, G.G., Mathew, S., Schroeder, C.A., *et al.* (2001) Training status influences T-cell responses in women following acute resistance exercise. *Journal of Strength and Conditioning Research* 15, 185–191.

Proske, U. and Morgan. D.L. (2001) Muscle damage from eccentric exercise, mechanism, mechanical signs, adaptation and clinical applications. *Journal of Physiology* 537, 333–345.

Przybyla, B., Gurley, C., Harvey, J.F., Bearden, E., Kortebein, P., *et al.* (2006) Aging alters macrophage properties in human skeletal muscle both at rest and in response to acute resistance exercise. *Experimental Gerontology* 41, 320–327.

Pyne, D.B. (1994) Regulation of neutrophil function during exercise. *Sports Medicine* 17, 245–258.

Raastad, T. and Hallen, J. (2000) Recovery of skeletal muscle contractility after high- and moderate-intensity strength exercise. *European Journal of Applied Physiology* 82, 206–214.

Raastad, T., Risoy, B.A., Benestad, H.B., Fjeld, J.G. and Hallen, J. (2003) Temporal relation between leukocyte accumulation in muscles and halted recovery 10-20 h after strength exercise. *Journal of Applied Physiology* 95, 2503–2509.

Rainer, T.H., Chan, T.Y.F. and Cocks, R.A. (1999) Do peripheral blood counts have any prognostic value following trauma? *Injury* 30, 179–185.

Ramel, A., Wagner, K.H. and Elmadfa, I. (2003) Acute impact of submaximal resistance exercise on immunological and hormonal parameters in young men. *Journal of Sports Science* 21, 1001–1008.

Rankin, J.A. (2004) Biological mediators of acute inflammation. *American Association of Critical Nurses Clinical Issues* 15, 3–17.

Reid, M.B. and Li, Y.P. (2001) Tumor necrosis factor-alpha and muscle wasting, a cellular perspective. *Respiratory Research* 2, 269–272.

Risøy, B.A., Raastad, T., Hallen, J., Lappegard, K.T., Baeverfjord, K., *et al.* (2003) Delayed leukocytosis after hard strength and endurance exercise, aspects of regulatory mechanisms. *BMC Physiology* 3, 14.

Round, J.M., Jones, D.A. and Cambridge, G. (1987) Cellular infiltrates in human skeletal muscle, exercise induced damage as a model for inflammatory muscle disease? *Journal of Neurological Science* 82, 1–11.

Saxton, J.M., Claxton, D., Winter, E. and Pockley, A.G. (2003) Peripheral blood leucocyte functional responses to acute eccentric exercise in humans are influenced by systemic stress, but not by exercise-induced muscle damage. *Clinical Science (Lond)* 104, 69–77.

Schmid-Schonbein, G.W. (2006) Analysis of inflammation. *Annual Review of Biomedical Engineering* 8, 93–131.

Schneider, B.S. and Tiidus, P.M. (2007) Neutrophil infiltration in exercise-injured skeletal muscle: how do we resolve the controversy? *Sports Medicine* 37, 837–856.

Scott, A., Khan, K.M., Roberts, C.R., Cook, J.L. and Duronio, V. (2004) What do we mean by the term "inflammation"? A contemporary basic science update for sports medicine. *British Journal of Sports Medicine* 38, 372–380.

Shephard, R.J. (2001) Sepsis and mechanisms of inflammatory response, is exercise a good model? *British Journal of Sports Medicine* 35, 223–230.

Shephard, R.J. (2002) Cytokine responses to physical activity, with particular reference to IL-6, sources, actions, and clinical implications. *Critical Reviews in Immunology* 22, 165–182.

Shephard, R.J. (2003) Adhesion molecules, catecholamines and leucocyte redistribution during and following exercise. *Sports Medicine* 33, 261–284.

Shephard, R.J., Verde, T.J., Thomas, S.G. and Shek, P. (1991) Physical activity and the immune system. *Canadian Journal of Sport Science* 16, 169–185.

Simonson, S.R. (2001) The immune response to resistance exercise. *Journal of Strength and Conditioning Research* 15, 378–384.

Simonson, S.R. and Jackson, C.G. (2004) Leukocytosis occurs in response to resistance exercise in men. *Journal of Strength and Conditioning Research* 18, 266–271.

Simpson, R.J., Florida-James, G.D., Whyte, G.P. and Guy, K. (2006) The effects of intensive, moderate and downhill treadmill running on human blood lymphocytes expressing the adhesion/activation molecules CD54 (ICAM-1), CD18 (beta2 integrin) and CD53. *European Journal of Applied Physiology* 97, 109–121.

Smith, L.L., Anwar, A., Fragen, M., Rananto, C., Johnson, R., *et al.* (2000) Cytokines and cell adhesion molecules associated with high-intensity eccentric exercise. European Journal of Applied Physiology 82, 61–67.

Smith, L.L., McKune, A.J., Semple, S.J., Sibanda, E., Steel, H., *et al.* (2007) Changes in serum cytokines after repeated bouts of downhill running. *Applied Physiology, Nutrition and Metabolism* 32, 233–240.

Spiering, B.A., Kraemer, W.J., Anderson, J.M., Armstrong, L.E., Nindl, *et al.* (2008) Resistance exercise biology, manipulation of resistance exercise programme variables determines the responses of cellular and molecular signalling pathways. *Sports Medicine* 38, 527–540.

Staron, R.S., Hikida, R.S., Murray, T.F., Nelson, M.M., Johnson, P., *et al.* (1992) Assessment of skeletal muscle damage in successive biopsies from strength-trained and untrained men and women. *European Journal of Applied Physiology and Occupational Physiology* 65, 258–264.

Stauber, W.T. (1989) Eccentric action of muscles, physiology, injury, and adaptation. *Exercise and Sport Science Review* 17, 157–185.

Stock, C., Schaller, K., Baum, M., Liesen, H. and Weiss, M. (1995) Catecholamines, lymphocyte subsets, and cyclic adenosine monophosphate production in mononuclear cells and CD4+ cells in response to submaximal resistance exercise. *European Journal of Applied Physiology and Occupational Physiology* 71, 166–172.

Stupka, N., Tarnopolsky, M.A., Yardley, N.J. and Phillips, S.M. (2001) Cellular adaptation to repeated eccentric exercise-induced muscle damage. *Journal of Applied Physiology* 91, 1669–1678.

Suzuki, K., Nakaji, S., Yamada, M., Totsuka, M., Sato, K., *et al.* (2002) Systemic inflammatory response to exhaustive exercise. Cytokine kinetics. *Exercise Immunology Review* 8, 6–48.

Suzuki, K., Nakaji, S., Yamada, M., Liu, Q., Kurakake, S., *et al.* (2003) Impact of a competitive marathon race on systemic cytokine and neutrophil responses. *Medicine and Science in Sports and Exercise* 35, 348–355.

Tee, J.C., Bosch, A.N. and Lambert, M.I. (2007) Metabolic consequences of exercise-induced muscle damage. *Sports Medicine* 37, 827–836.

Tesch, P.A., Colliander, E.B. and Kaiser, P. (1986) Muscle metabolism during intense, heavy-resistance exercise. *European Journal of Applied Physiology and Occupational Physiology* 55, 362–366.

Tidball, J.G. (2005) Inflammatory processes in muscle injury and repair. *American Journal of Physiology Regulatory, Integrative and Comparative Physiology* 288, R345–R353.

Toumi, H., F'guyer, S. and Best, T.M. (2006) The role of neutrophils in injury and repair following muscle stretch. *Journal of Anatomy* 208, 459–470.

Trenerry, M.K., Carey, K.A., Ward, A.C. and Cameron-Smith, D. (2007) STAT3 signaling is activated in human skeletal muscle following acute resistance exercise. *Journal of Applied Physiology* 102, 1483–1489.

Trenerry, M.K., Della Gatta, P.A., Larsen, A.E., Garnham, A.P. and Cameron-Smith, D. (2011) Impact of resistance exercise training on interleukin-6 and JAK/STAT in young men. *Muscle and Nerve* 43, 385–392.

Uchiyama, S., Tsukamoto, H., Yoshimura, S. and Tamaki, T. (2006) Relationship between oxidative stress in muscle tissue and weight-lifting-induced muscle damage. *Pflugers Archive* 452, 109–116.

van Eeden, S.F., Granton, J., Hards, J.M., Moore, B. and Hogg, J.C. (1999) Expression of the cell adhesion molecules on leukocytes that demarginate during acute maximal exercise. *Journal of Applied Physiology* 86, 970–976.

Vandenburgh, H.H. (1987) Motion into mass, how does tension stimulate muscle growth? *Medicine and Science in Sports and Exercise* 19, S142–S149.

Verde, T., Thomas, S. and Shephard, R.J. (1992) Potential markers of heavy training in highly trained distance runners. *British Journal of Sports Medicine* 26, 167–175.

Walsh, N.P., Gleeson, M., Pyne, D.B., Nieman, D.C., Dhabhar, F.S., *et al.* (2011a) Position statement. Part two, Maintaining immune health. *Exercise Immunology Review* 17, 64–103.

Walsh, N.P., Gleeson, M., Shephard, R.J., Gleeson, M., Woods, J.A., *et al.* (2011b) Position statement. Part one, Immune function and exercise. *Exercise Immunology Review* 17, 6–63.

Wang, J., Song, H., Tang, X., Yang, Y., Vieira, V.J., *et al.* (2011) Effect of exercise training intensity on murine T-regulatory cells and vaccination response. *Scandinavian Journal of Medicine and Science in Sports* doi:10.1111/j.1600-0838.2010.01288.x

Warren, G.L., Lowe, D.A. and Armstrong, R.B. (1999) Measurement tools used in the study of eccentric contraction-induced injury. *Sports Medicine* 27, 43–59.

Wernbom, M., Augustsson, J. and Thomee, R. (2007) The influence of frequency, intensity, volume and mode of strength training on whole muscle cross-sectional area in humans. *Sports Medicine* 37, 225–264.

Wernbom, M., Augustsson, J. and Raastad, T. (2008) Ischemic strength training, a low-load alternative to heavy resistance exercise? *Scandinavian Journal of Medicine and Science in Sports* 18, 401–416.

Willoughby, D.S., McFarlin, B. and Bois, C. (2003) Interleukin-6 expression after repeated bouts of eccentric exercise. *International Journal of Sports Medicine* 24, 15–21.

Yamada, M., Suzuki, K., Kudo, S., Totsuka, M., Nakaji, S., *et al.* (2002) Raised plasma G-CSF and IL-6 after exercise may play a role in neutrophil mobilization into the circulation. *Journal of Applied Physiology* 92, 1789–1794.

Zaldivar, F., Wang-Rodriguez, J., Nemet, D., Schwindt, C., Galassetti, P., *et al.* (2006) Constitutive pro- and anti-inflammatory cytokine and growth factor response to exercise in leukocytes. *Journal of Applied Physiology* 100, 1124–1133.

11 Endurance Exercise and Inflammation

J.M. Peake*[,1,2,3] and J.S. Coombes[1]

[1]*School of Human Movement Studies and* [2]*Centre for Military and Veterans' Health, The University of Queensland, Brisbane, Australia;* [3]*Centre of Excellence for Applied Sport Science Research, Queensland Academy of Sport, Brisbane, Australia*

* Corresponding author, jpeake@hms.uq.edu.au

Introduction

The effects of physical activity on the immune system are important to consider for several reasons. Firstly, regular physical activity can potentially prevent and treat a variety of diseases that are associated with lifestyle-related factors and chronic inflammation. These include metabolic syndrome related disorders (e.g. insulin resistance, type 2 diabetes, dyslipidemia, hypertension, obesity), cardiovascular diseases (e.g. coronary artery disease, chronic heart failure, peripheral artery disease) and muscle, bone and joint diseases (e.g. osteoarthritis, osteoporosis, fibromyalgia). Secondly, physical activity is important for treating other diseases linked to significant immune dysfunction. These include human immunodeficiency virus or acquired immunodeficiency syndrome (HIV/AIDS), rheumatoid arthritis, multiple sclerosis and cancer. Thirdly, physical activity can potentially slow the rate of decline in immune function that occurs with ageing. Lastly, physical activity can modify resistance to upper respiratory illnesses. Understanding how physical activity affects immune function is therefore important to prescribe safe exercise guidelines that maximize the benefits of exercise, while minimizing the possible adverse effects of excessive exercise on the immune system.

The immune response to exercise is complex, and is specific to the various components of the immune system. For example, cells of the adaptive branch of the immune system (i.e. T lymphocytes and B cells) respond differently to cells of the innate (nonspecific) branch of the immune system (i.e. monocytes, granulocytes and natural killer cells) and soluble factors (i.e. immunoglobulins, cytokines, acute-phase proteins, complement). Factors such as the intensity, duration and mode of exercise also regulate immune responses to exercise. Intense and/or prolonged exercise stimulates the release of stress hormones (e.g. catecholamines, growth hormone, ACTH, cortisol, β-endorphin), cytokines (e.g. tumour necrosis factor-α, interferon-γ, interleukins 1β, 6, 10) and chemokines (e.g. interleukin 8, monocyte chemotactic protein 1, granulocyte-colony stimulating factor). In turn, these hormones, cytokines and chemokines mediate the mobilization and activity of leucocytes in the circulation. Exercise-induced muscle damage also stimulates leucocyte trafficking and activity. Other factors that influence immune responses to exercise include level of fitness, environmental temperature and diet (e.g. carbohydrate, antioxidants).

In this chapter we describe the inflammatory responses to endurance exercise. Endurance exercise refers to exercise lasting at least 30 min at submaximal intensities. Acute exercise refers to a single exercise session, as opposed chronic exercise that comprises multiple exercise sessions over a period of weeks to months. Immune responses to exercise are diverse. Although many cells of the immune system mediate inflammation to some extent, it is beyond the scope of this chapter to describe the effects of endurance exercise on all cells and soluble factors of the immune system. We have therefore focused predominantly on changes in neutrophils, monocytes, cytokines and acute-phase proteins following endurance exercise in young, healthy humans.

Neutrophils

Neutrophil number

Neutrophils comprise the greatest proportion of circulating leucocytes (60–70%; 3.0–6.0 cells × 10^9/l of blood), and form the first line of defence against infection. Their main function is to engulf and destroy foreign pathogens or damaged tissue through the processes of phagocytosis, degranulation and respiratory burst activity. Exercise-induced changes in neutrophil number and activity are summarized in Table 11.1.

Acute exercise and neutrophil number

During exercise, neutrophil number rises rapidly, decreases slightly in the hour after exercise and then increases further 1–3 h post-exercise (McCarthy *et al.*, 1992; Cross *et al.*, 1996; Rhind *et al.*, 1999; Suzuki *et al.*, 1999). Neutrophil number may remain elevated for up to 8 h after exercise (Ronsen *et al.*, 2001; Kakanis *et al.*, 2010). Neutrophils present in the circulation in the hours after exercise

Table 11.1. Summary of circulating neutrophil responses to endurance exercise and training.

Regulatory factor	Cell number	Chemotaxis	Phagocytosis	Degranulation	Oxidative burst
Acute exercise		↔, ↑, ↓	↔, ↑, ↓	↑, ↓	↔, ↑, ↓
Intensity	↑↑↑	Unknown	Unknown	↑↑	↔, ↑, ↓
Duration	↑	Unknown	Unknown	↑↑	↔, ↑, ↓
Environment		Unknown	Unknown		
Heat	↑↑			↑	Unknown
Cold	Unknown			Unknown	Unknown
Altitude	↑			Unknown	↓
Repeated exercise					
≥2 Sessions versus 1 session/day	↑	Unknown	Unknown	↓	↑
Diet supplements		Unknown			
Carbohydrate	↓		↔, ↓	↔, ↓	↔, ↓
Antioxidants	↔		↔	↔	↔, ↑
Omega-3 fatty acids	↔		↔	Unknown	Unknown
Glutamine	↔		Unknown	↔	Unknown
Caffeine	↔, ↑		Unknown	Unknown	↔, ↓
Training					
At rest	↔, ↓	↔, ↓	↔, ↓	Unknown	↔, ↓
Acute exercise	↓	Unknown	Unknown	↓	↓

↑ = increase; ↓ = attenuation; ↔ = no substantial effect.

are classified morphologically as immature 'segmented' neutrophils that are probably mobilized from the marginated pools in the lungs and bone marrow (Suzuki *et al.*, 1996b, 2003b). Neutrophil number rises with increasing exercise intensity (Fry *et al.*, 1992a; Moyna *et al.*, 1996; Peake *et al.*, 2004), exercise duration (Robson *et al.*, 1999), ambient temperature (Cross *et al.*, 1996; Rhind *et al.*, 1999) and altitude (Niess *et al.*, 2003b; Chouker *et al.*, 2005). The exercise-induced neutrophilia is greater during the afternoon compared with the morning (Li and Gleeson, 2004). In response to repeated sessions of exercise on one day, the exercise-induced neutrophilia is greater following a second session of exercise compared with the first session (Ronsen *et al.*, 2001; Li and Gleeson, 2004). The increase in neutrophil number is also greater when two exercise sessions are separated by 3 h versus 6 h (Boyum *et al.*, 2002).

The post-exercise neutrophilia represents a nonspecific immune response to a rise in blood flow and body temperature, which is in turn mediated by stress hormones. After exercise, neutrophil number correlates with the concentration of circulating catecholamines, growth hormone, cortisol, interleukin (IL)-6, IL-8 and granulocyte-colony stimulating factor (G-CSF) (Suzuki *et al.*, 1996b, 1999; Rhind *et al.*, 1999; Yamada *et al.*, 2002; Peake *et al.*, 2004; Laing *et al.*, 2008). Infusion studies provide more direct evidence of a mechanistic link between these factors and neutrophil mobilization during exercise (Kappel *et al.*, 1993; Terashima *et al.*, 1998; Suwa *et al.*, 2000; Steensberg *et al.*, 2001, 2003; Semerad *et al.*, 2002).

Dietary supplements and neutrophil number

Carbohydrate supplementation during endurance exercise (Nieman *et al.*, 1997a, 1998, 2003; Henson *et al.*, 2000; Peake *et al.*, 2005a; Scharhag *et al.*, 2006) and a high carbohydrate diet in the days before exercise (Mitchell *et al.*, 1998; Bishop *et al.*, 2001b) attenuate exercise-induced changes in neutrophil number. The lower post-exercise neutrophilia following exercise and carbohydrate supplementation occurs as a result of a simultaneous decrease in the release of stress hormones and cytokines that mediate neutrophil mobilization (Nieman *et al.*, 2001). One study reported that caffeine increases post-exercise neutrophil number (Bassini-Cameron *et al.*, 2007), whereas other research does not indicate any effect of caffeine on neutrophil number (Walker *et al.*, 2006, 2007, 2008). Supplementation with glutamine, antioxidant vitamins (Nieman *et al.*, 1997b, 2002; Petersen *et al.*, 2001), omega-3 fatty acids (Toft *et al.*, 2000) and polyphenol compounds (Nieman *et al.*, 2007c) do not alter neutrophil number following exercise.

Endurance training and neutrophil number

A large 10-year retrospective study identified low resting neutrophil number in 5% of athletes in a variety of sports, 17% of endurance cyclists and 16% of triathletes (Horn *et al.*, 2010). In contrast, cross-sectional comparisons of athletes and non-athletes (Nieman *et al.*, 2000) and prospective studies conducted over a period of several weeks (Mackinnon *et al.*, 1997), months (Pyne *et al.*, 1995; Shing *et al.*, 2007) or years (Diaz *et al.*, 2011) report no long-term changes in circulating neutrophil number at rest in athletes. The reasons for these inconsistent findings are unclear, but might include differences in training loads, and/or the period between the end of the previous training session and the time of blood sampling.

Short periods of intense training suppress circulating neutrophil number at rest (Hack *et al.*, 1994; Suzuki *et al.*, 1996a) and in response to acute exercise (Blannin *et al.*, 1996; Suzuki *et al.*, 1996a, 1999). These neutrophil responses might result from alterations in the secretion of stress hormones. Neutrophil number in sputum is elevated in runners (Bonsignore *et al.*, 2001), swimmers (Helenius *et al.*, 1998) and rowers (Morici *et al.*, 2004), and correlates with weekly training load, suggesting that exercise training may cause chronic inflammation of the airways (Belda *et al.*, 2008). The clinical significance of elevated neutrophils in sputum is uncertain, however. This response might represent training adaptation rather than poor respiratory health (Bonsignore *et al.*, 2003). Alternatively, other research indicates that neutrophil number in sputum (at rest) is higher in athletes with asthma, and correlates with bronchial hyper-responsiveness, most notably in athletes involved in water sports (Belda *et al.*, 2008).

Neutrophil chemotaxis

Chemotaxis involves the migration of neutrophils towards the site of infection or tissue damage. This process is important because it ensures that neutrophils rapidly mount a defence against invading pathogens. Chemotaxis is assessed *in vitro* by incubating neutrophils in a chamber separated from chemotactic stimuli (e.g. N-formylmethionine leucyl-phenylalanine [f-MLP], IL-8, complement 5a) in another chamber. Chemotaxis is quantified by measuring the distance cells move in a given time or the number of cells that move a given distance in a certain time.

Acute exercise and neutrophil chemotaxis

The small number of studies investigating changes in blood neutrophil chemotaxis after endurance exercise have reported equivocal findings (Hack *et al.*, 1992; Suzuki *et al.*, 1996a; Wolach *et al.*, 1998, 2000, 2005; Gavrieli *et al.*, 2008; Ortega *et al.*, 2009). This disparity may be due in part to differences in exercise protocol, post-exercise blood-sampling points, and the fitness level of participants. Müns *et al.* (1996) demonstrated that neutrophil chemotaxis increases in nasal lavage fluid following endurance exercise. This response could explain observations of elevated neutrophil number in the sputum of athletes (Helenius *et al.*, 1998; Bonsignore *et al.*, 2001; Belda *et al.*, 2008).

Endurance training and neutrophil chemotaxis

Neutrophil chemotaxis at rest or after acute exercise either remains unchanged or decreases following regular endurance training (Espersen *et al.*, 1991; Hack *et al.*, 1992; Wolach *et al.*, 2000; Hill *et al.*, 2007).

Neutrophil phagocytosis

Phagocytosis involves engulfing pathogens or cellular debris to form an internal phagosome. Proteolytic enzymes released within neutrophils and monocytes then degrade these pathogens or tissue fragments. The phagocytic capacity of neutrophils and monocytes is assessed *in vitro* by incubating cells with fragments of bacteria (e.g. *Staphylococcus aureus*, *Candida albicans*) or yeast cells (e.g. zymosan) and fluorescently labelled beads. The amount of ingested cellular material or beads is then quantified either histologically or using flow cytometry.

Acute exercise and neutrophil phagocytosis

The effects of acute exercise on blood neutrophil phagocytic activity are variable, with reports that phagocytic activity increases (Hack *et al.*, 1992; Nieman *et al.*, 1997a; Henson *et al.*, 2000; Ortega *et al.*, 2005, 2006), decreases (Hack *et al.*, 1994; Gabriel *et al.*, 1995; Wolach *et al.*, 1998; Krause *et al.*, 2001; Kakanis *et al.*, 2010) or remains unchanged (Benoni *et al.*, 1995b; Gabriel *et al.*, 1995; Suzuki *et al.*, 1996b; Nieman *et al.*, 1998; Wolach *et al.*, 2000; Scharhag *et al.*, 2005). Again, this variation may be attributed to differences in exercise protocol, post-exercise blood-sampling points, the fitness level of participants and methods for assessing neutrophil phagocytosis. These inconsistent findings preclude any definitive conclusions regarding exercise-induced changes in neutrophil phagocytosis.

Müns (1994) has reported that acute endurance exercise suppresses the phagocytic activity of neutrophils in the upper airways. In the long term, this suppression could partially account for observations of upper respiratory illnesses in athletes. The factors that regulate exercise-induced changes in neutrophil phagocytosis are not well known, but might involve noradrenaline and/or heat shock protein 72 (Ortega *et al.*, 2005; Giraldo *et al.*, 2010). The effects of exercise intensity and duration and ambient heat on neutrophil phagocytosis are also unknown.

Dietary supplements and neutrophil phagocytosis

The effects of carbohydrate supplementation are variable (Nieman *et al.*, 1997a; Henson *et al.*, 2000), whereas vitamin C supplementation does not influence neutrophil phagocytosis during acute endurance exercise (Krause *et al.*, 2001).

Endurance training and neutrophil phagocytosis

Some (Ortega *et al.*, 1993; Benoni *et al.*, 1995a,b), but not all (Hack *et al.*, 1992; Blannin *et al.*, 1996) research indicates that regular exercise training increases neutrophil phagocytosis at rest. Regular training attenuates neutrophil phagocytic responses to acute exercise (Hack *et al.*, 1994; Blannin *et al.*, 1996).

Neutrophil degranulation

Neutrophil degranulation involves the release of enzymes from intracellular granules. Two key enzymes released during degranulation are elastase and myeloperoxidase. Elastase is a potent proteolytic enzyme that degrades pathogens and cellular debris. Myeloperoxidase catalyses the conversion of hydrogen peroxide (H_2O_2) to hypochlorous acid (HOCl), which also assists in destroying pathogens and damaged tissue. This process is important because it is an intermediate step between phagocytosis and the formation of reactive oxygen species during the neutrophil oxidative burst. Neutrophil degranulation is assessed by measuring: (i) elastase production in cell culture supernatants following 'spontaneous' degranulation or stimulation with lipopolysaccharide (LPS); (ii) the intracellular content of myeloperoxidase using flow cytometry; and (iii) the plasma concentrations of elastase and myeloperoxidase.

Acute exercise and neutrophil degranulation

The plasma concentrations of elastase and myeloperoxidase generally rise following endurance exercise (Peake, 2002; Nieman *et al.*, 2007c, 2009). Neutrophil degranulation is particularly evident following intense exercise (Pyne *et al.*, 2000; Peake *et al.*, 2004; Nakajima *et al.*, 2010) and exercise in hot conditions (Peake *et al.*, 2007a). Conversely, elastase production per neutrophil decreases after exercise (Bishop *et al.*, 2002; Li and Cheng, 2007;

Laing *et al.*, 2008). These findings indicate that higher plasma elastase concentration results from more neutrophils in the circulation after exercise rather than increased cellular release of elastase. The factors that mediate exercise-induced changes in neutrophil degranulation are unclear, but may include IL-1β, IL-8 and complement 5a (Topham *et al.*, 1998; Binder *et al.*, 1999). Plasma myeloperoxidase concentration correlates with the plasma concentrations of endotoxin and complement protein C5a after exercise (Camus *et al.*, 1994, 1998), which suggests a possible mechanistic interaction between these factors. Neutrophil degranulation decreases in response to repeated bouts of endurance exercise on the same day (Li and Gleeson, 2004).

Dietary supplements and neutrophil degranulation

One study has reported that acute carbohydrate supplementation attenuates the exercise-induced decline in neutrophil elastase production (Bishop *et al.*, 2002). In contrast, other studies indicate no changes in neutrophil degranulation following exercise and acute supplementation with carbohydrate (Bishop *et al.*, 1999, 2001a), glutamine (Walsh *et al.*, 2000), quercetin (Nieman *et al.*, 2007c) or omega-3 fatty acids (Nieman *et al.*, 2009).

Endurance training and neutrophil degranulation

Little is known concerning the effects of training on neutrophil degranulation at rest. Four weeks of intensified training decreases LPS-induced elastase release on a per cell basis (Robson-Ansley *et al.*, 2006). Exercise-induced increases in plasma elastase and myeloperoxidase concentrations decrease over consecutive days of exercise (Suzuki *et al.*, 1999; Nieman *et al.*, 2007c).

Neutrophil oxidative burst activity

A nicotinamide adenine dinucleotide phosphate (NADPH) oxidase enzyme complex within the cell membrane of neutrophils regulates the production of reactive oxygen species (ROS). NADPH oxidase produces superoxide anions ($O_2\cdot^-$) from oxygen. The $O_2\cdot^-$ is converted to H_2O_2, which then either forms unstable hydroxyl radicals (OH·) in the Fenton reaction catalysed by Fe^{2+}/Fe^{3+}, or is converted to HOCl. OH· and HOCl are the primary agents that assist neutrophils in breaking down pathogens and cellular debris by oxidizing thiols within lipid structures, proteins and nucleic acids. These ROS provide a potent and efficient means of destroying pathogens and cellular debris; however, they act non-discriminately. Consequently, when produced in excess, OH· and HOCl may damage bystander tissues.

Neutrophil oxidative burst activity is measured in several ways. Neutrophils are typically incubated *in vitro* with soluble stimulants (e.g. phorbol 12-myristate 13-acetate; PMA) or particulate stimulants (e.g. N-formylmethionine leucyl-phenylalanine, *S. aureus*, zymosan). These stimulants activate signal transduction pathways that regulate NADPH oxidase activity and the formation of ROS. ROS production is then measured using spectrophotometric assays (e.g. reduction of tetrazolium salts), chemiluminescence assays (e.g. oxidation of luminol or lucigenin) or fluorescent assays (e.g. oxidation of 2′7′dichlorodihydrofluorescein or dihydrorhodamine 123).

Acute exercise and neutrophil oxidative burst activity

Within the research on the effects of exercise on neutrophil function, most studies have focused on neutrophil oxidative burst activity. Similar to other neutrophil functions, exercise-induced changes in neutrophil oxidative burst activity are variable. There are reports that oxidative burst activity increases, decreases or remains unchanged after exercise (Nieman *et al.*, 1997a, 2007c; Wolach *et al.*, 1998, 2000; Hessel *et al.*, 2000; Boyum *et al.*, 2002; Peake, 2002; Quindry *et al.*, 2003; Nielsen *et al.*, 2004; Peake *et al.*, 2004; Scharhag *et al.*, 2005; Walker *et al.*, 2006, 2007; Li and Cheng, 2007; Kakanis *et al.*, 2010). Other studies report different alterations in neutrophil oxidative burst activity following exercise, depending on blood sampling time points and assay methods (Nieman *et al.*, 1997b, 1998;

Henson *et al.*, 2000; Peake *et al.*, 2004). Neutrophil oxidative burst activity is similar after prolonged running and cycling (Nieman *et al.*, 1998). Two bouts of exercise in a day increase neutrophil oxidative burst activity to a greater extent compared with one bout (Boyum *et al.*, 2002). Furthermore, neutrophil oxidative burst activity does not return to normal when the recovery period between exercise bouts is 3 h or less (Boyum *et al.*, 2002).

In vitro, catecholamines and glucocorticoids inhibit cell-signalling pathways that regulate neutrophil oxidative burst activity (Dandona *et al.*, 2001; Tintinger *et al.*, 2001). Following exercise, plasma adrenaline concentration correlates negatively with neutrophil oxidative burst activity (Hack *et al.*, 1994; Suzuki *et al.*, 1999), whereas no such relationship exists for plasma cortisol concentration. Post-exercise plasma concentrations of growth hormone and IL-6 correlate positively with neutrophil oxidative burst activity (Smith *et al.*, 1996; Suzuki *et al.*, 1999), which suggests that these factors stimulate this activity during exercise. Some researchers have proposed that exercise-induced changes in neutrophil oxidative burst activity depend on exercise intensity (Smith *et al.*, 1992). Existing research does not support this concept, however (Robson *et al.*, 1999; Pyne *et al.*, 2000; Peake *et al.*, 2004).

Dietary supplements and neutrophil oxidative burst activity

The effects of acute supplementation with carbohydrate or caffeine on neutrophil oxidative burst activity following exercise are variable. Several studies demonstrate no effects (Nieman *et al.*, 1997a, 1998; Henson *et al.*, 2000; Walker *et al.*, 2008), whereas other research demonstrates that carbohydrate and caffeine attenuate the exercise-induced decline in neutrophil oxidative burst activity (Walker *et al.*, 2006, 2007). The effects of antioxidant supplementation are also inconsistent. Vitamin C supplementation does not alter neutrophil oxidative burst activity following exercise (Nieman *et al.*, 1997b; Krause *et al.*, 2001). In contrast, supplementation with a cocktail of β-carotene and vitamins C and E enhances neutrophil oxidative burst activity after exercise (Robson *et al.*, 2003). These inconsistent findings are most likely due to differences in the dose and duration of supplementation, exercise protocols, assay procedures and blood sampling time points. Zinc supplementation reduces neutrophil oxidative burst activity following exercise (Singh *et al.*, 1994).

Endurance training and neutrophil oxidative burst activity

Some (Smith *et al.*, 1990; Baj *et al.*, 1994; Pyne *et al.*, 1995) but not all (Hack *et al.*, 1992; Nieman *et al.*, 2000) research indicates that at rest, neutrophil oxidative burst activity is lower in athletes compared with non-athletes. Three to seven days of consecutive exercise tends to attenuate neutrophil oxidative burst activity (Suzuki *et al.*, 1996a, 1999). This trend may persist for several months (Hack *et al.*, 1994; Pyne *et al.*, 1995). These observations suggest that regular training reduces the capacity of neutrophils to respond to an infectious challenge. This response could account, in part, for the higher incidence of upper respiratory illnesses in athletes compared with non-athletes (Nieman *et al.*, 1989a, 1990; Spence *et al.*, 2007). Alternatively, this may be an adaptive response to minimize ROS-induced tissue damage (Smith, 1994).

Summary of neutrophil responses to endurance exercise

Short-term increases in circulating neutrophil number after exercise may represent a mild inflammatory response, or an 'immuno-surveillance' response to pathogens present in the upper respiratory tract. In general, circulating neutrophil number at rest is clinically normal in athletes and/or does not change following a period of exercise training. These observations suggest that such changes are not functionally significant. Variable alterations in neutrophil chemotaxis, phagocytosis and oxidative burst activity following exercise make it difficult to establish whether such changes are beneficial or harmful. Lower neutrophil chemotaxis, phagocytosis and oxidative burst activity in response to regular training might serve to limit nonspecific damage to skeletal muscle.

Monocytes

Monocyte number

Monocytes make up 10–15% of the circulating leucocyte pool, with a normal clinical range of 0.15–0.60 cells × 10^9/l of blood. Monocytes circulate in the blood and then differentiate into macrophages when they enter tissues. Similar to neutrophils, monocytes/macrophages play a key role in defence against bacterial infection. Their main functions include phagocytosis, production of reactive oxygen and nitrogen species, antigen presentation and cytokine synthesis. Exercise-induced changes in monocyte number and activity are summarized in Table 11.2.

Acute exercise and monocyte number

Similar to neutrophils, monocyte number increases during exercise relative to the intensity and duration of exercise (Fry *et al.*, 1992a; Tvede *et al.*, 1993; Shek *et al.*, 1995; Moyna *et al.*, 1996). Subpopulations of monocytes respond to exercise in different ways. Specifically, the number of 'pro-inflammatory' $CD14^+CD16^+$ monocytes increases after exercise, whereas the number of 'classic' $CD14^+CD16^-$ monocytes decreases or remains unchanged (Steppich *et al.*, 2000; Selkirk *et al.*, 2009; Simpson *et al.*, 2009). Monocytes display distinct responses to exercise when compared with neutrophils. Firstly, monocytes do not show a biphasic response to exercise. Rather, monocyte number return to baseline within 2 h of short duration exercise (Fry *et al.*, 1992a; Moyna *et al.*, 1996), whereas they remain elevated for several hours after prolonged exercise (Shek *et al.*, 1995). Secondly, monocyte number increases similarly during exercise in temperate and hot conditions (Cross *et al.*, 1996; Rhind *et al.*, 1999), and also at simulated altitude versus sea level (Niess *et al.*, 2003b). Lastly, monocyte number does not increase cumulatively in response to repeated bouts of exercise on the same day (Nielsen *et al.*, 1996; Rohde *et al.*, 1998). $CD14^+CD16^+$ monocytes may express more cell-surface

Table 11.2. Summary of circulating monocyte responses to endurance exercise and training.

Regulatory factor	Cell number	Chemotaxis	Phagocytosis	Cytokine synthesis	Oxidative burst
Acute exercise		Unknown	↔, ↑	↓	↔, ↑, ↓
Intensity	↑↑		Unknown	Unknown	Unknown
Duration	↑↑		Unknown	Unknown	Unknown
Environment		Unknown	Unknown		Unknown
Heat	↔			↔	
Cold	Unknown			Unknown	
Altitude	↔			Unknown	
Repeated exercise					
≥2 Sessions versus 1 session/day	↔	Unknown	Unknown	Unknown	↑
Diet supplements		Unknown			
Carbohydrate	↓		↔, ↓	↔	↓
Antioxidants	↔		↔	↔, ↑	Unknown
Omega-3 fatty acids	↔		↔	Unknown	Unknown
Glutamine	↔		Unknown	Unknown	Unknown
Caffeine	↔		Unknown	Unknown	Unknown
Training			Unknown		Unknown
At rest	↔, ↓	↓		↔, ↑, ↓	
Acute exercise	↔, ↑	Unknown		Unknown	

↑ = increase; ↓ = attenuation; ↔ = no substantial effect.

adhesion/activation receptors, which could account for why they are mobilized during exercise (Simpson *et al.*, 2009). Cortisol mediates monocyte chemotaxis *ex vivo*, whereas its role in regulating monocyte trafficking during exercise is less certain (Okutsu *et al.*, 2008). Stronger evidence exists that adrenaline stimulates monocyte release during exercise (Tvede *et al.*, 1994).

Dietary supplements and monocyte number

Carbohydrate supplementation attenuates exercise-induced changes in monocyte number (Nieman *et al.*, 1997a, 1998, 2003; Henson *et al.*, 2000; Scharhag *et al.*, 2006). In contrast, glutamine (Krzywkowski *et al.*, 2001), vitamin C (Nieman *et al.*, 2002), omega-3 fatty acids (Nieman *et al.*, 2009) and non-steroidal anti-inflammatory drugs (Nieman *et al.*, 2006b) do not alter monocyte number after exercise.

Endurance training and monocyte number

Similar to neutrophil number, the effect of regular endurance training on resting monocyte number is variable. A retrospective study of around 2200 athletes conducted over 10 years reported monocyte numbers below the clinical reference range in 2% of all athletes, 5% of gymnasts and 5% of triathletes (Horn *et al.*, 2010). In contrast, other cross-sectional studies report that monocyte number in athletes generally falls within the clinical reference range (Mackinnon *et al.*, 1997; Nieman *et al.*, 1997a, 1998, 2000). Prospective training studies report no change (Fry *et al.*, 1992b; Bury *et al.*, 1998; Shing *et al.*, 2007), an increase (Baum *et al.*, 1994) or a decrease (Ndon *et al.*, 1992; Mackinnon *et al.*, 1997) in monocyte number following chronic endurance training. Some of this disparity might be due to differences in the timing of blood sampling after the last exercise session. The effect of chronic endurance training on changes in monocyte number after acute exercise is variable, with reports of no change (Ndon *et al.*, 1992; Eliakim *et al.*, 1997) or an increase (Selkirk *et al.*, 2009) in monocyte number.

Monocyte/macrophage chemotaxis

No research has directly examined the effects of acute endurance exercise on monocyte/macrophage chemotaxis in humans. Post-exercise plasma increases monocyte chemotaxis *ex vivo* and cortisol regulates this response (Okutsu *et al.*, 2008). Chronic endurance training reduces monocyte chemotaxis at rest (Czepluch *et al.*, 2011).

Monocyte/macrophage phagocytosis

Studies of exercise-induced changes in the phagocytic activity of monocytes/macrophages are variable, with reports that phagocytic activity increases (Nieman *et al.*, 1997a, 1998; Fehr *et al.*, 1989) or remains unchanged (Scharhag *et al.*, 2005) after exercise. Exercise stimulates tissue macrophages to produce lysosomal enzymes that augment macrophage bactericidal activity (Fehr *et al.*, 1989). Corticosterone, prolactin and thyroid hormones regulate macrophage phagocytosis *in vitro* (Ortega *et al.*, 1996), but it remains to be confirmed whether these hormones also mediate monocyte/macrophage phagocytosis during exercise. The effect of acute supplementation with carbohydrate on exercise-induced changes in the phagocytic activity of monocytes is variable, with reports of a decrease (Nieman *et al.*, 1998) or no change (Nieman *et al.*, 1997a). These equivocal findings might be due to differences in exercise, protocol, training status of participants and assay protocols. The effect of chronic endurance training on monocyte/macrophage phagocytosis in humans is unknown.

Monocyte oxidative burst activity

Studies of alterations in monocyte oxidative burst activity following endurance exercise are inconsistent, with reports that oxidative burst activity increases (Nieman *et al.*, 1998; Wang *et al.*, 2006), decreases (Moir *et al.*, 2010) or remains unchanged (Nieman *et al.*, 1997a; Scharhag *et al.*, 2005; Wang *et al.*, 2006). Carbohydrate supplementation attenuates monocyte oxidative burst activity after exercise, possibly by suppressing cortisol release (Nieman *et al.*, 1998). No research has investigated changes in monocyte oxidative burst activity following chronic endurance training.

Monocyte cytokine production

Monocytes and macrophages synthesize a variety of cytokines, chemokines and growth factors. IL-1β, tumour necrosis factor (TNF)-α and IL-6 are the major monocyte-derived cytokines.

Acute exercise and monocyte cytokine production

Endurance exercise increases the number of circulating monocytes that produce IL-1β, IL-6 and TNF-α (Starkie *et al.*, 2000, 2001b, 2005). 'Pro-inflammatory' $CD14^+CD16^+$ monocytes seem to produce more cytokines compared with 'classic' $CD14^+CD16^-$ monocytes after exercise (Selkirk *et al.*, 2009). Changes in the *amount* of cytokines produced following exercise are variable, however, with reports that monocyte cytokine production increases, decreases or remains unchanged after exercise (Starkie *et al.*, 2000, 2001b, 2005; Rhind *et al.*, 2001; Selkirk *et al.*, 2009). Other research demonstrates that endurance exercise also reduces *ex vivo* cytokine production in whole blood (Drenth *et al.*, 1995, 1998; Baum *et al.*, 1997; Weinstock *et al.*, 1997; Smits *et al.*, 1998; Nieman *et al.*, 2002) and isolated mononuclear cells (Kvernmo *et al.*, 1992; Bassit *et al.*, 2002). These discrepant findings may be due to differences in exercise protocols, post-exercise blood sampling times and assay methods used to measure monocyte cytokine production.

The mechanisms by which exercise suppresses monocyte cytokine production are unclear. One plausible mechanism is that catecholamines and glucocorticoids released during exercise reduce the capacity of T helper 1 lymphocytes to synthesise cytokines such as IL-2, TNF-α and interferon (IFN)-γ, which in turn regulate monocyte cytokine synthesis (Elenkov and Chrousos, 2002). Evidence against this concept, however, is that carbohydrate supplementation reduces plasma adrenaline concentration but does not prevent the decline in monocyte cytokine production during exercise (Starkie *et al.*, 2000). Glucocorticoids may exert a stronger inhibitory effect on monocyte cytokine production during exercise but this requires confirmation. The decreased monocyte production of IL-1β, IL-6 and TNF-α during exercise might promote humoral immune responses following exercise that are linked to allergic reactions and possibly asthma (Suzuki *et al.*, 2002).

Dietary supplements and monocyte cytokine production

Supplementation with carbohydrate (Starkie *et al.*, 2000) or vitamin C (Nieman *et al.*, 2002) does not alter monocyte cytokine production following exercise. In contrast, supplementation with a combination of vitamins E, C, A, allopurinol and *N*-acetylcysteine seems to increase monocyte production of IL-1β, IL-6 and TNF-α following endurance exercise (Toumpanakis *et al.*, 2009).

Endurance training and monocyte cytokine production

The effects of chronic endurance training on cellular cytokine production at rest are unclear. Baum *et al.* (1999) reported that LPS-stimulated production of IL-1β and IL-6 (but not IL-2 or IFN-γ) was higher in whole blood cultures of athletes compared with non-athletes. Pool *et al.* (2002) observed that spontaneous (i.e. unstimulated) production of IL-6 was higher, whereas LPS-stimulated production of IL-6 was lower in whole blood cultures of athletes compared with non-athletes. Sloan *et al.* (2007) found that LPS-stimulated production of TNF-α decreased after high-intensity, but not moderate-intensity endurance training. This disparity might be due to differences in the training status of participants and assay protocols to assess cytokine production. Whole blood and mononuclear cells consist of mixed cell populations. Therefore, it is difficult to determine whether the cytokine responses described above specifically reflect changes in monocyte cytokine production; however, this is plausible.

Other monocyte functions

Monocytes also produce tissue factor and eicosanoids such as leucotrienes, thromboxanes and prostaglandins. These agents regulate blood clotting, mast cell activity, leucocyte chemotaxis and oxidative burst activity. LPS-stimulated tissue factor activity in monocytes increases following intense exercise (Kvernmo *et al.*, 1992; Lund *et al.*, 1998) and repeated exercise bouts on the same day (Degerstrom and Osterud, 2006). Although monocytes and eicosanoids are implicated in exercise-induced bronchospasm (Parsons *et al.*, 2008), few studies have examined exercise-induced changes in the synthesis of eicosanoids. In healthy athletes, exercise suppresses monocyte production of leucotriene B_4 (Degerstrom and Osterud, 2006), whereas it increases monocyte production of thromboxane B_2 (Degerstrom and Osterud, 2006) and prostaglandin E_2 (Cannon *et al.*, 1991), monocyte cyclo-oxygenase expression (Kim *et al.*, 2009), and the plasma concentrations of leucotriene B_4 and prostaglandin E_2 increase (Peake *et al.*, 2005b). In asthmatics, exercise increases neutrophil production of leucotriene B_4 and the concentration of cysteinyl leucotrienes in sputum (Mickleborough *et al.*, 2006). Endurance training reduces monocyte tissue factor activity both at rest and in response to acute exercise (Lund *et al.*, 1998).

Summary of monocyte responses to endurance exercise

The transient increase in circulating monocyte number after endurance may facilitate communication between the innate and adaptive branches of the immune system so as to clear and destroy pathogens in the upper respiratory tract and circulation. Most evidence suggests that resting monocyte number decreases after a period of training, but this response is unlikely to increase the risk of infection. The inconsistent changes in monocyte phagocytosis, cytokine synthesis and oxidative burst activity following both acute exercise and long-term training preclude any definitive conclusions concerning the functional significance of such changes.

Leucocyte Gene Profiles

A number of studies have used gene microarrays to assess the patterns of changes in gene expression in blood leucocytes following exercise. These studies reveal that exercise stimulates changes in leucocyte genes involved in a wide range of functions, including inflammation. It is beyond the scope of this chapter to discuss the findings of these studies in any great detail, but we refer interested readers to the following literature for more information: Northoff *et al.* (2008), Connolly *et al.* (2004), Buttner *et al.* (2007), Radom-Aizik *et al.* (2008, 2010), Nakamura *et al.* (2010) and Matthews *et al.* (2009).

Cytokines

Cytokines are protein hormones that regulate communication between the innate and adaptive branches of the immune system. Cytokines are broadly classified according to the following functions: (i) mediators of natural immunity (e.g. IL-1β, TNF-α, IL-6, IL-8, monocyte chemotactic protein [MCP]-1); (ii) regulators of lymphocyte activation, growth and differentiation (e.g. IL-2, IL-4, IL-17, transforming growth factor [TGF]-β); (iii) regulators of immune-mediated inflammation (e.g. IFN-γ, IL-5, IL-10, IL-12); and (iv) inducers of haematopoiesis (e.g. G-CSF, monocyte-colony stimulating factor [M-CSF]). Many cytokines are coupled with soluble receptors. Cytokines are synthesized by muscle cells, monocytes, T lymphocytes, endothelial cells and fibroblasts, and act on a range of cell types and organs of the body. As discussed previously, IL-1β, TNF-α and IL-6 are produced rapidly in response to infection and tissue damage. These cytokines increase body temperature and blood flow while inducing the release of acute-phase proteins from the liver. Subsequently, IL-8 and MCP-1 attract neutrophils and monocytes to sites of infection or tissue damage. Other cytokines are then synthesized, as required, to induce proliferation and differentiation of specific cell types, or to restrict pro-inflammatory responses. Exercise-induced changes in cytokines are summarized in Table 11.3.

Acute cytokine responses to exercise

The acute cytokine response to exercise is likened to the cytokine response to sepsis, whereby TNF-α increases rapidly in the circulation, followed by IL-1β and IL-6 (Petersen and Pedersen, 2005). Unlike sepsis, however, during exercise circulating IL-6 increases dramatically, whereas TNF-α and IL-1β increase only slightly (if at all) in the bloodstream (Suzuki *et al.*, 2002; Nieman *et al.*, 2003, 2005b, 2006b, 2007a; Suzuki *et al.*, 2003b; Mastaloudis *et al.*, 2004; Starkie *et al.*, 2005). IL-6 inhibits the synthesis of TNF-α during exercise (Starkie *et al.*, 2003), possibly by stimulating cortisol release and the synthesis of anti-inflammatory cytokines (Steensberg *et al.*, 2003). For these reasons, IL-6 is typically considered to act in an anti-inflammatory fashion during exercise (Petersen and Pedersen, 2005).

Whereas exercise does not induce substantial systemic release of IL-1β and TNF-α, mRNA expression of these cytokines increases in skeletal muscle following endurance exercise (Nieman *et al.*, 2003, 2005a, 2007a). The functional significance of this response is uncertain. Transient expression of IL-1β and TNF-α in skeletal muscle after exercise might assist in breaking down damaged tissue (Frost *et al.*, 1997, 2003; Williamson *et al.*, 2005; Li *et al.*, 2009) so that muscle can regenerate efficiently (Warren *et al.*, 2002). The cellular sources of circulating IL-1β and TNF-α during exercise are uncertain because, as discussed previously, exercise induces variable changes in monocyte production of these cytokines.

Among all the cytokines and chemokines, most research has focused on exercise-induced changes in IL-6. Plasma IL-6 concentration increases during exercise in response to exercise intensity (Helge *et al.*, 2003; Peake *et al.*, 2004), exercise duration (Suzuki *et al.*, 1999, 2003b; Yamada *et al.*, 2002)

Table 11.3. Summary of cytokine responses to endurance exercise and training.

Regulatory factor	IL-1β, TNF-α	IL-1ra, IL-6, IL-10	IL-8, MCP-1
Acute exercise			
Intensity	↔	↑↑↑	↑
Duration	↑	↑↑↑	↑
Environment			
Heat	↑	↑	Unknown
Cold	Unknown	Unknown	Unknown
Altitude	Unknown	↑	↔
Repeated exercise			
≥2 Sessions v 1 session/day	Unknown	↑	Unknown
Diet supplements			
Carbohydrate	↔	↓	↓
Antioxidants	↔	↓, ↔	↔
Omega-3 fatty acids	↔	↔	↔
Glutamine	Unknown	↑	Unknown
Caffeine	Unknown	Unknown	Unknown
Training			
At rest	↓	↑, ↔	Unknown
Acute exercise	↓, ↔	↓, ↔	Unknown

↑ = increase; ↓ = attenuation; ↔ = no substantial effect. IL, interleukin; MCP, monocyte chemotactic protein; TNF α, tumour necrosis factor-α.

and core temperature (Rhind *et al.*, 2004; Laing *et al.*, 2008; Selkirk *et al.*, 2008). Plasma IL-6 concentration is higher following exercise in hypoxia compared with normoxia (Niess *et al.*, 2003b), and increases in response to repeated exercise sessions in one day (Ronsen *et al.*, 2002). Although IL-6 increases substantially after prolonged running (Nieman *et al.*, 2003, 2006b; Suzuki *et al.*, 2003b; Mastaloudis *et al.*, 2004), it is unlikely that muscle damage is a major factor driving IL-6 responses to exercise (Peake *et al.*, 2005c).

During exercise, IL-6 is mainly produced and released from skeletal muscle into the circulation (Steensberg *et al.*, 2000, 2002). Other sources of IL-6 during exercise include leucocytes (Degerstrom and Osterud, 2006), peritendinous tissue (Langberg *et al.*, 2002), the brain (Nybo *et al.*, 2002) and adipose tissue (Lyngso *et al.*, 2002). Muscle glycogen depletion is the main cause of IL-6 synthesis in muscle during exercise (Keller *et al.*, 2001). The factors that regulate IL-6 production in muscle (and other tissues) include nitric oxide (Steensberg *et al.*, 2007) and calcineurin (Keller *et al.*, 2006). Nuclear factor κB (NFκB) is proposed to regulate IL-6 expression in muscle but this requires confirmation (Pedersen, 2009). Adrenaline also induces a mild systemic IL-6 response but probably plays a limited role during exercise (Steensberg *et al.*, 2001). During exercise, the primary functions of IL-6 are to increase hepatic glucose production (Febbraio *et al.*, 2004), whole body lipolysis (van Hall *et al.*, 2003), glucose uptake and fatty acid oxidation (Carey *et al.*, 2006).

The plasma concentrations of chemokines IL-8 and MCP-1 increase during endurance exercise (Suzuki *et al.*, 2002; Nieman *et al.*, 2003, 2005b, 2006b, 2007a; Suzuki *et al.*, 2003b; Peake *et al.*, 2005b, 2007a; Okutsu *et al.*, 2008). Endurance exercise increases mRNA (Nieman *et al.*, 2003, 2005a, 2007a; Chan *et al.*, 2004) and protein expression of IL-8 (Akerstrom *et al.*, 2005). Similar to IL-6, IL-8 is responsive to muscle glycogen depletion (Nieman *et al.*, 2003, 2005a, 2007a; Chan *et al.*, 2004). IL-8 may also play a role in regulating angiogenesis in skeletal muscle (Akerstrom *et al.*, 2005). Unlike IL-6, IL-8 is not released from muscle into the circulation during exercise (Akerstrom *et al.*, 2005). Blood leucocytes are the most likely source of circulating IL-8 during exercise (Degerstrom and Osterud, 2006; Nieman *et al.*, 2006a, 2007a).

Anti-inflammatory cytokines such as IL-1ra and IL-10, and soluble TNF-α receptors are released into the circulation in the hours after exercise (Suzuki *et al.*, 2002; Nieman *et al.*, 2003, 2005b, 2006b, 2007a). IL-1ra and IL-10 respond to exercise intensity (Peake *et al.*, 2005b) and core temperature (Rhind *et al.*, 2004; Peake *et al.*, 2007a; Selkirk *et al.*, 2008). IL-1ra and IL-10 are probably released into the circulation after exercise in response to earlier increases in IL-6 (Steensberg *et al.*, 2003) and (to a lesser extent) adrenaline (Sondergaard *et al.*, 2000) during exercise. Blood leucocytes are the most likely source of circulating IL-1ra and IL-10 during exercise (Nieman *et al.*, 2006a, 2007a). IL-1ra and IL-10 may assist in regulating the pro-inflammatory effects of IL-1β and TNF-α (Suzuki *et al.*, 2002). Exercise increases mRNA expression of IL-10 (but not IL-1ra) in skeletal muscle (Nieman *et al.*, 2003). In contrast with the rise in circulating IL-1ra and IL-10 after endurance exercise, other anti-inflammatory cytokines such as IL-4, IL-5 and IL-13 are barely detectable in blood before and after endurance exercise (Suzuki *et al.*, 2003a; Peake *et al.*, 2005b). Endurance exercise also does not influence IL-4 and IL-5 mRNA expression in skeletal muscle (Nieman *et al.*, 2003).

Other cytokines and growth factors (e.g. IL-12, IL-15, G-CSF, M-CSF, brain-derived neurotrophic factor) are released into the circulation and/or expressed in skeletal muscle after endurance exercise (Suzuki *et al.*, 2002, 2006; Peake *et al.*, 2005b; Nieman *et al.*, 2006b; Matthews *et al.*, 2009). Less is known, however, about the factors that regulate these cytokines and growth factors, and their functional role during endurance exercise.

Dietary supplements and cytokines

Clear evidence exists that carbohydrate supplementation attenuates exercise-induced changes in the plasma concentrations of IL-1ra, IL-6, IL-8 and IL-10 (Nieman *et al.*, 1998,

2001; Henson *et al.*, 2000; Starkie *et al.*, 2001a; Bishop *et al.*, 2002). Carbohydrate loading in the days before exercise reduces exercise-induced alterations in circulating IL-1ra, IL-6 and IL-10 (Bishop *et al.*, 2001c). Carbohydrate supplementation reduces mRNA expression of IL-6 and IL-8 in skeletal muscle following prolonged running (Nieman *et al.*, 2003) but not prolonged cycling (Starkie *et al.*, 2001a; Febbraio *et al.*, 2003; Nieman *et al.*, 2005a). Differences in exercise intensity and duration might explain this discrepancy. In contrast with carbohydrate supplementation, glutamine supplementation increases plasma IL-6 concentration after exercise (Hiscock *et al.*, 2003). The effects of antioxidant supplements on circulating and intramuscular cytokine responses to exercise are variable, largely owing to a wide variation in antioxidant supplement and exercise protocols (Nieman *et al.*, 2007a,b,c; Peake *et al.*, 2007b). Omega-3 fatty acids do not alter plasma cytokine concentrations after exercise (Toft *et al.*, 2000; Nieman *et al.*, 2009).

Chronic endurance training and cytokines

Little is known about the long-term effects of endurance training on plasma cytokines at rest. One study has reported that plasma IL-6 concentration is persistently elevated after 4 weeks of intensified training, suggesting that IL-6 is a possible cause of fatigue in athletes (Robson-Ansley *et al.*, 2006). In contrast, other research indicates no significant changes in the plasma concentrations of TNF-α and IL-6 after 6 weeks of fluctuating training load (Halson *et al.*, 2003). Following several days to weeks of endurance training, cytokine responses to acute exercise generally decrease (Kvernmo *et al.*, 1992; Gokhale *et al.*, 2007; Nieman *et al.*, 2007a; Selkirk *et al.*, 2008; Croft *et al.*, 2009) or remain unchanged (Selkirk *et al.*, 2008; Limongelli *et al.*, 2010).

Summary of cytokine responses to endurance exercise

Transient increases in circulating cytokines during exercise may serve to regulate glucose and lipid metabolism. A shift in the balance of T helper 1:T helper 2 cytokines towards T helper 2 cytokines may reduce resistance to viral infection and increase the risk of allergic reaction. Evidence of long-term changes in cytokines with training is lacking. However, if IL-6 remains elevated in the circulation for several days or weeks, then this might contribute to perceptions of fatigue in athletes.

Acute-phase Proteins

Acute-phase proteins are proteins produced by the liver that increase ('positive' acute-phase protein) or decrease ('negative' acute-phase protein) in the circulation following infection and tissue damage. Acute-phase proteins are classified according to their function. They induce neuroendocrine, haematopoietic, metabolic and hepatic changes within the body. Complement is a group of more than 20 acute-phase proteins that play a fundamental role in inflammation and defence against infection. Complement proteins are activated in a cascade-like sequence. They can kill pathogens directly by disrupting the ionic gradient across their outer membrane. Alternatively, they can recruit phagocytic cells to sites of infection or inflammation, where these cells then break down cellular debris and/or pathogens. Other common acute-phase proteins include cytokines such as IL-1β, TNF-α and IL-6, the opsonins C-reactive protein (CRP) and serum amyloid A, the protease inhibitors α_1-antitrypsin and α_2-macroglobulin, and the iron-binding proteins ferritin, haptoglobin and ceruloplasmin. These acute-phase proteins help to regulate inflammatory reactions to infection and tissue damage.

Acute exercise and acute-phase proteins

Reports of exercise-induced alterations in the plasma concentrations of complement proteins C3, C4 and C5a after exercise are variable. Some studies report an increase following both short-duration (Camus *et al.*,

1994) and long-duration running (Dufaux and Order, 1989a; Camus *et al.*, 1997; Romeo *et al.*, 2008), whereas other research indicates that these complement proteins remain unchanged (Pyne *et al.*, 1997; Suzuki *et al.*, 2000; Fallon, 2001) or decrease (Wolach *et al.*, 1998) after similar forms of exercise. Some of this disparity is probably due to variations in blood sampling times after exercise and/or conditioning of study participants.

The serum concentrations of CRP and serum amyloid A do not increase after ≤1 h of exercise (Pyne *et al.*, 1997; Drenth *et al.*, 1998; Niess *et al.*, 2003a; Romeo *et al.*, 2008), whereas they increase for several days after ≥2 h of exercise (Jeukendrup *et al.*, 2000; Fallon, 2001; Peters *et al.*, 2001; Fischer *et al.*, 2004; Nieman *et al.*, 2006b; Suzuki *et al.*, 2006; Papassotiriou *et al.*, 2008). The greater increase in CRP following prolonged exercise is most likely due to the IL-6 release from skeletal muscle during later stages of exercise (Steensberg *et al.*, 2002, 2003). The protease inhibitors α_1-antitrypsin and α_2-macroglobulin either increase (Liesen *et al.*, 1977; Dufaux and Order, 1989b) or remain unchanged (Liesen *et al.*, 1977; Fallon, 2001) in the circulation after prolonged exercise. The iron-binding proteins haptoglobin, ferritin and ceruloplasmin all increase in blood following prolonged exercise (Liesen *et al.*, 1977; Fallon *et al.*, 1999; Fallon, 2001). Albumin, which provides a source of amino acids for synthesizing acute-phase proteins in the liver, either increases (Jeukendrup *et al.*, 2000; Suzuki *et al.*, 2006) or remains unchanged (Liesen *et al.*, 1977; Fallon, 2001) in the bloodstream in response to prolonged exercise.

Dietary supplements and acute-phase proteins

Vitamin C supplementation increases serum CRP concentration after ultra-endurance exercise (Peters *et al.*, 2001), whereas the effects of other dietary supplements on acute-phase proteins following exercise are unknown.

Chronic endurance training and acute-phase proteins

The serum concentrations of C4, CRP and α_1-antitrypsin increase cumulatively during 3 weeks of competitive exercise (Semple *et al.*, 2006). These short-term changes in acute-phase proteins might assist in regulating inflammatory responses to tissue injury. In contrast, long-term endurance training reduces the resting concentrations of serum CRP, C3, C4 and tissue plasminogen activator (Liesen *et al.*, 1977; Nieman *et al.*, 1989b; Kvernmo and Osterud, 1997; Mattusch *et al.*, 2000; Stewart *et al.*, 2007). The basal concentration of these acute-phase proteins may decline in the long term as athletes adapt to the stress of regular exercise.

Summary of acute-phase protein responses to endurance exercise

The inconsistent changes in acute-phase proteins following exercise make it difficult to establish whether such changes are beneficial or harmful. As athletes adapt to the regular stress of training, the synthesis of acute-phase proteins tends to decrease, which may help prevent excessive inflammatory responses to tissue damage.

Summary and Conclusions

Interest in the effects of endurance exercise on the immune system has increased substantially during the past two to three decades. Initially, most attention focused on how athletes respond to acute exercise and adapt to chronic training. More recently, research has focused more broadly on how exercise-induced immune changes are implicated in treating the elderly and patients with chronic diseases in clinical populations. In general, single sessions of exercise generate a robust inflammatory response. In contrast, regular exercise training over several weeks to months may help to reduce basal inflammation. The effectiveness of exercise training as a countermeasure against inflammation probably depends on the severity of basal inflammation, however. Through its effect on the immune system, exercise has the potential to modify the risk of disease, reverse existing morbidity and improve the functional capacity of most individuals. Despite intensive research activity, variation in the experimental approach to investigating exercise-induced changes in immune function has yielded many inconsistencies. Although we have developed a clear understanding about some aspects of exercise immunology, other aspects remain uncertain. Ongoing research is required to increase our knowledge base of how the immune system interacts with other systems of the body during exercise. Future research endeavours should also be directed toward enhancing our understanding of how the combination of diet and exercise influences the immune system. This information will inform clinicians, exercise physiologists, sport scientists and coaches about how to optimize exercise guidelines for competitive athletes, recreational exercisers and patients with chronic disease to maintain good health and minimize the risk of musculoskeletal injury.

References

Akerstrom, T., Steensberg, A., Keller, P., Keller, C., Penkowa, M., *et al.* (2005) Exercise induces interleukin-8 expression in human skeletal muscle. *Journal of Physiology* 563, 507–516.

Baj, Z., Kantorski, J., Majewska, E., Zeman, K., Pokoca, L., *et al.* (1994) Immunological status of competitive cyclists before and after the training season. *International Journal of Sports Medicine* 15, 319–324.

Bassini-Cameron, A., Sweet, E., Bottino, A., Bittar, C., Veiga, C., *et al.* (2007) Effect of caffeine supplementation on haematological and biochemical variables in elite soccer players under physical stress conditions. *British Journal of Sports Medicine* 41, 523–530.

Bassit, R.A., Sawada, L.A., Bacurau, R.F., Navarro, F., Martins, E., Jr, *et al.* (2002) Branched-chain amino acid supplementation and the immune response of long-distance athletes. *Nutrition* 18, 376–379.

Baum, M., Liesen, H. and Enneper, J. (1994) Leucocytes, lymphocytes, activation parameters and cell adhesion molecules in middle-distance runners under different training conditions. *International Journal of Sports Medicine* 15 Suppl 3, S122–S126.

Baum, M., Muller-Steinhardt, M., Liesen, H. and Kirchner, H. (1997) Moderate and exhaustive endurance exercise influences the interferon- gamma levels in whole-blood culture supernatants. *European Journal of Applied Physiology* 76, 165–169.

Baum, M., Klopping-Menke, K., Muller-Steinhardt, M., Liesen, H. and Kirchner, H. (1999) Increased concentrations of interleukin 1-beta in whole blood cultures supernatants after 12 weeks of moderate endurance exercise. *European Journal of Applied Physiology* 79, 500–503.

Belda, J., Ricart, S., Casan, P., Giner, J., Bellido-Casado, J., *et al.* (2008) Airway inflammation in the elite athlete and type of sport. *British Journal of Sports Medicine* 42, 244-248; discussion 248–249.

Benoni, G., Bellavite, P., Adami, A., Chirumbolo, S., Lippi, G., *et al.* (1995a) Changes in several neutrophil functions in basketball players before, during and after the sports season. *International Journal of Sports Medicine* 16, 34–37.

Benoni, G., Bellavite, P., Adami, A., Chirumbulo, S., Lippi, G., *et al.* (1995b) Effect of acute exercise on some haematological parameters and neutrophil functions in active and inactive subjects. *European Journal of Applied Physiology* 70, 187–191.

Binder, R., Kress, A., Kan, G., Herrmann, K. and Kirschfink, M. (1999) Neutrophil priming by cytokines and vitamin D binding protein (Gc- globulin): impact on C5a-mediated chemotaxis, degranulation and respiratory burst. *Molecular Immunology* 36, 885–892.

Bishop, N., Blannin, A., Robson, P., Walsh, N. and Gleeson, M. (1999) The effects of carbohydrate supplementation on immune responses to a soccer-specific exercise protocol. *Journal of Sports Science* 17, 787–796.

Bishop, N.C., Blannin, A.K., Walsh, N.P. and Gleeson, M. (2001a) Carbohydrate beverage ingestion and neutrophil degranulation responses following cycling to fatigue at 75% VO2 max. *International Journal of Sports Medicine* 22, 226–231.

Bishop, N.C., Walsh, N.P., Haines, D.L., Richards, E.E. and Gleeson, M. (2001b) Pre-exercise carbohydrate status and immune responses to prolonged cycling: I. Effect on neutrophil degranulation. *International Journal of Sport Nutrition and Exercise Metabolism* 11, 490–502.

Bishop, N.C., Walsh, N.P., Haines, D.L., Richards, E.E. and Gleeson, M. (2001c) Pre-exercise carbohydrate status and immune responses to prolonged cycling: II. Effect on plasma cytokine concentration. *International Journal of Sport Nutrition and Exercise Metabolism* 11, 503–512.

Bishop, N.C., Gleeson, M., Nicholas, C.W. and Ali, A. (2002) Influence of carbohydrate supplementation on plasma cytokine and neutrophil degranulation responses to high intensity intermittent exercise. *International Journal of Sport Nutrition and Exercise Metabolism* 12, 145–156.

Blannin, A.K., Chatwin, L.J., Cave, R. and Gleeson, M. (1996) Effects of submaximal cycling and long-term endurance training on neutrophil phagocytic activity in middle aged men. *British Journal of Sports Medicine* 30, 125–129.

Bonsignore, M.R., Morici, G., Riccobono, L., Insalaco, G., Bonanno, A., *et al.* (2001) Airway inflammation in nonasthmatic amateur runners. *American Journal of Physiology Lung Cellular and Molecular Physiology* 281, L668–L676.

Bonsignore, M.R., Morici, G., Vignola, A.M., Riccobono, L., Bonanno, A., *et al.* (2003) Increased airway inflammatory cells in endurance athletes: what do they mean? *Clinical and Experimental Allergy* 33, 14–21.

Boyum, A., Ronsen, O., Tennfjord, V.A., Tollefsen, S., Haugen, A.H., *et al.* (2002) Chemiluminescence response of granulocytes from elite athletes during recovery from one or two intense bouts of exercise. *European Journal of Applied Physiology* 88, 20–28.

Bury, T., Marechal, R., Mahieu, P. and Pirnay, F. (1998) Immunological status of competitive football players during the training season. *International Journal of Sports Medicine* 19, 364–368.

Buttner, P., Mosig, S., Lechtermann, A., Funke, H. and Mooren, F.C. (2007) Exercise affects the gene expression profiles of human white blood cells. *Journal of Applied Physiology* 102, 26–36.

Camus, G., Duchateau, J., Deby-Dupont, G., Pincemail, J., Deby, C., *et al.* (1994) Anaphylatoxin C5a production during short-term submaximal dynamic exercise in man. *International Journal of Sports Medicine* 15, 32–35.

Camus, G., Poortmans, J., Nys, M., Deby-Dupont, G., Duchateau, J., *et al.* (1997) Mild endotoxaemia and the inflammatory response induced by a marathon race. *Clinical Science* 92, 415–422.

Camus, G., Nys, M., Poortmans, J., Venneman, I., Monfils, T., *et al.* (1998) Possible in vivo tolerance of human polymorphonuclear neutrophil to low- grade exercise-induced endotoxaemia. *Mediators of Inflammation* 7, 413–415.

Cannon, J., Meydani, S., Fielding, R., Fiatarone, M., Meydani, M., *et al.* (1991) Acute phase response in exercise. II. Associations between vitamin E, cytokines and muscle proteolysis. *American Journal of Physiology Regulatory, Integrative and Comparative Physiology* 260, R1235–R1240.

Carey, A.L., Steinberg, G.R., Macaulay, S.L., Thomas, W.G., Holmes, A.G., *et al.* (2006) Interleukin-6 increases insulin-stimulated glucose disposal in humans and glucose uptake and fatty acid oxidation in vitro via AMP-activated protein kinase. *Diabetes* 55, 2688–2697.

Chan, M.H., Carey, A.L., Watt, M.J. and Febbraio, M.A. (2004) Cytokine gene expression in human skeletal muscle during concentric contraction: evidence that IL-8, like IL-6, is influenced by glycogen availability. *American Journal of Physiology Regulatory, Integrative and Comparative Physiology* 287, R322–R327.

Chouker, A., Demetz, F., Martignoni, A., Smith, L., Setzer, F., *et al.* (2005) Strenuous physical exercise inhibits granulocyte activation induced by high altitude. *Journal of Applied Physiology* 98, 640–647.

Connolly, P.H., Caiozzo, V.J., Zaldivar, F., Nemet, D., Larson, J., *et al.* (2004) Effects of exercise on gene expression in human peripheral blood mononuclear cells. *Journal of Applied Physiology* 97, 1461–1469.

Croft, L., Bartlett, J.D., Maclaren, D.P., Reilly, T., Evans, L., *et al.* (2009) High-intensity interval training attenuates the exercise-induced increase in plasma IL-6 in response to acute exercise. *Applied Physiology, Nutrition and Metabolism* 34, 1098–1107.

Cross, M.C., Radomski, M.W., Vanhelder, W.P., Rhind, S.G. and Shephard, R.J. (1996) Endurance exercise with and without a thermal clamp: effects on leukocytes and leukocyte subsets. *Journal of Applied Physiology* 81, 822–829.

Czepluch, F.S., Barres, R., Caidahl, K., Olieslagers, S., Krook, A., *et al.* (2011) Strenuous physical exercise adversely affects monocyte chemotaxis. *Thrombosis and Haemostasis* 105, 122–130.

Dandona, P., Aljada, A., Ghanim, H., Mohanty, P., Hamouda, W., *et al.* (2001) Acute suppressive effect of hydrocortisone on p47(phox) subunit of nicotinamide adenine dinucleotide phosphate oxidase. *Metabolism* 50, 548–552.

Degerstrom, J. and Osterud, B. (2006) Increased inflammatory response of blood cells to repeated bout of endurance exercise. *Medicine and Science in Sports and Exercise* 38, 1297–1303.

Diaz, V., Montalvo, Z. and Banfi, G. (2011) White blood cell counts in elite triathletes over four consecutive seasons. *European Journal of Applied Physiology* 111, 893–894.

Drenth, J., Van Uum, S., Van Deuren, M., Gj, P., Van Der Ven-Jongekrijg, J., *et al.* (1995) Endurance run increases circulating IL-6 and IL-1ra but downregulates ex vivo TNF-alpha and IL-1 beta production. *Journal of Applied Physiology* 79, 1497–1503.

Drenth, J.P., Krebbers, R.J., Bijzet, J. and Van Der Meer, J.W. (1998) Increased circulating cytokine receptors and ex vivo interleukin-1 receptor antagonist and interleukin-1beta production but decreased tumour necrosis factor-alpha production after a 5-km run. *European Journal of Clinical Investigation* 28, 866–872.

Dufaux, B. and Order, U. (1989a) Complement activation after prolonged exercise. *Clinica Chimica Acta* 179, 45–49.

Dufaux, B. and Order, U. (1989b) Plasma elastase-$\alpha\lambda\pi\eta\alpha$–1-antitrypsin, neopterin, tumor necrosis factor, and soluble interleukin-2 receptor after prolonged exercise. *International Journal of Sports Medicine* 10, 434–438.

Elenkov, I.J. and Chrousos, G.P. (2002) Stress hormones, proinflammatory and antiinflammatory cytokines, and autoimmunity. *Annals of the New York Academy of Sciences* 966, 290–303.

Eliakim, A., Wolach, B., Kodesh, E., Gavrieli, R., Radnay, J., *et al.* (1997) Cellular and humoral immune response to exercise among gymnasts and untrained girls. *International Journal of Sports Medicine* 18, 208–212.

Espersen, G., Toft, E., Ernst, E., Kaalund, S. and Grunnet, N. (1991) Changes of polymorphonuclear granulocyte migration and lymphocyte proliferative responses in elite runners undergoing intense exercise. *Scandinavian Journal of Medicine and Science in Sports* 1, 158–162.

Fallon, K.E. (2001) The acute phase response and exercise: the ultramarathon as prototype exercise. *Clinical Journal of Sports Medicine* 11, 38–43.

Fallon, K.E., Sivyer, G., Sivyer, K. and Dare, A. (1999) The biochemistry of runners in a 1600 km ultramarathon. *British Journal of Sports Medicine* 33, 264–269.

Febbraio, M.A., Steensberg, A., Keller, C., Starkie, R.L., Nielsen, H.B., *et al.* (2003) Glucose ingestion attenuates interleukin-6 release from contracting skeletal muscle in humans. *Journal of Physiology* 549, 607–612.

Febbraio, M., Hiscock, N., Sacchetti, M., Fischer, C. and Pedersen, B. (2004) Interleukin-6 is a novel factor mediating glucose homeostasis during skeletal muscle contraction. *Diabetes* 53, 1643–1648.

Fehr, H.G., Lotzerich, H. and Michna, H. (1989) Human macrophage function and physical exercise: phagocytic and histochemical studies. *European Journal of Applied Physiology Occupational Physiology* 58, 613–617.

Fischer, C., Hiscock, N., Penkowa, M., Basu, S., Vessby, B., *et al.* (2004) Vitamin C and E supplementation inhibits the release of interleukin-6 from contracting human skeletal muscle. *Journal of Physiology* 558, 633–645.

Frost, R., Lang, C. and Gelato, M. (1997) Transient exposure of human myoblasts to TNFalpha inhibits serum and IGF-I stimulated protein synthesis. *Endocrinology* 138, 4153–4159.

Frost, R.A., Nystrom, G. and Lang, C.H. (2003) Tumor necrosis factor-alpha decreases insulin like growth factor-I messenger ribonucleic acid expression in C2C12 myoblasts via a Jun N-terminal kinase pathway. *Endocrinology* 144, 1770–1779.

Fry, R., Morton, A., Crawford, G. and Keast, D. (1992a) Cell numbers and in vitro responses of leucocytes and lymphocyte subpopulations following maximal exercise and interval training sessions of different intensities. *European Journal of Applied Physiology* 64, 218–227.

Fry, R.W., Morton, A.R., Garcia-Webb, P., Crawford, G.P. and Keast, D. (1992b) Biological responses to overload training in endurance sports. *European Journal of Applied Physiology Occupational Physiology* 64, 335–344.

Gabriel, H., Muller, H.J., Kettler, K., Brechtel, L., Urhausen, A., *et al.* (1995) Increased phagocytic capacity of the blood, but decreased phagocytic activity per individual circulating neutrophil after an ultradistance run. *European Journal of Applied Physiology Occupational Physiology* 71, 281–284.

Gavrieli, R., Ashlagi-Amiri, T., Eliakim, A., Nemet, D., Zigel, L., *et al.* (2008) The effect of aerobic exercise on neutrophil functions. *Medicine and Science in Sports and Exercise* 40, 1623–1628.

Giraldo, E., Martin-Cordero, L., Garcia, J.J., Gerhmann, M., Multhoff, G. *et al.* (2010) Exercise-induced extracellular 72 kDa heat shock protein (Hsp72) stimulates neutrophil phagocytic and fungicidal capacities via TLR-2. *European Journal of Applied Physiology* 108, 217–225.

Gokhale, R., Chandrashekara, S. and Vasanthakumar, K.C. (2007) Cytokine response to strenuous exercise in athletes and non-athletes–an adaptive response. *Cytokine* 40, 123–127.

Hack, V., Strobel, G., Rau, J.-P. and Weicker, H. (1992) The effect of maximal exercise on the activity of neutrophil granulocytes in highly trained athletes in a moderate training period. *European Journal of Applied Physiology* 65, 520–524.

Hack, V., Strobel, G., Weiss, M. and Weicker, H. (1994) PMN cell counts and phagocytic activity of highly trained athletes depend on training period. *Journal of Applied Physiology* 77, 1731–1735.

Halson, S.L., Lancaster, G.I., Jeukendrup, A.E. and Gleeson, M. (2003) Immunological responses to overreaching in cyclists. *Medicine and Science in Sports and Exercise* 35, 854–861.

Helenius, I.J., Rytila, P., Metso, T., Haahtela, T., Venge, P., *et al.* (1998) Respiratory symptoms, bronchial responsiveness, and cellular characteristics of induced sputum in elite swimmers. *Allergy* 53, 346–352.

Helge, J.W., Stallknecht, B., Pedersen, B.K., Galbo, H., Kiens, B., *et al.* (2003) The effect of graded exercise on IL-6 release and glucose uptake in human skeletal muscle. *Journal of Physiology* 546, 299–305.

Henson, D., Nieman, D., Nehlsen-Cannarella, S., Fagoaga, O., Shannon, M., *et al.* (2000) Influence of carbohydrate on cytokine and phagocytic responses to 2 h of rowing. *Medicine and Science in Sports and Exercise* 32, 1384–1389.

Hessel, E., Haberland, A., Muller, M., Lerche, D. and Schimke, I. (2000) Oxygen radical generation of neutrophils: a reason for oxidative stress during marathon running? *Clinica Chimica Acta* 298, 145–156.

Hill, A.M., Worthley, C., Murphy, K.J., Buckley, J.D., Ferrante, A., *et al.* (2007) n-3 Fatty acid supplementation and regular moderate exercise: differential effects of a combined intervention on neutrophil function. *British Journal of Nutrition* 98, 300–309.

Hiscock, N., Petersen, E.W., Krzywkowski, K., Boza, J., Halkjaer-Kristensen, J., *et al.* (2003) Glutamine supplementation further enhances exercise-induced plasma IL-6. *Journal of Applied Physiology* 95, 145–148.

Horn, P.L., Pyne, D.B., Hopkins, W.G. and Barnes, C.J. (2010) Lower white blood cell counts in elite athletes training for highly aerobic sports. *European Journal of Applied Physiology* 110, 925–932.

Jeukendrup, A.E., Vet-Joop, K., Sturk, A., Stegen, J., Senden, J., *et al.* (2000) Relationship between gastrointestinal complaints and endotoxaemia, cytokine release and the acute-phase reaction during and after a long-distance triathlon in highly trained men. *Clinical Science* 98, 47–55.

Kakanis, M.W., Peake, J., Brenu, E.W., Simmonds, M., Gray, B., *et al.* (2010) The open window of susceptibility to infection after acute exercise in healthy young male elite athletes. *Exercise Immunology Review* 16, 119–137.

Kappel, M., Hansen, M.B., Diamant, M., Jorgensen, J.O., Gyhrs, A., *et al.* (1993) Effects of an acute bolus growth hormone infusion on the human immune system. *Hormone and Metabolism Research* 25, 579–585.

Keller, C., Steensberg, A., Pilegaard, H., Osada, T., Saltin, B., *et al.* (2001) Transcriptional activation of the IL-6 gene in human contracting skeletal muscle: influence of muscle glycogen content. *FASEB J* 15, 2748–2750.

Keller, C., Hellsten, Y., Steensberg, A. and Pedersen, B.K. (2006) Differential regulation of IL-6 and TNF-alpha via calcineurin in human skeletal muscle cells. *Cytokine* 36, 141–147.

Kim, S.Y., Jun, T.W., Lee, Y.S., Na, H.K., Surh, Y.J., *et al.* (2009) Effects of exercise on cyclooxygenase-2 expression and nuclear factor-kappaB DNA binding in human peripheral blood mononuclear cells. *Annals of the New York Academy of Sciences* 1171, 464–471.

Krause, R., Patruta, S., Daxbock, F., Fladerer, P., Biegelmayer, C., *et al.* (2001) Effect of vitamin C on neutrophil function after high-intensity exercise. *European Journal of Clinical Investigation* 31, 258–263.

Krzywkowski, K., Petersen, E.W., Ostrowski, K., Kristensen, J.H., Boza, J., *et al.* (2001) Effect of glutamine supplementation on exercise-induced changes in lymphocyte function. *American Journal of Physiology Cell Physiology* 281, C1259–C1265.

Kvernmo, H.D. and Osterud, B. (1997) The effect of physical conditioning suggests adaptation in procoagulant and fibrinolytic potential. *Thrombosis Research* 87, 559–569.

Kvernmo, H., Olsen, J.O. and Osterud, B. (1992) Changes in blood cell response following strenuous physical exercise. *European Journal of Applied Physiology and Occupational Physiology* 64, 318–322.

Laing, S.J., Jackson, A.R., Walters, R., Lloyd-Jones, E., Whitham, M., *et al.* (2008) Human blood neutrophil responses to prolonged exercise with and without a thermal clamp. *Journal of Applied Physiology* 104, 20–26.

Langberg, H., Olesen, J.L., Gemmer, C. and Kjaer, M. (2002) Substantial elevation of interleukin-6 concentration in peritendinous tissue, in contrast to muscle, following prolonged exercise in humans. *Journal of Physiology* 542, 985–990.

Li, T.L. and Cheng, P.Y. (2007) Alterations of immunoendocrine responses during the recovery period after acute prolonged cycling. *European Journal of Applied Physiology* 101, 539–546.

Li, T.L. and Gleeson, M. (2004) The effect of single and repeated bouts of prolonged cycling on leukocyte redistribution, neutrophil degranulation, IL-6, and plasma stress hormone responses. *International Journal of Sport Nutrition and Exercise Metabolism* 14, 501–516.

Li, W., Moylan, J.S., Chambers, M.A., Smith, J.D. and Reid, M.B. (2009) Interleukin-1 stimulates catabolism in C2C12 myotubes. *American Journal of Physiology Cell Physiology* 284, C706–C714.

Liesen, H., Dufaux, B. and Hollman, W. (1977) Modifications of serum glycoproteins the days following a prolonged physical exercise and the influence of physical training. *European Journal of Applied Physiology Occupational Physiology* 37, 243–254.

Limongelli, G., Calabro, P., Maddaloni, V., Russo, A., Masarone, D., *et al.* (2010) Cardiotrophin-1 and TNF-alpha circulating levels at rest and during cardiopulmonary exercise test in athletes and healthy individuals. *Cytokine* 50, 245–247.

Lund, T., Kvernmo, H.D. and Osterud, B. (1998) Cellular activation in response to physical exercise: the effect of platelets and granulocytes on monocyte reactivity. *Blood Coagulation and Fibrinolysis* 9, 63–69.

Lyngso, D., Simonsen, L. and Bulow, J. (2002) Interleukin-6 production in human subcutaneous abdominal adipose tissue: the effect of exercise. *Journal of Physiology* 543, 373–378.

Mackinnon, L.T., Hooper, S.L., Jones, S., Gordon, R.D. and Bachmann, A.W. (1997) Hormonal, immunological, and hematological responses to intensified training in elite swimmers. *Medicine and Science in Sports and Exercise* 29, 1637–1645.

Mastaloudis, A., Morrow, J., Hopkins, D., Devaraj, S. and Traber, M. (2004) Antioxidant supplementation prevents exercise-induced lipid peroxidation, but not inflammation, in ultramarathon runners. *Free Radical Biology and Medicine* 15, 1329–1341.

Matthews, V.B., Astrom, M.B., Chan, M.H., Bruce, C.R., Krabbe, K.S., *et al.* (2009) Brain-derived neurotrophic factor is produced by skeletal muscle cells in response to contraction and enhances fat oxidation via activation of AMP-activated protein kinase. *Diabetologia* 52, 1409–1418.

Mattusch, F., Dufaux, B., Heine, O., Mertens, I. and Rost, R. (2000) Reduction of the plasma concentration of C-reactive protein following nine months of endurance training. *International Journal of Sports Medicine* 21, 21–24.

Mccarthy, D., Macdonald, I., Grant, M., Marbut, M. and Watling, M. (1992) Studies on the immediate and delayed leucocytosis elicited by brief (30 min) strenuous exercise. *European Journal of Applied Physiology* 64, 513–517.

Mickleborough, T.D., Lindley, M.R., Ionescu, A.A. and Fly, A.D. (2006) Protective effect of fish oil supplementation on exercise-induced bronchoconstriction in asthma. *Chest* 129, 39–49.

Mitchell, J.B., Pizza, F.X., Paquet, A., Davis, B.J., Forrest, M.B., *et al.* (1998) Influence of carbohydrate status on immune responses before and after endurance exercise. *Journal of Applied Physiology* 84, 1917–1925.

Moir, H., Hughes, M.G., Potter, S., Sims, C., Butcher, L.R., *et al.* (2010) Exercise-induced immunosuppression: roles of reactive oxygen species and 5 -AMP-activated protein kinase dephosphorylation within immune cells. *Journal of Applied Physiology* 108, 1284–1292.

Morici, G., Bonsignore, M.R., Zangla, D., Riccobono, L., Profita, M., *et al.* (2004) Airway cell composition at rest and after an all-out test in competitive rowers. *Medicine and Science in Sports and Exercise* 36, 1723–1729.

Moyna, N.M., Acker, G.R., Weber, K.M., Fulton, J.R., Goss, F.L., *et al.* (1996) The effects of incremental submaximal exercise on circulating leukocytes in physically active and sedentary males and females. *European Journal of Applied Physiology Occupational Physiology* 74, 211–218.

Muns, G. (1994) Effect of long-distance running on polymorphonuclear neutrophil phagocytic function of the upper airways. *International Journal of Sports Medicine* 15, 96–99.

Muns, G., Rubinstein, I. and Singer, P. (1996) Neutrophil chemotactic activity is increased in nasal secretions of long-distance runners. *International Journal of Sports Medicine* 17, 56–59.

Nakajima, T., Kurano, M., Hasegawa, T., Takano, H., Iida, H., *et al.* (2010) Pentraxin3 and high-sensitive C-reactive protein are independent inflammatory markers released during high-intensity exercise. *European Journal of Applied Physiology* 110, 905–913.

Nakamura, S., Kobayashi, M., Sugino, T., Kajimoto, O., Matoba, R., *et al.* (2010) Effect of exercise on gene expression profile in unfractionated peripheral blood leukocytes. *Biochemical Biophysical Research Communications* 391, 846–851.

Ndon, J.A., Snyder, A.C., Foster, C. and Wehrenberg, W.B. (1992) Effects of chronic intense exercise training on the leukocyte response to acute exercise. *International Journal of Sports Medicine* 13, 176–182.

Nielsen, H.B., Secher, N.H., Christensen, N.J. and Pedersen, B.K. (1996) Lymphocytes and NK cell activity during repeated bouts of maximal exercise. *American Journal of Physiology Reagulatory, Integrative and Comparative Physiology* 271, R222–R227.

Nielsen, H.G., Hagberg, I.A. and Lyberg, T. (2004) Marathon running leads to partial exhaustion of ROS-generating capacity in leukocytes. *Medicine and Science in Sports and Exercise* 36, 68–73.

Nieman, D.C., Johanssen, L.M. and Lee, J.W. (1989a) Infectious episodes in runners before and after a roadrace. *Journal of Sports Medicine and Physical Fitness* 29, 289–296.

Nieman, D.C., Tan, S.A., Lee, J.W. and Berk, L.S. (1989b) Complement and immunoglobulin levels in athletes and sedentary controls. *International Journal of Sports Medicine* 10, 124–128.

Nieman, D.C., Johanssen, L.M., Lee, J.W. and Arabatzis, K. (1990) Infectious episodes in runners before and after the Los Angeles Marathon. *Journal of Sports Medicine and Physical Fitness* 30, 316–328.

Nieman, D., Fagoaga, O., Butterworth, D., Warren, B., Utter, A., *et al.* (1997a) Carbohydrate supplementation affects blood granulocyte and monocyte trafficking but not function following 2.5 hours of running. *American Journal of Clinical Nutrition* 66, 153–159.

Nieman, D., Henson, D., Butterworth, D., Warren, B., Davis, J., *et al.* (1997b) Vitamin C supplementation does not alter the immune response to 2.5 hours of running. *International Journal of Sport Nutrition* 7, 173–184.

Nieman, D.C., Nehlsen-Cannarella, S.L., Fagoaga, O.R., Henson, D.A., Utter, A., *et al.* (1998) Effects of mode and carbohydrate on the granulocyte and monocyte response to intensive, prolonged exercise. *Journal of Applied Physiology* 84, 1252–1259.

Nieman, D.C., Nehlsen-Cannarella, S.L., Fagoaga, O.R., Henson, D.A., Shannon, M., *et al.* (2000) Immune function in female elite rowers and non-athletes. *British Journal of Sports Medicine* 34, 181–187.

Nieman, D.C., Henson, D.A., Smith, L.L., Utter, A.C., Vinci, D.M., *et al.* (2001) Cytokine changes after a marathon race. *Journal of Applied Physiology* 91, 109–114.

Nieman, D.C., Henson, D.A., Mcanulty, S., Mcanulty, L., Swick, N., *et al.* (2002) Influence of vitamin C supplementation on oxidative and immune changes after an ultramarathon. *Journal of Applied Physiology* 92, 1970–1977.

Nieman, D.C., Davis, J.M., Henson, D.A., Walberg-Rankin, J., Shute, M., *et al.* (2003) Carbohydrate ingestion influences skeletal muscle cytokine mRNA and plasma cytokine levels after a 3–h run. *Journal of Applied Physiology* 94, 1917–1925.

Nieman, D.C., Davis, J.M., Henson, D.A., Gross, S.J., Dumke, C.L., *et al.* (2005a) Muscle cytokine mRNA changes after 2.5 h of cycling: influence of carbohydrate. *Medicine and Science in Sports and Exercise* 37, 1283–1290.

Nieman, D.C., Dumke, C.L., Henson, D.A., Mcanulty, S.R., Gross, S.J. *et al.* (2005b) Muscle damage is linked to cytokine changes following a 160-km race. *Brain Behavior and Immunity* 19, 398–403.

Nieman, D.C., Henson, D.A., Davis, J.M., Dumke, C.L., Utter, A.C., *et al.* (2006a) Blood leukocyte mRNA expression for IL-10, IL-1Ra, and IL-8, but not IL-6, increases after exercise. *Journal of Interferon and Cytokine Research* 26, 668–674.

Nieman, D.C., Henson, D.A., Dumke, C.L., Oley, K., Mcanulty, S.R., *et al.* (2006b) Ibuprofen use, endotoxemia, inflammation, and plasma cytokines during ultramarathon competition. *Brain, Behavior and Immunity* 20, 578–584.

Nieman, D.C., Henson, D.A., Davis, J.M., Angela Murphy, E., Jenkins, D.P., *et al.* (2007a) Quercetin's influence on exercise-induced changes in plasma cytokines and muscle and leukocyte cytokine mRNA. *Journal of Applied Physiology* 103, 1728–1735.

Nieman, D.C., Henson, D.A., Davis, J.M., Dumke, C.L., Gross, S.J., *et al.* (2007b) Quercetin ingestion does not alter cytokine changes in athletes competing in the Western States Endurance Run. *Journal of Interferon and Cytokine Research* 27, 1003–1011.

Nieman, D.C., Henson, D.A., Gross, S.J., Jenkins, D.P., Davis, J.M., *et al.* (2007c) Quercetin reduces illness but not immune perturbations after intensive exercise. *Medicine and Science in Sports and Exercise* 39, 1561–1569.

Nieman, D.C., Henson, D.A., Mcanulty, S.R., Jin, F. and Maxwell, K.R. (2009) n-3 polyunsaturated fatty acids do not alter immune and inflammation measures in endurance athletes. *International Journal of Sport Nutrition and Exercise Metabolism* 19, 536–546.

Niess, A.M., Fehrenbach, E., Lehmann, R., Opavsky, L., Jesse, M., *et al.* (2003a) Impact of elevated ambient temperatures on the acute immune response to intensive endurance exercise. *European Journal of Applied Physiology* 89, 344–351.

Niess, A.M., Fehrenbach, E., Strobel, G., Roecker, K., Schneider, E.M., *et al.* (2003b) Evaluation of stress responses to interval training at low and moderate altitudes. *Medicine and Science in Sports and Exercise* 35, 263–269.

Northoff, H., Symons, S., Zieker, D., Schaible, E.V., Schafer, K., *et al.* (2008) Gender- and menstrual phase dependent regulation of inflammatory gene expression in response to aerobic exercise. *Exercise Immunology Review* 14, 86–103.

Nybo, L., Nielsen, B., Pedersen, B.K., Moller, K. and Secher, N.H. (2002) Interleukin-6 release from the human brain during prolonged exercise. *Journal of Physiology* 542, 991–995.

Okutsu, M., Suzuki, K., Ishijima, T., Peake, J. and Higuchi, M. (2008) The effects of acute exercise-induced cortisol on CCR2 expression on human monocytes. *Brain, Behavior and Immunity* 22, 1066–1071.

Ortega, E., Barriga, C. and De La Fuente, M. (1993) Study of the phagocytic process in neutrophils from elite sportswomen. *European Journal of Applied Physiology and Occupational Physiology* 66, 37–42.

Ortega, E., Rodriguez, M.J., Barriga, C. and Forner, M.A. (1996) Corticosterone, prolactin and thyroid hormones as hormonal mediators of the stimulated phagocytic capacity of peritoneal macrophages after high-intensity exercise. *International Journal of Sports Medicine* 17, 149–155.

Ortega, E., Marchena, J.M., Garcia, J.J., Barriga, C. and Rodriguez, A.B. (2005) Norepinephrine as mediator in the stimulation of phagocytosis induced by moderate exercise. *European Journal of Applied Physiology* 93, 714–718.

Ortega, E., Giraldo, E., Hinchado, M.D., Martinez, M., Ibanez, S., *et al.* (2006) Role of Hsp72 and norepinephrine in the moderate exercise-induced stimulation of neutrophils' microbicide capacity. *European Journal of Applied Physiology* 98, 250–255.

Ortega, E., Hinchado, M.D., Martin-Cordero, L. and Asea, A. (2009) The effect of stress-inducible extracellular Hsp72 on human neutrophil chemotaxis: a role during acute intense exercise. *Stress* 12, 240–249.

Papassotiriou, I., Alexiou, V.G., Tsironi, M., Skenderi, K., Spanos, A., *et al.* (2008) Severe aseptic inflammation caused by long distance running (246 km) does not increase procalcitonin. *European Journal of Clinical Investigation* 38, 276–279.

Parsons, J.P., Baran, C.P., Phillips, G., Jarjoura, D., Kaeding, C., *et al.* (2008) Airway inflammation in exercise-induced bronchospasm occurring in athletes without asthma. *Journal of Asthma* 45, 363–367.

Peake, J.M. (2002) Exercise-induced alterations in neutrophil degranulation and respiratory burst activity: possible mechanisms of action. *Exercise Immunology Review* 8, 49–100.

Peake, J.M., Wilson, G., Hordern, M., Suzuki, K., Nosaka, K., *et al.* (2004) Changes in neutrophil receptor expression, degranulation and respiratory burst activity after moderate and high intensity exercise. *Journal of Applied Physiology* 97, 612–618.

Peake, J., Wilson, G., Mackinnon, L. and Coombes, J.S. (2005a) Carbohydrate supplementation and alterations in neutrophils, and plasma cortisol and myoglobin concentration after intense exercise. *European Journal of Applied Physiology* 93, 672–678.

Peake, J.M., Suzuki, K., Hordern, M., Wilson, G., Nosaka, K., *et al.* (2005b) Plasma cytokine changes in relation to exercise intensity and muscle damage. *European Journal of Applied Physiology* 95, 514–521.

Peake, J.M., Suzuki, K., Wilson, G., Hordern, M., Yamaya, K., *et al.* (2005c) Exercise-induced muscle damage, plasma cytokines and markers of neutrophil activation. *Medicine and Science in Sports and Exercise* 37, 737–745.

Peake, J., Peiffer, J., Abbiss, C., Nosaka, K., Laursen, P., *et al.* (2007a) Body temperature and its effect on leukocyte mobilisation, cytokines and markers of neutrophil activation. *European Journal of Applied Physiology* 102, 391–401.

Peake, J.M., Suzuki, K. and Coombes, J.S. (2007b) The influence of antioxidant supplementation on markers of inflammation and the relationship to oxidative stress after exercise. *Journal of Nutrtional Biochemistry* 18, 357–371.

Pedersen, B.K. (2009) Edward F. Adolph distinguished lecture: muscle as an endocrine organ: IL-6 and other myokines. *Journal of Applied Physiology* 107, 1006–1014.

Peters, E.M., Anderson, R. and Theron, A.J. (2001) Attenuation of increase in circulating cortisol and enhancement of the acute phase protein response in vitamin C-supplemented ultramarathoners. *International Journal of Sports Medicine* 22, 120–126.

Petersen, A.M. and Pedersen, B.K. (2005) The anti-inflammatory effect of exercise. *Journal of Applied Physiology* 98, 1154–1162.

Petersen, E.W., Ostrowski, K., Ibfelt, T., Richelle, M., Offord, E., *et al.* (2001) Effect of vitamin supplementation on cytokine response and on muscle damage after strenuous exercise. *American Journal of Physiology Cell Physiology* 280, C1570–C1575.

Pool, E.J., Robson, P.J., Smith, C., Van Wyk, J.H. and Myburgh, K.H. (2002) In vitro interleukin-6 release in whole blood cultures in samples taken at rest from triathletes and professional rugby players. *European Journal of Applied Physiology* 87, 233–237.

Pyne, D., Baker, M., Fricker, P., Macdonald, W., Telford, R. *et al.* (1995) Effects of an intensive 12-wk training program by elite swimmers on neutrophil oxidative activity. *Medicine and Science in Sports and Exercise* 27, 536–542.

Pyne, D.B., Baker, M.S., Telford, R.D. and Weidermann, M.J. (1997) A treadmill protocol to investigate independently the metabolic and mechanical stress of exercise. *Australian Journal of Science and Medicine in Sport* 29, 77–82.

Pyne, D., Smith, J., Baker, M., Telford, R. and Weidemann, M. (2000) Neutrophil oxidative activity is differentially affected by exercise intensity and type. *Journal of Science and Medicine in Sport,* 3, 44–54.

Quindry, J., Stone, W., King, J. and Broeder, C. (2003) The effects of acute exercise on neutrophils and plasma oxidative stress. *Medicine and Science in Sports and Exercise,* 35, 1139–1145.

Radom-Aizik, S., Zaldivar, F., Jr, Leu, S.Y., Galassetti, P. and Cooper, D.M. (2008) Effects of 30 min of aerobic exercise on gene expression in human neutrophils. *Journal of Applied Physiology* 104, 236–243.

Radom-Aizik, S., Zaldivar, F., Jr, Oliver, S., Galassetti, P. and Cooper, D.M. (2010) Evidence for microRNA involvement in exercise-associated neutrophil gene expression changes. *Journal of Applied Physiology* 109, 252–261.

Rhind, S.G., Gannon, G.A., Shek, P.N., Brenner, I.K., Severs, Y., *et al.* (1999) Contribution of exertional hyperthermia to sympathoadrenal-mediated lymphocyte subset redistribution. *Journal of Applied Physiology* 87, 1178–1185.

Rhind, S.G., Castellani, J.W., Brenner, I.K., Shephard, R.J., Zamecnik, J., *et al.* (2001) Intracellular monocyte and serum cytokine expression is modulated by exhausting exercise and cold exposure. *American Journal of Physiology Regulatory, Integrative and Comparative Physiology* 281, R66–R75.

Rhind, S.G., Gannon, G.A., Shephard, R.J., Buguet, A., Shek, P.N. *et al.* (2004) Cytokine induction during exertional hyperthermia is abolished by core temperature clamping: neuroendocrine regulatory mechanisms. *International Journal of Hyperthermia* 20, 503–516.

Robson, P., Blannin, A., Walsh, N., Castell, L. and Gleeson, M. (1999) Effects of exercise intensity, duration and recovery on *in vitro* neutrophil function in male athletes. *International Journal of Sports Medicine* 20, 128–135.

Robson, P., Bouic, P. and Myburgh, K. (2003) Antioxidant supplementation enhances neutrophil oxidative burst in trained runners following prolonged exercise. *International Journal of Sport Nutrition and Exercise Metabolism* 13, 369–381.

Robson-Ansley, P.J., Blannin, A. and Gleeson, M. (2006) Elevated plasma interleukin-6 levels in trained male triathletes following an acute period of intense interval training. *European Journal of Applied Physiology* 99, 353–360.

Rohde, T., Maclean, D.A. and Pedersen, B.K. (1998) Effect of glutamine supplementation on changes in the immune system induced by repeated exercise. *Medicine and Science in Sports and Exercise* 30, 856–862.

Romeo, J., Jimenez-Pavon, D., Cervantes-Borunda, M., Warnberg, J., Gomez-Martinez, S., *et al.* (2008) Immunological changes after a single bout of moderate-intensity exercise in a hot environment. *Journal of Physiology and Biochemistry* 64, 197–204.

Ronsen, O., Pedersen, B.K., Oritsland, T.R., Bahr, R. and Kjeldsen-Kragh, J. (2001) Leukocyte counts and lymphocyte responsiveness associated with repeated bouts of strenuous endurance exercise. *Journal of Applied Physiology* 91, 425–434.

Ronsen, O., Lea, T., Bahr, R. and Pedersen, B.K. (2002) Enhanced plasma IL-6 and IL-1ra responses to repeated vs. single bouts of prolonged cycling in elite athletes. *Journal of Applied Physiology* 92, 2547–2553.

Scharhag, J., Meyer, T., Gabriel, H.H., Schlick, B., Faude, O. *et al.* (2005) Does prolonged cycling of moderate intensity affect immune cell function? *British Journal of Sports Medicine* 39, 171–177.

Scharhag, J., Meyer, T., Auracher, M., Gabriel, H.H. and Kindermann, W. (2006) Effects of graded carbohydrate supplementation on the immune response in cycling. *Medicine and Science in Sports and Exercise* 38, 286–292.

Selkirk, G.A., Mclellan, T.M., Wright, H.E. and Rhind, S.G. (2008) Mild endotoxemia, NF-kappaB translocation, and cytokine increase during exertional heat stress in trained and untrained individuals. *American Journal of Physiology Regulatory, Integrative and Comparative Physiology* 295, R611–R623.

Selkirk, G.A., Mclellan, T.M., Wright, H.E. and Rhind, S.G. (2009) Expression of intracellular cytokines, HSP72, and apoptosis in monocyte subsets during exertional heat stress in trained and untrained individuals. *American Journal of Physiology Regulatory, Integrative and Comparative Physiology* 296, R575–R586.

Semerad, C.L., Liu, F.L., Gregory, A.D., Stumpf, K. and Link, D.C. (2002) G-CSF is an essential regulator of neutrophil trafficking from the bone marrow to the blood. *Immunity* 17, 413–423.

Semple, S.J., Smith, L.L., Mckune, A.J., Hoyos, J., Mokgethwa, B., *et al.* (2006) Serum concentrations of C reactive protein, alpha1 antitrypsin, and complement (C3, C4, C1 esterase inhibitor) before and during the Vuelta a Espana. *British Journal of Sports Medicine* 40, 124–127.

Shek, P.N., Sabiston, B.H., Buguet, A. and Radomski, M.W. (1995) Strenuous exercise and immunological changes: a multiple-time-point analysis of leukocyte subsets, CD4/CD8 ratio, immunoglobulin production and NK cell response. *International Journal of Sports Medicine* 16, 466–474.

Shing, C., Peake, J., Suzuki, K., Okutsu, M., Pereira, R., *et al.* (2007) Effects of bovine colostrum supplementation on immune variables in highly trained cyclists. *Journal of Applied Physiology* 102, 1113–1122.

Simpson, R.J., Mcfarlin, B.K., Mcsporran, C., Spielmann, G., Hartaigh, B.O., *et al.* (2009) Toll-like receptor expression on classic and pro-inflammatory blood monocytes after acute exercise in humans. *Brain, Behavior and Immunity* 23, 232–239.

Singh, A., Failla, M.L. and Deuster, P.A. (1994) Exercise-induced changes in immune function: effects of zinc supplementation. *Journal of Applied Physiology* 76, 2298–2303.

Sloan, R., Shapiro, P., De Meersman, R., Mckinley, P., Tracey, K., *et al.* (2007) Aerobic exercise attenuates inducible TNF production in humans. *Journal of Applied Physiology* 103, 1007–1011.

Smith, J. (1994) Neutrophils, host defense, and inflammation: a double-edged sword. *Journal of Leukocyte Biology* 56, 672–686.

Smith, J., Telford, R., Mason, I. and Weidemann, M. (1990) Exercise, training and neutrophil microbicidal activity. *International Journal of Sports Medicine* 11, 179–187.

Smith, J., Mckenzie, S., Telford, R. and Weidemann, M. (1992) Why does moderate exercise enhance, but intense training depress immunity? In: Husband, E. (ed.) *Behaviour and Immunity.* CRC, Boca Raton, Florida.

Smith, J., Gray, A., Pyne, D., Baker, M., Telford, R., *et al.* (1996) Moderate exercise triggers both priming and activation of neutrophil subpopulations. *American Journal of Physiology Regulatory, Integrative and Comparative Physiology* 270, R838–R845.

Smits, H.H., Grunberg, K., Derijk, R.H., Sterk, P.J. and Hiemstra, P.S. (1998) Cytokine release and its modulation by dexamethasone in whole blood following exercise. *Clinical and Experimental Immunology* 111, 463–468.

Sondergaard, S.R., Ostrowski, K., Ullum, H. and Pedersen, B.K. (2000) Changes in plasma concentrations of interleukin-6 and interleukin-1 receptor antagonists in response to adrenaline infusion in humans. *European Journal of Applied Physiology* 83, 95–98.

Spence, L., Brown, W.J., Pyne, D.B., Nissen, M.D., Sloots, T.P., *et al.* (2007) Incidence, etiology, and symptomatology of upper respiratory illness in elite athletes. *Medicine and Science in Sports and Exercise* 39, 577–586.

Starkie, R.L., Angus, D.J., Rolland, J., Hargreaves, M. and Febbraio, M.A. (2000) Effect of prolonged, submaximal exercise and carbohydrate ingestion on monocyte intracellular cytokine production in humans. *Journal of Physiology* 528, 647–655.

Starkie, R.L., Arkinstall, M.J., Koukoulas, I., Hawley, J.A. and Febbraio, M.A. (2001a) Carbohydrate ingestion attenuates the increase in plasma interleukin-6, but not skeletal muscle interleukin-6 mRNA, during exercise in humans. *Journal of Physiology* 533, 585–591.

Starkie, R.L., Rolland, J., Angus, D.J., Anderson, M. and Febbraio, M.A. (2001b) Circulating monocytes are not the source of elevations in plasma IL-6 and TNF-alpha levels after prolonged running. *American Journal of Physiology Cell Physiology* 280, C769–C774.

Starkie, R., Ostrowski, S.R., Jauffred, S., Febbraio, M. and Pedersen, B.K. (2003) Exercise and IL-6 infusion inhibit endotoxin-induced TNF-alpha production in humans. *FASEB J* 17, 884–886.

Starkie, R.L., Hargreaves, M., Rolland, J. and Febbraio, M. (2005) Heat stress, cytokines and the immune response to exercise. *Brain, Behavior and Immunity* 19, 404–412.

Steensberg, A., Van Hall, G., Osada, T., Sacchetti, M., Saltin, B., *et al.* (2000) Production of interleukin-6 in contracting human skeletal muscles can account for the exercise-induced increase in plasma interleukin-6. *Journal of Physiology* 529, 237–242.

Steensberg, A., Toft, A.D., Schjerling, P., Halkjaer-Kristensen, J. and Pedersen, B.K. (2001) Plasma interleukin-6 during strenuous exercise: role of epinephrine. *American Journal of Physiology Cell Physiology* 281, C1001–C1004.

Steensberg, A., Keller, C., Starkie, R., Osada, T., Febbraio, M., *et al.* (2002) IL-6 and TNF-alpha expression in, and release from, contracting human skeletal muscle. *American Journal of Physiology Endocrinology and Metabolism* 283, E1272–E1278.

Steensberg, A., Fischer, C.P., Keller, C., Moller, K. and Pedersen, B.K. (2003) IL-6 enhances plasma IL-1ra, IL-10, and cortisol in humans. *American Journal of Physiology Endocrinology and Metabolism* 285, E433–E437.

Steensberg, A., Keller, C., Hillig, T., Frosig, C., Wojtaszewski, J.F., *et al.* (2007) Nitric oxide production is a proximal signaling event controlling exercise-induced mRNA expression in human skeletal muscle. *FASEB J* 21, 2683–2694.

Steppich, B., Dayyani, F., Gruber, R., Lorenz, R., Mack, M., *et al.* (2000) Selective mobilization of $CD14^{+}CD16^{+}$monocytes by exercise. *American Journal of Physiology Cell Physiology* 279, C578–C586.

Stewart, L.K., Flynn, M.G., Campbell, W.W., Craig, B.A., Robinson, J.P., *et al.* (2007) The influence of exercise training on inflammatory cytokines and C-reactive protein. *Medicine and Science in Sports and Exercise* 39, 1714–1719.

Suwa, T., Hogg, J.C., English, D. and Van Eeden, S.F. (2000) Interleukin-6 induces demargination of intravascular neutrophils and shortens their transit in marrow. *American Journal of Physiology Heart and Circulatory Physiology* 279, H2954–H2960.

Suzuki, K., Naganuma, S., Totsuka, M., Suzuki, K.J., Mochizuki, M., *et al.* (1996a) Effects of exhaustive endurance exercise and its one-week daily repetition on neutrophil count and functional status in untrained men. *International Journal of Sports Medicine* 17, 205–212.

Suzuki, K., Sato, H., Kikuchi, T., Abe, T., Nakaji, S., *et al.* (1996b) Capacity of circulating neutrophils to produce reactive oxygen species after exhaustive exercise. *Journal of Applied Physiology* 81, 1213–1222.

Suzuki, K., Totsuka, M., Nakaji, S., Yamada, M., Kudoh, S., *et al.* (1999) Endurance exercise causes interaction among stress hormones, cytokines, neutrophil dynamics, and muscle damage. *Journal of Applied Physiology* 86, 1360–1367.

Suzuki, K., Yamada, M., Kurakake, S., Okamura, N., Yamaya, K., *et al.* (2000) Circulating cytokines and hormones with immunosuppressive but neutrophil-priming potentials rise after endurance exercise in humans. *European Journal of Applied Physiology* 81, 281–287.

Suzuki, K., Nakaji, S., Yamada, M., Totsuka, M., Sato, K., *et al.* (2002) Systemic inflammatory response to exhaustive exercise. Cytokine kinetics. *Exercise Immunology Review* 8, 6–48.

Suzuki, K., Nakaji, S., Kurakake, S., Totsuka, M., Sato, K., *et al.* (2003a) Exhaustive exercise and type-1/type-2 cytokine balance with special focus on interleukin-12 p40/p70. *Exercise Immunology Review* 9, 48–57.

Suzuki, K., Nakaji, S., Yamada, M., Liu, Q., Kurakake, S., Okamura, N., Kumae, T., Umeda, T. and Sugawara, K. (2003b) Impact of a competitive marathon race on systemic cytokine and neutrophil responses. *Medicine and Science in Sports and Exercise* 35, 348–355.

Suzuki, K., Peake, J., Nosaka, K., Okutsu, M., Laursen, P., *et al.* (2006) Changes in markers of muscle damage, inflammation and HSP70 after an Ironman triathlon race. *European Journal of Applied Physiology* 98, 525–534.

Terashima, T., English, D., Hogg, J.C. and Van Eeden, S.F. (1998) Release of polymorphonuclear leukocytes from the bone marrow by interleukin-8. *Blood* 92, 1062–1069.

Tintinger, G., Theron, A., Anderson, R. and Ker, J. (2001) The anti-inflammatory interactions of epinephrine with human neutrophils in vitro are achieved by cyclic AMP-mediated accelerated resequestration of cytosolic calcium. *Biochemistry and Pharmacology* 61, 1319–1328.

Toft, A.D., Thorn, M., Ostrowski, K., Asp, S., Moller, K., *et al.* (2000) N-3 polyunsaturated fatty acids do not affect cytokine response to strenuous exercise. *Journal of Applied Physiology* 89, 2401–2406.

Topham, M., Carveth, H., Mcintyre, T., Prescott, S. and Zimmerman, G. (1998) Human endothelial cells regulate polymorphonuclear leukocyte degranulation. *FASEB J* 12, 733–746.

Toumpanakis, D., Karatza, M.H., Katsaounou, P., Roussos, C., Zakynthinos, S., *et al.* (2009) Antioxidant supplementation alters cytokine production from monocytes. *Journal of Interferon and Cytokine Research* 29, 741–748.

Tvede, N., Kappel, M., Halkjaer-Kristensen, J., Galbo, H. and Pedersen, B.K. (1993) The effect of light, moderate and severe bicycle exercise on lymphocyte subsets, natural and lymphokine activated killer cells, lymphocyte proliferative response and interleukin 2 production. *International Journal of Sports Medicine* 14, 275–282.

Tvede, N., Kappel, M., Klarlund, K., Duhn, S., Halkjaer-Kristensen, J., *et al.* (1994) Evidence that the effect of bicycle exercise on blood mononuclear cell proliferative responses and subsets is mediated by epinephrine. *International Journal of Sports Medicine* 15, 100–104.

Van Hall, G., Steensberg, A., Sacchetti, M., Fischer, C., Keller, C., *et al.* (2003) Interleukin-6 stimulates lipolysis and fat oxidation in humans. *Journal of Clinical Endocrinology and Metabolism* 88, 3005–3010.

Walker, G.J., Caudwell, P., Dixon, N. and Bishop, N.C. (2006) The effect of caffeine ingestion on neutrophil oxidative burst responses following prolonged cycling. *International Journal of Sport Nutrition and Exercise Metabolism* 16, 24–35.

Walker, G.J., Finlay, O., Griffiths, H., Sylvester, J., Williams, M. *et al.* (2007) Immunoendocrine response to cycling following ingestion of caffeine and carbohydrate. *Medicine and Science in Sports and Exercise* 39, 1554–1560.

Walker, G.J., Dziubak, A., Houghton, L., Prendergast, C., Lim, L., *et al.* (2008) The effect of caffeine ingestion on human neutrophil oxidative burst responses following time-trial cycling. *Journal of Sports Science* 26, 611–619.

Walsh, N., Blannin, A., Bishop, N., Robson, P. and Gleeson, M. (2000) Effect of oral glutamine supplementation on human neutrophil lipopolysaccharide-stimulated degranulation following prolonged exercise. *International Journal of Sport Nutrition and Exercise Metabolism* 10, 39–50.

Wang, J.S., Lee, T. and Chow, S.E. (2006) Role of exercise intensities in oxidized low-density lipoprotein-mediated redox status of monocyte in men. *Journal of Applied Physiology* 101, 740–744.

Warren, G.L., Hulderman, T., Jensen, N., Mckinstry, M., Mishra, M., *et al.* (2002) Physiological role of tumor necrosis factor alpha in traumatic muscle injury. *FASEB J* 16, 1630–1632.

Weinstock, C., Konig, D., Harnischmacher, R., Keul, J., Berg, A. *et al.* (1997) Effect of exhaustive exercise stress on the cytokine response. *Medicine and Science in Sports and Exercise* 29, 345–354.

Williamson, D., Kimball, S. and Jefferson, L. (2005) Acute treatment with TNF-alpha attenuates insulin-stimulated protein synthesis in cultures of C2C12 myotubes through a MEK1-sensitive mechanism. *American Journal of Physiology Endocrinology and Metabolism* 289, E95–E104.

Wolach, B., Eliakim, A., Gavrieli, R., Kodesh, E., Yarom, Y., *et al.* (1998) Aspects of leukocyte function and the complement system following aerobic exercise in young female gymnasts. *Scandinavian Journal of Medicine and Science in Sports* 8, 91–97.

Wolach, B., Falk, B., Gavrieli, R., Kodesh, E. and Eliakim, A. (2000) Neutrophil function response to aerobic and anaerobic exercise in female judoka and untrained subjects. *British Journal of Sports Medicine* 34, 23–28.

Wolach, B., Gavrieli, R., Ben-Dror, S.G., Zigel, L., Eliakim, A., *et al.* (2005) Transient decrease of neutrophil chemotaxis following aerobic exercise. *Medicine and Science in Sports and Exercise* 37, 949–954.

Yamada, M., Suzuki, K., Kudo, S., Totsuka, M., Nakaji, S., *et al.* (2002) Raised plasma G-CSF and IL-6 after exercise may play a role in neutrophil mobilization into the circulation. *Journal of Applied Physiology* 92, 1789–1794.

12 Obesity and Inflammation

M. Bulló* and M. Garcia-Aloy
*Human Nutrition Unit, Faculty of Medicine & Health Sciences,
Rovira i Virgili University, Reus, Spain*

Introduction

Obesity is defined as a condition of abnormal or excessive fat accumulation in adipose tissue that may impair health. This metabolic condition has reached epidemic proportions globally and it has a deep negative impact on public health. According to World Health Organization (WHO) data (2006), in 2005 approximately 1.6 billion adults over 15 years old were overweight and at least 400 million adults were obese worldwide. More recently, WHO (2010) revealed that the prevalence of obesity ranges from less than 5% in India

* Corresponding author, monica.bullo@urv.cat

and other Asian countries to more than 30% in the USA, and exceeds 50% in the Pacific Islands. Furthermore, while WHO (2006) predicts that worldwide 2.3 billion adults will be overweight and more than 700 million will be obese by 2015, the International Obesity Task Force (IOTF) estimates that the prevalence rate of obesity by 2025 could be as high as 45–50% in the USA, 30–40% in Australia, England and Mauritius, and more than 20% in Brazil (IOTF Secretariat, 2002). A recent review showed that adult obesity is present and rising in both developed and developing countries (Low *et al.*, 2009). In developing countries, obesity is more prevalent in rural areas and females than in urban areas and males, and increases with age, reaching maximum rates of prevalence between 40 and 60 years of age (Low *et al.*, 2009). It is noteworthy that developing countries are facing a 'double burden' of disease: obesity and undernutrition (WHO, 2006).

The spiraling global epidemic of obesity has a considerable healthcare cost. In the USA this cost reached 1.2% of the gross domestic product (GDP) (Yach *et al.*, 2006), whereas in Europe 10.4 billion Euros were spent on obesity-related healthcare, accounting for 0.09–0.61% of GDP (Muller-Riemenschneider *et al.*, 2008).

Factors contributing to the development of obesity

The etiology of obesity is characterized by its multifactorial nature and involves complex interactions among the genetic background, metabolism, and socioeconomic, cultural and environmental factors such as sedentary lifestyle and unhealthy dietary habits (WHO, 2006). In terms of energy metabolism, obesity is the consequence of a positive energy balance caused by a high energy intake and/or a low energy expenditure mediated by physiological adjustments and maintained over time. Biological (age, sex, hormones and genetics) and psychological (habits, emotions, attitudes, beliefs and cognitions) factors as well as the physical, economic and sociocultural environment are the main influences on this energy imbalance (Egger and Swinburn, 1997). Several studies have reported a marked shift in dietary patterns worldwide toward a higher energy density diet with a greater intake of fat and added sugars, considerable increases in animal-derived food consumption, and a reduced intake of complex carbohydrates, dietary fibre, fruits and vegetables (WHO, 2003). These dietary changes have taken place in parallel with reduced physical activity at work and during leisure time, thus contributing to the worldwide obesity epidemic (Yang *et al.*, 2007; Brock *et al.*, 2009). Furthermore, the lack of physical activity is often accompanied by increased food intake (e.g. while people watch television they also consume food and beverages, most of which are high-density products) (Cleland *et al.*, 2008).

Obesity as a cardiometabolic risk factor

Excess body weight is the most important modifiable risk factor in the development of several highly prevalent diseases, such as cardiovascular diseases, type 2 diabetes, many cancers and other health problems, which can lead to further morbidity and mortality (Brown *et al.*, 2009). It has been demonstrated that overweight and obesity are the most important risk factors of type 2 diabetes (Hu *et al.*, 2001) and, as obesity becomes more prevalent worldwide, so the incidence of diabetes is also on the increase (Mokdad *et al.*, 2003). Recently, a meta-analysis of 89 studies examining the relative risk of obesity-related co-morbidities showed that the strongest association was with type 2 diabetes mellitus (Guh *et al.*, 2009). Obesity also predisposes to hypertension or imbalanced lipid profile, thus contributing to a higher cardiovascular risk. In the Multi-Ethnic Study of Atherosclerosis, which analysed more than 6000 people between 45 and 84 years old, a higher body-mass index (BMI) was associated with higher blood pressure, higher levels of lipoproteins and fasting glucose and higher prevalence of hypertension (Burke *et al.*, 2008). Another study in an Asia Pacific cohort showed that a 1 standard deviation increase in BMI was associated with a 17% increase in the risk of ischaemic heart disease (Asia Pacific Cohort

Studies Collaboration, 2006). Finally, obesity has also been widely reported to be associated with cancer: data from a meta-analysis estimated that the relative risk of various cancers across categories of BMI ranged from 1.05 to 3.22 (Guh *et al.*, 2009) and these associations have been supported by data from both the World Cancer Research Fund (WCRF) and the American Institute for Cancer Research (2007). These data also suggest that abdominal fat is a risk factor of colon cancer and probably increases the risk of breast and endometrium cancers.

Weight loss as a driving force in reducing the risk of cardiometabolic diseases

Population-based strategies for preventing excess weight gain are of great interest for those international organizations that have raised worldwide awareness of the increasing prevalence of obesity and the impact that it has on morbidity, mortality, quality of life and the economic costs of healthcare. If such strategies are to be developed and implemented, the contributing target factors must be identified and understood so that they can be modulated by effective large-scale action plans. These strategies focus on lifestyle changes on the personal, environmental and socio-economic level, and are designed to actively involve stakeholders and other major parties (Sacks *et al.*, 2009).

Many secondary prevention strategies have been designed to reduce excess weight in adults. These include weight control, reduction of excess body fat, maintenance of weight loss and other measures to control associated risk factors. The most common strategies involve a reduced calorie diet, exercise or a combination of both as recommended by the EU Platform for Action on Diet, Physical Activity and Health (Lachat *et al.*, 2005) and the WHO global strategy on diet, physical activity and health (Waxman and World Health Assembly, 2004). Lifestyle intervention programmes encouraging weight loss through a combination of dietary changes and increased physical activity have demonstrated significant short-term weight reduction and improvements in cardiovascular risk factors in moderate to severely obese subjects (Pan *et al.*, 1997; Tuomilehto *et al.*, 2001; Knowler *et al.*, 2002; Esposito *et al.*, 2003; Kosaka *et al.*, 2005; Ratner *et al.*, 2005; Ramachandran *et al.*, 2006; Ryan *et al.*, 2010). Increased physical activity also has positive metabolic effects other than weight reduction (Eriksson *et al.*, 1997). Obesity-related conditions have also been improved by surgery (Pories *et al.*, 1992; Sjostrom *et al.*, 2004; Navarro-Diaz *et al.*, 2006). Several long-term clinical trials designed to evaluate the effect of intensive lifestyle intervention programmes on incidence of diabetes or cardiovascular diseases also reported significant weight loss in subjects in the active treatment arms (Lindstrom *et al.*, 2006; Li *et al.*, 2008; Harwell *et al.*, 2011; Vanderwood *et al.*, 2011). Because a considerable proportion of these participants regained weight during follow-up, however, the question arises of whether these strategies are effective in the long term.

It is widely accepted that body weight control is the long-term outcome of the energy balance equation and thermodynamic laws. Food intake, then, is controlled by several mechanisms that adjust energy intake and energy expenditure of which the satiety mechanisms are particularly important. To lose body weight, energy intake must be lower than energy expenditure, and this can be achieved with a hypocaloric diet and an increase in physical activity. However, after weight loss, a new energy equilibrium is reached. Weight stabilizes again and more weight loss requires more changes in lifestyle (Saltzman and Roberts, 1995). Maintaining weight after weight loss is even more difficult than losing weight (Saltzman and Roberts, 1995). Moreover, the physiological state of negative energy balance can disrupt a number of processes within the body, including inflammation, which contributes to adipose tissue deposition and weight regain (Lumeng and Saltiel, 2011). Thus, the effects of dietary manipulation on inflammation could be of great interest.

There is increasing evidence that obesity in humans is associated with chronic low-level inflammation characterized by altered cytokine production and activation of inflammatory signalling pathways. It has been suggested that this could link obesity and co-morbid diseases (O'Rourke, 2009). Given the evidence that elevated levels of obesity-related inflammatory markers may cause the development of associated comorbidities, it has been hypothesized that the lower risk of disease after weight loss could be the result of an improved inflammatory profile. In addition to diet, physical activity is a major modifiable risk factor of obesity and can be a useful therapeutic approach for modulating low-grade inflammation. This chapter reviews epidemiological and intervention studies on the effect of diet or physical activity on the modulation of inflammation in obesity.

Inflammation and Obesity

Adipose tissue and inflammation

Since the discovery of leptin in 1994, the perception of the physiological role of white adipose tissue has changed dramatically. In the past, fat was believed to play a passive role in the development of obesity and thought to be simply stored in the adipocytes. Adipose tissue is now recognized as a major endocrine organ with an important role in regulating energy metabolism. Adipose tissue is a matrix of different cell types and mature adipocytes make up no more than half of the total cell content of white fat. The remaining components contain pre-adipocytes, fibroblasts, endothelial cells and macrophages (Weisberg *et al.*, 2003). Moreover, the plasticity between different types of cells is well documented (Zhang *et al.*, 1996) and macrophages have been reported to infiltrate from peripheral blood during fat mass expansion (Weisberg *et al.*, 2003; Curat *et al.*, 2004). In this regard, the relative gene expression of several proteins in adipocytes versus non-fat cells of human adipose tissue has recently been reported, showing that most classical inflammatory proteins were significantly more expressed in the non-fat cells of adipose tissue (Fain, 2010) This functional homology between adipocytes and non-fat cells of adipose tissue with cells from the immune system reinforces the relationship between adipose tissue and immunity (Stallone, 1994).

Obesity as a chronic inflammatory state

There is increasing evidence that obesity is associated with low-grade inflammation, and this leads to the development of health complications. In fact, it has been reported that in the circulation of obese subjects at least 24 adipokines are elevated in obese humans. Some of these adipokines such as C-reactive protein (CRP), haptoglobin and amyloid A are acute-phase proteins primarily released by the liver in response to the inflammatory state associated with obesity. Most of the remaining adipokines are inflammatory proteins, but it is unclear which tissues could be responsible for their elevated concentrations in obese subjects (Fain, 2010). Finally, some of these adipokines actually have anti-inflammatory effects and circulate at higher levels in obesity as a counter-regulatory mechanism against the upregulation of inflammatory markers. For example, adiponectin has anti-inflammatory properties, and the decrease in production and expression of adiponectin in the obese state exacerbates inflammation. Other adipokines seem to exert a dual effect such as interleukin (IL)-10 (Mocellin *et al.*, 2003) or even IL-6, which enhances insulin action in muscle (Kim *et al.*, 2009).

Most adipokines have also been related to metabolic derangements associated with obesity, such as type 2 diabetes and cardiovascular disease. Indeed, several adipokines affect insulin sensitivity or modulate adhesion molecules in endothelial cells, findings that help to explain their relationship to hypertension or atherogenic diseases.

Several clinical studies have demonstrated that abdominal fat distribution, rather than the amount of fat, is more strongly related to inflammation. Furthermore, differences have been reported in adipokine expression and production between visceral and subcutaneous fat depots. Although the relationship between inflammation and obesity has increasingly been the subject of research, whether the inflammatory state is the cause or the consequence of obesity remains to be elucidated.

Inflammation and weight loss

Weight-loss intervention programmes have revealed a connection between obesity and inflammation. If adipose tissue from obese subjects overexpresses adipokines, weight loss should restore inflammatory levels because adipose mass is reduced. This should improve insulin resistance and other cardiovascular risk factors. Most studies on weight loss focusing on diet, physical activity, combined diet and physical activity or surgical interventions have reported a significant decrease in the inflammatory state. There are, however, some discrepancies in terms of inflammation during the weight-maintenance phase after weight loss. The effect of diet- and exercise-induced weight loss will be discussed in the next section.

Dietary Modulation of Inflammation in Obesity

Diet-induced weight loss

Dietary habits are one of the key determinants of energy balance and influence the overall inflammatory process in obesity and chronic diseases. The effects of dietary restriction on obesity-induced inflammation have been investigated in various studies. Considine *et al.* (1996) found that serum leptin concentrations were significantly reduced following a diet-induced 10% weight loss. Leptin concentrations slightly increased, however, during the 4-week weight maintenance phase, although they still remained significantly lower than the baseline levels. In contrast, Keogh *et al.* (2007) found that after 12 weeks of energy-restricted diet, CRP concentrations did not decrease and adiponectin levels did not increase significantly. But after 1 year of follow-up with a maintained weight loss of 6%, adiponectin concentrations were significantly greater. In a 6-week low-calorie diet conducted by our group, a weight loss of 9% was associated with a significant improvement in IL-6 and CRP concentrations. After a 2-week weight-maintenance phase, however, plasma IL-6 increased but remained significantly lower than baseline. CRP levels rose sharply to higher concentrations than that at baseline (Salas-Salvado *et al.*, 2006). We concluded that the systemic inflammatory status is restored after weight loss. This effect, however, seems to be largely due to energy restriction rather than adipose mass loss, because inflammation levels tended to return to baseline soon after the body weight stabilized. Furthermore, a negative energy balance is associated with an increase in the mRNA expression of several cytokines in subcutaneous adipose tissue, which might be considered to favour fat mobilization. This restoration of inflammatory levels may be explained not only by the lipolytic activity attributed to several pro-inflammatory cytokines but also by the lower infiltration of macrophages in adipose tissue after weight loss and changes in its distribution. More randomized, controlled intervention studies are required, however, to determine the duration of weight loss needed in order to improve long-term inflammatory status.

Other dietary components

Dietary habits are probably one of the main determinants that influence the inflammatory process in obesity and other chronic conditions. There is evidence to suggest that food components such as eicosapentanoic acid (EPA), docosohexanoic acid (DHA), butyrate, curcumin, resveratrol, lutein, quercetin or oleuropein can modulate the inflammatory process. For example, IL-6 and IL-1β production in THP-1 cells was reduced after incubation with DHA or α-linolenic acid (ALA) (Zhao *et al.*, 2005). Phenolic compounds from extra-virgin olive oil also exerted anti-inflammatory effects on human whole blood cultures (Miles *et al.*, 2005). In a similar way, such dietary components as resveratrol in red grapes or wine, the butyrate generated from the colonic microbiota metabolism and curcumin in curry spice can suppress tumour necrosis factor alpha (TNF-α) induced activation of nuclear factor kappa B (NFκB) and cyclooxygenase-2 expression *in vitro* and *in vivo*.

Cereals, fibre and glycaemic response

The consumption of refined starches and sugars is associated with a rapid increase in blood glucose and insulin levels and a subsequent decrease in glycaemia, leading to hunger and decreasing fat oxidation. Higher plasma levels of adiponectin were observed in a subgroup of overweight and obese subjects from the Health Professional's Follow-up study with diets low in glycemic load and high in dietary fibre (Qi *et al.*, 2006), and plasma levels of CRP have been observed to be negatively related to total fibre intake in subjects with diabetes, hypertension or obesity (Ajani *et al.*, 2004). Moreover, in a study conducted on adults with diabetes, hypertension or obesity in the National Health and Nutrition Examination Survey (NHANES), after controlling for demographic factors, BMI, cardiovascular risk factors and total calorie intake, subjects in the lowest quartile of fibre consumption with two or more risk conditions had a greater risk of elevated CRP than those in the highest quartile of fibre consumption (King *et al.*, 2005). The results of clinical trials are inconsistent, however. Whereas King *et al.* (2007) observed some changes in CRP levels in obese hypertensive individuals taking a physillium-fibre supplement for 3 weeks, the physillium supplementation for 3 months in overweight or obese subjects did not significantly reduce CRP, IL-6, fibrinogen or white blood cell count (WBC) (King *et al.*, 2008). Moreover, mildly overweight and hypercholesterolemic subjects who were randomized to consume muesli, oat-β-glucan muesli or a combination of muesli for 4 weeks did not differ in TNF-α, IL-6 or IL-8 production by peripheral blood mononuclear cells and whole blood after lipopolysaccharide stimulation (Theuwissen *et al.*, 2009). Nevertheless, the few clinical trials evaluating the effect of dietary glycaemic index or glycaemic load on inflammation have reported a controversial effect on CRP circulating levels (Wolever *et al.*, 2008; Hartman *et al.*, 2010; Vrolix and Mensink, 2010) and no effect on TNF-α or IL-6 (Pittas *et al.*, 2006; Wolever *et al.*, 2008; Vrolix and Mensink, 2010).

Fish and omega-3 fatty acids

Omega-3 fatty acids, especially EPA and DHA, are probably one of the most commonly studied dietary constituents. Omega-3 fatty acids decrease the cellular membrane content of arachidonic acid, which results in the synthesis of 3-series eicosanoids with fewer inflammatory properties than those synthesized from omega-6 fatty acids. Plasma levels of omega-3 fatty acids have been inversely associated with circulating pro-inflammatory cytokines and endothelial markers in healthy and obese subjects (Ferrucci *et al.*, 2006; Kalogeropoulos *et al.*, 2010). Some interventional studies have also demonstrated that dietary fish oil and ALA decrease CRP, IL-6 and IL-18 in normal weight and obese subjects (Bemelmans *et al.*, 2004; Troseid *et al.*, 2009). More recently, in a randomized clinical trial conducted on 27 overweight subjects following an 8-week fatty fish (FF), lean fish (LF) or control diet, those subjects allocated to the LF diet showed a significant decrease in soluble intercellular adhesion molecule-1 (ICAM-1) (de Mello *et al.*, 2009). Recently, in a cross-sectional study conducted on 2848 adults from the MESA study (Multi-Ethnic Study of Atherosclerosis) it has been observed that obesity modifies the relationship between plasma polyunsaturated fatty acids (PUFAs) and sICAM-1 and IL-6 (Steffen, *et al.*, 2011). Therefore, prospective studies are needed to determine whether omega-3 fatty acids and other PUFAs influence inflammation and risk for several diseases in obese subjects.

Trans and saturated fatty acids

Several epidemiological studies and clinical trials in humans have suggested that diets rich in *trans* or saturated fatty acids are closely related to inflammation, although some of the published results have raised controversy. Subjects consuming a diet enriched in *trans* fatty acids showed higher levels of CRP, IL-6, soluble TNF-R2, E-selectin, soluble ICAM-1 and vascular cell adhesion molecule-1 (VCAM-1) than those subjects allocated to the lowest quintile of *trans* fatty acid consumption (Lopez-Garcia *et al.*, 2005). However, 6% substitution of *trans* fatty acid in a standard fat diet containing 30% fat had no effects on CRP in moderately hypercholesterolemic subjects, although a significant increase in TNF-α and IL-6 was observed (Lichtenstein *et al.*, 2003).

Virgin olive oil and nuts

Virgin olive oil (VOO) and nuts are foods with important anti-inflammatory properties. VOO is rich in monounsaturated fatty acids (MUFAs) and phenolic compounds that have important antioxidant and anti-inflammatory properties. Recent epidemiological and clinical trials have sustained the positive role of olive oil in inflammation, extending results observed *in vitro*. Out of a total of 772 elderly subjects at high cardiovascular disease risk from the PREDIMED cohort study, those with the highest consumption of VOO and nuts showed the lowest concentrations of VCAM-1, ICAM-1, IL-6 and CRP (Salas-Salvado *et al.*, 2008).

The effect of nut consumption on inflammation has been studied in several cross-sectional and prospective epidemiologic studies and in different population groups (healthy subjects, obese subjects, subjects with type 2 diabetes and those at high cardiovascular disease risk). Nuts are rich in fibre (Salas-Salvado *et al.*, 2006), phenolic compounds and other anti-inflammatory and antioxidant molecules (Blomhoff, *et al.*, 2006). They also contain sizeable amounts of L-arginine, a precursor of the endogenous vasodilator nitric oxide (Cooke *et al.*, 1993; Fitzpatrick *et al.*, 1993). Nut consumption was inversely associated with peripheral concentrations of CRP, IL-6 and fibrinogen in overweight subjects from the MESA study (Jiang *et al.*, 2006). A cross-sectional analysis of diabetic women from the Nurses' Health Study showed that greater adherence to a Mediterranean diet was associated with higher concentrations of plasma adiponectin, a potent anti-inflammatory cytokine originating in adipose tissue, although this association was attenuated after adjustment for several covariates (Mantzoros *et al.*, 2006). The PREDIMED cohort study reported that subjects in the highest tertiles of nut consumption showed the lowest VCAM-1, ICAM-1, CRP and IL-6 serum concentrations, although the association was only significant for ICAM-1 (Salas-Salvado *et al.*, 2008). Also, clinical trials of nut consumption have reported decreases in inflammatory markers and improvements in the endothelial function (Rajaram *et al.*, 2011).

Fruits and vegetables

Fruits and vegetables are rich in antioxidants and phytochemicals with anti-inflammatory properties. Indeed, inverse relationships have been observed between fruit and vegetable intakes and some biomarkers of inflammation, such CRP (Esmaillzadeh *et al.*, 2006) or hs-CRP (Oliveira *et al.*, 2009). In the Boston Puerto Rican Health Study cohort, Bhupathiraju and Tucker (2011) observed, however, that fruit and vegetable variety, but not quantity, was negatively associated with inflammation. Furthermore, several interventional studies with fruit or vegetables, or their individual compounds have demonstrated their anti-inflammatory properties. In an intervention study, α-tocopherol supplementation for 3 months in obese and type 2 diabetic subjects lowered levels of CRP and IL-6 (Devaraj and Jialal, 2000).

Wine and alcohol

Epidemiological and experimental studies support that regular moderate wine consumption is associated with reduced morbidity and mortality from a variety of chronic diseases in which inflammation is involved. Wine contains polyphenolic compounds and flavonoids and also different ethanol contents, and nowadays there is still controversy over whether it is the alcohol or the polyphenol content that most contributes to the health benefits of regular moderate wine consumption (Walzem, 2008). Although the down-regulatory effect of resveratrol on the synthesis and release of pro-inflammatory cytokines has been demonstrated (Marier *et al.*, 2005; Rahman *et al.*, 2006), moderate alcohol intake has also been associated with beneficial effects on inflammatory markers independently of the bioactive compounds of grapes (Rimm and Stampfer, 2002). No specific studies evaluating the effect of wine consumption on inflammation have been conducted in obese subjects, however.

Healthy dietary patterns

Considering the evidence on diet and inflammation, the best diet for obesity prevention would be high in fibre-rich cereals, fruits, vegetables, fish, VOO and nuts, moderate in wine, and low in meat, processed meats and *trans* fatty acids. Along these lines, the results from the Nurses' Health Study I Cohort reported that the levels of inflammatory markers associated to a prudent pattern were lower than those of a Western dietary pattern (Lopez-Garcia *et al.*, 2004). Moreover, a Mediterranean-type diet characterized by the above-mentioned foods has been associated with a lower risk of cardiovascular disease (Estruch *et al.*, 2006) probably because inflammation improves (Salas-Salvado *et al.*, 2008).

Physical Activity and Modulation of Inflammation in Obesity

Physical activity, energy balance and weight

A better understanding of the energy balance in obesity might provide some insight into the etiology of the disease. As has been discussion in the previous section, overweight and obesity are the result of a persistent positive imbalance between energy intake and energy expenditure. Whereas energy intake is provided by the chemical energy of food, energy expenditure consists of three major components: the basal metabolic rate (BMR), the thermal effect of food and activity energy expenditure (AEE). On the energy expenditure side of the equation, the major contributor is BMR, but the most easily modified component is AEE. A negative energy balance is required for weight loss and an increase in AEE contributes to this. The concept of AEE involves exercise-related and non-exercise aspects. The latter makes a considerable contribution to the inter- and the intra-personal variability in energy expenditure. It includes the energy expenditure of occupation, leisure and talking, among other things (Levine, 2004).

Several studies have assessed the importance of energy expenditure in the energy imbalance that results in obesity. The main hypotheses have focused on low BMR (Ravussin, 1995; Tataranni *et al.*, 2003) or low AEE (Levine *et al.*, 1999; Esparza, *et al.*, 2000; Johannsen *et al.*, 2008), leading to a low energy expenditure (Ravussin *et al.*, 1988; Roberts *et al.*, 1988; Esparza *et al.*, 2000).

Some studies, however, have disputed the association between obesity or weight gain and low energy expenditure (Prentice *et al.*, 1996; Westerterp, 2010) as a consequence of a decreased BMR (Flatt, 2007; Johannsen *et al.*, 2008) or low AEE (Tataranni, *et al.*, 2003; Westerterp and Speakman, 2008; Luke *et al.*, 2009). Firstly, it has been hypothesized that the higher BMR observed in obese subjects is probably a consequence of an increase of lean body mass (LBM) associated with the expansion of adipose tissue. Therefore, there are more energy demands, i.e. a higher BMR. On the other hand, even though it has been shown that obese subjects move less than non-obese subjects, the energy required to move a larger body mass is higher, also explaining why obese subjects engage in less physical activity. Finally, it is interesting to point out that weight reduction improves energy efficiency during physical exercise (Levine, 2004).

Physical activity for preventing weight gain

There is compelling evidence of a strong inverse dose–response association between physical activity and body weight and obesity, although this association varies between age and sex groups (Westerterp and Goran, 1997; Ekelund *et al.*, 2005b). In the EPIC-PANACEA cohort study, containing more than 400,000 men and women from nine European countries, a strong inverse association between total physical activity and

BMI and waist circumference was observed, independent of age, energy intake and sex (Besson *et al.*, 2009). However, prospective cohort studies in which body weight or obesity is measured at baseline are more useful in determining causal associations. A systematic review by Fogelholm and Kukkonen-Harjula (2000) of 16 prospective cohort studies conducted between 1980 and 2000, ranging from 210 to 79,236 subjects with a mean follow-up of 7 years, found a significant inverse relationship between baseline physical activity and gain in body weight in three studies. In one study, the inverse association was only observed in men. Two more studies observed a positive association and four studies suggested that higher levels of physical activity at follow-up were associated with less weight gain. The authors concluded that the evidence of a predictive effect of baseline physical activity on body weight gain was inconsistent. An update of this review published in 2005, which identified 14 additional studies in adults on the prospective association between physical activity and gain in body weight, reported that more studies, but not all, showed an association in the expected direction (Wareham *et al.*, 2005). More recently, a prospective cohort study involving 34,079 healthy US women, aged 54.2 years and followed up for 13 years concluded that those women carrying out 150 to 420 min/week of moderate-intensity physical activity gain significantly more weight than the most active group. Moreover, in a prospective cohort of the EPIC study conducted in 288,498 men and women, higher levels of physical activity significantly predicted a lower waist circumference in men and in women, independently of baseline body weight, baseline waist circumference and other confounding variables (Ekelund *et al.*, 2011). Overall, results suggest an inverse relationship between baseline levels of physical activity and gain in body weight and abdominal obesity. The magnitude of the effect is small, however, probably because of the high degree of measurement error when physical activity is assessed by self-report.

Few studies using objective measurements of physical activity energy expenditure have been published and their results do not support the notion that low levels of physical activity contribute to gain in body weight, which makes it tempting to speculate that energy intake plays a greater role than physical activity in weight gain (Tataranni *et al.*, 2003; Ekelund *et al.*, 2005a; Luke *et al.*, 2009). It is important to note that these studies have been conducted in small samples and large prospective cohort studies should be conducted in order to clarify the detailed association between physical activity and weight gain.

Physical activity in obesity treatment

Several randomized clinical trials between 4 and 16 months in duration have evaluated the effect of moderate physical activity on weight loss in overweight and obese subjects (Anderssen *et al.*, 1995; Cox *et al.*, 2004; Stewart *et al.*, 2005; Catenacci and Wyatt, 2007). They all showed a trend towards some degree of weight loss or prevention of weight gain in exercise groups in comparison with control groups. However, the magnitude of the differences in weight outcomes between groups was small, between 0.1 kg and 5.2 kg, with most studies showing a weight loss of 1–3 kg. It is important to consider the role of fat-free mass (FFM) when physical activity is used as a strategy for weight loss. Physical activity increases FFM, which might explain the relatively small levels of weight loss observed in these studies compared with the dietary strategies for obesity. Therefore, although physical activity is important for controlling weight loss, most short-term behavioural weight loss programmes show that loss is most significant when diet and exercise are combined (Jakicic *et al.*, 2001; Jakicic and Otto, 2006; Catenacci and Wyatt, 2007; Donnelly *et al.*, 2009) (Table 12.1).

Once weight has been lost, the focus shifts to maintaining the loss. Several studies have also evaluated the role of physical activity in weight maintenance after weight reduction. In these studies, a strong association between physical activity and weight-loss maintenance has been observed (Catenacci and Wyatt, 2007) (Table 12.2).

Table 12.1. Randomized, controlled trials for weight loss in diet alone versus diet and exercise.

Reference	Duration (months)	Total n (completed diet)	Study design	Weight change in diet-only groups	Weight change in diet + exercise groups	Significance[a]
Anderssen *et al.*, 1995	12	219 M/F (209)	C vs D vs E vs (D+E)	–4 kg	(D+E) –5.6 kg	NS
Ashutosh *et al.*, 1997	12	37 F (31)	D vs (D+AE) vs (D+RE) vs (D+AE+RE)	–14.5 kg	(D+AE) –15.0 kg (D+RE) –15.1 kg (D+AE+RE) –17.3 kg	NS NS NS
Bertram *et al.*, 1990	4	45 F (36)	D vs (D+E) vs (D+BT)	–9.3 kg	(D+E) –7 kg	NS
Cox *et al.*, 2004	4	60 M (51)	C vs D vs E vs (D+E)	–10.88 kg	(D+E) –11.66 kg	NS
Hammer *et al.*, 1989	4	36 F (26)	D1 vs D2 vs (D1+E) vs (D2+E)[b]	D1 –5.8 kg D2 –9.5 kg	(D1+E) –6.7 kg (D2+E) –12.9 kg	P <0.05 NS
Hellenius *et al.*, 1993	6	158 M (157)	C vs D vs E vs (D+E)	–0.3 BMI	(D+E) –0.6 BMI	NS
Layman *et al.*, 2005	4	48 F (48)	D1 vs D2 vs (D1+E) vs (D2+E)[c]	–8.7 kg –7.8 kg	(D1+E) –9.8 kg (D2+E) –6.7 kg	NS
Lemons *et al.*, 1989	4	60 F (60)	D vs AE vs RE vs (D+AE) vs (D+RE) vs (D+AE or RE)[d]	–12.8 kg	(D+AE) –12.2 (D+RE) –11.3 (D+AE or RE) –13.1	NS
Marks, *et al.*, 1995	5	67 F (44)	C vs D vs (D+AE) vs (D+RE) vs (D+AE) + RE	–3.7 kg	(D+AE) –4.5 kg (D+RE) –3.5 kg (D+AE+RE) –5.4 kg	NS NS NS
Nicklas *et al.*, 1997	6	28 F (20)	D vs (D+E)	–9.8 kg	(D+E) –6.6 kg	NS
Ross *et al.*, 1995	4	33 F (24)	D vs (D+E)	–10 kg	(D+E) –11.7 kg	NS
Ross *et al.*, 1996	4	33 M (33)	D vs (D+AE) vs (D+RE)	–11.9 kg	(D+AE) –11.6 kg (D+RE) –13.2 kg	NS NS

Stefanick *et al.*, 1998	12	377 M/F (367)	C vs D vs E vs (D+E)	−2.7 kg (male) −2.8 kg (female)	(D+E) −3.1 kg (female) (D+E) −4.2 kg (male)	NS NS
Sweeney *et al.*, 1993	6	47 F (30)	D1 vs D2 vs (D1+AE) vs (D1+AE+RE) vs (D2+AE) vs (D2+AE+RE)[e]	−13.5 kg	(D1 or D2+AE) −14.5 kg (D1 or D2+AE+RE) −11.5 kg	NS
Van Aggel-Leijssen *et al.*, 2002	12	37 M (29)	D vs (D+E)	−7.1 kg	(D+E) −8.9 kg	NS
Wadden *et al.*, 1997	11	128 F (99)	D vs (D+AE) vs (D+RE) vs (D+AE+RE)	−15.3 kg	(D+AE) −13.5 kg (D+RE) −17.3 kg (D+AE+RE) −16.6 kg	NS
Wood *et al.*, 1991	12	264 M/F (227)	C vs D vs D + E	−5.1 kg (male) −4.1 kg (female)	(D+E) −8.7 kg (male) (D+E) −5.1 kg (female)	P <0.05 NS

[a]*P* <0.05 was considered significant for difference in weight changes in exercise group versus (vs) weight change in control groups. [b]Comparison of the interaction of two diets (D1 low fat ad libitum diet vs D 2800 kcal low fat) with exercise in a 2 × 2 factorial design. [c]Comparison of the interaction of two diets (D1 high protein vs D2 high carbohydrate) with exercise in a 2 × 2 factorial design. [d]Comparison of diet alone with diet + AE, diet + RE, diet + 8 weeks AE followed by 8 weeks RE, AE only, and RE only. [e]Comparison of two diets (D1 severe energy restriction versus D2 moderate energy restriction) with no exercise, AE only, or AE and RE in a 2 × 3 factorial design. Abbreviations: AE, aerobic exercise; BT, behavioural therapy; C, control; D, diet; E, exercise; F, female; M, male; NS, not significant; RE, resistance exercise.

Table 12.2. Randomized, controlled trials for weight-loss maintenance with minimal supervision after exercise intervention of weight loss.

Reference	Weight-loss intervention	Supervised follow-up duration	Total n (completed diet)	Study design	Weight change for diet only	Weight change for diet + exercise	Significance[a]
Pavlou *et al.*, 1989	8 weeks	18 months, unsupervised	160 (110)	VLCD vs (VLCD+E)	–3 kg	–11 kg	P <0.05
Perri *et al.*, 1986	20 weeks	18 months, randomized to no contact vs 12-month maintenance programme[b]	90 M/F (67)	BT vs (BT+E)	4.9 kg	+5.1 kg	NS
Sikand *et al.*, 1988	20 weeks	2 years, unsupervised	30 (15)	D vs (D+E)	–0.8 kg	–9.1 kg	NS
Skender *et al.*, 1996	1 year	1 year, unsupervised	127 M/F (61)	D vs E vs (D+E)	–6.8 kg (after 1 year)	–8.9 kg (after 1 year)	NS
					+0.9 kg (after 2 years)	–2.2 kg (after 2 years)	NS
van Dale *et al.*, 1990	12/14 weeks	18–42 months, unsupervised	54 M/F (36)	D vs (D+E)	–7.7 kg	–14.4 kg	P <0.05
Wadden *et al.*, 1998	48 weeks	12 months, unsupervised	99 F (77)	D + BT vs	100 weeks	100 weeks	NS
				D + AE,	–6.9 kg	–8.5 kg	NS
				D + RE, or		–10.1 kg	NS
				D + AE + RE		–8.6 kg	
Wing *et al.*, 1988	10 weeks	1 year (monthly visits for initial 6 months)	25 M/F (19)	Study 1: D vs (D+E)	–4.0 kg	–7.8 kg	NS
	10 weeks	1 year (weekly visits for 10 weeks then monthly)	30 M/F (28)	Study 2: D vs (D+E)	–3.8 kg	–7.9 kg	P <0.05
Wing *et al.*, 1998	1 year	1 year (two 6-week refresher courses)	154 M/F (129)	C vs D vs E vs (D+E)	–5.5 kg (after 1 year)	–7.4 kg (after 1 year)	NS
					–2.1 kg (after 2 years)	–2.5 kg (after 2 years)	NS

[a]*P* <0.05 was considered significant for difference in weight changes in exercise group versus weight change in control groups. [b]Multicomponent maintenance programme included peer self-help groups, mail and telephone therapist contact for 1 year; therapist support was tailored to the individual client's initial treatment condition.
Abbreviations: AE, aerobic exercise; BT, behavioural therapy; C, control; D, diet; E, exercise; F, female; M, male; NS, not significant; RE, resistance exercise; VLCD, very-low-calorie diet.

Physical activity and inflammation

It is widely accepted that physical activity has favourable effects on the circulating lipid profile, blood pressure, glucose tolerance, platelet function, fibrinolysis and endothelial dysfunction (Hambrecht *et al.*, 2000; Thompson *et al.*, 2003; Braith and Stewart, 2006). Although the mechanisms involved in these effects are not well defined, growing evidence from epidemiological and clinical trials suggests that physical activity could explain at least some of these cardiometabolic effects. The inflammatory response to physical activity seems to depend, however, on the type of exercise (King *et al.*, 2003).

Epidemiological studies

Most epidemiological studies evaluating the association between inflammatory markers and acute physical activity levels have reported lower levels of inflammatory markers in active subjects than in sedentary individuals (Table 12.3). A cross-sectional association between physical activity levels and markers of inflammation was assessed in a cohort of 5888 men and women aged up to 65 years from the Cardiovascular Health Study. Those subjects allocated to the highest quartile of physical activity (≥2270 kcal/week) had 19%, 6%, 4% and 3% lower concentrations of CRP, WBC, fibrinogen and Factor VIII activity, respectively, than

Table 12.3. Associations between physical activity and markers of inflammation.

Marker of inflammation	Association with physical activity	References
Amyloid-A	↓	Pitsavos *et al.*, 2003; Rothenbacher *et al.*, 2003; Panagiotakos *et al.*, 2005; Pitsavos *et al.*, 2005
	No association	Verdaet *et al.*, 2004
CRP	↓	Geffken *et al.*, 2001; Abramson and Vaccarino, 2002; Ford, 2002; King *et al.*, 2003; Pitsavos *et al.*, 2003; Reuben *et al.*, 2003; Rothenbacher *et al.*, 2003; Tomaszewski *et al.*, 2003; Colbert *et al.*, 2004; Stauffer *et al.*, 2004; Panagiotakos *et al.*, 2005; Pitsavos *et al.*, 2005; Lavoie *et al.*, 2010
	No association	Manns *et al.*, 2003; Pischon *et al.*, 2003; Fredrikson *et al.*, 2004; Jankord and Jemiolo, 2004; Verdaet *et al.*, 2004
Fibrinogen	↓	Geffken *et al.*, 2001; Ford, 2002; King *et al.*, 2003; Panagiotakos *et al.*, 2005; Pitsavos *et al.*, 2005
	No association	Abramson and Vaccarino, 2002; Rothenbacher *et al*, 2003; Verdaet *et al.*, 2004
IL-6	↓	Bruunsgaard *et al.*, 2003; Reuben *et al.*, 2003; Rothenbacher *et al.*, 2003; Colbert *et al.*, 2004; Jankord and Jemiolo, 2004; Panagiotakos *et al.*, 2005; Pitsavos *et al.*, 2005
	No association	Pischon *et al.*, 2003; Tomaszewski *et al.*, 2003; Lavoie *et al.*, 2010
TNF-α	↓	Bruunsgaard *et al.*, 2003; Panagiotakos *et al.*, 2005; Pitsavos *et al.*, 2005
	No association	Rothenbacher *et al.*, 2003; Colbert *et al.*, 2004
WBC	↓	Geffken *et al.*, 2001; Abramson and Vaccarino, 2002; Ford, 2002; King *et al.*, 2003; Pitsavos *et al.*, 2003; Panagiotakos *et al.*, 2005; Pitsavos *et al.*, 2005
	No association	Rothenbacher *et al.*, 2003; Lavoie *et al.*, 2010

CRP, C-reactive protein; IL-6, interleukin 6; TNF-α, tumour necrosis factor α; WBC, white blood cells.

those in the lowest quartile (<367.5 kcal/week) after adjustment for gender, the presence of cardiovascular disease, age, race, smoking, BMI, diabetes and hypertension (Geffken *et al.*, 2001). Similar results were subsequently observed in a cohort of 1514 men and 1528 women from the ATTICA study. In this study, those subjects allocated to the physically active group (>7 kcal/min expended) showed significantly lower levels of CRP, WBC, serum amyloid-A, TNF-α, IL-6 and fibrinogen than sedentary subjects, after controlling for potential confounders (Panagiotakos *et al.*, 2005). Similar results have been reported elsewhere (Abramson and Vaccarino, 2002; Ford, 2002; Pitsavos *et al.*, 2003; Reuben *et al.*, 2003; Colbert *et al.*, 2004; Elosua *et al.*, 2005; Pitsavos *et al.*, 2005; McFarlin *et al.*, 2006), although in some cases these associations disappeared after adjustment for body mass measures (Manns *et al.*, 2003; Pischon *et al.*, 2003; Verdaet *et al.*, 2004). The relationship between physical activity and inflammation has usually been assessed by comparing active subjects with sedentary subjects. Lavoie *et al.* (2010) studied a group of 152 overweight/obese sedentary subjects and reported that those women allocated to the highest tertile of physical activity energy expenditure (1276 kcal/day) had lower concentrations of CRP and haptoglobin than those in the lowest tertile (587 kcal/day). Additionally, physical activity energy expenditure explained the 14% and 5% variations in CRP and haptoglobin, respectively, thus supporting the role of physical activity in reducing subclinical inflammation. It has been hypothesized that the intensity and duration of exercise might be responsible for this controversy among activity types (King *et al.*, 2003).

Randomized clinical trials

Several studies have evaluated the effect of an exercise intervention programme on inflammatory markers (Table 12.4). Most showed

Table 12.4. Effect of physical activity on markers of inflammation.

Marker of inflammation	Effect	References
Adiponectin	↑	Kondo *et al.*, 2006; Olson *et al.*, 2007
	No effect	Kadoglou *et al.*, 2007; Rokling-Andersen *et al.*, 2007; Devries *et al.*, 2008
CRP	↓	Tisi *et al.*, 1997; Mattusch *et al.*, 2000; Okita *et al.*, 2004; Goldhammer *et al.*, 2005; Kondo *et al.*, 2006; Kadoglou *et al.*, 2007; Olson *et al.*, 2007; Campbell *et al.*, 2009
	No effect	Tisi *et al.*, 1997; Nicklas *et al.*, 2004; Giannopoulou *et al.*, 2005; Dekker *et al.*, 2007; Campbell *et al.*, 2008; Devries *et al.*, 2008; Huffman *et al.*, 2008
Fibrinogen	No effect	Tisi *et al.*, 1997
IL-6	↓	Gielen *et al.*, 2003; Goldhammer *et al.*, 2005; Dekker *et al.*, 2007
	No effect	Larsen *et al.*, 2001; Conraads *et al.*, 2002; Nicklas *et al.*, 2004; Olson *et al.*, 2007; Devries *et al.*, 2008; Huffman *et al.*, 2008; Campbell *et al.*, 2009
IL-10	↑	Goldhammer *et al.*, 2005; Kadoglou *et al.*, 2007
	No effect	Huffman *et al.*, 2008
IL-18	↓	Kadoglou *et al.*, 2007
	No effect	Larsen *et al.*, 2001; Leick *et al.*, 2007
SAA	↓	Tisi *et al.*, 1997
	No effect	Campbell *et al.*, 2009
TNF-α	↑	Rokling-Andersen *et al.*, 2007
	↓	Tsukui *et al.*, 2000; Larsen *et al.*, 2001; Straczkowski *et al.*, 2001; Gielen *et al.*, 2003; Kondo *et al.*, 2006
	No effect	Conraads *et al.*, 2002; Giannopoulou *et al.*, 2005; Kadoglou *et al.*, 2007; Huffman *et al.*, 2008

CRP, C-reactive protein; IL, interleukin; SAA, serum amyloid A; TNF-α, tumour necrosis factor α.

an improvement in systemic inflammation after an exercise intervention programme, in healthy subjects (Mattusch *et al.*, 2000; Tsukui *et al.*, 2000; Okita *et al.*, 2004) and patients with overweight or obesity (Straczkowski *et al.*, 2001; Kondo *et al.*, 2006; Kadoglou *et al.*, 2007; Olson *et al.*, 2007; Campbell *et al.*, 2009), coronary heart disease (Goldhammer *et al.*, 2005), claudication (Tisi *et al.*, 1997) or chronic heart failure (Gielen *et al.*, 2003). In some trials, however, an exercise intervention programme had no significant effect on systemic inflammation (Nicklas *et al.*, 2004; Leick *et al.*, 2007; Devries *et al.*, 2008; Huffman *et al.*, 2008; Campbell *et al.*, 2009). It has been postulated that the combination of muscle injury and muscle contraction is responsible for a rise in IL-6. Recent research has demonstrated that IL-6 mRNA is upregulated in contracting skeletal muscle (Jonsdottir *et al.*, 2000; Steensberg *et al.*, 2001) and that IL-6, but not TNF-α, is released from skeletal muscle during exercise (Steensberg *et al.*, 2001). Increased IL-6 may exert inhibitory effects on TNF-α and IL-1 cell production, thus contributing to anti-inflammatory effects. Moreover, acute physical activity has also been related to the elevation of other anti-inflammatory markers, such as IL-10 and IL-1RA, and inhibitors of pro-inflammatory markers, thus contributing to the counter-regulation of inflammatory process during acute exercise. A study of 90 runners demonstrated significant increases in blood cell count and CRP levels immediately and 24h after a marathon (Weight *et al.*, 1991). Other studies have found similar results. Overall, the finding that regular training reduces CRP levels suggests that physical activity as such might suppress low-grade inflammation (Mattusch *et al.*, 2000; Fallon *et al.*, 2001).

Again, the effect of an exercise intervention programme also seems to be dependent on frequency, intensity and duration (Bruunsgaard *et al.*, 2003; Tziomalos *et al.*, 2010). Table 12.4 shows that the effects of exercise on CRP and TNF-α are controversial, but that most reports on adiponectin and IL-6 show no changes after a training programme. As proposed by Lehman *et al.* (1997), acute resistance training (RT) response may differ from long-term resistance training response. During acute response, muscular damage plays a major role, whereas during long-term RT changes take place in body composition, metabolism and organ function, even though cell antioxidant capacity increases. Most studies evaluating the effect of RT on inflammatory markers have reported a significant increase in inflammatory markers (Smith *et al.*, 2000; MacIntyre *et al.*, 2001; Hirose *et al.*, 2004; Peake *et al.*, 2005; Phillips *et al.*, 2010). The results obtained after long-term RT depend, however, on the intervals at which samples were taken and if pre- and post-training comparisons were made in the resting state or after an acute bout of RT (Calle and Fernandez, 2010).

Finally, different forms of exercise can also have different effects on markers of inflammation (King *et al.*, 2003; Reuben *et al.*, 2003; Rothenbacher *et al.*, 2003; Colbert *et al.*, 2004). It is still unclear, however, whether these differences can exert differential effects on cardiometabolic risk.

Summary and Conclusions

Obesity is a common, serious and growing problem worldwide, with a mutifactorial ethiology. Nowadays, excess body weight has been recognized as the most important modifiable risk factor in the development of several highly prevalent diseases that can lead to further morbidity and mortality. In the past couple of decades, inflammation has had a growing role in the pathophysiology of obesity and, nowadays, obesity is considered as a chronic low-level inflammatory disease, suggesting that this could be the link with co-morbid diseases related to obesity. Dietary modulation of inflammatory status or even inflammatory modulation mediated by physical activity could therefore be reasonable strategies to prevent and to treat weight gain. In this chapter, we focused on those studies conducted on obese people, evaluating the relationship of specific dietary compounds and physical activity strategies used to modulate inflammation. There is evidence to suggest that some food components can modulate the inflammatory process. For this reason, it has been hypothesized that dietary habits are probably one of the main determinants that influence the inflammatory process in obesity. Regarding physical activity, several epidemiological and clinical studies have shown an inverse relationship between the levels of inflammatory markers and the physical activity level. More randomized, controlled intervention studies are thus required to elucidate the relationships between the inflammatory process and the strategies used to reduce the prevalence of obesity co-morbidities.

References

Abramson, J.L. and Vaccarino, V. (2002) Relationship between physical activity and inflammation among apparently healthy middle-aged and older US adults. *Archives of Internal Medicine* 162, 1286–1292.

Ajani, U.A., Ford, E.S. and Mokdad, A.H. (2004) Dietary fiber and C-reactive protein: findings from national health and nutrition examination survey data. *The Journal of Nutrition* 134, 1181–1185.

Anderssen, S., Holme, I., Urdal, P. and Hjermann, I. (1995) Diet and exercise intervention have favourable effects on blood pressure in mild hypertensives: the Oslo Diet and Exercise Study (ODES). *Blood Pressure* 4, 343–349.

Ashutosh, K., Methrotra, K. and Fragale-Jackson, J. (1997) Effects of sustained weight loss and exercise on aerobic fitness in obese women. *The Journal of Sports Medicine and Physical Fitness* 37, 252–257.

Asia Pacific Cohort Studies Collaboration (2006) Central obesity and risk of cardiovascular disease in the Asia Pacific Region. *Asia Pacific Journal of Clinical Nutrition* 15, 287–292.

Bemelmans, W.J., Lefrandt, J.D., Feskens, E.J., van Haelst, P.L., Broer, J., *et al.* (2004) Increased alpha-linolenic acid intake lowers C-reactive protein, but has no effect on markers of atherosclerosis. *European Journal of Clinical Nutrition* 58, 1083–1089.

Bertram, S.R., Venter, I. and Stewart, R.I. (1990) Weight loss in obese women–exercise v. dietary education. *South African Medical Journal = Suid-Afrikaanse Tydskrif Vir Geneeskunde* 78, 15–18.

Besson, H., Ekelund, U., Luan, J., May, A.M., Sharp, S., *et al.* (2009) A cross-sectional analysis of physical activity and obesity indicators in European participants of the EPIC-PANACEA study. *International Journal of Obesity* (2005) 33, 497–506.

Blomhoff, R., Carlsen, M.H., Andersen, L.F. and Jacobs, D.R., Jr (2006) Health benefits of nuts: potential role of antioxidants. *The British Journal of Nutrition* 96 Suppl 2, S52–S60.

Braith, R.W. and Stewart, K.J. (2006) Resistance exercise training: its role in the prevention of cardiovascular disease. *Circulation* 113, 2642–2650.

Brock, D.W., Thomas, O., Cowan, C.D., Allison, D.B., Gaesser, G.A. and Hunter, G.R. (2009) Association between insufficiently physically active and the prevalence of obesity in the United States. *Journal of Physical Activity & Health* 6, 1–5.

Brown, W.V., Fujioka, K., Wilson, P.W. and Woodworth, K.A. (2009) Obesity: why be concerned? *The American Journal of Medicine* 122(4 Suppl 1), S4–S11.

Bruunsgaard, H., Ladelund, S., Pedersen, A.N., Schroll, M., Jorgensen, T. and Pedersen, B.K. (2003) Predicting death from tumour necrosis factor-alpha and interleukin-6 in 80-year-old people. *Clinical and Experimental Immunology* 132, 24–31.

Burke, G.L., Bertoni, A.G., Shea, S., Tracy, R., Watson, K.E., *et al.* (2008) The impact of obesity on cardiovascular disease risk factors and subclinical vascular disease: the Multi-Ethnic Study of Atherosclerosis. *Archives of Internal Medicine* 168, 928–935.

Calle, M.C. and Fernandez, M.L. (2010) Effects of resistance training on the inflammatory response. *Nutrition Research and Practice* 4, 259–269.

Campbell, K.L., Campbell, P.T., Ulrich, C.M., Wener, M., Alfano, C.M., *et al.* (2008) No reduction in C-reactive protein following a 12-month randomized controlled trial of exercise in men and women. Cancer Epidemiology, Biomarkers & Prevention. *A Publication of the American Association for Cancer Research, Cosponsored by the American Society of Preventive Oncology* 17, 1714–1718.

Campbell, P.T., Campbell, K.L., Wener, M.H., Wood, B.L., Potter, J.D., *et al.* (2009) A yearlong exercise intervention decreases CRP among obese postmenopausal women. *Medicine and Science in Sports and Exercise* 41, 1533–1539.

Catenacci, V.A. and Wyatt, H.R. (2007) The role of physical activity in producing and maintaining weight loss. *Nature Clinical Practice. Endocrinology & Metabolism* 3, 518–529.

Ciubotaru, I., Lee, Y.S. and Wander, R.C. (2003) Dietary fish oil decreases C-reactive protein, interleukin-6, and triacylglycerol to HDL-cholesterol ratio in postmenopausal women on HRT. *The Journal of Nutritional Biochemistry* 14, 513–521.

Cleland, V.J., Schmidt, M.D., Dwyer, T. and Venn, A.J. (2008) Television viewing and abdominal obesity in young adults: is the association mediated by food and beverage consumption during viewing time or reduced leisure-time physical activity? *The American Journal of Clinical Nutrition* 87, 1148–1155.

Colbert, L.H., Visser, M., Simonsick, E.M., Tracy, R.P., Newman, A.B., *et al.* (2004) Physical activity, exercise, and inflammatory markers in older adults: findings from the Health, Aging and Body Composition Study. *Journal of the American Geriatrics Society* 52, 1098–1104.

Conraads, V.M., Beckers, P., Bosmans, J., De Clerck, L.S., Stevens, W.J., *et al.* (2002) Combined endurance/resistance training reduces plasma TNF-alpha receptor levels in patients with chronic heart failure and coronary artery disease. *European Heart Journal* 23, 1854–1860.

Cooke, J.P., Tsao, P., Singer, A., Wang, B.Y., Kosek, J. and Drexler, H. (1993) Anti-atherogenic effect of nuts: is the answer NO? *Archives of Internal Medicine* 153, 896, 899, 902.

Cox, K.L., Burke, V., Morton, A.R., Beilin, L.J. and Puddey, I.B. (2004) Independent and additive effects of energy restriction and exercise on glucose and insulin concentrations in sedentary overweight men. *The American Journal of Clinical Nutrition* 80, 308–316.

Curat, C.A., Miranville, A., Sengenes, C., Diehl, M., Tonus, C., *et al.* (2004) From blood monocytes to adipose tissue-resident macrophages: induction of diapedesis by human mature adipocytes. *Diabetes* 53, 1285–1292.

de Mello, V.D., Erkkila, A.T., Schwab, U.S., Pulkkinen, L., Kolehmainen, M., *et al.* (2009) The effect of fatty or lean fish intake on inflammatory gene expression in peripheral blood mononuclear cells of patients with coronary heart disease. *European Journal of Nutrition* 48, 447–455.

Dekker, M.J., Lee, S., Hudson, R., Kilpatrick, K., Graham, T.E., *et al.* (2007) An exercise intervention without weight loss decreases circulating interleukin-6 in lean and obese men with and without type 2 diabetes mellitus. *Metabolism: Clinical and Experimental* 56, 332–338.

Devaraj, S. and Jialal, I. (2000) Alpha tocopherol supplementation decreases serum C-reactive protein and monocyte interleukin-6 levels in normal volunteers and type 2 diabetic patients. *Free Radical Biology & Medicine* 29, 790–792.

Devries, M.C., Hamadeh, M.J., Glover, A.W., Raha, S., Samjoo, I.A. and Tarnopolsky, M.A. (2008) Endurance training without weight loss lowers systemic, but not muscle, oxidative stress with no effect on inflammation in lean and obese women. *Free Radical Biology & Medicine* 45, 503–511.

Donnelly, J.E., Blair, S.N., Jakicic, J.M., Manore, M.M., Rankin, J.W., *et al.* (2009) American College of Sports Medicine Position Stand. Appropriate physical activity intervention strategies for weight loss and prevention of weight regain for adults. *Medicine and Science in Sports and Exercise* 41, 459–471.

Egger, G. and Swinburn, B. (1997) An "ecological" approach to the obesity pandemic. *British Medical Journal (Clinical Research Edn)* 315, 477–480.

Ekelund, U., Brage, S., Franks, P.W., Hennings, S., Emms, S. and Wareham, N.J. (2005a) Physical activity energy expenditure predicts progression toward the metabolic syndrome independently of aerobic fitness in middle-aged healthy Caucasians: the Medical Research Council Ely Study. *Diabetes Care* 28, 1195–1200.

Ekelund, U., Brage, S., Franks, P.W., Hennings, S., Emms, S., *et al.* (2005b) Physical activity energy expenditure predicts changes in body composition in middle-aged healthy whites: effect modification by age. *The American Journal of Clinical Nutrition* 81, 964–969.

Ekelund, U., Besson, H., Luan, J., May, A.M., Sharp, S.J., *et al.* (2011) Physical activity and gain in abdominal adiposity and body weight: prospective cohort study in 288,498 men and women. *The American Journal of Clinical Nutrition* 93, 826–835.

Elosua, R., Bartali, B., Ordovas, J.M., Corsi, A.M., Lauretani, F., *et al.* (2005) Association between physical activity, physical performance, and inflammatory biomarkers in an elderly population: the InCHIANTI study. *The Journals of Gerontology. Series A, Biological Sciences and Medical Sciences* 60, 760–767.

Eriksson, J., Taimela, S. and Koivisto, V.A. (1997) Exercise and the metabolic syndrome. *Diabetologia* 40, 125–135.

Esparza, J., Fox, C., Harper, I.T., Bennett, P.H., Schulz, L.O., *et al.* (2000) Daily energy expenditure in Mexican and USA Pima indians: low physical activity as a possible cause of obesity. International Journal of Obesity and Related Metabolic Disorders. *Journal of the International Association for the Study of Obesity* 24, 55–59.

Esposito, K., Pontillo, A., Di Palo, C., Giugliano, G., Masella, M., *et al.* (2003) Effect of weight loss and lifestyle changes on vascular inflammatory markers in obese women: a randomized trial. *JAMA: The Journal of the American Medical Association* 289, 1799–1804.

Estruch, R., Martinez-Gonzalez, M.A., Corella, D., Salas-Salvado, J., Ruiz-Gutierrez, V., *et al.* (2006) Effects of a Mediterranean-style diet on cardiovascular risk factors: a randomized trial. *Annals of Internal Medicine* 145, 1–11.

Fain, J.N. (2010) Release of inflammatory mediators by human adipose tissue is enhanced in obesity and primarily by the nonfat cells: a review. *Mediators of Inflammation* 2010513948.

Fallon, K.E., Fallon, S.K. and Boston, T. (2001) The acute phase response and exercise: court and field sports. *British Journal of Sports Medicine* 35, 170–173.

Fitzpatrick, D.F., Hirschfield, S.L. and Coffey, R.G. (1993) Endothelium-dependent vasorelaxing activity of wine and other grape products. *The American Journal of Physiology* 265(2 Pt 2), H774–H778.

Flatt, J.P. (2007) Differences in basal energy expenditure and obesity. *Obesity (Silver Spring)* 15, 2546–2548.

Fogelholm, M. and Kukkonen-Harjula, K. (2000) Does physical activity prevent weight gain–a systematic review. *Obesity Reviews: An Official Journal of the International Association for the Study of Obesity* 1, 95–111.

Ford, E.S. (2002) Does exercise reduce inflammation? Physical activity and C-reactive protein among U.S. adults. *Epidemiology (Cambridge)* 13, 561–568.

Fredrikson, G.N., Hedblad, B., Nilsson, J.A., Alm, R., Berglund, G., *et al.* (2004) Association between diet, lifestyle, metabolic cardiovascular risk factors, and plasma C-reactive protein levels. *Metabolism: Clinical and Experimental* 53, 1436–1442.

Geffken, D.F., Cushman, M., Burke, G.L., Polak, J.F., Sakkinen, P.A., *et al.* (2001) Association between physical activity and markers of inflammation in a healthy elderly population. *American Journal of Epidemiology* 153, 242–250.

Giannopoulou, I., Fernhall, B., Carhart, R., Weinstock, R.S., Baynard, T., *et al.* (2005) Effects of diet and/or exercise on the adipocytokine and inflammatory cytokine levels of postmenopausal women with type 2 diabetes. *Metabolism: Clinical and Experimental* 54, 866–875.

Gielen, S., Adams, V., Mobius-Winkler, S., Linke, A., Erbs, S., *et al.* (2003) Anti-inflammatory effects of exercise training in the skeletal muscle of patients with chronic heart failure. *Journal of the American College of Cardiology* 42, 861–868.

Goldhammer, E., Tanchilevitch, A., Maor, I., Beniamini, Y., *et al.* (2005) Exercise training modulates cytokines activity in coronary heart disease patients. *International Journal of Cardiology* 100, 93–99.

Guh, D.P., Zhang, W., Bansback, N., Amarsi, Z., Birmingham, C.L., *et al.* (2009) The incidence of co-morbidities related to obesity and overweight: a systematic review and meta-analysis. *BMC Public Health* 988.

Hambrecht, R., Wolf, A., Gielen, S., Linke, A., Hofer, J., *et al.* (2000) Effect of exercise on coronary endothelial function in patients with coronary artery disease. *The New England Journal of Medicine* 342, 454–460.

Hammer, R.L., Barrier, C.A., Roundy, E.S., Bradford, J.M. and Fisher, A.G. (1989) Calorie-restricted low-fat diet and exercise in obese women. *The American Journal of Clinical Nutrition* 49, 77–85.

Hartman, T.J., Albert, P.S., Zhang, Z., Bagshaw, D., Kris-Etherton, P.M., *et al.* (2010) Consumption of a legume-enriched, low-glycemic index diet is associated with biomarkers of insulin resistance and inflammation among men at risk for colorectal cancer. *The Journal of Nutrition* 140, 60–67.

Harwell, T.S., Vanderwood, K.K., Hall, T.O., Butcher, M.K., Helgerson, S.D. and the Montana Cardiovascular Disease and Diabetes Prevention Workgroup (2011) Factors associated with achieving a weight loss goal among participants in an adapted Diabetes Prevention Program. *Primary Care Diabetes* 5, 125–128.

Hellenius, M.L., de Faire, U., Berglund, B., Hamsten, A. and Krakau, I. (1993) Diet and exercise are equally effective in reducing risk for cardiovascular disease. Results of a randomized controlled study in men with slightly to moderately raised cardiovascular risk factors. *Atherosclerosis* 103, 81–91.

Hirose, L., Nosaka, K., Newton, M., Laveder, A., Kano, M., *et al.* (2004) Changes in inflammatory mediators following eccentric exercise of the elbow flexors. *Exercise Immunology Review* 1075–1090.

Hu, F.B., Manson, J.E., Stampfer, M.J., Colditz, G., Liu, S., *et al.* (2001) Diet, lifestyle, and the risk of type 2 diabetes mellitus in women. *The New England Journal of Medicine* 345, 790–797.

Huffman, K.M., Slentz, C.A., Bales, C.W., Houmard, J.A. and Kraus, W.E. (2008) Relationships between adipose tissue and cytokine responses to a randomized controlled exercise training intervention. *Metabolism: Clinical and Experimental* 57, 577–583.

International Obesity Task Force Secretariat (2002) The global challenge of obesity and the International Obesity Task Force. Available at: http://www.iuns.org/features/obesity/obesity.htm. (Accessed: 14 December 2010).

Jakicic, J.M. and Otto, A.D. (2006) Treatment and prevention of obesity: what is the role of exercise? *Nutrition Reviews* 64, S57–S61.

Jakicic, J.M., Clark, K., Coleman, E., Donnelly, J.E., Foreyt, J., *et al.* (2001) American College of Sports Medicine position stand. Appropriate intervention strategies for weight loss and prevention of weight regain for adults. *Medicine and Science in Sports and Exercise* 33, 2145–2156.

Jankord, R. and Jemiolo, B. (2004) Influence of physical activity on serum IL-6 and IL-10 levels in healthy older men. *Medicine and Science in Sports and Exercise* 36, 960–964.

Jiang, R., Jacobs, D.R., Jr, Mayer-Davis, E., Szklo, M., Herrington, D., *et al.* (2006) Nut and seed consumption and inflammatory markers in the multi-ethnic study of atherosclerosis. *American Journal of Epidemiology* 163, 222–231.

Johannsen, D.L., Welk, G.J., Sharp, R.L. and Flakoll, P.J. (2008) Differences in daily energy expenditure in lean and obese women: the role of posture allocation. *Obesity (Silver Spring)* 16, 34–39.

Jonsdottir, I.H., Schjerling, P., Ostrowski, K., Asp, S., Richter, E.A., *et al.* (2000) Muscle contractions induce interleukin-6 mRNA production in rat skeletal muscles. *The Journal of Physiology* 528, 157–163.

Kadoglou, N.P., Iliadis, F., Angelopoulou, N., Perrea, D., Ampatzidis, G., *et al.* (2007) The anti-inflammatory effects of exercise training in patients with type 2 diabetes mellitus. *European Journal of Cardiovascular Prevention and Rehabilitation: Official Journal of the European Society of Cardiology, Working Groups on Epidemiology & Prevention and Cardiac Rehabilitation and Exercise Physiology* 14, 837–843.

Kim, J.H., Bachmann, R.A. and Chen, J. (2009) Interleukin-6 and insulin resistance. *Vitamins and Hormones* 80, 613–633.

King, D.E., Carek, P., Mainous, A.G., 3rd and Pearson, W.S. (2003) Inflammatory markers and exercise: differences related to exercise type. *Medicine and Science in Sports and Exercise* 35, 575–581.

King, D.E., Mainous, A.G., 3rd, Egan, B.M., Woolson, R.F. and Geesey, M.E. (2005) Fiber and C-reactive protein in diabetes, hypertension, and obesity. *Diabetes Care* 28, 1487–1489.

King, D.E., Egan, B.M., Woolson, R.F., Mainous, A.G., 3rd, Al-Solaiman, Y., *et al.* (2007) Effect of a high-fiber diet vs a fiber-supplemented diet on C-reactive protein level. *Archives of Internal Medicine* 167, 502–506.

King, D.E., Mainous, A.G., 3rd, Egan, B.M., Woolson, R.F. and Geesey, M.E. (2008) Effect of psyllium fiber supplementation on C-reactive protein: the trial to reduce inflammatory markers (TRIM). *Annals of Family Medicine* 6, 100–106.

Knowler, W.C., Barrett-Connor, E., Fowler, S.E., Hamman, R.F., Lachin, J.M., *et al.* (2002) Reduction in the incidence of type 2 diabetes with lifestyle intervention or metformin. *The New England Journal of Medicine* 346, 393–403.

Kondo, T., Kobayashi, I. and Murakami, M. (2006) Effect of exercise on circulating adipokine levels in obese young women. *Endocrine Journal* 53, 189–195.

Kosaka, K., Noda, M. and Kuzuya, T. (2005) Prevention of type 2 diabetes by lifestyle intervention: a Japanese trial in IGT males. *Diabetes Research and Clinical Practice* 67, 152–162.

Lachat, C., Van Camp, J., De Henauw, S., Matthys, C., Larondelle, Y., *et al.* (2005) A concise overview of national nutrition action plans in the European Union Member States. *Public Health Nutrition* 8, 266–274.

Larsen, A.I., Aukrust, P., Aarsland, T. and Dickstein, K. (2001) Effect of aerobic exercise training on plasma levels of tumor necrosis factor alpha in patients with heart failure. *The American Journal of Cardiology* 88, 805–808.

Lavoie, M.E., Rabasa-Lhoret, R., Doucet, E., Mignault, D., Messier, L., *et al.* (2010) Association between physical activity energy expenditure and inflammatory markers in sedentary overweight and obese women. *International Journal of Obesity* (2005) 34, 1387–1395.

Layman, D.K., Evans, E., Baum, J.I., Seyler, J., Erickson, D.J., *et al.* (2005) Dietary protein and exercise have additive effects on body composition during weight loss in adult women. *The Journal of Nutrition* 135, 1903–1910.

Lehmann, M.J., Lormes, W., Opitz-Gress, A., Steinacker, J.M., Netzer, N., *et al.* (1997) Training and overtraining: an overview and experimental results in endurance sports. *The Journal of Sports Medicine and Physical Fitness* 37, 7–17.

Leick, L., Lindegaard, B., Stensvold, D., Plomgaard, P., Saltin, B., *et al.* (2007) Adipose tissue interleukin-18 mRNA and plasma interleukin-18: effect of obesity and exercise. *Obesity (Silver Spring)* 15, 356–363.

Lemons, A.D., Kreitzman, S.N., Coxon, A. and Howard, A. (1989) Selection of appropriate exercise regimens for weight reduction during VLCD and maintenance. *International Journal of Obesity* 13 Suppl 2, 119–123.

Levine, J.A. (2004) Non-exercise activity thermogenesis (NEAT). *Nutrition Reviews* 62, S82–S97.

Levine, J.A., Eberhardt, N.L. and Jensen, M.D. (1999) Role of nonexercise activity thermogenesis in resistance to fat gain in humans. *Science* 283, 212–214.

Li, G., Zhang, P., Wang, J., Gregg, E.W., Yang, W., *et al.* (2008) The long-term effect of lifestyle interventions to prevent diabetes in the China Da Qing Diabetes Prevention Study: a 20-year follow-up study. *Lancet* 371, 1783–1789.

Lichtenstein, A.H., Erkkila, A.T., Lamarche, B., Schwab, U.S., Jalbert, S.M., *et al.* (2003) Influence of hydrogenated fat and butter on CVD risk factors: remnant-like particles, glucose and insulin, blood pressure and C-reactive protein. *Atherosclerosis* 171, 97–107.

Lindstrom, J., Ilanne-Parikka, P., Peltonen, M., Aunola, S., Eriksson, J.G., *et al.* (2006) Sustained reduction in the incidence of type 2 diabetes by lifestyle intervention: follow-up of the Finnish Diabetes Prevention Study. *Lancet* 368, 1673–1679.

Lopez-Garcia, E., Schulze, M.B., Manson, J.E., Meigs, J.B., Albert, C.M., *et al.* (2004) Consumption of (n-3) fatty acids is related to plasma biomarkers of inflammation and endothelial activation in women. *The Journal of Nutrition* 134, 1806–1811.

Lopez-Garcia, E., Schulze, M.B., Meigs, J.B., Manson, J.E., Rifai, N., *et al.* (2005) Consumption of trans fatty acids is related to plasma biomarkers of inflammation and endothelial dysfunction. *The Journal of Nutrition* 135, 562–566.

Low, S., Chin, M.C. and Deurenberg-Yap, M. (2009) Review on epidemic of obesity. *Annals of the Academy of Medicine* 38, 57–59.

Luke, A., Dugas, L.R., Ebersole, K., Durazo-Arvizu, R.A., Cao, G., *et al.* (2009) Energy expenditure does not predict weight change in either Nigerian or African American women. *The American Journal of Clinical Nutrition* 89, 169–176.

MacIntyre, D.L., Sorichter, S., Mair, J., Berg, A. and McKenzie, D.C. (2001) Markers of inflammation and myofibrillar proteins following eccentric exercise in humans. *European Journal of Applied Physiology* 84, 180–186.

Manns, P.J., Williams, D.P., Snow, C.M. and Wander, R.C. (2003) Physical activity, body fat, and serum C-reactive protein in postmenopausal women with and without hormone replacement. *American Journal of Human Biology* 15, 91–100.

Mantzoros, C.S., Williams, C.J., Manson, J.E., Meigs, J.B. and Hu, F.B. (2006) Adherence to the Mediterranean dietary pattern is positively associated with plasma adiponectin concentrations in diabetic women. *The American Journal of Clinical Nutrition* 84, 328–335.

Marier, J.F., Chen, K., Prince, P., Scott, G., del Castillo, J.R. and Vachon, P. (2005) Production of ex vivo lipopolysaccharide-induced tumor necrosis factor-alpha, interleukin-1beta, and interleukin-6 is suppressed by trans-resveratrol in a concentration-dependent manner. *Canadian Journal of Veterinary Research = Revue Canadienne De Recherche Veterinaire* 69, 151–154.

Marks, B.L., Ward, A., Morris, D.H., Castellani, J. and Rippe, J.M. (1995) Fat-free mass is maintained in women following a moderate diet and exercise program. *Medicine and Science in Sports and Exercise* 27, 1243–1251.

Mattusch, F., Dufaux, B., Heine, O., Mertens, I. and Rost, R. (2000) Reduction of the plasma concentration of C-reactive protein following nine months of endurance training. *International Journal of Sports Medicine* 21, 21–24.

McFarlin, B.K., Flynn, M.G., Campbell, W.W., Craig, B.A., Robinson, J.P., *et al.* (2006) Physical activity status, but not age, influences inflammatory biomarkers and toll-like receptor 4. *The Journals of Gerontology. Series A, Biological Sciences and Medical Sciences* 61, 388–393.

Miles, E.A., Zoubouli, P. and Calder, P.C. (2005) Differential anti-inflammatory effects of phenolic compounds from extra virgin olive oil identified in human whole blood cultures. *Nutrition* 21, 389–394.

Mocellin, S., Panelli, M.C., Wang, E., Nagorsen, D. and Marincola, F.M. (2003) The dual role of IL-10. *Trends in Immunology* 24, 36–43.

Mokdad, A.H., Ford, E.S., Bowman, B.A., Dietz, W.H., Vinicor, F., *et al.* (2003) Prevalence of obesity, diabetes, and obesity-related health risk factors, 2001. *The Journal of the American Medical Association* 289, 76–79.

Muller-Riemenschneider, F., Reinhold, T., Berghofer, A. and Willich, S.N. (2008) Health-economic burden of obesity in Europe. *European Journal of Epidemiology* 23, 499–509.

Navarro-Diaz, M., Serra, A., Romero, R., Bonet, J., Bayes, B., *et al.* (2006) Effect of drastic weight loss after bariatric surgery on renal parameters in extremely obese patients: long-term follow-up. *Journal of the American Society of Nephrology* 17, S213–S217.

Nicklas, B.J., Rogus, E.M. and Goldberg, A.P. (1997) Exercise blunts declines in lipolysis and fat oxidation after dietary-induced weight loss in obese older women. *The American Journal of Physiology* 273, E149–E155.

Nicklas, B.J., Ambrosius, W., Messier, S.P., Miller, G.D., Penninx, B.W., *et al.* (2004) Diet-induced weight loss, exercise, and chronic inflammation in older, obese adults: a randomized controlled clinical trial. *The American Journal of Clinical Nutrition* 79, 544–551.

Okita, K., Nishijima, H., Murakami, T., Nagai, T., Morita, N., *et al.* (2004) Can exercise training with weight loss lower serum C-reactive protein levels? *Arteriosclerosis, Thrombosis, and Vascular Biology* 24, 1868–1873.

Olson, T.P., Dengel, D.R., Leon, A.S. and Schmitz, K.H. (2007) Changes in inflammatory biomarkers following one-year of moderate resistance training in overweight women. *International Journal of Obesity* 31, 996–1003.

O'Rourke, R.W. (2009) Inflammation in obesity-related diseases. *Surgery* 145, 255–259.

Pan, X.R., Yang, W.Y., Li, G.W. and Liu, J. (1997) Prevalence of diabetes and its risk factors in China, 1994. National Diabetes Prevention and Control Cooperative Group. *Diabetes Care* 20, 1664–1669.

Panagiotakos, D.B., Pitsavos, C., Chrysohoou, C., Kavouras, S., Stefanadis, C. and ATTICA Study (2005) The associations between leisure-time physical activity and inflammatory and coagulation markers related to cardiovascular disease: the ATTICA Study. *Preventive Medicine* 40, 432–437.

Pavlou, K.N., Krey, S. and Steffee, W.P. (1989) Exercise as an adjunct to weight loss and maintenance in moderately obese subjects. *The American Journal of Clinical Nutrition* 49, 1115–1123.

Peake, J.M., Suzuki, K., Hordern, M., Wilson, G., Nosaka, K., *et al.* (2005) Plasma cytokine changes in relation to exercise intensity and muscle damage. *European Journal of Applied Physiology* 95, 514–521.

Perri, M.G., McAdoo, W.G., McAllister, D.A., Lauer, J.B. and Yancey, D.Z. (1986) Enhancing the efficacy of behavior therapy for obesity: effects of aerobic exercise and a multicomponent maintenance program. *Journal of Consulting and Clinical Psychology* 54, 670–675.

Phillips, M.D., Mitchell, J.B., Currie-Elolf, L.M., Yellott, R.C. and Hubing, K.A. (2010) Influence of commonly employed resistance exercise protocols on circulating IL-6 and indices of insulin sensitivity. *Journal of Strength and Conditioning Research / National Strength & Conditioning Association* 24, 1091–1101.

Pischon, T., Hankinson, S.E., Hotamisligil, G.S., Rifai, N. and Rimm, E.B. (2003) Leisure-time physical activity and reduced plasma levels of obesity-related inflammatory markers. *Obesity Research* 11, 1055–1064.

Pitsavos, C., Chrysohoou, C., Panagiotakos, D.B., Skoumas, J., Zeimbekis, A., *et al.* (2003) Association of leisure-time physical activity on inflammation markers (C-reactive protein, white cell blood count, serum amyloid A, and fibrinogen) in healthy subjects (from the ATTICA study). *The American Journal of Cardiology* 91, 368–370.

Pitsavos, C., Panagiotakos, D.B., Chrysohoou, C., Kavouras, S. and Stefanadis, C. (2005) The associations between physical activity, inflammation, and coagulation markers, in people with metabolic syndrome: the ATTICA study. *European Journal of Cardiovascular Prevention and Rehabilitation: Official Journal of the European Society of Cardiology, Working Groups on Epidemiology & Prevention and Cardiac Rehabilitation and Exercise Physiology* 12, 151–158.

Pittas, A.G., Roberts, S.B., Das, S.K., Gilhooly, C.H., Saltzman, E., *et al.* (2006) The effects of the dietary glycemic load on type 2 diabetes risk factors during weight loss. *Obesity* 14, 2200–2209.

Pories, W.J., MacDonald, K.G., Jr, Morgan, E.J., Sinha, M.K., Dohm, G.L., *et al.* (1992) Surgical treatment of obesity and its effect on diabetes: 10-y follow-up. *The American Journal of Clinical Nutrition* 55, 582S–585S.

Prentice, A.M., Black, A.E., Coward, W.A. and Cole, T.J. (1996) Energy expenditure in overweight and obese adults in affluent societies: an analysis of 319 doubly-labelled water measurements. *European Journal of Clinical Nutrition* 50, 93–97.

Qi, L., Meigs, J.B., Liu, S., Manson, J.E., Mantzoros, C., *et al.* (2006) Dietary fibers and glycemic load, obesity, and plasma adiponectin levels in women with type 2 diabetes. *Diabetes Care* 29, 1501–1505.

Rahman, I., Biswas, S.K. and Kirkham, P.A. (2006) Regulation of inflammation and redox signaling by dietary polyphenols. *Biochemical Pharmacology* 72, 1439–1452.

Rajaram, S., Connell, K.M. and Sabate, J. (2010) Effect of almond-enriched high-monounsaturated fat diet on selected markers of inflammation: a randomised, controlled, crossover study. *The British Journal of Nutrition* 103, 907–912.

Ramachandran, A., Snehalatha, C., Mary, S., Mukesh, B., Bhaskar, A.D., *et al.* (2006) The Indian Diabetes Prevention Programme shows that lifestyle modification and metformin prevent type 2 diabetes in Asian Indian subjects with impaired glucose tolerance (IDPP-1). *Diabetologia* 49, 289–297.

Ratner, R., Goldberg, R., Haffner, S., Marcovina, S., Orchard, T., *et al.* (2005) Impact of intensive lifestyle and metformin therapy on cardiovascular disease risk factors in the diabetes prevention program. *Diabetes Care* 28, 888–894.

Ravussin, E. (1995) Low resting metabolic rate as a risk factor for weight gain: role of the sympathetic nervous system. *International Journal of Obesity and Related Metabolic Disorders: Journal of the International Association for the Study of Obesity* 19 Suppl 7, S8–S9.

Ravussin, E., Lillioja, S., Knowler, W.C., Christin, L., Freymond, D., *et al.* (1988) Reduced rate of energy expenditure as a risk factor for body-weight gain. *The New England Journal of Medicine* 318, 467–472.

Reuben, D.B., Judd-Hamilton, L., Harris, T.B., Seeman, T.E. and MacArthur Studies of Successful Aging (2003) The associations between physical activity and inflammatory markers in high-functioning older persons: MacArthur Studies of Successful Aging. *Journal of the American Geriatrics Society* 51, 1125–1130.

Rimm, E.B. and Stampfer, M.J. (2002) Wine, beer, and spirits: are they really horses of a different color? *Circulation* 105, 2806–2807.

Roberts, S.B., Savage, J., Coward, W.A., Chew, B. and Lucas, A. (1988) Energy expenditure and intake in infants born to lean and overweight mothers. *The New England Journal of Medicine* 318, 461–466.

Rokling-Andersen, M.H., Reseland, J.E., Veierod, M.B., Anderssen, S.A., Jacobs, D.R., Jr, *et al.* (2007) Effects of long-term exercise and diet intervention on plasma adipokine concentrations. *The American Journal of Clinical Nutrition* 86, 1293–1301.

Ross, R., Rissanen, J., Pedwell, H., Clifford, J. and Shragge, P. (1996) Influence of diet and exercise on skeletal muscle and visceral adipose tissue in men. *Journal of Applied Physiology* 81, 2445–2455.

Ross, R., Pedwell, H. and Rissanen, J. (1995) Effects of energy restriction and exercise on skeletal muscle and adipose tissue in women as measured by magnetic resonance imaging. *The American Journal of Clinical Nutrition* 61, 1179–1185.

Rothenbacher, D., Hoffmeister, A., Brenner, H. and Koenig, W. (2003) Physical activity, coronary heart disease, and inflammatory response. *Archives of Internal Medicine* 163, 1200–1205.

Ryan, D.H., Johnson, W.D., Myers, V.H., Prather, T.L., McGlone, M.M., *et al.* (2010) Nonsurgical weight loss for extreme obesity in primary care settings: results of the Louisiana Obese Subjects Study. *Archives of Internal Medicine* 170, 146–154.

Sacks, G., Swinburn, B. and Lawrence, M. (2009) Obesity Policy Action framework and analysis grids for a comprehensive policy approach to reducing obesity. *Obesity Reviews: An Official Journal of the International Association for the Study of Obesity* 10, 76–86.

Salas-Salvado, J., Bullo, M., Garcia-Lorda, P., Figueredo, R., Del Castillo, D., *et al.* (2006a) Subcutaneous adipose tissue cytokine production is not responsible for the restoration of systemic inflammation markers during weight loss. *International Journal of Obesity* 30, 1714–1720.

Salas-Salvado, J., Bullo, M., Perez-Heras, A. and Ros, E. (2006b) Dietary fibre, nuts and cardiovascular diseases. The *British Journal of Nutrition* 96 Suppl 2, S46–S51.

Salas-Salvado, J., Garcia-Arellano, A., Estruch, R., Marquez-Sandoval, F., Corella, D., *et al.* (2008) Components of the Mediterranean-type food pattern and serum inflammatory markers among patients at high risk for cardiovascular disease. *European Journal of Clinical Nutrition* 62, 651–659.

Sikand, G., Kondo, A., Foreyt, J.P., Jones, P.H. and Gotto, A.M., Jr (1988) Two-year follow-up of patients treated with a very-low-calorie diet and exercise training. *Journal of the American Dietetic Association* 88, 487–488.

Sjostrom, L., Lindroos, A.K., Peltonen, M., Torgerson, J., Bouchard, C., *et al.* (2004) Lifestyle, diabetes, and cardiovascular risk factors 10 years after bariatric surgery. *The New England Journal of Medicine* 351, 2683–2693.

Skender, M.L., Goodrick, G.K., Del Junco, D.J., Reeves, R.S., Darnell, L., *et al.* (1996) Comparison of 2-year weight loss trends in behavioral treatments of obesity: diet, exercise, and combination interventions. *Journal of the American Dietetic Association* 96, 342–346.

Smith, L.L., Anwar, A., Fragen, M., Rananto, C., Johnson, R., *et al.* (2000) Cytokines and cell adhesion molecules associated with high-intensity eccentric exercise. *European Journal of Applied Physiology* 82, 61–67.

Stallone, D.D. (1994) The influence of obesity and its treatment on the immune system. *Nutrition Reviews* 52, 37–50.

Stauffer, B.L., Hoetzer, G.L., Smith, D.T. and DeSouza, C.A. (2004) Plasma C-reactive protein is not elevated in physically active postmenopausal women taking hormone replacement therapy. *Journal of Applied Physiology* 96, 143–148.

Steensberg, A., Febbraio, M.A., Osada, T., Schjerling, P., van Hall, G., *et al.* (2001) Interleukin-6 production in contracting human skeletal muscle is influenced by pre-exercise muscle glycogen content. *The Journal of Physiology* 537, 633–639.

Stefanick, M.L., Mackey, S., Sheehan, M., Ellsworth, N., Haskell, W.L., *et al.* (1998) Effects of diet and exercise in men and postmenopausal women with low levels of HDL cholesterol and high levels of LDL cholesterol. *The New England Journal of Medicine* 339, 12–20.

Stewart, K.J., Bacher, A.C., Turner, K., Lim, J.G., Hees, P.S., *et al.* (2005) Exercise and risk factors associated with metabolic syndrome in older adults. *American Journal of Preventive Medicine* 28, 9–18.

Straczkowski, M., Kowalska, I., Dzienis-Straczkowska, S., Stepien, A., Skibinska, E., *et al.* (2001) Changes in tumor necrosis factor-alpha system and insulin sensitivity during an exercise training program in obese women with normal and impaired glucose tolerance. *European Journal of Endocrinology / European Federation of Endocrine Societies* 145, 273–280.

Sweeney, M.E., Hill, J.O., Heller, P.A., Baney, R. and DiGirolamo, M. (1993) Severe vs moderate energy restriction with and without exercise in the treatment of obesity: efficiency of weight loss. *The American Journal of Clinical Nutrition* 57, 127–134.

Tataranni, P.A., Harper, I.T., Snitker, S., Del Parigi, A., Vozarova, B., *et al.* (2003) Body weight gain in free-living Pima Indians: effect of energy intake vs expenditure. *International Journal of Obesity and Related Metabolic Disorders: Journal of the International Association for the Study of Obesity* 27, 1578–1583.

Theuwissen, E., Plat, J. and Mensink, R.P. (2009) Consumption of oat beta-glucan with or without plant stanols did not influence inflammatory markers in hypercholesterolemic subjects. *Molecular Nutrition & Food Research* 53, 370–376.

Thompson, P.D., Buchner, D., Pina, I.L., Balady, G.J., Williams, M.A., *et al.* (2003) Exercise and physical activity in the prevention and treatment of atherosclerotic cardiovascular disease: a statement from the Council on Clinical Cardiology (Subcommittee on Exercise, Rehabilitation, and Prevention) and the Council on Nutrition, Physical Activity, and Metabolism (Subcommittee on Physical Activity). *Circulation* 107, 3109–3116.

Tisi, P.V., Hulse, M., Chulakadabba, A., Gosling, P. and Shearman, C.P. (1997) Exercise training for intermittent claudication: does it adversely affect biochemical markers of the exercise-induced inflammatory response? *European Journal of Vascular and Endovascular Surgery: The Official Journal of the European Society for Vascular Surgery* 14, 344–350.

Tomaszewski, M., Charchar, F.J., Przybycin, M., Crawford, L., Wallace, A.M., *et al.* (2003) Strikingly low circulating CRP concentrations in ultramarathon runners independent of markers of adiposity: how low can you go? *Arteriosclerosis, Thrombosis, and Vascular Biology* 23, 1640–1644.

Troseid, M., Seljeflot, I., Hjerkinn, E.M. and Arnesen, H. (2009) Interleukin-18 is a strong predictor of cardiovascular events in elderly men with the metabolic syndrome: synergistic effect of inflammation and hyperglycemia. *Diabetes Care* 32, 486–492.

Tsukui, S., Kanda, T., Nara, M., Nishino, M., Kondo, T. and Kobayashi, I. (2000) Moderate-intensity regular exercise decreases serum tumor necrosis factor-alpha and HbA1c levels in healthy women. *International Journal of Obesity and Related Metabolic Disorders: Journal of the International Association for the Study of Obesity* 24, 1207–1211.

Tuomilehto, J., Lindstrom, J., Eriksson, J.G., Valle, T.T., Hamalainen, H., *et al.* (2001) Prevention of type 2 diabetes mellitus by changes in lifestyle among subjects with impaired glucose tolerance. *The New England Journal of Medicine* 344, 1343–1350.

Tziomalos, K., Dimitroula, H.V., Katsiki, N., Savopoulos, C. and Hatzitolios, A.I. (2010) Effects of lifestyle measures, antiobesity agents, and bariatric surgery on serological markers of inflammation in obese patients. *Mediators of Inflammation* DOI: 10.1155/2010/364957.

Van Aggel-Leijssen, D.P., Saris, W.H., Hul, G.B. and Van Baak, M.A. (2002) Long-term effects of low-intensity exercise training on fat metabolism in weight-reduced obese men. *Metabolism: Clinical and Experimental* 51, 1003–1010.

van Dale, D., Saris, W.H. and ten Hoor, F. (1990) Weight maintenance and resting metabolic rate 18-40 months after a diet/exercise treatment. *International Journal of Obesity* 14, 347–359.

Vanderwood, K.K., Hall, T.O., Harwell, T.S., Arave, D., Butcher, M.K., *et al.* (2011) Factors associated with the maintenance or achievement of the weight loss goal at follow-up among participants completing an adapted diabetes prevention program. *Diabetes Research and Clinical Practice* 91, 141–147.

Verdaet, D., Dendale, P., De Bacquer, D., Delanghe, J., Block, P., *et al.* (2004) Association between leisure time physical activity and markers of chronic inflammation related to coronary heart disease. *Atherosclerosis* 176, 303–310.

Vrolix, R. and Mensink, R.P. (2010) Effects of glycemic load on metabolic risk markers in subjects at increased risk of developing metabolic syndrome. *The American Journal of Clinical Nutrition* 92, 366–374.

Wadden, T.A., Vogt, R.A., Andersen, R.E., Bartlett, S.J., Foster, G.D., *et al.* (1997) Exercise in the treatment of obesity: effects of four interventions on body composition, resting energy expenditure, appetite, and mood. *Journal of Consulting and Clinical Psychology* 65, 269–277.

Wadden, T.A., Vogt, R.A., Foster, G.D. and Anderson, D.A. (1998) Exercise and the maintenance of weight loss: 1-year follow-up of a controlled clinical trial. *Journal of Consulting and Clinical Psychology* 66, 429–433.

Walzem, R.L. (2008) Wine and health: state of proofs and research needs. *Inflammopharmacology* 16(6), 265–271.

Wareham, N.J., van Sluijs, E.M. and Ekelund, U. (2005) Physical activity and obesity prevention: a review of the current evidence. *The Proceedings of the Nutrition Society* 64, 229–247.

Waxman, A. and World Health Assembly (2004) WHO global strategy on diet, physical activity and health. *Food and Nutrition Bulletin* 25, 292–302.

Weight, L.M., Alexander, D. and Jacobs, P. (1991) Strenuous exercise: analogous to the acute-phase response? *Clinical Science* 81, 677–683.

Weisberg, S.P., McCann, D., Desai, M., Rosenbaum, M., Leibel, R.L., *et al.* (2003) Obesity is associated with macrophage accumulation in adipose tissue. *The Journal of Clinical Investigation* 112, 1796–1808.

Westerterp, K.R. (2010) Physical activity, food intake, and body weight regulation: insights from doubly labeled water studies. *Nutrition Reviews* 68, 148–154.

Westerterp, K.R. and Goran, M.I. (1997) Relationship between physical activity related energy expenditure and body composition: a gender difference. *International Journal of Obesity and Related Metabolic Disorders: Journal of the International Association for the Study of Obesity* 21, 184–188.

Westerterp, K.R. and Speakman, J.R. (2008) Physical activity energy expenditure has not declined since the 1980s and matches energy expenditures of wild mammals. *International Journal of Obesity* (2005) 32(8), 1256–1263.

Wing, R.R., Epstein, L.H., Paternostro-Bayles, M., Kriska, A., Nowalk, M.P., *et al.* (1988) Exercise in a behavioural weight control programme for obese patients with Type 2 (non-insulin-dependent) diabetes. *Diabetologia* 31, 902–909.

Wing, R.R., Venditti, E., Jakicic, J.M., Polley, B.A. and Lang, W. (1998) Lifestyle intervention in overweight individuals with a family history of diabetes. *Diabetes Care* 21, 350–359.

Wolever, T.M., Gibbs, A.L., Mehling, C., Chiasson, J.L., Connelly, P.W., *et al.* (2008) The Canadian Trial of Carbohydrates in Diabetes (CCD), a 1-y controlled trial of low-glycemic-index dietary carbohydrate in type 2 diabetes: no effect on glycated hemoglobin but reduction in C-reactive protein. *The American Journal of Clinical Nutrition* 87, 114–125.

Wood, P.D., Stefanick, M.L., Williams, P.T. and Haskell, W.L. (1991) The effects on plasma lipoproteins of a prudent weight-reducing diet, with or without exercise, in overweight men and women. *The New England Journal of Medicine* 325, 461–466.

World Cancer Research Fund and American Institute for Cancer Research (2007) Food, Nutrition, Physical Activity, and the Prevention of Cancer: a Global Perspective. AICR, Washington DC.

World Health Organization (2003) Diet, Nutrition and the Prevention of Chronic Diseases (WHO Technical Report Series n°916). Available at: http://whqlibdoc.who.int/trs/WHO_TRS_916.pdf

World Health Organization (2006) Fact sheet N°311: Obesity and overweight. Geneva: Available at: http://www.who.int/mediacentre/factsheets/fs311/en/index.html (Accessed: 31 October 2010).

Yach, D., Stuckler, D. and Brownell, K.D. (2006) Epidemiologic and economic consequences of the global epidemics of obesity and diabetes. *Nature Medicine* 12, 62–66.

Yang, X., Telama, R., Leskinen, E., Mansikkaniemi, K., Viikari, J. and Raitakari, O.T. (2007) Testing a model of physical activity and obesity tracking from youth to adulthood: the cardiovascular risk in young Finns study. *International Journal of Obesity* 31, 521–527.

Zhang, B., Berger, J., Hu, E., Szalkowski, D., White-Carrington, S., *et al.* (1996) Negative regulation of peroxisome proliferator-activated receptor-gamma gene expression contributes to the antiadipogenic effects of tumor necrosis factor-alpha. *Molecular Endocrinology* 10, 1457–1466.

Zhao, G., Etherton, T.D., Martin, K.R., Vanden Heuvel, J.P., Gillies, P.J., *et al.* (2005) Anti-inflammatory effects of polyunsaturated fatty acids in THP-1 cells. *Biochemical and Biophysical Research Communications* 336, 909–917.

13 Type 2 Diabetes and Inflammation

J. Lieffers, B. Hawkins, A. Hofstra, D. Cheung, L.L. McCargar and C.J. Field*
Alberta Diabetes Institute, University of Alberta, Canada

Introduction

Type 2 diabetes (T2D) and metabolic syndrome (MetS) are both associated with low-grade systemic inflammation (Pickup, 2004). Type 2 diabetes is a metabolic disorder characterized by chronic hyperglycaemia with disturbances of carbohydrate, fat and protein metabolism resulting from defects in insulin secretion, insulin action or both (Alberti and Zimmet, 1998). By 2030, the number of people with diabetes worldwide is predicted to be 366 million (Wild *et al.*, 2004), whereby 90–95% of these cases are people with T2D (Doria *et al.*, 2008).

* Corresponding author, catherine.field@ualberta.ca

The World Health Organization (WHO) clinical criteria for MetS include insulin resistance plus any two of the following: high blood pressure, plasma triglycerides >150 mg/dl, high-density lipoprotein (HDL) <35 mg/dl, body mass index (BMI) >30 kg/m^2 or urinary albumin excretion rate ≥20 µg/min or albumin: creatinine ratio ≥30 mg/g (Grundy *et al.*, 2004).

Chronic inflammation is characterized by a decrease in adiponectin (Duncan *et al.*, 2004) and an increase in the plasma/serum biomarkers C-reactive protein (CRP), interleukin 6 (IL-6) and tumour necrosis factor alpha (TNF-α) (Duncan *et al.*, 2003). Even though other inflammatory markers exist, these four biomarkers are the most commonly measured in research studies. Higher plasma concentrations of adiponectin have been associated with a lower incidence of diabetes (Duncan *et al.*, 2004), whereas higher TNF-α and elevated IL-6 concentrations have been suggested to induce insulin resistance in adipose tissue by inhibiting insulin signalling (Maachi *et al.*, 2004). A significant positive correlation between CRP concentrations and circulating IL-6 and TNF-α concentration has been reported (Maachi *et al.*, 2004). CRP is a commonly used biomarker for inflammation because there are not diurnal changes, and it is easily measured by highly sensitive assays (Libby and Ridker, 2004). It is now generally accepted that serum CRP concentrations are an independent risk factor for cardiovascular disease (CVD) such that <1.0 mg/l is low risk, 1.0–3.0 mg/l is average risk and high risk is >3.0 mg/l (Pearson *et al.*, 2003).

Diet and exercise can play a beneficial role in the prevention of diabetes (Eriksson and Lindgarde, 1991) as well as decreasing inflammatory markers in related conditions such as obesity (Bruun *et al.*, 2006). Thus, it is likely that these lifestyle factors could also reduce inflammatory markers in individuals with T2D or MetS. Although there is a growing body of literature to support this hypothesis, to our knowledge, there has not been a comprehensive review published to aid health professionals in making recommendations aimed at reducing chronic inflammation in individuals with T2D or MetS. The objective of the following chapter is to review the evidence for diet and exercise in inflammation in those with T2D or MetS.

Effects of Diet

Glycaemic index/load and fibre

Glycaemic index/load

Five studies (four cross-sectional and one randomized controlled trial [RCT]) have reported on the effect of glycaemic index (GI) and glycaemic load (GL) on inflammation in subjects with diabetes or metabolic syndrome (Table 13.1). In two cross-sectional studies, meals with increasing GI and GL were independently negatively associated with plasma adiponectin (Qi *et al.*, 2005, 2006a). Qi *et al.* (2006a) performed a cross-sectional analysis of 902 women with T2D from the Nurses' Health Study and Qi *et al.* (2005) studied 780 males with T2D from the Health Professionals Follow-up Study. In females, plasma adiponectin was 17% lower in the highest quintile of GL and 18% lower in the highest quintile of GI (Qi *et al.*, 2006a) compared with the lowest quintile after adjustment for covariates. In another study by the same authors, the same association of GI and GL with plasma adiponectin concentrations was reported. Plasma adiponectin was 13% and 18% lower in the highest quintiles of GI and GL, respectively, compared with the lowest quintile after adjustment for covariates (Qi *et al.*, 2005). In the same study, the additive effect of both cereal fibre and GL was examined. Males who had the highest GL and lowest cereal fibre intakes and males who consumed the lowest GL and highest cereal fibre intakes had the lowest and highest plasma adiponectin levels, respectively (difference of 3.7 µg/ml, $P = 0.0097$; Qi *et al.*, 2005).

Two cross-sectional studies examined associations between dietary GI/GL and inflammatory biomarkers (CRP and/or tumour necrosis factor receptor 2 [TNF-R2] concentrations) (Qi *et al.*, 2006b; Du *et al*, 2008). After adjusting for age, BMI, smoking, HbA1c, physical activity, dietary fibre, magnesium and fibre intake, Qi *et al* (2006b) observed significantly lower plasma CRP (5.05 mg/l versus 6.68 mg/l) and TNF-R2 (2387 pg/ml versus 2660 pg/ml) concentrations in the lowest quintile for dietary GI, compared with the highest in women with T2D from the Nurses'

Table 13.1. Summary of the studies that have examined the relationship/effect of dietary intake on inflammation in subjects with diabetes or MetS.

Author, year	Study design	Duration	Sample	Variable	Physical activity	Marker(s)	Results
Glycaemic index/load and fibre							
Qi *et al.*, 2006a	Cross-sectional analysis of a prospective cohort study	N/A	n = 902 women, T2D, 30–55 years	Dietary fibre (cereal fibre), glycaemic load, glycaemic index Fruit fibre	Adjusted for in analysis	Adiponectin	Cereal fibre: adiponectin concentration was 24% higher in highest intake quintile compared with the lowest quintile GI/GL: adiponectin 18% and 17% lower for the highest compared with lowest quintile for GI and GL, respectively No relationship with fruit fibre intake
Qi *et al.*, 2005	Cross-sectional analysis of a prospective cohort study	N/A	n = 780 men, T2D, 40–75 years	Cereal fibre, glycaemic load, glycaemic index	Adjusted for in analysis	Adiponectin	GI/GL: plasma adiponectin 13% and 18% lower in highest quintiles compared to the lowest quintile for GI and GL, respectively Cereal fibre: plasma adiponectin 19% higher in highest quintile compared to the lowest quintile - this diminished after adjustment for Mg
Qi *et al.*, 2006b	Cross-sectional analysis of a prospective cohort study	N/A	n = 902 women, T2D, 30–55 years	Whole grains, dietary cereal fibre, glycaemic index	Adjusted for in analysis	hs-CRP TNF-R2	CRP: decreasing trend with increasing quintiles of whole-grain, bran and cereal fibre TNF-R2: decreasing trend with increasing cereal fibre, and whole-grain intakes Cereal fibre: CRP 18% lower and TNF-R2 8% lower in highest quintile compared to the lowest quintile GI: CRP and TNF-R2 32% and 11% higher, respectively, in highest quintile compared to the lowest quintile

Continued

Table 13.1. Continued.

Author, year	Study design	Duration	Sample	Variable	Physical activity	Marker(s)	Results
Du *et al.*, 2008	Cross-sectional analysis of observational data from two studies	N/A	n = 974 (517 M, 457 F), 42–87 years with T2D or MetS	Glycaemic index, glycaemic load	Adjusted for in analysis	hs-CRP	GI: increase of 10 units (difference between the lowest and highest quintile) of GI intake was associated with a 29% increase in CRP concentration GL: no significant association
Wolever *et al.*, 2008	Randomized controlled clinical trial	1 year	n = 162, (74 M, 88 F), 35–75 years with T2D	Glycaemic index Randomized to one of three diets: high-CHO, high GI; high-CHO, low GI; low-CHO, MUFA (low-CHO)	Not reported	hs-CRP	Significant effect of diet CRP with low-GI diet was 29% less than with the high-GI diet. CRP decreased ≥20% by 12 months in low-GI diet compared with baseline High-GI diet, CRP increased by 40% and stabilized at 15–20% above baseline from 3–12 months
Jenkins *et al.*, 2002	Randomized cross-over study	3-month crossover, 8-week washout	n = 23 (16 M, 7 post-menopausal F), T2D, mean age 63 years	Wheat bran (19 g/day additional wheat bran cereal fibre)	Maintain regular level	hs-CRP	No treatment effect seen
Kallio *et al.*, 2008	Randomized controlled clinical trial	3 months	n = 47 (24 M, 23 F), MetS, mean age 55 years	Postprandial insulin response: oat and wheat bread and potato (high ppIR) versus rye bread and pasta (low ppIR)	Not reported	hs-CRP TNF-α TNF-α mRNA IL-6	hs-CRP unchanged TNF-α was not significantly different between the two groups TNF-α mRNA expression in subcutaneous adipose tissue was up-regulated in the high ppIR diet compared to baseline (1.24-fold upregulation of mRNA, $P = 0.024$) IL-6 change was borderline significant between the two groups ($P = 0.055$)

Mediterranean diet							
Mena *et al.*, 2009	Randomized controlled study	3 months	n = 106 (60 M, 46 F), mean age 68 years, T2D	3 groups: (i) Low fat diet (n = 36) (ii) Med Diet + virgin olive oil (n = 35) (iii) Med Diet + mixed nuts (n = 35)	Evaluated at baseline and after 3 months. No change observed	hs-CRP IL-6	IL-6 was reduced by >10% in both Med Diet groups compared to baseline. Low-fat diet increased IL-6 by >20% compared with baseline The Med Diet + virgin olive oil group decreased CRP by >30% compared with baseline. CRP did not significantly change in the other groups
Salas-Salvadó *et al.*, 2008	Cross-sectional analysis	N/A	n = 772 (339 M, 433 F), 55–80 years, T2D	Mediterranean diet	Not reported	hs-CRP IL-6 ICAM-1 VCAM-1	The highest tertile for both fruit and cereal consumption associated with a lower IL-6 by 4.2% and 11.7%, respectively, compared with the lowest tertile No association with IL-6 Higher consumption of nuts and olive oil associated with lower vCAM-1 and/or iCAM-1 Adherence score to Med diet did not significantly correlate with inflammatory markers
Esposito *et al.*, 2006	Randomized controlled clinical trial	24 months	n = 65 men (35 intervention, 30 control), MetS, mean age 44 years	Med diet and control diet (advised about healthy eating)	Recommend >30 min/day. Both groups increase PA	hs-CRP	CRP decreased significantly more in the Med Diet group compared with the control group (–0.9 mg/dl versus –0.1 mg/dl, $P < 0.01$)
Caffeine/caffeinated coffee							
Williams *et al.*, 2008	Cross-sectional analysis of a prospective cohort study	N/A	n = 982 women with T2D, mean ages for quartiles of caffeinated coffee ranged from 58.1–59.2 years	Caffeinated coffee intake	Adjusted for estimated physical activity exercise	Adiponectin	Those consuming ≥4 cups/day had significantly higher adiponectin concentrations ($P = 0.004$) than those who consumed <1 cup/week

Continued

Table 13.1. Continued.

Author, year	Study design	Duration	Sample	Variable	Physical activity	Marker(s)	Results
Lopez-Garcia *et al.*, 2006	Cross-sectional analysis of a prospective cohort: nested case-control	N/A	n = 663 women with T2D, mean ages for categories of caffeinated coffee consumption ranged from 57–59 years	Caffeinated coffee intake	Adjusted for estimated physical activity	hs-CRP TNF-αR2	Significant inverse association of caffeinated coffee with plasma CRP (the adjusted CRP change was –10.2% per 1 cup/day caffeinated coffee increase) Similar relationship for just caffeine intake No association of caffeinated coffee intake with TNF-αR2
Antioxidants							
Rytter *et al.*, 2010	Parallel randomized double-blind placebo-controlled trial	12 weeks	n = 40 (18 M, 22 F), randomly assigned to 3 groups (control group, single antioxidant dose, double antioxidant dose), mean age 62 years T2D	Antioxidant supplement (extracted from fruits, berries and vegetables)	Asked to keep physical activity levels stable	hs-CRP IL-6	No changes in hs-CRP or IL-6
Devaraj and Jalal, 2000	Selective controlled trial Clinical trial	3 months	n = 72 (26 M, 46 F) with T2D who have (DM2-MV) (n = 23) or do not have (DM2) (n = 24) macro-vascular complications or matched healthy controls without T2D (n = 25). Middle-aged males and females	1200 IU/day of RRR-α tocopherol	Asked to not change PA levels	hs-CRP IL-6	DM2-MV had significantly higher hs-CRP levels at baseline compared with DM2 and controls. hs-CRP decreased (*P*<0.02) in all three groups DM2 and DM2-MV had significantly higher levels of IL-6 at baseline compared with the control group. IL-6 significantly decreased following supplementation in all three groups (*P*<0.02)

Asgard *et al.*, 2007	Cross-sectional study	N/A	n = 54 (25 M, 29 F), mean age 63 years T2D	Fruits and vegetables/ antioxidants measured using dietary records	Not reported	hs-CRP IL-6	Plasma carotenoids were negatively correlated with IL-6 Plasma γ-tocopherol was positively associated with CRP
Omega-3 fatty acids							
De Luis *et al.*, 2009	Open label trial	12 weeks	n = 30 (16 M, 14 F), T2D, mean age 55 years	Omega-3 fatty acids supplement (1.7 g DHA + EPA)	Not reported	hs-CRP TNF-α IL-6	CRP: significantly decreased (–34.8%) compared to baseline TNF-α: significantly decreased (–18.1%) compared to baseline IL-6: no significant changes
Wong *et al.*, 2010	Double blind randomized placebo-controlled trial	12 weeks	n = 97 (43 M, 54 F), T2D, mean age 60 years	Omega-3 fatty acids (2.7 g DHA + EPA) (4 g/day fish oil) or olive oil	Asked to not change lifestyle	hs-CRP	No treatment effect seen
Vitamin D							
Luo *et al.*, 2009	Cross-sectional design with a supplement intervention in those with low vitamin D status	3 months (open label trial)	n = 109 (52 M, 57 F), >50 years T2D, n = 21 for supplement trial	Vitamin D Vitamin D (2000 IU in supplement trial)	Not reported	hs-CRP	Cross-sectional study: No difference in CRP concentration between vitamin D deficient and replete participants Open label trial: No effect of vitamin D supplementation on CRP
Targher *et al.*, 2006	Cross-sectional design	N/A	n = 390 (253 M, 137 F) T2D, mean age 58 years	Vitamin D	Not reported	hs-CRP	Those with hypovitaminosis had significantly higher CRP (13.7%) compared to those without
Magnesium status							
Qi *et al.*, 2005	Cross-sectional analysis of a prospective cohort study	N/A	n = 780 men, T2D, 40–75 years	Magnesium intake	Adjusted for in analysis	Adiponectin	Magnesium intake had a positive association with adiponectin concentration (*P* for trend = 0.011)

Continued

Table 13.1. Continued.

Author, year	Study design	Duration	Sample	Variable	Physical activity	Marker(s)	Results
Evangelopoulos *et al.*, 2008	Case control	N/A	n = 117 (25 M, 92 F) MetS (n = 82) No MetS (n = 35) Mean age MetS: 67 years, No MetS: 65 years	Serum magnesium	Adjusted for in analysis: 4 MetS and 2 No MetS participants had light physical activity (20–30 mins 3/week) All others were sedentary	hs-CRP/CRP	MetS subjects had 9% lower serum Mg (P<0.001) and 110% higher hs-CRP (P<0.001) compared with control subjects Serum Mg was inversely correlated with CRP
Guerrero-Romero and Rodriquez-Moran, 2006	Case control	N/A	n = 441 MetS (63 M, 84 F) Healthy control (131 M, 163 W) Mean age MetS 44.0 years, No MetS 43.0 years	Serum magnesium	Not reported	hs-CRP	Hypomagnesemia was significantly associated with CRP and with MetS When controlling for malondialdehyde levels there was no relationship between CRP and MetS After adjusting for magnesium levels, CRP remained associated to MetS
Red wine							
Marfella *et al.*, 2006	Randomized secondary prevention trial	1 year	n = 115 (57 intervention, 58 control), T2D, <70 years (mean: intervention group 36.5 years, controls: 35.1 years)	Red wine (118ml/day)	Encouraged to walk 1 h 3 times a week	hs-CRP TNF-α IL-6	Control group had significantly higher concentrations of TNF-α, IL-6 and CRP compared with the red wine group at the end of the intervention

CHO, carbohydrate; DM2-MV, type 2 diabetes with macrovascular disease; F, female; GI, glycaemic index; GL, glycaemic load; hs-CRP, high-sensitivity CRP; ICAM-1, intercellular adhesion molecule 1; M, male; MetS, metabolic syndrome; MUFA, monounsaturated fatty acid; ppIR, postprandial insulin response; T2D, type 2 diabetes; TNF-R2, tumour necrosis factor receptor 2; VCAM-1, vascular cell adhesion molecule 1.

Health Study. Du *et al.* (2008) conducted a cross-sectional analysis of males and females (n = 974) from the Dutch population. They found similar associations to Qi *et al.* (2006b), and reported that an increase of 10 units of GI intake (difference between the highest and lowest quintiles) was associated with a 29% increase in serum CRP, even after adjusting for covariates. Glycaemic load was not found to be associated with CRP or TNF-R2 in these studies (Qi *et al.*, 2006b; Du *et al.*, 2008). These results are consistent with studies that have reported an association between the GI and CRP concentrations in a non-diabetic population (Liu *et al.*, 2002).

One RCT investigated the relationship between serum CRP concentration and GI in 162 participants (Wolever *et al.*, 2008). Those who consumed a high-carbohydrate, low-GI diet for 1 year had a >20% CRP reduction from baseline, and a mean CRP concentration 29% less than participants consuming a high-carbohydrate, high-GI diet. These results support the findings from the cross-sectional studies.

Fibre

Five studies (three nested cross-sectional studies and two clinical trials) have examined the relationship between cereal fibre intake and inflammatory markers in diabetes or metabolic syndrome (Table 13.1). Two cross-sectional studies observed a significant increasing trend of adiponectin when comparing the highest quintile of dietary cereal fibre intake with the lowest in males (n = 780, 19% difference; Qi *et al.*, 2005) and women (n = 902, 24% difference; Qi *et al.*, 2006a) after adjusting for both GL and other potential covariables. In females, those with a BMI <25 kg/m^2 with the highest cereal fibre intakes tended to have the highest adiponectin concentrations, whereas those who were obese (BMI >30 kg/m^2) and had the lowest cereal fibre intakes had the lowest plasma adiponectin concentrations after adjusting for covariates (Qi *et al.*, 2006a). This suggests that physical activity and BMI modify the relationship between cereal fibre intake and adiponectin concentrations in males. Consistent with this, the association between cereal fibre and plasma adiponectin concentrations was significantly stronger in those with a lower BMI or those who were more physically active than those with a higher BMI or low physical activity levels (Qi *et al.*, 2005). Intakes of total fibre, vegetable fibre and fruit fibre were not significantly associated with plasma adiponectin after adjusting for covariates including BMI in males and females (Qi *et al.*, 2005, 2006a).

The relationships between whole grain, wheat-germ and bran intakes on TNF-R2 and CRP were studied in a cross-sectional study of female participants with T2D from the Nurses' Health study (Qi *et al.*, 2006b). All analyses included adjustments for covariates, including GI and BMI. A significant decreasing trend of CRP concentration with increasing quintiles of whole grain and bran intakes was reported. CRP concentrations were 18% lower and TNF-R2 was 8% lower in the highest quintile of cereal fibre intake compared with the lowest quintile (Qi *et al.*, 2006b). Wheat-germ intake was not associated with levels of CRP or TNF-R2.

In contrast with results from the cross-sectional studies, clinical trial data do not support a relationship between cereal fibre intake and CRP concentrations. Feeding a diet rich in cereal fibre did not reduce serum CRP concentration in 23 participants with T2D (Jenkins *et al.*, 2002). In this 12-week randomized cross-over study, subjects were supplemented with breakfast cereals high in cereal fibre (+19 g cereal fibre/day) and compared with a low-fibre diet (+4 g cereal fibre/day). Several factors in this study may have influenced study results, such as a short study duration, small sample size, and the inclusion of subjects with both a lower BMI and low baseline CRP concentrations compared with those subjects included in the cross-sectional studies. Another 12-week RCT by Kallio *et al.* (2008) randomized 47 participants to one of two different replacement bread/pasta diets differing in postprandial insulin responses (ppIR) (oat, wheat and potato for the high ppIR diet, and rye and pasta for the low ppIR diet). They observed no change in plasma high-sensitivity (hs)-CRP and a borderline significant change in IL-6 ($P = 0.055$) concentrations between the two groups (IL-6 increased in the high ppIR group compared with the low ppIR group). A longer intervention might be needed to see changes in serum markers because TNF-α mRNA expression in subcutaneous adipose tissue was 1.24-fold higher ($P = 0.024$) from baseline in those who had consumed the high-ppIR diet (Kallio *et al.*, 2008). This suggests that the diet had an effect on inflammatory markers in adipose tissue.

In summary, the results of four cross-sectional studies suggest that consuming a low GI diet is associated with higher adiponectin concentration and lower inflammatory markers (CRP and TNF-R2) in plasma (Qi *et al.*, 2005, 2006a, b; Du *et al.*, 2008). This beneficial effect of a low GI diet on inflammatory markers was confirmed in a 1-year trial (Wolever *et al.*, 2008). There is also evidence from cross-sectional studies that consuming a diet rich in cereal fibres has beneficial effects on plasma inflammatory markers but this may be complicated by physical activity and BMI. Clinical trials have yet to confirm this association.

Mediterranean diet

Three studies (two RCTs and one cross-sectional) have examined the effect of the Mediterranean diet on at least one marker of inflammation (Table 13.1). The three-month RCT by Mena *et al.* (2009) compared 106 participants randomized to one of 3 groups: (i) a low-fat diet, or a Mediterranean diet supplemented with either (ii) mixed nuts or (iii) virgin olive oil (VOO). Both Mediterranean diet groups were advised to increase intake of vegetable oils and fats and the low-fat diet group was advised to decrease intake of all types of fat (Mena *et al.*, 2009). In both Mediterranean diet groups there was a significant decrease in IL-6 by >10%, whereas IL-6 concentrations increased by >20% in the low-fat diet group compared with baseline. Concentrations of CRP significantly decreased by >30% in the VOO group; however, there was no significant change in the other groups. Esposito *et al.* (2006) conducted a 24 month RCT in 65 males with MetS and fed either a Mediterranean diet or a control diet. Feeding the Mediterranean diet significantly reduced CRP concentrations by ~38% compared with baseline; there was no change in the control group. In a cross-sectional study, Salas-Salvado *et al.* (2008) evaluated the association between components of the Mediterranean diet and markers of inflammation in 772 participants who completed a questionnaire that measured adherence to the Mediterranean diet. For each Mediterranean dietary component, participants were placed in one of three tertiles (high, average or low) on the basis of their self-reported adherence. Inflammatory markers were then compared between tertiles for each food segment. The highest tertile for both fruit and cereal consumption was associated with the lowest IL-6 concentrations. There was, however, no effect of overall Mediterranean diet adherence on IL-6 concentrations.

The study by Esposito *et al.* (2006) provides the most convincing support for the benefits of a Mediterranean diet on reducing inflammation biomarkers in blood. This RCT included subjects who had CRP concentrations in the lower risk range (~2.4 mg/l) and demonstrated a significant decrease in CRP concentrations. A limitation of this and most of the studies of the Mediterranean diet pattern is the inability to determine whether it is one or more of the individual components or the total pattern that has beneficial effects on inflammatory markers (Esposito *et al.*, 2006). The results of the study by Mena *et al.* (2009) suggest that olive oil may be one of the bioactive components and the study by Salas-Salvado *et al.* (2008) suggests that the dietary fibre intake might be responsible for a large portion of the effect. Future studies systematically isolating the various components of the Mediterranean diet pattern might provide more insights into the beneficial components.

Antioxidants

Three studies (two clinical trials and one cross-sectional survey) have examined the inflammatory response to antioxidant supplementation in diabetes (Table 13.1). In a cross-sectional study of 54 T2D patients, Asgard *et al.* (2007) reported a significant positive correlation between dietary intake of fruits and vegetables and several antioxidants (e.g. β-carotene, α-tocopherol, vitamin E, vitamin C and selenium) with plasma antioxidant concentrations (e.g. α-tocopherol, α-carotene, β-carotene, ascorbate and lycopene). They observed a significant inverse correlation between plasma carotenoids, lutein and lycopene and plasma IL-6 concentration.

The effects of supplementation on high-sensitivity (hs)-CRP and plasma IL-6 concentration were investigated in two clinical trials, with conflicting results (Devaraj and Jialal, 2000; Rytter *et al.*, 2010). Supplementation with two different doses of antioxidant capsules made from a fruit, berry and vegetable extract was conducted in a 12-week parallel randomized, double-blind, placebo-controlled trial (n = 40; Rytter *et al.*, 2010). Antioxidant treatment significantly increased plasma concentrations of all measured antioxidants (with the exception of α-tocopherol) compared with the control group (Rytter *et al.*, 2010) but did not significantly change plasma hs-CRP or IL-6 concentrations. Devaraj and Jialal (2000) performed a controlled trial in 75 age-, sex- and BMI-matched men and women who they divided into three groups: those who had T2D with or without macrovascular complications, and a group of non-diabetic control subjects. Baseline plasma hs-CRP concentrations were significantly elevated in those with T2D and macrovascular complications (~12 mg/l) compared with those with T2D without macrovascular complications (~8mg/l) or the control subjects (~6 mg/l). Baseline monocyte IL-6 concentrations were significantly higher in both T2D groups compared to controls. After all groups were supplemented daily for 3 months with 1200 IU/day of RRR-α-tocopherol, there was a significant decrease in plasma hs-CRP and monocyte IL-6 concentrations (P <0.02) in all three groups compared to baseline. Unlike the first trial reviewed, during supplementation, plasma and mononuclear cell α-tocopherol significantly increased 2- to 2.5-fold, suggesting that this may be the important antioxidant. There were several other differences between the two clinical trials, including baseline concentrations of inflammatory markers and antioxidant supplementation doses, which might also have contributed to the different results. Rytter *et al.* (2010) studied a sample who had lower baseline CRP and IL-6 concentrations compared with the population studied by Devaraj and Jialal (2000). The combination of antioxidants supplemented by Rytter *et al.* (2010) provided 40 and 80 mg/day of α-tocopherol for the single-and double-dose groups, much lower than the 1200 IU (or 804 mg) of α-tocopherol supplemented in the study by Devaraj and Jialal (2000). Rytter *et al.* (2010) did not observe a significant difference in plasma α-tocopherol with supplementation of any dose compared with the control group, suggesting that this combination antioxidant supplement was not enough to increase plasma levels and impact inflammation.

In summary, there is evidence from an epidemiological study that diets high in antioxidants are associated with lower biomarkers of inflammation in diabetes. Clinical interventions suggest that supplementation of antioxidants, particularly those that increase plasma α-tocopherol concentrations, to individuals with T2D and elevated inflammatory biomarkers is effective in reducing plasma inflammation (CRP and IL-6 concentrations).

Caffeine

Two nested case-control analyses of the Nurses' Health Study data have reported an association between caffeinated coffee intake and plasma adiponectin and CRP (Table 13.1). Williams *et al.* (2008) studied 982 women with T2D and found that after adjusting for numerous covariates including age, BMI, smoking and physical activity, those who consumed more than 4 cups/day of caffeine-containing coffee had significantly higher concentrations of plasma adiponectin (7.7 μg/ml) than those who drank <1 cup per week (6.1 μg/ml). The relationship remained after further adjustment for dietary factors such as glycaemic load, dietary fibre and the Mediterranean diet pattern. In 663 women with T2D, Lopez-Garcia *et al.* (2006) observed a significant inverse association between caffeinated coffee intake, adjusted for other dietary factors and CRP concentration; the adjusted CRP change was -10.2% per 1 cup/day caffeinated coffee increase. There was no association between sTNF-R2 and caffeinated coffee intake in this study (Lopez-Garcia *et al.*, 2006). There were no associations between decaffeinated coffee intakes on adiponectin or CRP concentrations, strongly suggesting that caffeine was the compound responsible for the association (Lopez-Garcia *et al.*, 2006; Williams *et al.*, 2008). At least in this cohort, coffee, more specifically caffeine intake, is associated with reduced markers of inflammation in those with T2D. Clinical trials are required to support the findings.

Red wine

A randomized, secondary controlled trial examined the effects of red wine intake on inflammation in individuals with T2D following an acute myocardial infarction (Table 13.1). Marfella *et al.* (2006) randomized 115 participants to a diet similar to the Mediterranean diet with or without 118 ml of red wine each day. At the end of the 12-month intervention, the group consuming red wine had significantly lower TNF-α, IL-6 and CRP concentrations than the control group. More studies are needed to confirm this finding and to study the various compounds (e.g. resveratrol) in red wine that might have anti-inflammatory properties.

Omega-3 fatty acids

Two studies (one open label study and one RCT) have examined the effects of supplementation with omega-3 fatty acids on inflammatory biomarkers in individuals with T2D (Table 13.1). De Luis *et al.* (2009) conducted an open label trial with 30 participants who were supplemented with 930 mg eicosapentaenoic acid (EPA) and 750 mg docosahexaenoic acid (DHA) (total 1680 mg omega-3 fatty acids) a day. After 12 weeks, they found a significant decrease in plasma CRP (−34.8%) and serum TNF-α (−18.1%) but not serum IL-6 concentrations. In a 12-week double-blind, placebo-controlled trial with 97 participants, however, daily supplementation with 4 g of fish oil (containing 2.7 g DHA + EPA) did not have a significant effect on CRP concentrations compared with those who were supplemented with olive oil capsules (Wong *et al.*, 2010). These two studies differed in population characteristics. The De Luis *et al.* (2009) study population were obese at baseline (mean BMI 31.2) and had elevated CRP concentrations, suggesting that omega-3 fatty acid supplementation might be more effective in those with CVD risk factors.

Vitamin D

Two studies (one cross-sectional survey and one intervention trial) have examined the association between vitamin D and inflammatory markers in individuals with T2D (Table 13.1). A cross-sectional study by Targher *et al.* (2006) separated 390 T2D participants into those with vitamin D deficiency (serum 25(OH)D ≤37.5 nmol/l) and those without. Participants with hypovitaminosis D had a small but statistically higher mean CRP concentration (4.98mg/l versus 4.30mg/l, P = 0.001) compared with the group without. In an intervention study involving 109 Chinese participants with T2D, Luo *et al.* (2009) found no differences in hs-CRP concentrations in those they defined as hypovitaminosis D (serum 25(OH)D ≤ 50 nmol/l) compared with those with normal vitamin D status. In addition, Luo *et al.* (2009) treated a subset of 21 of those with hypovitaminosis D with vitamin D3 (2000 IU cholecalciferol) daily for 3 months. While vitamin D concentrations doubled, hs-CRP concentrations were unchanged (Luo *et al.*, 2009).

Both studies used serum 25(OH) vitamin D to define baseline vitamin D status; however, there were some differences between the two studies. The definition of hypovitaminosis D differed between studies. The Luo *et al.* (2009) study defined hypovitaminosis D as serum 25(OH)D ≤50 nmol/l, whereas Targher *et al.* (2006) defined hypovitaminosis D as serum 25(OH)D ≤37.5 nmol/l. The differences might also be due to dissimilar study populations, however. In the study by Luo *et al.* (2009), participants were Chinese immigrants with normal CRP concentrations (mean ~1.0 mg/l; Pearson *et al.*, 2003) and median BMI in the normal weight range, whereas the individuals from the Targher *et al.* (2006) study had higher CRP concentrations (mean concentrations of 4–5 mg/l; Pearson *et al.*, 2003) and a mean BMI in the overweight range.

Magnesium status

Two case control studies and one cross-sectional study have examined the association between magnesium status and inflammation in diabetes (Table 13.1). Evangelopoulos *et al.* (2008) reported that serum magnesium concentrations were significantly lower (9%), and hs-CRP concentrations were significantly higher (110%) in those with MetS compared with those without (Evangelopoulos *et al.*, 2008). They also reported an inverse relationship between serum magnesium concentrations and CRP in participants with MetS. However, another study by Guerrero-Romero and Rodriquez-Moran (2006), found a relationship between metabolic syndrome and serum magnesium, but hypomagnesemia was not strongly associated with CRP concentrations. In yet another study, Qi *et al.* (2005) reported, in a cross-sectional study of 780 males with T2D, that adiponectin concentrations were positively related to higher quintiles of magnesium intake. More research is needed to establish the relationship between dietary magnesium, magnesium status and inflammation.

Conclusions

The relationships between dietary components and inflammatory biomarkers in individuals with T2D and MetS are summarized in Fig. 13.1 and Table 13.2. The main conclusions are:

1. A low-GI diet and a Mediterranean diet pattern have more conclusive results for significantly improving or being associated with improved plasma inflammatory markers in diabetes and MetS (Fig. 13.1). RCTs indicate that following a low-GI diet or a Mediterranean dietary pattern is effective in decreasing CRP concentrations. Cross-sectional studies also support associations between consumption of a low-GI diet and lower CRP, TNF-α and increased adiponectin concentrations. Mediterranean diets high in fruits and cereals are associated with decreased IL-6 concentrations. The small number of studies in these categories indicates, however, a need for further research to assist in confirming the nutrient or combination of nutrients that contribute to the anti-inflammatory properties of these dietary patterns.

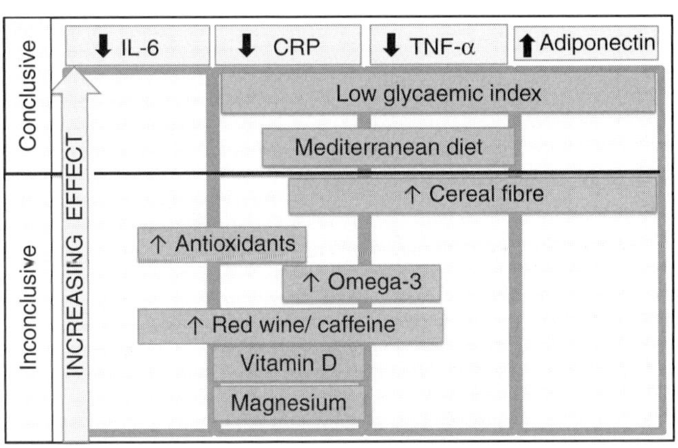

Fig. 13.1. Summary of the effects of diet on inflammation in diabetes. IL, interleukin; CRP, C-reactive protein; TNF-α, tumour necrosis factor-α.

Table 13.2. Summary of the relationship between diet and inflammatory markers in studies of subjects with diabetes or MetS.

Diet/nutrient	Study design	Number of papers	Inflammatory marker (plasma/serum) hs-CRP/CRP	TNF-α	IL-6	Adiponectin
Glycaemic index/load (GI/GL) and cereal fibre (CF)	Cross-sectional	4	Inverse relationship[a] 18% lower in higher CF (2/2)	Inverse relationship[a] 8% lower in high CF/WG (1/1)	Not studied	Direct relationship[a] 19–24% higher in higher CF (2/2)
			Direct relationship ↑29% with 10↑ unit GI[a] (2/2)	Direct relationship[a] 11% higher in higher GI (1/1)	Not studied	Inverse relationship[a] 13–18% lower in higher GI/GL (2/2)
	RCT	2	>20% decrease in low GI (1/2)	Not studied	Not studied	Not studied
Post-prandial insulin response (ppIR)	RCT	1	No effect	No effect	No effect	Not studied
Antioxidants	Cross-sectional	1	Direct relationship (plasma γ-tocopherol) (1/1)	Not studied	Inverse relationship (plasma carotenoids) (1/1)	Not studied
	RCT/selective trials	2	↓Decrease (α-tocopherol) (1/2)	Not studied	↓Decrease (α-tocopherol) (1/2)	Not studied
Caffeinated coffee/ caffeine intake	Cross-sectional	2	Inverse relationship lower 10.2% with every 1 cup/d increased intake (1/1)	No significant effect	Not studied	Direct relationship (1/1)
Omega-3 fatty acids	Open trial/ double blind placebo control	2	↓Decrease (1/2)	↓Decrease (1/1)	No effect	Not studied
Vitamin D	Intervention	1	No significant effect	Not studied	Not studied	Not studied
	Cross-sectional	2	Inverse relationship 13.7% increase with hypovitaminosis D (1/2)	Not studied	Not studied	Not studied
Magnesium	Cross-sectional	3	Inverse relationship higher with hypomagnesemia (1/2)	Not studied	Not studied	Positive relationship[a] (1/1)
Red wine	Randomized prevention trial	1	↓Decrease (1/1)	↓Decrease (1/1)	↓Decrease (1/1)	Not studied
Mediterranean diet	RCT/ controlled trial	2	↓Decrease (2/2)	Not studied	↓Decrease (1/1)	Not studied
	Cross-sectional	1	No significant relationship	Not studied	Inverse relationship[b] 4.2% and 11.7% with fruits and cereals (1/1)	Not studied

↓ (decreased/lower in clinical trials, $P < 0.05$); ↑ (increased/higher in clinical trials, $P < 0.05$). [a]Significant trend for increasing quintiles of intake. [b]Significant trend for increasing tertiles of intake. Number of studies with a significant result/number of studies with a measurement of the marker shown in parentheses.
IL, interleukin; RCT, randomized, controlled trial; TNF-α, tumour necrosis factor α.

2. In the other diet categories, omega-3 fatty acids, cereal fibre, caffeine, red wine, vitamin D, magnesium and antioxidants were not found to have consistent, significant effects on inflammatory biomarkers. More research, especially RCTs, is needed to establish the effect of these factors on inflammation.
3. In order to increase the strength of the evidence on diet, consideration of physical activity or exercise interventions should be included in all dietary studies. Other factors such as baseline levels of inflammatory markers and habitual diet need to be measured, and all dietary nutrients that could potentially alter inflammatory status should be considered in the analysis or design of intervention studies. The research shows potential for diet to be used to modulate inflammation in those with T2D, but presently there is insufficient data to make strong evidence-based clinical recommendations for those with T2D or MetS.

Effects of Exercise

Resistance exercise

Two resistance exercise studies have been conducted in T2D or MetS (Table 13.3). An intervention study by Praet *et al.* (2008) investigated the effect of a 10-week resistance exercise protocol on plasma hs-CRP, TNF-α and adiponectin in 11 male subjects. There were no significant changes after the intervention. An RCT by Brooks *et al.* (2007) randomized 62 Hispanic individuals to either 16 weeks of resistance training and standard care or standard care alone. On average, the resistance training group had a 20% decrease in CRP and 30% increase in adiponectin concentrations, whereas the control group experienced an increase in CRP concentrations and a decrease in adiponectin concentrations. Adiponectin concentrations were, however, dissimilar between the groups at baseline (intervention: 5.1 μg/ml, control 8.3 μg/ml). Both of these studies used a 45-min resistance exercise protocol completed three times a week, and both studies looked at the exercise impact through muscle biopsies (Brooks *et al.*, 2007; Praet *et al.*, 2008). These two studies differed in many other aspects, however (e.g. sample size, exercise intensity, study duration). When comparing the changes in muscle strength, the results from Brooks *et al.* (2007) showed significant changes to upper and lower body muscle strength, increases in whole body lean tissue mass, and hypertrophy of type 1 and 2 muscle fibres. On the other hand, Praet *et al.* (2008) observed no changes in type 1 and 2 muscle distribution and cross-sectional area following the intervention. It is possible that the intensity and duration of the exercise are potential factors that might explain the different results.

To summarize, only one long-term (16 week) RCT by Brooks *et al.* (2007) showed a beneficial effect of high-intensity resistance exercise on inflammation (i.e. decreasing CRP and increasing adiponectin concentrations). Future research studies are warranted to: (i) apply the same resistance exercise protocol from Brooks *et al.* (2007) to both younger and older adult populations; (ii) control for the confounding variable of diet; (iii) control for the potential confounding factor of extracurricular physical activities; and (iv) determine whether a longer study duration will continue to promote a beneficial effect on these biomarkers or whether a plateau effect will occur (Brooks *et al.*, 2007; Praet *et al.*, 2008).

Aerobic exercise

Seven studies (five RCTs and two open label trials) have examined the effects of aerobic exercise on inflammation in individuals with T2D or MetS (Giannopoulou *et al.*, 2005; Zoppini *et al.*, 2006; Dekker *et al.*, 2007; Kadoglou *et al.*, 2007a,b; Balducci *et al.*, 2010a; Palomo *et al.*, 2010) (Table 13.3). Six of the seven studies found a significant decrease in at least one inflammatory marker after completing an aerobic exercise intervention. All studies incorporated an aerobic intervention that was within a 50–85% maximal oxygen uptake (VO_2 max) range, with the exception of Palomo *et al.* (2010), whose subjects started at a lower VO_2 max (40%) but progressed to 80% VO_2 max after the first month. Six trials (four RCTs and two open label trials)

Table 13.3. Summary of the studies that have examined the relationship/effect of exercise on inflammation in subjects with diabetes.

Author, year	Study design and sample	Exercise type/intensity	Exercise duration	Diet	Marker(s)	Results
Resistance exercise						
Brooks *et al.*, 2007	Randomized controlled clinical trial n = 62 Hispanic individuals with T2D, ≥55 years, randomly assigned to intervention group (n = 31; 21 M, 10 F) or control group (n = 31, 19 M, 12 F)	Strength training: use of 5 pneumatic machines (chest press, upper back, leg press, knee extension, knee flexion) with 3 sets of 8 repetitions on each machine/exercise Intensity was 60–80% of baseline 1-repetition maximum in first 8 weeks; after 8 weeks, intensity increased to 70–80% of mid-study 1 RM	3 times a week for 16 weeks 45 min/session (35 min strength training, 5 min warm up, 5 min cool down)	Not reported	hs-CRP/CRP Adiponectin	CRP serum concentrations significantly decreased by 20% in the exercise group, but increased by 17% in the control group Adiponectin serum concentrations significantly increased in the exercise group by approximately 30%, but decreased by nearly 20% in the control group
Praet *et al.*, 2008	Intervention study n = 11 males, T2D, mean age 59 years	Progressive resistance with high intensity training to supplement After 5 months, intensity increase from 50 to 60% 1 RM for PRT and remained at 50–60% Wmax for HIT	3 times a week for 10 weeks 45 min/session	30 g of CHO and 5 g protein given before exercise if low blood glucose	hs-CRP/CRP TNF-α Adiponectin	No significant changes in plasma concentrations of hs-CRP, adiponectin, or TNF-α

Aerobic exercise						
Baldducci *et al.*, 2010a	Randomized controlled clinical trial n = 82 (34 F, 48 M), T2D and MetS, 40–75 years, randomly assigned to control (Group A, n = 20) or 3 exercise groups (Group B, n = 20; Group C, n = 20; Group D, n = 22)	Group B: low intensity aerobic exercise Group C: high intensity aerobic exercise (70–80% of VO_2 max) Group D: high intensity aerobic exercise (40 min aerobic exercise at 70–80% of VO_2 max and 20 min resistance exercise at 80% 1 RM)	2 times a week for 12 months supervised sessions of 60 min	Standard diabetes dietary prescription	hs-CRP/CRP TNF-α Adiponectin IL-6	hs-CRP decreased by 28% in Group C and by 54% in Group D compared to baseline 50% of Group C and D participants moved into lower risk levels of hs-CRP based on AHA classifications IL-6 decreased by 59% in Group D and by 41% in Group C compared to baseline TNF-α decreased by 44% in Group D compared to baseline Adiponectin concentrations increased by 36% in Group C and by 38% in Group D compared to baseline
Dekker *et al.*, 2007	Intervention trial (no control) n = 24 Caucasian men (8 lean, 8 obese, 8 T2D), 48–51 years	Light walking at 60% of VO_2 max	5 times a week for 12 weeks 60 min sessions	Weight- maintaining diet of 55–60% CHO, 15–20% protein, 20–25% fat	hs-CRP/CRP IL-6	IL-6 concentrations decreased significantly in all groups with the T2D group having the largest decrease (–52%) compared to baseline No effect on CRP concentrations

Continued

Table 13.3. Continued.

Author, year	Study design and sample	Exercise type/intensity	Exercise duration	Diet	Marker(s)	Results
Giannopoulou *et al.*, 2005	Randomized controlled clinical trial n = 33 women, 50–70 years T2D, randomly assigned to a Diet (D) group, a Diet and Exercise (D+E) group, or an Exercise (E) group	Walking at 65–70% of VO_2 max and expending 1050 to 1250 kJ/session	3–4 times a week for 14 weeks 60 min sessions	For the D and D+E groups: 40% fat (30% MUFA, 5% PUFA, 5% SFA), 40% CHO (15% simple, 25% complex CHO), 20% protein	hs-CRP/CRP TNF-α Adiponectin IL-6	CRP decreased significantly by 10–18% in all groups; there were no significant differences between the groups Trend for IL-6 to decrease in all 3 groups ($P = 0.07$) No effect on TNF-α, IL-6 or plasma adiponectin
Kadoglou *et al.*, 2007a	Randomized controlled clinical trial n = 54 men and women, T2D, randomly assigned to a control group (n = 26; 11 M, 15 F; mean age 62 years) or an exercise group (n = 28; 12 M, 16 F; mean age 57 years)	Aerobic exercise at 50–85% of VO_2 max	4 times a week for 16 weeks 45–60 min sessions	Not reported (retained eating patterns)	hs-CRP/CRP IL-6	hs-CRP decreased by 37% compared to baseline in the exercise group IL-6 concentrations were 34% lower compared to baseline in the exercise group
Kadoglou *et al.*, 2007b	Randomized controlled clinical trial n = 56 men and women, mean age 62 years T2D, randomly assigned to exercise group (n = 29) or control group (n = 27)	Aerobic exercise at 50–75% VO_2 max	4 times a week for 6 months 45–60 min/session (10 min warm up, 30–45 min exercise, 5 min cool down)	Not reported	hs-CRP/CRP TNF-α Adiponectin	CRP decreased by 37% in the exercise group No effect on adiponectin and TNF-α concentrations
Palomo *et al.*, 2010	Randomized controlled clinical trial n = 51 men and women with MetS, 39–62 years, randomly assigned to an intervention group (n = 27; 9 M, 18 F) or a non-intervention group (n = 24; 12 M, 12 F)	Aerobic exercise at 40% of max HR for 1 month, and increasing to 80% of max HR	3 times a week for 18 weeks 60 min/session	Not reported	TNF-α	Serum TNF-α concentrations decreased significantly by 53% in the intervention group compared to baseline

Zoppini *et al.*, 2006	Intervention trial (no control) n = 16 men and women, mean age 66 years	Progressive aerobic exercise training at 50–70% HRR	2 times a week for 6 months 70 min/session (10 min warm up, 40 min aerobic exercise, 10 min cool down)	Advised not to change their diet	hs-CRP/CRP TNF-α	No effect on plasma hs-CRP or sTNF-α concentrations after exercise intervention
Combined exercise						
Balducci *et al.*, 2010a	Randomized controlled clinical trial n = 82 (34 F, 48 M), T2D and MetS, 40–75 years, randomly assigned to a control group (Group A, n = 20) or 3 exercise groups (Group B, n = 20; Group C, n = 20; Group D, n = 22)	Group B: low intensity aerobic exercise Group C: high intensity aerobic exercise (70–80% of VO_2 max) Group D: high intensity aerobic exercise (40 min aerobic exercise at 70-80% of VO_2 max and 20 min resistance exercise at 80% 1 RM)	2 times a week for 12 months supervised sessions of 60 min	Not reported (standard diabetes dietary prescription)	hs-CRP/CRP TNF-α Adiponectin IL-6	hs-CRP decreased by 28% in Group C and by 54% in Group D compared to baseline 50% of Group C and D participants moved into lower risk levels of hs-CRP based on AHA classifications IL-6 decreased by 59% in Group D and by 41% in Group C compared to baseline TNF-α decreased by 44% in Group D compared with baseline Adiponectin concentrations increased by 36% in Group C and by 38% in Group D compared with baseline
Balducci *et al.*, 2010b	Randomized controlled clinical trial n = 563 men and women, T2D, randomly assigned to an exercise intervention group (n = 288; 173 M, 115 F; 152 <60 years, 136 ≥60 years) or a control (counselling only) group (n = 275; 156 M, 119 F; 147 <60 years, 128 ≥60 years)	Not reported other than intensity was adjusted based on improvements	2 times a week for 12 months 75 min/session	Diet of 500 kcal/days lower than daily energy expenditure and was within the range of 55% CHO, 30% fat, and 15% protein	hs-CRP/CRP	hs-CRP concentrations decreased significantly by 29% (from 2.8 mg/l to 2 mg/l) in the exercise group.

Continued

Table 3.3. Continued.

Author year	Study design and sample	Exercise type/intensity	Exercise duration	Diet	Marker(s)	Results
Oberbach *et al.*, 2006	Intervention trial (no control) n = 60 Caucasian men and women, mean age 45 years, classified (based on ADA) as having normal glucose tolerance (NGT; n = 20; 9 M, 11 F), impaired glucose tolerance (IGT; n = 20; 9 M, 11 F), or T2D (n = 20; 11 M, 9 F)	Not reported	3 times a week for 4 weeks 60 min/session (20 min warm up/cool down, 20 min biking or running, 20 min power training), plus an extra day of swimming for 60 min	NGT: CHO M: 45%, F: 50%, fat: M: 35%, F: 31%, protein M: 20%, F: 19% IGT: CHO M: 39%, F: 46% fat M: 44%, F: 35%, protein M: 18%, F: 18% T2D: CHO M: 42%, F: 43%, fat: M: 40%, F: 39% protein M:18%, F: 17%	hs-CRP/CRP Adiponectin IL-6	CRP concentrations decreased significantly from baseline in all groups Adiponectin concentrations significantly increased baseline in the T2D and IGT groups There was no significant effect of exercise on IL-6 concentrations
Troseid *et al.*, 2004	Randomized controlled clinical trial n= 32 men with MetS (n = 11) or T2D (n = 21), 20–75 years, randomly assigned to a control group (n = 6), a pravastatin only group (n = 8), an exercise only group (n = 9), or a pravastatin and exercise group (n = 9)	Endurance exercise -light jogging and strength training	3 times a week for 12 weeks 45–60 min/session (40% dedicated to aerobic and 60% dedicated to resistance/strength training)	Not reported	hs-CRP/CRP TNF-α IL-6	No significant changes occurred for CRP, TNF-α, or IL-6, in any group

CHO, carbohydrate; hs-CRP, high-sensitivity C reactive protein; IL, interleukin; RM, repetition maximum; TNF-α, tumour necrosis factor α; VO_2 max, maximal oxygen uptake.

examined the effect of aerobic exercise on serum CRP concentrations (Giannopoulou *et al.*, 2005; Zoppini *et al.*, 2006; Dekker *et al.*, 2007; Kadoglou *et al.*, 2007a,b; Balducci *et al.*, 2010a). All four RCTs reported significant decreases (10–37%) in CRP concentrations with aerobic exercise, whereas the two open label trials found no significant effect. Five trials (four RCTs and one open label trial) investigated the effect of aerobic exercise on TNF-α concentrations (Giannopoulou *et al.*, 2005; Zoppini *et al.*, 2006; Kadoglou *et al.*, 2007b; Balducci *et al.*, 2010a; Palomo *et al.*, 2010;). Only the RCT by Palomo *et al.* (2010) reported an effect of aerobic exercise on TNF-α concentrations, which decreased by 53% compared with baseline in the intervention group. The effect of aerobic exercise on serum IL-6 concentrations was investigated in four trials (three RCTs and one open label trial; Giannopoulou *et al.*, 2005; Dekker *et al.*, 2007; Kadoglou *et al.*, 2007a; Balducci *et al.*, 2010a). In all four trials, IL-6 concentrations were reduced with aerobic exercise; however, the decrease failed to reach statistical significance ($P = 0.07$) in the study by Giannopoulou *et al.* (2005). Three RCTs examined the effect of aerobic exercise on plasma adiponectin concentrations (Giannopoulou *et al.*, 2005; Kadoglou *et al.*, 2007b; Balducci *et al.*, 2010a). Only the trial by Balducci *et al.* (2010a) reported an effect of aerobic exercise on adiponectin concentrations, which increased by 36% among participants in the high-intensity exercise group. Although this study had the lowest exercise frequency (2 sessions/week), it had the longest study duration (12 months) and largest study population (n = 82), and incorporated the highest exercise intensity, supporting an effect of long-term, high-intensity aerobic exercise on plasma adiponectin concentrations.

In summary, evidence from these studies indicates that older adults (>40 years) can show decreases in IL-6 and CRP and an increase in adiponectin when undergoing a long-term (12 months), high-intensity (70–80% VO_2 max) aerobic exercise intervention. Future studies are again warranted to: (i) investigate the effect of long term (>1 year) aerobic interventions like that used by Balducci *et al.* (2010a) in younger and older adults to determine whether biomarkers continue to improve or plateau; (ii) limit confounding factors by controlling for a balanced diet; and (iii) possibly categorize different groups by baseline CRP concentrations because the aerobic studies varied from 2.5 to 15 mg/l CRP at baseline.

Combined exercise

Four studies (three RCTs and one open label trial) examined a combined exercise intervention (i.e. a mix of resistance and aerobic exercise) (Troseid *et al.*, 2004; Oberbach *et al.*, 2006; Balducci *et al.*, 2010a,b) (Table 13.3). Three studies found a significant and beneficial change in at least one biomarker (Oberbach *et al.*, 2006; Balducci *et al.*, 2010a,b). Participants ranged in age from 40 to 75 years, and sample sizes ranged from 60 to 563 men and women. The total number of hours of exercise per week ranged from 120–180 min/week; each intervention had a different split between the aerobic and resistance exercise portion.

As mentioned earlier, Balducci *et al.* (2010a) studied 82 males and females who were split into one of four groups (control, low-intensity aerobic, high-intensity aerobic and high-intensity combined), where each group did 2 sessions per week, at 60 min (combined: 40 min of aerobic, 70–80% VO_2 max and 20 min of resistance, 80% 1 RM) for 12 months with no diet control. Oberbach *et al.* (2006) studied 60 Caucasian males and females who were split according to ADA classifications: normal glucose tolerance (NGT), impaired glucose tolerance (IGT) and T2D. Each group incorporated 3 sessions per week, at 60 min (20 min warm up/cool down, 20 min aerobic, 20 min power training) for 4 weeks while on a constant diet. The individuals in both studies had elevated baseline CRP concentrations of approximately 3.4 mg/l (Balducci *et al.*, 2010a) and approximately 0.8 mg/dl (Oberbach *et al.*, 2006), which showed significant decreases in the intervention groups at 54% and 44%, respectively, and a 38% and 58% increase in adiponectin concentrations, respectively, at the end of the study. TNF-α was not studied and IL-6 concentrations did not change significantly in the study by Oberbach *et al.* (2006), whereas Balducci *et al.* (2010a) showed a 44% and 59% decrease in those biomarkers, respectively. The lack of change in IL-6 concentrations from Oberbach *et al.* (2006) might be due to a higher baseline concentration (~7.5 pg/ml) compared with Balducci *et al.* (2010a) (~2.3pg/ml). The 12-week RCT study by Troseid *et al.* (2004) divided 32 males and females into four groups (control, pravastatin only, pravastatin and exercise, and exercise). Individuals in the exercise arms underwent a 45–60 min combined exercise intervention three times per week. There was no significant effect on hs-CRP, TNF-α and IL-6.

The study by Balducci *et al.* (2010a) demonstrated a significant relationship between combined exercise and a decrease in inflammatory markers and an increase in adiponectin. This study had the fewest sessions per week (two compared with three of Oberbach *et al.*, 2006), did not factor in diet and had a session duration of 60 min. However, Balducci *et al.* (2010a) had the larger study population (82 compared with 60 by Oberbach *et al.*, 2006) and had a very high intensity of 70–80% VO_2 max and 80% 1 RM, which was a factor not mentioned by Oberbach *et al.* (2006). The results of this study were supported, specifically for the decrease in CRP concentrations from the larger study done by Balducci *et al.* (2010b). This particular study population was the largest of all exercise papers (563 males and females) and though the intervention was 2 times/week, it had one of the longest exercise protocols at 75 min/session and one of the longest study durations at 1 year (Oberbach *et al.*, 2006; Balducci *et al.*, 2010a,b).

To summarize, these studies suggest that a long-term (12 months), combined exercise intervention (40 min of aerobic at 70–80% VO_2 max and 20 min of resistance exercise at 80% 1 RM twice a week) is beneficial in lowering CRP, IL-6 and TNF-α concentrations while also increasing adiponectin concentrations in males and females of 40–75 years of age with T2D or MetS. Some potential areas of future research/study include: (i) categorizing individuals on the basis of their baseline biomarkers; (ii) controlling for diet because it was only measured in two out of four studies; and (iii) more studies on both younger and older adult populations.

Conclusions

The relationships between the various forms of exercise and inflammatory biomarkers in individuals with T2D and MetS are summarized in Table 13.4 and Fig. 13.2. The main conclusions are:

1. All exercise types suggested some beneficial effect on inflammation, with the common finding being the decrease in CRP and increase in adiponectin concentrations as indicated by the centre overlap in the Venn diagram (Fig. 13.2). Resistance exercise

Table 13.4: A summary of the effect of exercise on inflammatory markers in studies of subjects with diabetes.

Exercise type	Number of papers	Inflammatory marker (plasma/serum)			
		hs-CRP	TNF-α	IL-6	Adiponectin
Resistance	2	↓ 20% (1/2)[a]	Not studied	Not studied	↑ 30% (1/2)[a]
Aerobic	7	↓ 10–37% (4/6)[a]	↓ 53% (1/5)[a]	↓ 34–52% (3/4)[a]	↑ 36% (1/3)[a]
Combined	4	↓ 29–54% (3/4)[a]	↓ 44% (1/2)[a]	↓ 59% (1/3)[a]	↑ >38% (2/2)[a]

↓ Significant decrease, $P<0.05$; ↑ significant increase, $P<0.05$. [a]Number of studies with a significant result/number of studies with a measurement of the marker.

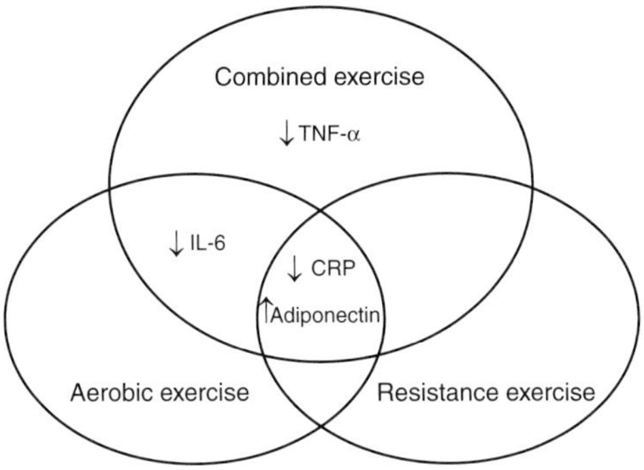

Fig. 13.2. Summary of the effects of exercise on inflammation in diabetes. IL, interleukin; CRP, C-reactive protein; TNF-α, tumour necrosis factor-α.

showed a beneficial effect on inflammation by decreasing CRP (20%) and increasing adiponectin (30%) concentrations at higher intensity levels (70–80% mid 1 RM) in 16-week studies with older adults (males and females) over the age of 55 years. Long-term (12 months) aerobic exercise showed decreases in CRP (28%), IL-6 (41%) and increases in adiponectin (36%) in older adults (>40 years), whereas long-term (12 months), combined high-intensity exercise interventions (40 min of aerobic at 70–80% VO_2 max and 20 min of resistance exercise at 80% 1 RM) is beneficial in lowering CRP (54%), IL-6 (59%) and TNF-α concentrations (44%) while also increasing adiponectin (38%) concentrations in adults (men and women) over 40 years of age with T2D or MetS.

2. Although the summary of studies to date shows a link between exercise and improvements in the inflammatory response, more studies that incorporate some of the suggestions provided in this chapter (long-term RCTs on young and older adults, controlling for diet, organizing based on biomarkers) are needed to understand potential benefits.

Relationship between Inflammation and Clinical Outcomes

A major limitation in studies that have examined the relationship between diet and inflammation in individuals with T2D has been the failure or inability to measure clinical outcomes. There is, however, considerable evidence that chronic inflammation plays a key role in the development and progression of T2D. Cross-sectional and prospective studies have described elevated circulating levels of acute-phase proteins (such as CRP, haptoglobin, fibrinogen, plasminogen activator inhibitor and serum amyloid A), as well as cytokines and chemokines, in patients with T2D (Donath and Shoelson, 2011). Elevated concentrations of some inflammatory biomarkers, including CRP, IL-6 and IL-1β, are predictive of those with MetS and/or obesity progressing to T2D (Manabe, 2011). It is well established that high concentrations of CRP are an independent risk factor for cardiovascular disease, perhaps even stronger in those with T2D, and chronic inflammation has been found to be associated with β-cell dysfunction and poorer insulin sensitivity (Manabe, 2011). These findings strongly suggest that chronic inflammation plays a critical role in both the development, metabolic control and the development of complications in T2D. There is a growing body of evidence that suggests that strategies aimed at reducing inflammation result in improved glycaemic control and reduced cardiovascular complications in those with T2D (Garcia *et al*, 2010). These findings suggest that dietary and exercise strategies that help reduce inflammatory biomarkers would be beneficial to those with T2D.

Summary and Conclusions

High concentrations of CRP have been related to increased risk of CVD in persons with MetS and T2D (Malik *et al.*, 2005). Diet and lifestyle therapies are important aspects of the prevention and management of individuals with T2D and MetS. Since 2000, a growing number of studies investigating the effect of/association of lifestyle variables such as diet and exercise with inflammatory biomarkers in those with T2D or MetS have been published. To our knowledge, this is the first review done in a systematic way reviewing the role of diet and exercise on inflammation in T2D or MetS populations. The first objective of this review was to 'review and analyse the current data'. According to the evidence presented in this review, following a low-GI diet or a Mediterranean diet pattern showed evidence of a beneficial effect on plasma biomarkers of inflammation. Current data indicates that, based on the results of the RCTs done on these two diets, a low-GI diet can be expected to promote a 20% decrease in CRP. Future studies will hopefully better define the dietary regimen that will promote the greatest effect on inflammatory biomarkers. Although there is inconclusive evidence for other dietary factors, there is emerging evidence that omega-3 fatty acids, red wine, vitamin D and a variety of dietary antioxidants may have some beneficial effects in individuals with T2D or MetS. The effect of exercise on inflammatory status has been more conclusively studied in a number of RCTs. Anaerobic and aerobic exercise, particularly when combined, have been consistently demonstrated to reduce plasma inflammatory markers in those with T2D and MetS. Because of the limited number of studies available for this review, there still remain many questions that need to be answered to design the optimal lifestyle intervention to reduce chronic inflammation in those with or at risk for T2D. Future studies will help establish the specific intensity and/or duration of exercise that is most effective at producing a beneficial inflammatory profile. These studies will need to control for, or consider, the definition of baseline inflammatory status, carefully measure diet and physical activity, and design studies in a way that can clearly identify individual and combined lifestyle factor(s) that influence inflammatory status.

Acknowledgements

The authors would like to thank Patricia Biondo for her assistance in the editing of this chapter.

References

Alberti, K.G. and Zimmet, P.Z. (1998) Definition, diagnosis and classification of diabetes mellitus and its complications. Part 1: diagnosis and classification of diabetes mellitus provisional report of a WHO consultation. *Diabetic Medicine: a Journal of the British Diabetic Association* 15, 539–553.

Asgard, R., Rytter, E., Basu, S., Abramsson-Zetterberg, L., Mueller, L., *et al.* (2007) High intake of fruit and vegetables is related to low oxidative stress and inflammation in a group of patients with type 2 diabetes. *Scandinavian Journal of Food and Nutrition* 51, 149–158.

Balducci, S., Zanuso, S., Nicolucci, A., Fernando, F., Cavallo, S., *et al.* (2010a) Anti-inflammatory effect of exercise training in subjects with type 2 diabetes and the metabolic syndrome is dependent on exercise modalities and independent of weight loss. *Nutrition, Metabolism and Cardiovascular Diseases* 20, 608–617.

Balducci, S., Zanuso, S., Nicolucci, A., De Feo, P., Cavallo, S., *et al.* (2010b) Effect of an intensive exercise intervention strategy on modifiable cardiovascular risk factors in subjects with type 2 diabetes mellitus. A randomized controlled trial: the Italian Diabetes and Exercise Study (IDES). *Archives of Internal Medicine* 170, 1794–1803.

Brooks, N., Layne, J.E., Gordon, P.L., Roubenoff, R., Nelson, M.E., *et al.* (2007) Strength training improves muscle quality and insulin sensitivity in Hispanic older adults with type 2 diabetes. *International Journal of Medical Sciences* 4, 19–27.

Bruun, J.M., Helge, J.W., Richelsen, B. and Stallknecht, B. (2006) Diet and exercise reduce low-grade inflammation and macrophage infiltration in adipose tissue but not in skeletal muscle in severely obese subjects. *American Journal of Physiology, Endocrinology and Metabolism* 290, E961–E9627.

De Luis, D.A., Conde, R., Aller, R., Izaola, O., Gonzalez Sagrado, M., *et al.* (2009) Effect of omega-3 fatty acids on cardiovascular risk factors in patients with type 2 diabetes mellitus and hypertriglyceridemia: an open study. *European Review for Medical and Pharmacological Sciences* 13, 51–55.

Dekker, M.J., Lee, S., Hudson, R., Kilpatrick, K., Graham, T.E., *et al.* (2007) An exercise intervention without weight loss decreases circulating interleukin-6 in lean and obese men with and without type 2 diabetes mellitus. *Metabolism Clinical and Experimental* 56, 332–338.

Devaraj, S. and Jialal, I. (2000) Alpha tocopherol supplementation decreases serum C-reactive protein and monocyte interleukin-6 levels in normal volunteers and type 2 diabetic patients. *Free Radical Biology and Medicine* 29, 790–792.

Donath, M.Y. and Shoelson, S.E. (2011) Type 2 diabetes as an inflammatory disease. *Nature Reviews Immunology* 11, 98–107.

Doria, A., Patti, M.E. and Kahn, C.R. (2008) The emerging genetic architecture of type 2 diabetes. *Cell Metabolism* 8, 186–200.

Du, H., Van, D.A., Van Bakel, M.M.E., Van Der Kallen, C.J.H., Blaak, E.E., *et al.* (2008) Glycemic index and glycemic load in relation to food and nutrient intake and metabolic risk factors in a Dutch population. *American Journal of Clinical Nutrition* 87, 655–661.

Duncan, B.B., Schmidt, M.I., Pankow, J.S., Ballantyne, C.M., Couper, D., *et al.,* and Atherosclerosis Risk in Communities Study (2003) Low-grade systemic inflammation and the development of type 2 diabetes: the atherosclerosis risk in communities study. *Diabetes* 52, 1799–1805.

Duncan, B.B., Schmidt, M.I., Pankow, J.S., Bang, H., Couper, D., *et al.* (2004) Adiponectin and the development of type 2 diabetes: the atherosclerosis risk in communities study. *Diabetes* 53, 2473–2478.

Eriksson, K.F. and Lindgarde, F. (1991) Prevention of type 2 (non-insulin-dependent) diabetes mellitus by diet and physical exercise. The 6-year Malmo feasibility study. *Diabetologia* 34, 891–898.

Esposito, K., Ciotola, M., Giugliano, F., De Sio, M., Giugliano, G., *et al.* (2006) Mediterranean diet improves erectile function in subjects with the metabolic syndrome. *International Journal of Impotence Research* 18, 405–410.

Evangelopoulos, A.A., Vallianou, N.G., Panagiotakos, D.B., Georgiou, A., Zacharias, G.A., *et al.* (2008) An inverse relationship between cumulating components of the metabolic syndrome and serum magnesium levels. *Nutrition Research* 28, 659–663.

Garcia, C., Feve, B., Ferre, P., Halimi, S., Baizri, H., *et al.* (2010) Diabetes and inflammation: fundamental aspects and clinical implications. *Diabetes and Metabolism* 36, 327–338.

Giannopoulou, I., Fernhall, B., Carhart, R., Weinstock, R.S., Baynard, T., *et al.* (2005) Effects of diet and/or exercise on the adipocytokine and inflammatory cytokine levels of postmenopausal women with type 2 diabetes. *Metabolism Clinical and Experimental* 54, 866–875.

Grundy, S.M., Brewer, H.B.,Jr, Cleeman, J.I., Smith, S.C.,Jr, Lenfant, C. and National Heart, Lung, and Blood Institute and American Heart Association (2004) Definition of metabolic syndrome: report of the National Heart, Lung, and Blood Institute/American Heart Association conference on scientific issues related to definition. *Arteriosclerosis, Thrombosis, and Vascular Biology* 24, E13–E18.

Guerrero-Romero, F. and Rodriguez-Moran, M. (2006) Hypomagnesemia, oxidative stress, inflammation, and metabolic syndrome. *Diabetes/Metabolism Research and Reviews* 22, 471–476.

Jenkins, D.J.A., Kendall, C.W.C., Augustin, L.S.A., Martini, M.C., Axelsen, M., *et al.* (2002) Effect of wheat bran on glycemic control and risk factors for cardiovascular disease in type 2 diabetes. *Diabetes Care* 25, 1522–1528.

Kadoglou, N., Perrea, D., Iliadis, F., Angelopoulou, N., Llapis, C. and Alevizos, M. (2007a) Exercise reduces resistin and inflammatory cytokines in patients with type 2 diabetes. *Diabetes Care* 30, 719–721.

Kadoglou, N.P.E., Iliadis, F., Angelopoulou, N., Perrea, D., Ampatzidis, G., Liapis, C.D. and Alevizos, M. (2007b) The anti-inflammatory effects of exercise training in patients with type 2 diabetes mellitus. *The European Society of Cardiology* 14, 837–843.

Kallio, P., Kolehmainen, M., Laaksonen, D.E., Pulkkinen, L., Atalay, M., *et al.* (2008) Inflammation markers are modulated by responses to diets differing in postprandial insulin responses in individuals with the metabolic syndrome. *American Journal of Clinical Nutrition* 87, 1497–1503.

Libby, P. and Ridker, P.M. (2004) Inflammation and atherosclerosis: role of C-reactive protein in risk assessment. *American Journal of Medicine* 116, 9S–16S.

Liu, S., Manson, J.E., Buring, J.E., Stampfer, M.J., Willett, W.C., *et al.* (2002) Relation between a diet with a high glycemic load and plasma concentrations of high-sensitivity C-reactive protein in middle-aged women. *American Journal of Clinical Nutrition* 75, 492–498.

Lopez-Garcia, E., van Dam, R.M., Qi, L. and Hu, F.B. (2006) Coffee consumption and markers of inflammation and endothelial dysfunction in healthy and diabetic women. *American Journal of Clinical Nutrition* 84, 888–893.

Luo, C., Wong, J., Brown, M., Hooper, M., Molyneaux, L., *et al.* (2009) Hypovitaminosis D in Chinese type 2 diabetes: Lack of impact on clinical metabolic status and biomarkers of cellular inflammation. *Diabetes and Vascular Disease Research,* 6, 194–199.

Maachi, M., Pieroni, L., Bruckert, E., Jardel, C., Fellahi, S., *et al.* (2004) Systemic low-grade inflammation is related to both circulating and adipose tissue TNFalpha, leptin and IL-6 levels in obese women. *International Journal of Obesity and Related Metabolic Disorders* 28, 993–997.

Malik, S., Wong, N.D., Franklin, S., Pio, J., Fairchild, C., *et al.* (2005). Cardiovascular disease in U.S. patients with metabolic syndrome, diabetes, and elevated C-reactive protein. *Diabetes Care* 28, 690–693.

Manabe, I. (2011) Chronic inflammation links cardiovascular, metabolic and renal diseases. *Circulation Journal* 75, 2739–2748.

Marfella, R., Cacciapuoti, F., Siniscalchi, M., Sasso, F.C., Marchese, F., *et al.* (2006) Effect of moderate red wine intake on cardiac prognosis after recent acute myocardial infarction of subjects with Type 2 diabetes mellitus. *Diabetic Medicine* 23, 974–981.

Mena, M.P., Sacanella, E., Vazquez-Agell, M., Morales, M., Fito, M., *et al.* (2009) Inhibition of circulating immune cell activation: a molecular antiinflammatory effect of the Mediterranean diet. *American Journal of Clinical Nutrition* 89, 248–256.

Oberbach, A., Tonjes, A., Kloting, N., Fasshauer, M., Kratzsch, J., *et al.* (2006) Effect of a 4 week physical training program on plasma concentrations of inflammatory markers in patients with abnormal glucose tolerance. *European Journal of Endocrinology* 154, 577–585.

Palomo, I., Herrera, J., Cancino, V., Alarco´n, M., Mujica, V., *et al.* (2010) Physical activity reduces circulating TNF-alpha but not pro-thrombotic factors levels in patients with metabolic syndrome. *Diabetes & Metabolic Syndrome: Clinical Research and Reviews* 4, 234–238.

Pearson, T.A., Mensah, G.A., Alexander, R.W., Anderson, J.L., Cannon III, R.O., *et al.* (2003) Markers of inflammation and cardiovascular disease: application to clinical and public health practice: a statement for healthcare professionals from the Centers for Disease Control and Prevention and the American Heart Association. *Circulation* 107, 499–511.

Pickup, J.C. (2004) Inflammation and activated innate immunity in the pathogenesis of type 2 diabetes. *Diabetes Care* 27, 813–823.

Praet, S.F.E., Jonkers, R.A.M., Schep, G., Stehouwer, C.D.A., Kuipers, H., *et al.* (2008) Long-standing, insulin-treated type 2 diabetes patients with complications respond well to short-term resistance and interval exercise training. *European Journal of Endocrinology* 158, 163–172.

Qi, L., Rimm, E., Liu, S., Rifai, N. and Hu, F.B. (2005) Dietary glycemic index, glycemic load, cereal fiber, and plasma adiponectin concentration in diabetic men. *Diabetes Care* 28, 1022–1028.

Qi, L., Meigs, J.B., Liu, S., Manson, J.E., Mantzoros, C., *et al.* (2006a) Dietary fibers and glycemic load, obesity, and plasma adiponectin levels in women with type 2 diabetes. *Diabetes Care* 29, 1501–1505.

Qi, L., van Dam, R.M., Liu, S., Franz, M., Mantzoros, C., *et al.* (2006b) Whole-grain, bran, and cereal fiber intakes and markers of systemic inflammation in diabetic women. *Diabetes Care* 29, 207–211.

Rytter, E., Vessby, B., Asgard, R., Ersson, C., Moussavian, S., *et al.* (2010) Supplementation with a combination of antioxidants does not affect glycaemic control, oxidative stress or inflammation in type 2 diabetes subjects. *Free Radical Research* 44, 1445–1453.

Salas-Salvado, J., Garcia-Arellano, A., Estruch, R., Marquez-Sandoval, F., Corella, D., *et al.,* and PREDIMED Investigators (2008) Components of the Mediterranean-type food pattern and serum inflammatory markers among patients at high risk for cardiovascular disease. *European Journal of Clinical Nutrition* 62, 651–659.

Targher, G., Bertolini, L., Padovani, R., Zenari, L., Scala, L., *et al.* (2006) Serum 25-hydroxyvitamin D3 concentrations and carotid artery intima-media thickness among type 2 diabetic patients. *Clinical Endocrinology* 65, 593–597.

Trøseid, M., Lappegard, K.T., Claudi, T., Damas, J.K., Morkrid, L., *et al.* (2004) Exercise reduces plasma levels of the chemokines MCP-1 and IL-8 in subjects with the metabolic syndrome. *European Heart Journal* 25, 349–355.

Wild, S., Roglic, G., Green, A., Sicree, R. and King, H. (2004) Global prevalence of diabetes: estimates for the year 2000 and projections for 2030. *Diabetes Care* 27, 1047–1053.

Williams, C.J., Fargnoli, J.L., Hwang, J.J., van Dam, R.M., Blackburn, G.L., *et al.* (2008) Coffee consumption is associated with higher plasma adiponectin concentrations in women with or without type 2 diabetes: A prospective cohort study. *Diabetes Care* 31, 504–507.

Wolever, T.M.S., Gibbs, A.L., Mehling, C., Chiasson, J.L., Connelly, P.W., *et al.* (2008) The Canadian Trial of Carbohydrates in Diabetes (CCD), a 1-y controlled trial of low-glycemic-index dietary carbohydrate in type 2 diabetes: No effect on glycated hemoglobin but reduction in C-reactive protein. *American Journal of Clinical Nutrition* 87, 114–125.

Wong, C.Y., Yiu, K.H., Li, S.W., Lee, S., Tam, S., *et al.* (2010) Fish-oil supplement has neutral effects on vascular and metabolic function but improves renal function in patients with Type 2 diabetes mellitus. *Diabetic Medicine* 27, 54–60.

Zoppini, G., Targher, G., Zamboni, C., Venturi, C., Cacciatori, V., *et al.* (2006) Effects of moderate-intensity exercise training on plasma biomarkers of inflammation and endothelial dysfunction in older patients with type 2 diabetes. *Nutrition, Metabolism and Cardiovascular Diseases* 16, 543–549.

14 Cardiovascular Disease and Inflammation

A. Heather* **and K. McGrath**
School of Medical and Molecular Biosciences, University of Technology, Sydney, Australia

Introduction

Cardiovascular disease (CVD) is the leading cause of death in Australia. In 2008, CVD was responsible for 34% of all deaths in Australia and it currently affects more than 3.4 million Australians. Of these, 1.4 million people are prevented from living a full life because of disability (http://www.heartfoundation.org.au).

It has been promising that the death rate from CVD has steadily decreased during the past 30 years. This is largely attributable to the impact of cholesterol-lowering drugs and the improvements in treatments and interventions that allow people to survive their first cardiovascular event. This promising trend is, however, set to be reversed as current predictions are that CVD worldwide is escalating,

* Corresponding author, Alison.Heather@uts.edu.au

with rates in the USA alone expected to double during the next 50 years (Foot *et al.*, 2000). This dramatic increase in CVD is in line with the worldwide epidemic of obesity and type 2 diabetes. Australia has the highest rates of childhood obesity in the world (http://www.abs.gov.au/ausstats). So, although improvements in treatment and awareness have made tremendous impact on CVD death rates, this will not alleviate the future increase owing to lifestyle impact. This is alarming given that, in 2011, one Australian dies every 11 minutes from CVD (Fig. 14.1).

Atherosclerosis

CVD describes a number of diseases including hypertrophic cardiomyopathy, ventricular arrhythmias and atherosclerosis or coronary artery disease. Of these, atherosclerosis is the major CVD and the one that is very readily affected by lifestyle. Atherosclerosis is the build-up of fatty lesions in the arterial wall. These fatty lesions are initially quite small but, with age, they can develop into large lesions that protrude into the lumen of the artery and occlude blood flow.

Some lesions are inherently unstable and, with increased pressure within the vessel created by blood trying to squeeze through the narrow lumen, can lead to plaque rupture. A ruptured plaque will release its toxic lipid core and, once exposed to blood, will induce clot formation. This clot can completely occlude the artery causing a heart attack. If the artery involved is a carotid artery that supplied cerebral blood then the occluded blood flow will cause a stroke.

Inflammatory processes underlie atherosclerosis

Coronary arteries are tubular vessels, comprising an inner endothelium layer, a middle intimal layer and the tunica externa. The middle layer contains primarily smooth muscle cells that control vascular tone, whereas the outer layer contains connective tissue and the vasa vasorum. The innermost layer, or endothelium, lines the vessel and is in direct contact with blood. Accumulating research has shown that endothelial dysfunction plays a central role in all stages of atherosclerosis development and progression. Initial lesion development begins with focal endothelial cell dysfunction (Lusis, 2000; Hansson, 2005) induced by a chronic inflammatory process within the arterial wall. The inflammation is initiated by the trapping of low density lipoproteins (LDL) in the sub-endothelial layer of the arterial wall. The LDL is retained in the intima by

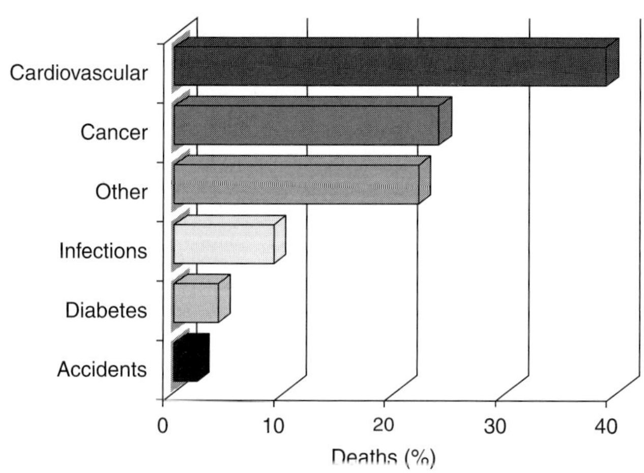

Fig. 14.1. Cardiovascular disease is the leading cause of mortality.

binding to proteoglycan and undergoes oxidative modification to oxLDL (Berliner *et al.*, 1997). The oxLDL induces a low-grade chronic inflammatory response in vascular cells that is characterized by expression of cell-adhesion molecules, chemokines and pro-inflammatory cytokines. The protein components of the LDL particle also undergo modification in the arterial wall. These modifications render the proteins antigenic, thereby inducing T lymphocyte recruitment (Stemme *et al.*, 1995). The expression of cell-adhesion molecules promotes the adhesion of blood monocytes to the endothelium and the increased secretion of chemokines such as MCP-1, and then promotes the migration of these monocytes into the intima and their subsequent differentiation into macrophages (Smith *et al.*, 1995; Qiao *et al.*, 1997).

Once resident in the intima, macrophages express scavenger receptors that allow them to engulf and modify oxLDL. In doing so, macrophages form the characteristic foam cells of an atherosclerotic plaque (Smith *et al.*, 1995; Qiao *et al.*, 1997). The macrophages perpetuate the chronic inflammatory response by secreting a number of cytokines such as interleukin (IL)-1, IL-6 and tumour necrosis factor α (TNF-α). These cytokines further activate endothelial dysfunction and enhance endothelial layer permeability that facilitates the entry of more LDL and monocytes. The infiltrating T lymphocytes secrete their own inflammatory cytokines such as γ-interferon and TNF-β that, in turn, further activate macrophages and endothelial cell dysfunction (Hansson, 1996). As the inflammatory response progresses, the macrophages and endothelial cells release fibrogenic mediators, including a variety of peptide growth factors that promote the transformation of the intimal smooth muscle cells from a quiescent, contractile to a migratory, synthetic phenotype. The smooth muscle cells begin to proliferate and migrate to the area of the early lesion and once in this region produce a dense extracellular matrix that acts as a cap that covers the accumulating lesions. The presence of a cap with an underlying lipid core represents a clinically advanced atherosclerotic lesion (Ross, 1999; Fig. 14.2).

The initial inflammatory response is sustained by the increasing levels of two major cytokines, namely IL-1 and TNF-α. These two cytokines stimulate the production of IL-6. IL-6 is a major player in perpetuating the inflammatory response because once released systemically it activates the generation of cytokines beyond the site of lesion formation, including hepatic synthesis of acute-phase cytokines such as C-reactive protein (CRP), fibrinogen and serum amyloid A (SAA).

Advanced atherosclerotic lesions may themselves not be stable owing to underlying inflammatory processes that contribute to lesion vulnerability and ruptured cap. For example, inflammatory cytokines decrease production of stabilizing collagen, whilst simultaneously increasing the expression and activity of matrix metalloproteinases that degrade the dense extracellular matrix of the lesion cap. IL-6 also stimulates expression of the potent procoagulant tissue factor that contributes to thrombus formation (Ross, 1999; Virmani *et al.*, 2000; Fig. 14.3).

Endothelium integrity and atherosclerosis

Endothelial cell integrity is central for maintaining healthy, lesion-free, arteries. Endothelial cells are involved in vasorelaxation, anticoagulation, and inhibit the binding of platelets and white blood cells to healthy arteries (Pearson, 2000). Endothelial dysfunction, as it pertains to atherosclerosis, is notarized by an adverse change in phenotype where the endothelium becomes vasoconstrictive, pro-coagulative, platelet-activating and anti-fibrinolytic (Mombouli and Vanhoutte, 1999; Constans and Conri, 2006). The dysfunctional endothelial cells secrete lower levels of vascular protective agents including nitric oxide, prostacyclin, thrombomodulin and tissue plasminogen activator, while increasing production of damaging factors including endothelin-1, angiotensin II, plasminogen activator inhibitor-1 (PAI-1) and von Willebrand factor (Corti *et al.*, 2004). All of these are

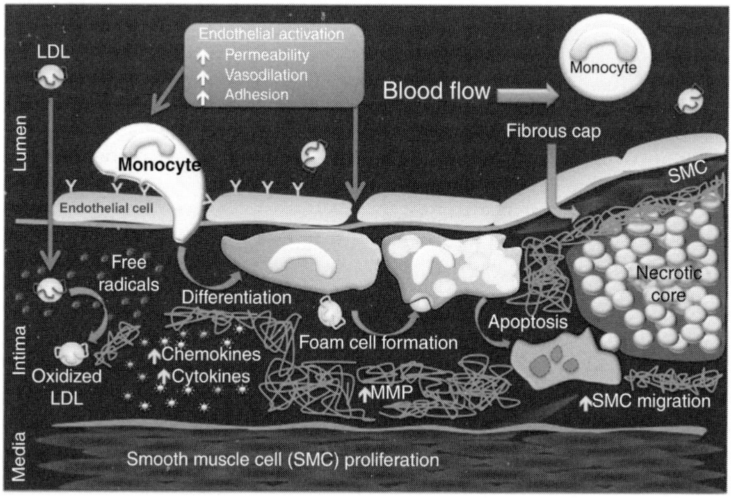

Fig. 14.2. Inflammation underlies the development of an atherosclerotic plaque. This figure schematizes the early inflammatory steps in the development of an atherosclerotic lesion. Normally, the healthy endothelium resists contact with monocytes, but the build-up of oxidized low-density lipoprotein (LDL) in the intima leads to endothelial cell activation. Activated endothelial cells express cell-adhesion molecules that facilitate the adhesion and migration of monocytes into the intima. The monocytes differentiate into macrophages that express chemokines and cytokines that further activate the endothelium. Dysfunctional endothelium is more permeable so more LDL diffuses into the intima. The proteoglycan secreted by the vascular cells binds the LDL and the free radicals secreted by the macrophages and activated endothelial cells leads to more oxidized LDL and so a chronic cycle of inflammation is established. The increase in chemokines and cytokines activates a smooth muscle phenotype change such that normally contractile cells become migratory and proliferate and move to form a cap over the developing lesion. The macrophages engulf oxidized LDL and this leads to their apoptosis, releasing their lipid content that forms the early streak. The smooth muscle cells (SMCs) that migrate to this fatty streak lay down extracellular matrix that forms a cap over the fatty streak and thus begins the development of an atherosclerotic lesion that can continue to enlarge and occlude the lumen. MMP, matrix metalloproteinase.

extremely important to vascular homeostasis, but of most importance is nitric oxide.

Nitric oxide and atherosclerosis

Nitric oxide is generated by the oxidation of L-arginine into L-citrulline by the action of an enzyme called endothelial nitric oxide synthase (eNOS). NO is central to the functional endothelium because it directly regulates vascular tone by increasing vasodilatation (widening of arteries), inhibits platelet aggregation (reducing blood clot formation), reduces leucocyte migration into the intima, and decreases the contractile to synthetic phenotypic change of smooth muscle cells. NO levels are reduced in atherosclerosis because reactive oxygen species that are formed and present in the inflammatory milieu interact with nitric oxide and convert it into a toxic by-product that causes damage to proteins, lipids and DNA. Macrophages present in the lesion especially generate substantial amounts of the reactive oxygen species. The decrease in nitric oxide levels and the accompanying increase in damaging ROS levels lead to oxidative stress. So, within the vicinity of the lesion there are high levels of mediators of both inflammatory and oxidative stress responses. This damaging milieu actually switches off protective antioxidant defences, such as the expression and activity of the enzymes, superoxide dismutase and glutathione peroxidase (Ennezat *et al.*, 2000).

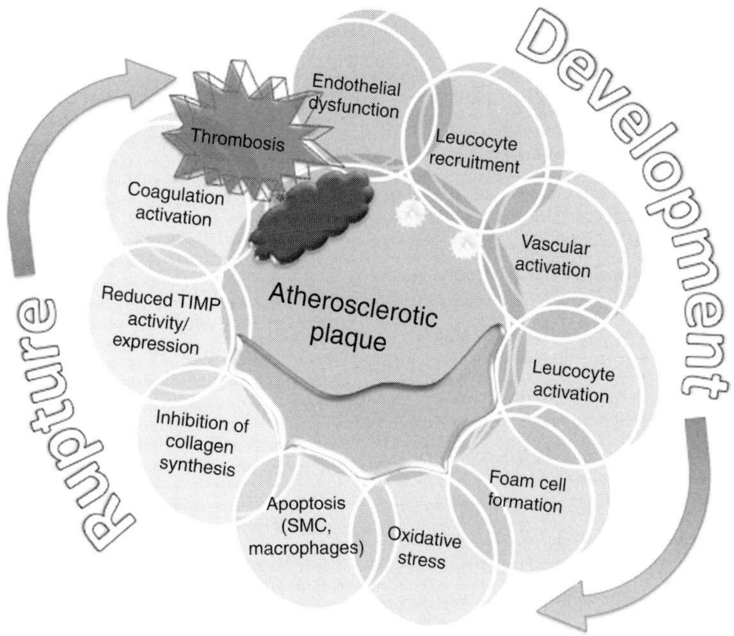

Fig. 14.3. Inflammation underlies all stages of atherosclerotic development and rupture. SMC, smooth muscle cell; TIMP, tissue inhibitor of metalloproteinase.

Inflammation and Biomarkers of Atherosclerosis

Given that inflammatory processes underlie the development of atherosclerosis, it has been investigated whether cytokines generated as part of the disease process might act as important biomarkers of atherosclerosis. Cytokines are proteins with relatively small molecular weights (Ait-Oufella *et al.*, 2011) and therefore when produced as part of an inflammatory response within the body can easily be secreted into blood. Thus, it follows that elevated circulating levels could be measured and act as a marker of atherosclerosis development. One cytokine that has been found to be particularly useful as a biomarker of atherosclerosis, and a strong predictor of coronary events (Torres and Ridker, 2003; Koenig *et al.*, 2006) is C-reactive protein (CRP). CRP is primarily produced by the liver in response to the inflammatory cytokines IL-6, IL-1 and TNF-α (Casas *et al.*, 2008; Blake and Ridker, 2002). CRP may be more than just a biomarker, with proposed roles in the development and progression of atherosclerosis. It has been proposed that CRP actively promotes LDL uptake by macrophages (Zwaka *et al.*, 2001; Libby and Ridker, 2004), increases expression of cell-adhesion molecules by endothelial cells and tissue factor by macrophages (Cermak *et al.*, 1993; Pasceri *et al.*, 2000; Pasceri *et al.*, 2001), induces plasminogen activator inhibitor-1 (PAI-1) expression (Devaraj *et al.*, 2003) and decreases nitric oxide generation by endothelial cells (Venugopal *et al.*, 2002).

CRP is easily measurable in the plasma of subjects using commercially available assays (Yeh and Willerson, 2003). Many clinical studies have demonstrated that CRP levels predict future cardiovascular events, with both men and women with elevated levels of CRP consistently showing high risk of a heart attack or stroke, even in the absence of high cholesterol levels (Ridker *et al.*, 1998; Albert *et al.*, 2002; Ridker, 2003).

Exercise, Inflammation and Atherosclerosis

Lifestyle modifications including diet, exercise and weight control are recommended for the treatment of atherosclerosis. In 2007, the American Heart Association (AHA) published guidelines for physical activity that could improve public health, with healthy hearts and low blood cholesterol as the primary goal (Williams *et al.*, 2007). The recommendation was walking briskly for 30 mins for 5 days, or a combination of jogging/vigorous physical activity for shorter time intervals. It was also recommended that every adult should perform activities that maintain or increase muscular strength and endurance for a minimum of 2 days each week. The studies that led to the AHA recommendations also demonstrated that there is a dose–response relationship between physical activity and health, so if the minimum recommendation was exceeded, this led to a proportional improvement in cholesterol levels and reduction in risk for atherosclerosis.

Indeed, it is well established from large population-based studies that regular physical exercise reduces the incidence and prevents the complications of atherosclerosis (Leon *et al.*, 1997; Manson *et al.*, 1999; Davey Smith *et al.*, 2000; Sesso *et al.*, 2000; Tanasescu *et al.*, 2002; Hamer and Chida, 2008). This is especially important for patients with coronary artery disease who have had a primary cardiovascular event because it has been shown from 48 trials and 8940 subjects that long-term exercise programmes significantly reduced cardiac mortality as well as mean cholesterol and triglyceride levels (Taylor *et al.*, 2004; Jolliffe *et al.*, 2001). The beneficial effects of exercise on cardiovascular risk may be due to weight loss, improved body fat distribution, increased insulin sensitivity, improved lipid profile and lowering of blood pressure (Mora *et al.*, 2007). It has also been clearly demonstrated, however, that exercise reduces inflammation and increases NO levels.

Exercise and nitric oxide

Low nitric oxide (NO) levels could represent one of the most important mechanisms explaining cardiovascular morbidity and mortality (Hambrecht *et al.*, 2000, 2003). Atherosclerotic coronary arteries exhibit a reduced ability to dilate in response to increased blood flow, which can cause a critical ischaemia even with only a moderate blockage of the artery. It has been shown that aerobic exercise increases nitric oxide levels via favourable adaptations in endothelial function. To test for endothelial function, the usual test is to measure vasoconstriction in response to acetylcholine, with more constriction indicating worse endothelial function. In a clinical study with coronary artery disease patients, intensive exercise training for 4 weeks decreased coronary artery vasoconstriction, in response to acetylcholine, by 54% (Hambrecht *et al.*, 2000). Moreover, the follow-up of those patients showed that, if the regular exercise was continued in a home-based programme, the beneficial effects on coronary endothelial function could be sustained (Gielen *et al.*, 2003a). Mechanistically, 4 weeks of regular exercise training in coronary artery disease patients led to increased eNOS levels and activity that generated increased NO. The improvement in NO levels was shown to improve blood flow in arteries during aerobic exercise. Regular exercise also increased levels of antioxidant defence enzymes, superoxide dismutase and glutathione peroxidase (Ennezat *et al.*, 2001).

In a separate study, patients scheduled for elective aortocoronary bypass grafting (CABG) were assigned to either 4 weeks of in-hospital regular aerobic exercise training or to an inactive control group. It was found that exercise training was accompanied by increased eNOS levels and activity (Hambrecht *et al.*, 2003).

Exercise and biomarkers of inflammation

The anti-inflammatory effect of exercise training has been assessed through the measurement of circulating levels of systemic biomarkers of inflammation, namely circulating cytokines and CRP. It has been demonstrated that 9 months of marathon training results in a 31% decrease in CRP (Mattusch *et al.*, 2000). Moreover, there was a 35% decrease in CRP after 6 months of exercise training in individuals with high risk for cardiovascular events (Smith *et al.*, 1999). Physical training also reduced plasma levels of the pro-inflammatory cytokines TNF-α and IL-1β in patients with chronic heart failure (Adamopoulos *et al.*, 2002). In a study of exercise effects on CAD, patients were randomized to either percutaneous intervention with a stent or aerobic exercise training. After 24 months of training, CRP levels were reduced by 41%, whereas there was no change in CRP measured in the percutaneous intervention group. The mechanisms proposed to underlie the decrease in CRP induced by exercise training are all related to a decrease in the production of IL-6, IL-1 and TNF-α (Kasapis and Thompson, 2005).

An even more exciting body of research demonstrates that individuals at risk of developing a heart attack can be protected from damage to the heart myocardium by regular exercise training. Firstly, 6 months of exercise training decreased systemic cytokine levels including TNF-α, IL-1β, interferon (IFN)-γ and CRP. Exercise training also reduces oxidative stress and LDL oxidation, which decreases vascular inflammation and endothelial dysfunction (Fukai *et al.*, 2000; Gielen *et al.*, 2003b; Lawler *et al.*, 2006). Experiments in rats have shown that physical activity induces biochemical alterations in cardiac muscle that include increased glycogen synthetase activity, increased glycogen stores and increased use of fats as an energy source (Scheuer and Tipton, 1977), all adaptations that would enhance energy availability and production in damaged myocardium. The clinical consequence was that the hearts of the exercise rats responded more effectively to sustained (1–3 days) pressure overload by aortic constriction because they could maintain or increase myocardial contractility whilst the sedentary rat control animals could not (Dowell *et al.*, 1976). In another study, rats that were exercised by swimming 1 h/day, 5 days/week for 5 weeks showed after acute ischaemia was induced by ligation of the left coronary artery that the size of the myocardial infarction was decreased by 30% (McElroy *et al.*, 1978). This was associated with an exercise-induced increase in capillary/muscle fibre ratio, suggesting an increase in myocardial vascularity helps to preserve the myocardium subjected to acute ischaemia.

Exercise and reduced atherosclerosis

Regular aerobic exercise can also reduce lesion size in animal models of atherosclerosis. Most studies have been completed in the ApoE-null mouse, a mouse that develops human-like atherosclerotic lesions by ~12–16 weeks of age. Studies using the ApoE-null mouse have shown that treadmill running (up to 6 km/day) or swimming (30 min, 3 times, 8 weeks) decreases lesion area (Pynn *et al.*, 2004; Okabe *et al.*, 2007; Shimada *et al.*, 2007). The lesion reductions were independent of weight loss or lipid profile but associated with reduced inflammatory markers. Using the same mouse model, it has been shown that the positive effects of exercise can be augmented when combined with a heart-healthy diet enriched in protein and unsaturated oils (Cesar *et al.*, 2011).

The decrease in lesion size in response to aerobic exercise may also be related to improved nitric oxide generation. ApoE mice that underwent exercise training involving 30 min swimming, 3 times a week for 8 weeks, showed decreased lesion size that could be completely abrogated if the exercising mice were treated with an inhibitor (L-NAME) of eNOS. These mice were unable to increase their production of NO, indicating that NO levels are crucial to the exercise-dependent effects on atherosclerosis (Okabe *et al.*, 2007).

Nutrition and Atherosclerosis

The high incidence of atherosclerosis in Australia and other Western societies is primarily driven by a diet high in saturated fats and processed foods with concurrent low intakes of polyunsaturated fatty acids (PUFAs), fruit, vegetables and fibre. Many epidemiological studies have reported strong associations between saturated fat and *trans* fatty acid intake, plasma cholesterol levels and death rates from atherosclerosis-related disease. It therefore follows that nutrition is one of the modifiable risk factors for atherosclerosis (Chiuve *et al.*, 2006, 2008; Fung *et al.*, 2009). Many studies have shown that changing dietary patterns or adding nutritional supplements to a healthy diet can significantly affect the development and progression of atherosclerosis (Keys *et al.*, 1984; Kromhout *et al.*, 1995; Knoops *et al.*, 2004; Mead *et al.*, 2006; Iqbal *et al.*, 2008; Mozaffarian *et al.*, 2010).

The current American Heart Association (AHA) and National Heart Foundation of Australia (NHF) suggest that a healthy lifestyle inclusive of regular physical activity and a diet rich in vegetables and fruits, whole grain high-fibre foods, fish at least twice a week, low saturated fat (<7% of energy), low *trans* fat (<1% of energy), fat-free or low-fat dairy products, minimal hydrogenated fats and minimal beverages with added sugar (Knoops *et al.*, 2004) protect against coronary heart disease. Although the general population is becoming increasingly aware of these recommendations, good nutrition remains a challenge. There are many different diets and supplements available and treating physicians often lack the knowledge about food composition and are not trained to give dietary advice (Wood *et al.*, 1998). Moreover, the tools that are used to evaluate diets are very complicated involving diet interviews, diet records and food-frequency questionnaires. Advice given about nutrition therefore remains quite varied with regards to timing, frequency, amount of certain food components and calorie intake.

Food groups and nutrients associated with atherosclerosis include salt, saturated fatty acids, monounsaturated fatty acids (MUFAs), omega-3 PUFAs, and fruit and vegetables.

Salt

There is substantial evidence for a causal relationship between salt intake and blood pressure. There is also increasing evidence that a high salt intake is directly related to left ventricular hypertrophy, an effect independent of blood pressure. Both raised blood pressure and left ventricular hypertrophy are risk factors for heart failure (He *et al.*, 2011). There have now been several studies that have shown that a reduction in salt intake is one of the most cost-effective interventions to reduce cardiovascular disease in the population (Selmer *et al.*, 2000; Asaria *et al.*, 2007; Joffres *et al.*, 2007; Palar and Sturm, 2009; Bibbins-Domingo *et al.*, 2010; Smith-Spangler *et al.*, 2010). In recognition of this, most developed countries, including Australia, are taking action to reduce salt intake (Karppanen and Mervaala, 2006).

The ancestors of humans, like all other mammals, consumed a very low salt diet (<0.5 g salt per day). Approximately 5000 years ago, however, it was discovered that salt could be used to preserve food and now our diet contains a large amount of highly salted processed foods. This high salt intake represents a major challenge to our kidneys that must filter and excrete these large salt concentrations. As a consequence, it is now common in our society to see a gradual increase in blood pressure with age (Intersalt Cooperative Research Group, 1988; He *et al.*, 2010) resulting from the high salt content in the diet. A study in chimpanzees showed that increasing salt consumption from 0.5 g/day to 10–15 g/day, which is close to the current salt intake in many countries (9–12 g/day), leads to a large increase in blood pressure (Denton *et al.*, 1995).

Salt intake is a major driver of blood pressure with age because communities that do not have a high salt intake have a lower adult blood pressure. For example, in an isolated tribe, the Yanomamo Indians, their blood pressure does not rise with age, associated with a low salt intake of <3 g/day (Manchilla-Carvalho *et al.* 1989). In an equally isolated tribe, however, the Qash'qai in Iran, that does have access to salt, adults do develop high blood pressure, very similar to that measured in Western communities (Page *et al.*, 1981). Intervention studies to reduce salt intake consistently show an improvement in blood pressure. It is currently recommended that salt intake is 5–6 g/day but a further reduction to 3–4 g/day has a much greater effect (MacGregor *et al.*, 1989; Sacks *et al.*, 2001). On the basis of the fall in blood pressure from a meta-analysis study of randomized salt reduction trials, it was suggested that reducing salt intake by 6 g/day (in a population where current salt intake is 9–12 g/day) would lead to a reduction in the incidence of stroke by 24% and heart attack by 18%, which would prevent ~2.5 million deaths worldwide (He and MacGregor, 2002). The extent of evidence that salt leads to increased blood pressure, atherosclerosis, stroke and heart failure is stronger than for any other dietary variable currently under consideration as important in the prevention of cardiovascular disease.

Saturated fatty acids

It has long been recognised that saturated fatty acids (SFAs) should be avoided. High intake levels of SFA increase blood cholesterol levels that directly accelerate atherosclerosis. In a major study, the Seven Countries Study, where 11,579 men, aged 40–49 years, were followed for 15 years, SFA was associated with increased risk of cardiovascular events or deaths (Keys *et al.*, 1986). In the Japanese Ni-Hon San Study, it was documented that men in Japan had very low saturated fat intake compared with Japanese immigrants in California. Associated with this, coronary heart disease, body weight and cholesterol levels were high in the Japanese men living in California, with very low coronary heart disease reported for the men living in Japan (Kato *et al.*, 1973).

Monounsaturated fatty acids

Foods that are high in MUFAs include olive oil and nuts, both important components of the Mediterranean diet that will be discussed later. Oleic acid, found in olive oil, is the primary MUFA in Western diets. Studies have investigated whether MUFA protect against atherosclerosis, with results showing only a small amount of, or no, protection (Garcia-Palmieri *et al.*, 1980; Kromhout and de Lezenne Coulander, 1984; Hu *et al.*, 1997). Olive oil contains other biologically active components, however, that make it more than just a MUFA fat (Perez-Jimenez *et al.*, 2005). Olive oil has been shown to improve the major risk factors for coronary heart disease, including lipoprotein and anti-thrombotic profiles, blood pressure, glucose metabolism and endothelial function. Olive oil has also been shown to exert anti-inflammatory and antioxidant properties (Perez-Jimenez *et al.*, 2005) such as decreased cell adhesion molecule expression via attenuated NFκB activation, decreased smooth muscle cell proliferation and decreased foam cell formation. One of the major bioactive components is hydroxytyrosol, which is a major antioxidant phenol. This component has been shown to inhibit lipid peroxidation, enhance cholesterol efflux and inhibit platelet aggregation (Covas *et al.*, 2006; Berrougui *et al.*, 2009).

Nuts are another major source of MUFA. Epidemiological studies have regularly demonstrated that frequent nut consumption is associated with reduced risk of coronary heart disease (Kelly and Sabate, 2006). Similar to olive oil, the major mechanism of protection is through improving the lipoprotein profile (Mukuddem-Petersen *et al.*, 2005); however, decreased inflammation and improved endothelial function also contribute to the protective effects of nuts. Because of their increasingly recognized cardiovascular benefits, nutritional guidelines often now include nut consumption (Johnson and Kennedy, 2000; Krauss *et al.*, 2000).

Polyunsaturated fats, omega-3

The benefits of omega-3 PUFA on coronary heart disease were first brought to light via an observation that coronary heart disease was only responsible for 3.5% of all deaths in Greenland Eskimos (The State of Health in Greenland, 1978). Investigations revealed that serum lipids of this population were enriched in omega-3 fatty acids (Bang *et al.*, 1971, Bang and Dyerberg, 1975) owing to their high consumption of oily fish (Dyerberg *et al.*, 1975; Bang *et al.*, 1980). Many studies have since confirmed the benefits of omega-3, with a very recent meta-analysis showing in 200,575 subjects that fish consumption was inversely associated with mortality from coronary heart disease (He *et al.*, 2004). Clinical data also support that omega-3 fatty acids protect against coronary heart disease. The Diet and Reinfarction Trial (DART) involved 2033 Welsh men that had all suffered a recent heart attack. These patients were assigned to two servings of fish per week, or equivalent in omega-3 supplement if fish intolerant, or no fish. After 2 years, there was a significant 29% decrease in cardiovascular mortality in those men that consumed fish. Similarly, in the largest clinical trial, the GISSI-Prevention Trial, omega-3 supplements for 3.5 years significantly reduced total death by 20% and non-fatal myocardial infarction and stroke by 15%. It is important to note that these supplements were provided in conjunction with a Mediterranean diet (GISSI-Prevenzione Trial, 1999). The Japanese population have low rates of coronary heart disease compared with the USA or Australia; however, even in this population the Japan EPA Lipid Prevention Study showed that in 18,645 patients with hypercholesteremia, treated with statins alone or statins and a high-dose highly purified EPA (1.8 g) for 5 years, the rate of major cardiovascular events was reduced by 19% in those taking EPA. Overall, the evidence is very strong that omega-3 are cardioprotective, with greater than 25 published trials showing that intake of fish oil is associated with decreased risk of cardiovascular events.

Given the strong evidence that omega-3 fatty acids are cardioprotective, the AHA guidelines now recommend that subjects without known coronary heart disease eat fish at least twice a week. For those patients with coronary heart disease, it is recommended that they take supplements (at least 1 g/day). Supplementation itself poses issues because the source of supplements is very important, on the basis of concerns about the method of processing and potential contamination by toxins including mercury. Pharmaceutical grade products that have undergone rigorous quality control testing are recommended (Hooper *et al.*, 2006; Wang *et al.*, 2006).

The mechanisms by which omega-3 fatty acids exert cardioprotective effects include decreased plasma triglycerides, decreased blood pressure, decreased platelet aggregation, improved endothelial function and improved cardiac rhythms (Kris-Etherton *et al.*, 2002; De Caterina and Zampolli, 2007). At the cellular level, omega-3 fatty acids decrease smooth muscle cell proliferation (Engler *et al.*, 2003) and decrease inflammation. Omega-3 fatty acids have been shown to reduce the expression of endothelial cell adhesion molecules (Collie *et al.*, 1996), cyclooxygenase-2 (COX-2), IL-6 and IL-8 (De Caterina *et al.*, 1994), macrophage colony stimulating factor (M-CSF) (Massaro *et al.*, 2002) and monocyte chemoattractant protein (MCP-1; Matsumoto *et al.*, 2008). The decreased expression of these molecules is associated with decreased binding of monocytes to cytokine-activated endothelium (De Caterina *et al.*, 1995). Omega-3 fatty acids also suppress superoxide generation (ROS) in endothelial cells through decreased assembly and activation of the key enzyme complex, NADPH oxidase (Massaro *et al.*, 2006), and therefore omega-3 fatty acids have an antioxidant function. Finally, it has been shown that omega-3 fatty acids can inhibit the secretion of metalloproteinases from macrophages, thus increasing plaque stability (Thies *et al.*, 2003).

Fruits and vegetables

'They should build houses, and inhabit them; and they shall plant vegetables, and eat the fruit of them' (Isaiah, 65:20–22). The prophet Isaiah suggested long ago that a diet full of fruit and vegetables was central to a healthful life. It is now estimated that an inadequate consumption of fruit and vegetables accounts for up to 2.64 million global deaths per year (Lock *et al.*, 2005). Following on, projections suggest that increasing consumption of fruit and vegetables by 600 g per day could decrease the global burden of coronary heart disease and stroke by 31% and 19%, respectively (Lock *et al.*, 2005). Meta-analysis showed that risk decreased by 4% for every portion of fruit or vegetable intake (Dauchet *et al.*, 2006). Another study, CARDIO2000, showed that consumption of >5 servings of fruit per day was associated with 72% lower risk, and consumption of vegetables more than 3 days per week was associated with a 70% lower risk of coronary heart disease, when compared with non-consumption (Panagiotakos *et al.*, 2003). Other more recent studies have confirmed the benefits of fruit and vegetable intake (Dauchet *et al.*, 2004, 2010). Despite this accumulating evidence, there are very few randomized control trials to show the protective role in coronary heart disease, and to determine the mechanisms by which fruit and vegetables exert their protective effects. One study, however, implicates anti-inflammatory mechanisms because fruit and vegetable intake was reported to be associated with lower circulating concentrations of CRP (Bhupathiraju and Tucker, 2011).

Vegetables and fruits, as well as cocoa, tea and wine, all contain polyphenols that are suggested to be cardioprotective (Kuhnau, 1976; Hertog *et al.*, 1993). A Finland study showed that very low intake of these polyphenols was associated with increased mortality from coronary heart disease (Knekt *et al.*, 1996). Myocardial infarction has been shown to be inversely associated with tea consumption (Peters *et al.*, 2001), although this is related to region. In the UK and Australia, where milk is commonly added to tea, the cardioprotection is lost.

Dietary patterns and atherosclerosis

A meal consists of a variety of foods with complex combinations of nutrients that could well have synergistic or interactive effects. One diet that incorporates many healthy individual components is the Mediterranean diet. This diet includes: (i) daily consumption of unrefined cereals and cereal products, vegetables (2–3 servings), fruit (4–6 servings), olive oil, dairy products (1–2 servings) and red or white wine (1–2 wine glasses); (ii) weekly consumption of potatoes (4–5 servings), fish (4–5 servings), olives, pulses and nuts (more than 4 servings) and eggs and sweets (1–3 servings); (iii) monthly consumption of red meat and meat products (4–5 servings) (Dontas *et al.*, 2007). There have now been a number of studies that show this type of diet is associated with a lower risk of coronary heart disease mortality (Panagiotakos *et al.*, 2008; Sofi *et al.*, 2008) and that there are inverse associations with cardiovascular risk factors including serum lipids, blood pressure, inflammatory and coagulation markers (Panagiotakos *et al.*, 2006).

Summary and Conclusions

There is no question that endothelial dysfunction and vascular wall inflammation underlie all stages of atherosclerosis. Exercise training represents a non-pharmacological treatment that reduces inflammation, improves endothelial function and importantly decreases atherosclerosis and protects against myocardial ischemia (Fig. 14.4). Exercise training increases nitric oxide

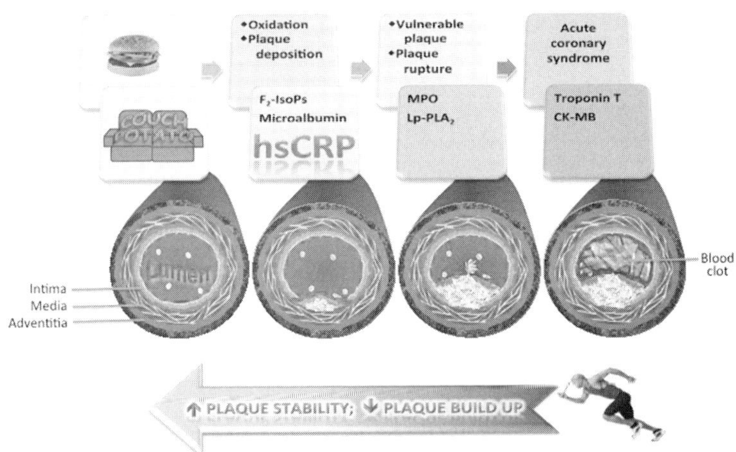

Fig. 14.4. Exercise can reduce the extent of atherosclerosis. Atherosclerosis is an inflammatory disease and a number of biomarkers have been identified that can predict atherosclerosis. C-reactive protein, or CRP, is the most powerful biomarker. Exercise studies completed in cycling, running and swimming show a decrease in inflammatory markers and exercise has been shown to reduce the extent of atherosclerosis. CK-MB, creatin kinase-MB; F2-IsoPs, F2-isoprostane; hs-CRP, high-sensitivity C-reactive protein; Lp-PLA2, lipoprotein-associated phospholipase; MPO, myeloperoxidase.

generation, which represents a major cardioprotective mechanism because it decreases cytokine production and increases antioxidant defences. It is highly likely that other mechanisms await discovery. Whatever the mechanisms, it remains that exercise training reduces the morbidity and mortality in patients with atherosclerosis and moreover improves the heart myocardium in non-cardiac patients such that exercise affords protection if there is a cardiovascular event. In addition to implementing an exercise regime, good nutrition practices are crucial. There is now strong evidence that some foods or food components can decrease cardiovascular risk, and/or improve coronary heart disease if it already exists. These nutrients include those found in fruits and vegetables and omega-3 PUFA that act via a variety of mechanisms, including reducing inflammation. A healthful lifestyle inclusive of exercise and nutrition plans should therefore be considered for coronary heart disease prevention and treatment.

References

Adamopoulos, S., Parissis, J., Karatzas, D., Kroupis, C., Georgiadis, M., *et al.* (2002) Physical training modulates proinflammatory cytokines and the soluble Fas/soluble Fas ligand system in patients with chronic heart failure. *Journal of American College of Cardiology* 39, 653–963.

Ait-Oufella, H., Taleb, S., Mallat, Z. and Tedgui, A. (2011) Recent advances on the role of cytokines in atherosclerosis. *Arteriosclerosis Thrombosis Vascular Biology* 31, 969–979.

Albert, C.M., Ma, J., Rifai, N., Stampfer, M.J. and Ridker, P.M. (2002) Prospective study of C-reactive protein, homocysteine, and plasma lipid levels as predictors of sudden cardiac death. *Circulation* 105, 2595–2599.

Asaria, P., Chisholm, D., Mathers, C., Ezzati, M. and Beaglehole, R. (2007) Chronic disease prevention: health effects and financial costs of strategies to reduce salt intake and control tobacco use. *Lancet* 370, 2044–2053.

Bang, H.O. and Dyerberg, J. (1972) Plasma lipids and lipoproteins in Greenlandic west coast Eskimos. *Acta Medica Scandinivica* 192, 85–94.

Bang, H.O., Dyerberg, J. and Nielsen, A.B. (1971) Plasma lipid and lipoprotein pattern in Greenlandic West-coast Eskimos. *Lancet* 1, 1143–1145.

Bang, H.O., Dyerberg, J. and Sinclair, H.M. (1980) The composition of the Eskimo food in north western Greenland. *American Journal of Clinical Nutrition* 33, 2657–2661.

Berliner, J., Leitinger, N., Watson, A., Huber, J., Fogelman, A., *et al.* (1997) Oxidized lipids in atherogenesis: formation, destruction and action. *Thrombosis and Haemostasis* 78, 195–199.

Berrougui, H., Grenier, G., Loued, S., Drouin, G. and Khalil, A. (2009) A new insight into resveratrol as an atheroprotective compound: inhibition of lipid peroxidation and enhancement of cholesterol efflux. *Atherosclerosis* 207, 420–427.

Bhupathiraju, S.N. and Tucker, K.L. (2011) Greater variety in fruit and vegetable intake is associated with lower inflammation in Puerto Rican adults. *American Journal of Clinical Nutrition* 93, 37–46.

Bibbins-Domingo, K., Chertow, G.M., Coxson, P.G., Moran, A., Lightwood, J.M., *et al.* (2010) Projected effect of dietary salt reductions on future cardiovascular disease. *New England Journal Medicine* 362, 590–599.

Blake, G.J. and Ridker, P.M. (2002) Inflammatory bio-markers and cardiovascular risk prediction. *Journal of Internal Medicine* 252, 283–294.

Casas, J.P., Shah, T., Hingorani, A.D., Danesh, J. and Pepys, M.B. (2008) C-reactive protein and coronary heart disease: a critical review. *Journal of Internal Medicine* 264, 295–314.

Cermak, J., Key, N.S., Bach, R.R., Balla, J., Jacob, H.S., *et al.* (1993) C-reactive protein induces human peripheral blood monocytes to synthesize tissue factor. *Blood* 82, 513–520.

Cesar, L., Suarez, S.V., Adi, J., Adi, N., Vazquez-Padron, R., *et al.* (2011) An essential role for diet in exercise-mediated protection against dyslipidemia, inflammation and atherosclerosis in ApoE/mice. *PLoS One* 6, e17263.

Chiuvo, S.E., Mccullough, M.L., Sacks, F.M. and Rimm, E.B. (2006) Healthy lifestyle factors in the primary prevention of coronary heart disease among men: benefits among users and nonusers of lipid-lowering and antihypertensive medications. *Circulation* 114, 160–167.

Chiuve, S.E., Rexrode, K.M., Spiegelman, D., Logroscino, G., Manson, J.E., *et al.* (2008) Primary prevention of stroke by healthy lifestyle. *Circulation* 118, 947–954.

Collie-Duguid, E.S. and Wahle, K.W. (1996) Inhibitory effect of fish oil N-3 polyunsaturated fatty acids on the expression of endothelial cell adhesion molecules. *Biochemical Biophysical Research Communications* 220, 969–974.

Constans, J. and Conri, C. (2006) Circulating markers of endothelial function in cardiovascular disease. *Clinical Chimica Acta* 368, 33–347.

Corti, R., Hutter, R., Badimon, J.J. and Fuster, V. (2004) Evolving concepts in the triad of atherosclerosis, inflammation and thrombosis. *Journal of Thrombosis and Thrombolysis* 17, 35–44.

Covas, M.I., De La Torre, K., Farre-Albaladejo, M., Kaikkonen, J., Fito, M., *et al.* (2006) Postprandial LDL phenolic content and LDL oxidation are modulated by olive oil phenolic compounds in humans. *Free Radical Biology Medicine* 40, 608–616.

Dauchet, L., Ferrieres, J., Arveiler, D., Yarnell, J.W., Gey, F., *et al.* (2004) Frequency of fruit and vegetable consumption and coronary heart disease in France and Northern Ireland: the PRIME study. *British Journal of Nutrition* 92, 963–972.

Dauchet, L., Amouyel, P., Hercberg, S. and Dallongeville, J. (2006) Fruit and vegetable consumption and risk of coronary heart disease: a meta-analysis of cohort studies. *Journal of Nutrition* 136, 2588–2593.

Dauchet, L., Montaye, M., Ruidavets, J.B., Arveiler, D., Kee, F., *et al.* (2010) Association between the frequency of fruit and vegetable consumption and cardiovascular disease in male smokers and non-smokers. *European Journal of Clinical Nutrition* 64, 578–586.

Davey Smith, G., Shipley, M.J., Batty, G.D., Morris, J.N. and Marmot, M. (2000) Physical activity and cause-specific mortality in the Whitehall study. *Public Health* 114, 308–315.

De Caterina, R. and Zampolli, A. (2007) Omega-3 fatty acids, atherogenesis, and endothelial activation. *Journal of Cardiovascular Medicine* (Hagerstown) 8 Supplementary 1, S11–S14.

De Caterina, R., Cybulsky, M.I., Clinton, S.K., Gimbrone, M.A., Jr and Libby, P. (1994) The omega-3 fatty acid docosahexaenoate reduces cytokine-induced expression of proatherogenic and proinflammatory proteins in human endothelial cells. *Arteriosclerosis and Thrombosis* 14, 1829–1836.

De Caterina, R., Cybulsky, M.A., Clinton, S.K., Gimbrone, M.A., Jr and Libby, P. (1995) Omega-3 fatty acids and endothelial leukocyte adhesion molecules. *Prostaglandins Leukotrienes Essential Fatty Acids* 52, 191–195.

De Caterina, R., Bernini, W., Carluccio, M.A., Liao, J.K. and Libby, P. (1998) Structural requirements for inhibition of cytokine-induced endothelial activation by unsaturated fatty acids. *Journal of Lipid Research* 39, 1062–1070.

Denton, D., Weisinger, R., Mundy, N.I., Wickings, E.J., Dixson, A., *et al.* (1995) The effect of increased salt intake on blood pressure of chimpanzees. *Nature Medicine* 1, 1009–1016.

Devaraj, S., Xu, D.Y. and Jialal, I. (2003) C-reactive protein increases plasminogen activator inhibitor-1 expression and activity in human aortic endothelial cells: implications for the metabolic syndrome and atherothrombosis. *Circulation* 107, 398–404.

Dontas, A.S., Zerefos, N.S., Panagiotakos, D.B., Vlachou, C. and Valis, D.A. (2007) Mediterranean diet and prevention of coronary heart disease in the elderly. *Journal of Clinical Interventions in Aging* 2, 109–115.

Dowell, R.T., Cutilletta, A.F., Rudnik, M.A. and Sodt, P.C. (1976) Heart functional responses to pressure overload in exercised and sedentary rats. *American Journal of Physiology* 230, 199–204.

Dyerberg, J., Bang, H.O. and Hjorne, N. (1975) Fatty acid composition of the plasma lipids in Greenland Eskimos. *American Journal of Clinical Nutrition* 28, 958–966.

Engler, M.M., Engler, M.B., Pierson, D.M., Molteni, L.B. and Molteni, A. (2003) Effects of docosahexaenoic acid on vascular pathology and reactivity in hypertension. *Experimental Biology Medicine* (Maywood) 228, 299–307.

Ennezat, P.V., Malendowicz, S.L., Testa, M., Colombo, P.C., Cohen-Solal, A., *et al.* (2001) Physical training in patients with chronic heart failure enhances the expression of genes encoding antioxidative enzymes. *Journal of the American College of Cardiology* 38, 194–198.

Foot, D.K., Lewis, R.P., Pearson, T.A. and Beller, G.A. (2000) Demographics and cardiology, 1950–2050. *Journal of American College of Cardiology* 35, 66B–80B.

Fukai, T., Siegfried, M.R., Ushio-Fukai, M., Cheng, Y., Kojda, G., *et al.* (2000) Regulation of the vascular extracellular superoxide dismutase by nitric oxide and exercise training. *Journal of Clinical Investigation* 105, 1631–1639.

Fung, T.T., Rexrode, K.M., Mantzoros, C.S., Manson, J.E., Willett, W.C., *et al.* (2009) Mediterranean diet and incidence of and mortality from coronary heart disease and stroke in women. *Circulation* 119, 1093–1100.

Garcia-Palmieri, M.R., Sorlie, P., Tillotson, J., Costas, R. Jr, Cordero, E. and Rodriguez, M. (1980) Relationship of dietary intake to subsequent coronary heart disease incidence: The Puerto Rico Heart Health Program. *American Journal of Clinical Nutrition* 33, 1818–1827.

Gielen, S., Erbs, S., Linke, A., Mobius-Winkler, S., Schuler, G., *et al.* (2003a) Home-based versus hospital-based exercise programs in patients with coronary artery disease: effects on coronary vasomotion. *American Heart Journal* 145, E3.

Gielen, S., Adams, V., Mobius-Winkler, S., Linke, A., Erbs, S., *et al.* (2003b) Anti-inflammatory effects of exercise training in the skeletal muscle of patients with chronic heart failure. *Journal of the American College of Cardiology* 42, 861–868.

Gruppo Italiano per lo Studio della Sopravvivenza nell'Infarto miocardico (1999) Dietary supplementation with n-3 polyunsaturated fatty acids and vitamin E after myocardial infarction: results of the GISSI-Prevenzione trial. *Lancet* 354, 447–455.

Hambrecht, R., Adams, V., Erbs, S., Linke, A., Krankel, N., *et al.* (2003) Regular physical activity improves endothelial function in patients with coronary artery disease by increasing phosphorylation of endothelial nitric oxide synthase. *Circulation* 107, 3152–3158.

Hambrecht, R., Wolf, A., Gielen, S., Linke, A., Hofer, J., *et al.* (2000) Effect of exercise on coronary endothelial function in patients with coronary artery disease. *New England Journal of Medicine* 342, 454–460.

Hamer, M. and Chida, Y. (2008) Walking and primary prevention: a meta-analysis of prospective cohort studies. *British Journal of Sports Medicine* 42, 238–243.

Hansson, G.K. (2005) Inflammation, atherosclerosis, and coronary artery disease. *New England Journal of Medicine* 352, 1685–1695.

He, F.J. and Macgregor, G.A. (2002) Effect of modest salt reduction on blood pressure: a meta-analysis of randomized trials. Implications for public health. *Journal of Human Hypertension* 16, 761–770.

He, F.J. and Macgregor, G.A. (2010) Reducing population salt intake worldwide: from evidence to implementation. *Progressive Cardiovascular Disease* 52, 363–382.

He, F.J., Burnier, M. and Macgregor, G.A. (2011) Nutrition in cardiovascular disease: salt in hypertension and heart failure. *European Heart Journal* 32, 3073–3080.

He, K., Song, Y., Daviglus, M.L., Liu, K., Van Horn, L., *et al.* (2004) Accumulated evidence on fish consumption and coronary heart disease mortality: a meta-analysis of cohort studies. *Circulation* 109, 2705–2711.

Hertog, M.G., Feskens, E.J., Hollman, P.C., Katan, M.B. and Kromhout, D. (1993) Dietary antioxidant flavonoids and risk of coronary heart disease: the Zutphen Elderly Study. *Lancet* 342, 1007–1011.

Hooper, L., Thompson, R.L., Harrison, R.A., Summerbell, C.D., Ness, A.R., *et al.* (2006) Risks and benefits of omega 3 fats for mortality, cardiovascular disease, and cancer: systematic review. *British Medical Journal* 332, 752–760.

Hu, F.B., Stampfer, M.J., Manson, J.E., Rimm, E., Colditz, G.A., *et al.* (1997) Dietary fat intake and the risk of coronary heart disease in women. *New England Journal of Medicine* 337, 1491–1499.

Intersalt Cooperative Research Group (1988) Intersalt: an international study of electrolyte excretion and blood pressure. Results for 24 hour urinary sodium and potassium excretion. *British Medical Journal* 297, 319–328.

Iqbal, R., Anand, S., Ounpuu, S., Islam, S., Zhang, X., *et al.* (2008) Dietary patterns and the risk of acute myocardial infarction in 52 countries: results of the INTERHEART study. *Circulation* 118, 1929–1937.

Joffres, M.R., Campbell, N.R., Manns, B. and Tu, K. (2007) Estimate of the benefits of a population-based reduction in dietary sodium additives on hypertension and its related health care costs in Canada. *Canadian Journal of Cardiology* 23, 437–443.

Johnson, R.K. and Kennedy, E. (2000) The 2000 Dietary Guidelines for Americans: what are the changes and why were they made? The Dietary Guidelines Advisory Committee. *Journal of the American Dietetic Association* 100, 769–774.

Jolliffe, J.A., Rees, K., Taylor, R.S., Thompson, D., Oldridge, N., *et al.* (2001) Exercise-based rehabilitation for coronary heart disease. *Cochrane Database Systemic Review* CD001800.

Karppanen, H. and Mervaala, E. (2006) Sodium intake and hypertension. *Progressive Cardiovascular Disease* 40, 59–75.

Kasapis, C. and Thompson, P.D. (2005) The effects of physical activity on serum C reactive protein and inflammatory markers: a systematic review. *Journal of the American College of Cardiology* 45, 1563–1569.

Kato, H., Tillotson, J., Nichaman, M.Z., Rhoads, G.G. and Hamilton, H.B. (1973) Epidemiologic studies of coronary heart disease and stroke in Japanese men living in Japan, Hawaii and California. *American Journal of Epidemiology* 97, 372–385.

Kelly, J.H., Jr and Sabate, J. (2006) Nuts and coronary heart disease: an epidemiological perspective. British Journal of Nutrition, 96 Supplement 2, S61–S67.

Keys, A., Menotti, A., Aravanis, C., Blackburn, H., Djordevic, B.S., *et al.* (1984) The seven countries study: 2,289 deaths in 15 years. *Preventative Medicine* 13, 141–154.

Keys, A., Menotti, A., Karvonen, M.J., Aravanis, C., Blackburn, H., *et al.* (1986) The diet and 15-year death rate in the seven countries study. American Journal of Epidemiology, 124, 903–915.

Knekt, P., Jarvinen, R., Reunanen, A. and Maatela, J. (1996) Flavonoid intake and coronary mortality in Finland: a cohort study. *British Medical Journal* 312, 478–481.

Knoops, K.T., De Groot, L.C., Kromhout, D., Perrin, A.E., Moreiras-Varela, O., *et al.* (2004) Mediterranean diet, lifestyle factors, and 10-year mortality in elderly European men and women: the HALE project. *Journal of the American Medical Association* 292, 1433–1439.

Koenig, W., Khuseyinova, N., Baumert, J., Thorand, B., Loewel, H., *et al.* (2006) Increased concentrations of C-reactive protein and IL-6 but not IL-18 are independently associated with incident coronary events in middle-aged men and women: results from the MONICA/KORA Augsburg case-cohort study, 1984–2002. *Arteriosclerosis, Thrombosis and Vascular Biology* 26, 2745–2751.

Krauss, R.M., Eckel, R.H., Howard, B., Appel, L.J., Daniels, S.R., *et al.* (2000) AHA Dietary Guidelines: revision 2000: A statement for healthcare professionals from the Nutrition Committee of the American Heart Association. *Circulation* 102, 2284–2299.

Kris-Etherton, P.M., Harris, W.S. and Appel, L.J. (2002) Fish consumption, fish oil, omega-3 fatty acids, and cardiovascular disease. *Circulation* 106, 2747–2757.

Kromhout, D. and De Lezenne Coulander, C. (1984) Diet, prevalence and 10-year mortality from coronary heart disease in 871 middle-aged men. The Zutphen Study. *American Journal of Epidemiology* 119, 733–741.

Kromhout, D., Menotti, A., Bloemberg, B., Aravanis, C., Blackburn, H., *et al.*. (1995) Dietary saturated and trans fatty acids and cholesterol and 25-year mortality from coronary heart disease: the Seven Countries Study. *Preventative Medicine* 24, 308–315.

Kuhnau, J. (1976) The flavonoids. A class of semi-essential food components: their role in human nutrition. *World Review of Nutrition and Dietetics* 24, 117–191.

Lawler, J.M., Kwak, H.B., Song, W. and Parker, J.L. (2006) Exercise training reverses downregulation of HSP70 and antioxidant enzymes in porcine skeletal muscle after chronic coronary artery occlusion. *American Journal of Physiology Regulatory Integrative and Comparative Physiology* 291, R1756–R1763.

Leon, A.S., Myers, M.J. and Connett, J. (1997) Leisure time physical activity and the 16-year risks of mortality from coronary heart disease and all-causes in the Multiple Risk Factor Intervention Trial (MRFIT). *International Journal of Sports Medicine* 18 Supplement 3, S208–S215.

Libby, P. and Ridker, P.M. (2004) Inflammation and atherosclerosis: role of C-reactive protein in risk assessment. *American Journal of Medicine* 116 Supplement 6A, 9S–16S.

Lock, K., Pomerleau, J., Causer, L., Altmann, D.R. and Mckee, M. (2005) The global burden of disease attributable to low consumption of fruit and vegetables: implications for the global strategy on diet. *Bulletin of the World Health Organisation* 83, 100–118.

Lusis, A.J. (2000) Atherosclerosis. *Nature* 407, 233–241.

Macgregor, G.A., Markandu, N.D., Sagnella, G.A., Singer, D.R. and Cappuccio, F.P. (1989) Double-blind study of three sodium intakes and long-term effects of sodium restriction in essential hypertension. *Lancet* 2, 1244–1247.

Mancilha-Carvalho, J.J., De Oliveira, R. and Esposito, R.J. (1989) Blood pressure and electrolyte excretion in the Yanomamo Indians, an isolated population. *Journal of Human Hypertension* 3, 309–314.

Manson, J.E., Hu, F.B., Rich-Edwards, J.W., Colditz, G.A., Stampfer, M.J., *et al.* (1999) A prospective study of walking as compared with vigorous exercise in the prevention of coronary heart disease in women. *New England Journal of Medicine* 341, 650–658.

Massaro, M., Basta, G., Lazzerini, G., Carluccio, M.A., Bosetti, F., *et al.* (2002) Quenching of intracellular ROS generation as a mechanism for oleate-induced reduction of endothelial activation and early atherogenesis. *Thrombosis and Haemostasis* 88, 335–344.

Massaro, M., Habib, A., Lubrano, L., Del Turco, S., Lazzerini, G., *et al.* (2006) The omega-3 fatty acid docosahexaenoate attenuates endothelial cyclooxygenase-2 induction through both NADP(H) oxidase and PKC epsilon inhibition. *Proceedings of the National Academy of Science USA* 103, 15184–15189.

Matsumoto, M., Sata, M., Fukuda, D., Tanaka, K., Soma, M., *et al.* (2008) Orally administered eicosapentaenoic acid reduces and stabilizes atherosclerotic lesions in ApoE-deficient mice. *Atherosclerosis* 197, 524–533.

Mattusch, F., Dufaux, B., Heine, O., Mertens, I. and Rost, R. (2000) Reduction of the plasma concentration of C-reactive protein following nine months of endurance training. *International Journal of Sports Medicine* 21, 21–24.

Mcelroy, C.L., Gissen, S.A. and Fishbein, M.C. (1978) Exercise-induced reduction in myocardial infarct size after coronary artery occlusion in the rat. *Circulation* 57, 958–962.

Mead, A., Atkinson, G., Albin, D., Alphey, D., Baic, S., *et al.* (2006) Dietetic guidelines on food and nutrition in the secondary prevention of cardiovascular disease - evidence from systematic reviews of randomized controlled trials (second update, January 2006). *Journal of Human Nutrition and Dietetics* 19, 401–419.

Mombouli, J.V. and Vanhoutte, P.M. (1999) Endothelial dysfunction: from physiology to therapy. *Journal of Molecular and Cellular Cardiology* 31, 61–74.

Mora, S., Cook, N., Buring, J.E., Ridker, P.M. and Lee, I.M. (2007) Physical activity and reduced risk of cardiovascular events: potential mediating mechanisms. *Circulation* 116, 2110–2118.

Mozaffarian, D., Micha, R. and Wallace, S. (2010) Effects on coronary heart disease of increasing polyunsaturated fat in place of saturated fat: a systematic review and meta-analysis of randomized controlled trials. *PLoS Medicine* 7, e1000252.

Mukuddem-Petersen, J., Oosthuizen, W. and Jerling, J.C. (2005) A systematic review of the effects of nuts on blood lipid profiles in humans. *Journal of Nutrition* 135, 2082–2089.

Okabe, T.A., Shimada, K., Hattori, M., Murayama, T., Yokode, M., *et al.* (2007) Swimming reduces the severity of atherosclerosis in apolipoprotein E deficient mice by antioxidant effects. *Cardiovascular Research* 74, 537–545.

Page, L.B., Vandevert, D.E., Nader, K., Lubin, N.K. and Page, J.R. (1981) Blood pressure of Qash'qai pastoral nomads in Iran in relation to culture, diet, and body form. *American Journal of Clinical Nutrition* 34, 527–538.

Palar, K. and Sturm, R. (2009) Potential societal savings from reduced sodium consumption in the U.S. adult population. *American Journal of Health Promotion* 24, 49–57.

Panagiotakos, D.B., Pitsavos, C., Kokkinos, P., Chrysohoou, C., Vavuranakis, M., *et al.* (2003) Consumption of fruits and vegetables in relation to the risk of developing acute coronary syndromes; the CARDIO2000 case-control study. *Nutrition Journal* 2, 2.

Panagiotakos, D.B., Pitsavos, C. and Stefanadis, C. (2006) Dietary patterns: a Mediterranean diet score and its relation to clinical and biological markers of cardiovascular disease risk. *Nutrition Metabolism and Cardiovascular Diseases* 16, 559–568.

Panagiotakos, D.B., Pitsavos, C., Chrysohoou, C., Skoumas, I. and Stefanadis, C. (2008) Five-year incidence of cardiovascular disease and its predictors in Greece: the ATTICA study. *Vascular Medicine* 13, 113–121.

Pasceri, V., Willerson, J.T. and Yeh, E.T. (2000) Direct proinflammatory effect of C-reactive protein on human endothelial cells. *Circulation* 102, 2165–2168.

Pasceri, V., Cheng, J.S., Willerson, J.T. and Yeh, E.T. (2001) Modulation of C-reactive protein-mediated monocyte chemoattractant protein-1 induction in human endothelial cells by anti-atherosclerosis drugs. *Circulation* 103, 2531–2534.

Pearson, J.D. (2000) Normal endothelial cell function. *Lupus* 9, 183–8.

Perez-Jimenez, F., Alvarez De Cienfuegos, G., Badimon, L., Barja, G., Battino, M., *et al.* (2005) International conference on the healthy effect of virgin olive oil. *European Journal of Clinical Investigation* 35, 421–424.

Peters, U., Poole, C. and Arab, L. (2001) Does tea affect cardiovascular disease? A meta-analysis. *American Journal of Epidemiology* 154, 495–503.

Pynn, M., Schafer, K., Konstantinides, S. and Halle, M. (2004) Exercise training reduces neointimal growth and stabilizes vascular lesions developing after injury in apolipoprotein e-deficient mice. *Circulation* 109, 386–392.

Qiao, J.H., Tripathi, J., Mishra, N.K., Cai, Y., Tripathi, S., *et al.* (1997) Role of macrophage colony-stimulating factor in atherosclerosis: studies of osteopetrotic mice. *American Journal of Pathology* 150, 1687–1699.

Ridker, P.M. (2003) Clinical application of C-reactive protein for cardiovascular disease detection and prevention. *Circulation* 107, 363–369.

Ridker, P.M., Glynn, R.J. and Hennekens, C.H. (1998) C-reactive protein adds to the predictive value of total and HDL cholesterol in determining risk of first myocardial infarction. *Circulation* 97, 2007–2011.

Ross, R. (1999) Atherosclerosis–an inflammatory disease. *New England Journal of Medicine* 340, 115–126.

Sacks, F.M., Svetkey, L.P., Vollmer, W.M., Appel, L.J., Bray, G.A., *et al.* (2001) Effects on blood pressure of reduced dietary sodium and the Dietary Approaches to Stop Hypertension (DASH) diet. DASH-Sodium Collaborative Research Group. *New England Journal of Medicine* 344, 3–10.

Scheuer, J. and Tipton, C.M. (1977) Cardiovascular adaptations to physical training. *Annual Review Physiology* 39, 221–251.

Selmer, R.M., Kristiansen, I.S., Haglerod, A., Graff-Iversen, S., Larsen, H.K., *et al.* (2000) Cost and health consequences of reducing the population intake of salt. *Journal of Epidemiology Community Health* 54, 697–702.

Sesso, H.D., Paffenbarger, R.S., Jr and Lee, I.M. (2000) Physical activity and coronary heart disease in men: The Harvard Alumni Health Study. *Circulation* 102, 975–980.

Shimada, K., Kishimoto, C., Okabe, T.A., Hattori, M., Murayama, T., *et al.* (2007) Exercise training reduces severity of atherosclerosis in apolipoprotein E knockout mice via nitric oxide. *Circulation Journal* 71, 1147–1151.

Smith, J.D., Trogan, E., Ginsberg, M., Grigaux, C., Tian, J. *et al.* (1995) Decreased atherosclerosis in mice deficient in both macrophage colony-stimulating factor (op) and apolipoprotein E. *Proceedings of the National Academy of Science USA* 92, 8264–8268.

Smith, J.K., Dykes, R., Douglas, J.E., Krishnaswamy, G. and Berk, S. (1999) Long-term exercise and atherogenic activity of blood mononuclear cells in persons at risk of developing ischemic heart disease. *Journal of the American Medical Association* 281, 1722–1727.

Smith-Spangler, C.M., Juusola, J.L., Enns, E.A., Owens, D.K. and Garber, A.M. (2010) Population strategies to decrease sodium intake and the burden of cardiovascular disease: a cost-effectiveness analysis. *Annals of Internal Medicine* 152, 481–487, W170–W173.

Sofi, F., Cesari, F., Abbate, R., Gensini, G.F. and Casini, A. (2008) Adherence to Mediterranean diet and health status: meta-analysis. *British Medical Journal* 337, a1344.

Stemme, S., Faber, B., Holm, J., Wiklund, O., Witztum, J.L., *et al.* (1995) T lymphocytes from human atherosclerotic plaques recognize oxidized low density lipoprotein. *Proceedings of the National Academy of Science USA* 92, 3893–3897.

Tanasescu, M., Leitzmann, M.F., Rimm, E.B., Willett, W.C., Stampfer, M.J., *et al.* (2002) Exercise type and intensity in relation to coronary heart disease in men. *Journal of the American Medical Association* 288, 1994–2000.

Taylor, R.S., Brown, A., Ebrahim, S., Jolliffe, J., Noorani, H., *et al.* (2004) Exercise-based rehabilitation for patients with coronary heart disease: systematic review and meta-analysis of randomized controlled trials. *American Journal of Medicine* 116, 682–692.

Thies, F., Garry, J.M., Yaqoob, P., Rerkasem, K., Williams, J., *et al.* (2003) Association of n-3 polyunsaturated fatty acids with stability of atherosclerotic plaques: a randomised controlled trial. *Lancet* 361, 477–485.

Torres, J.L. and Ridker, P.M. (2003) Clinical use of high sensitivity C-reactive protein for the prediction of adverse cardiovascular events. *Current Opinion in Cardiology* 18, 471–478.

Venugopal, S.K., Devaraj, S., Yuhanna, I., Shaul, P. and Jialal, I. (2002) Demonstration that C-reactive protein decreases eNOS expression and bioactivity in human aortic endothelial cells. *Circulation* 106, 1439–1441.

Virmani, R., Kolodgie, F.D., Burke, A.P., Farb, A. and Schwartz, S.M. (2000) Lessons from sudden coronary death: a comprehensive morphological classification scheme for atherosclerotic lesions. *Arteriosclerosis, Thrombosis and Vascular Biology* 20, 1262–1275.

Wang, C., Harris, W.S., Chung, M., Lichtenstein, A.H., Balk, E.M., *et al.* (2006) n-3 Fatty acids from fish or fish-oil supplements, but not alpha-linolenic acid, benefit cardiovascular disease outcomes in primary- and secondary-prevention studies: a systematic review. *American Journal of Clinical Nutrition* 84, 5–17.

Williams, M.A., Haskell, W.L., Ades, P.A., Amsterdam, E.A., Bittner, V., *et al.* (2007) Resistance exercise in individuals with and without cardiovascular disease: 2007 update: a scientific statement from the American Heart Association Council on Clinical Cardiology and Council on Nutrition, Physical Activity, and Metabolism. *Circulation* 116, 572–584.

Wood, D., De Backer, G., Faergeman, O., Graham, I., Mancia, G. *et al.* (1998) Prevention of coronary heart disease in clinical practice: recommendations of the Second Joint Task Force of European and other Societies on Coronary Prevention. *Atherosclerosis* 140, 199–270.

Yeh, E.T. and Willerson, J.T. (2003) Coming of age of C-reactive protein: using inflammation markers in cardiology. *Circulation* 107, 370–371.

Zwaka, T.P., Hombach, V. and Torzewski, J. (2001) C-reactive protein-mediated low density lipoprotein uptake by macrophages: implications for atherosclerosis. Circulation 103, 1194–1197.

15 Stress and Inflammation: An Emerging Story

F.R. Walker,* E. Nalivaiko and T.A. Day
School of Biomedical Sciences & Pharmacy, Priority Research Centre for Brain & Mental Health Research, University of Newcastle and Hunter Institute of Medical Research, Newcastle, Australia

Introduction

During the past decade, it has become increasingly apparent that enhanced levels of inflammation within the brain, most likely the result of chronic stress, are associated with significant changes in mood state and cognitive function. Indeed, these alterations are so similar to those observed in patients with depression that it has been proposed that inflammation might in fact represent a significant causal factor in this type of psychopathology. Given that nutraceuticals and dietary supplements, such as long-chain omega-3 fatty acid supplementation, as well as increased physical fitness, are increasingly being recommended by front-line health professionals to treat excessive or undesirable levels of inflammation, there is significant promise for their use as a treatment in the area of mental health. The aim of the current chapter is to introduce the reader to recent findings demonstrating the ability of stress to promote inflammation within the central nervous system and to critically evaluate the evidence linking these changes to alterations in mental health.

* Corresponding author, Rohan.walker@newcastle.edu.au

Stress: A Biological Mechanism to Meet Uncontrollable Unpredictable Threats

The body has evolved to deal with many challenges on a moment-by-moment basis, with some being routine (temperature fluctuation) while others are life threatening (predatory attack). Hans Selye, often referred to as the father of stress, was the first to explicitly formulate the idea that the body engages a non-selective response to any serious challenge, a response that serves to reorientate almost all of the organism's cognitive and physiological systems to deal with the impending challenge (Day, 2005). The theoretical foundation established by Selye has now been elaborated to differentiate between the event that causes a response in the body and the body's actual response to it. Specifically, it was accepted that a stressor is any stimulus (real or imagined) that substantially threatens the homeostatic balance that exists within the body, while by extension the stress response (often just shortened to stress) is the reaction of the body aimed at re-establishing homeostatic balance (Day, 2005). More recently, this conceptualization has been extended by the view that environmental events be considered stressors only if they are uncontrollable and/or unpredictable in nature (Koolhaas *et al.*, 2011). It would also be reasonable to add to this that an event must also be considered to be salient, as well as unpredictable and uncontrollable, to be considered a stressor (Day and Walker, 2007). The magnitude of the stress response is determined by the intensity of these three combined factors and the biological history of the organism.

Although the definition of a stressor as an event that is perceived to be threatening, unpredictable and uncontrollable is useful theoretically, it is also useful to place this definition within the context of actual life events. In this regard, for humans, actual or imminent unemployment, poverty, medical illness or disability, discord in marital or other intimate personal relationships, and loss are all frequently experienced stressors (Hammen, 2005). The intensity of these stressors can be significantly moderated by the individual's personality, coping strategies and level of social support (Hammen, 2005).

Why is stress clinically relevant?

From an evolutionary standpoint, the benefit of a biological mechanism that can rapidly provide the body with sufficient resources to deal with serious and immediate challenges appears obvious. Problems can arise, however, when the stress response is repeatedly engaged or inadequately terminated. With respect to humans, it is now well established that stress, and in particular chronic stress, is a major risk factor for a variety of diseases, including diabetes, cardiovascular diseases, autoimmune diseases and cancer. The strongest and most intensively investigated relationship between stress and disease has, however, been the one that exists between stress and mood disorders, notably depression (Checkley, 1996; Hammen, 2005). The strength of the relationship between the two has led many researchers to suggest that stress is a major cause of depression. Although some remain cautious about this view (Baune, 2009), it is widely and empirically well supported.

Overview of major physiological aspects of stress response

Once an event has been appraised by the brain as constituting a stressor, the stress response is initiated. On a biological level this involves substantial changes in the release of a variety of molecular mediators into the bloodstream (Fig. 15.1). Of these, the most significant are cortisol (CORT), released from the adrenal cortex by activation of the hypothalamic pituitary adrenal (HPA) axis, and catecholamines, released via activation of the sympathetic nervous system (SNS) (Ulrich-Lai and Herman, 2009). These two systems work in a complementary manner with the catecholamines released by the SNS acting to provide near instantaneous changes required for dealing with a challenge, and the slower acting effects of CORT working to mobilize the body's resources for more sustained action (Ulrich-Lai and Herman, 2009).

Activation of the SNS involves the centrally driven activation of preganglionic

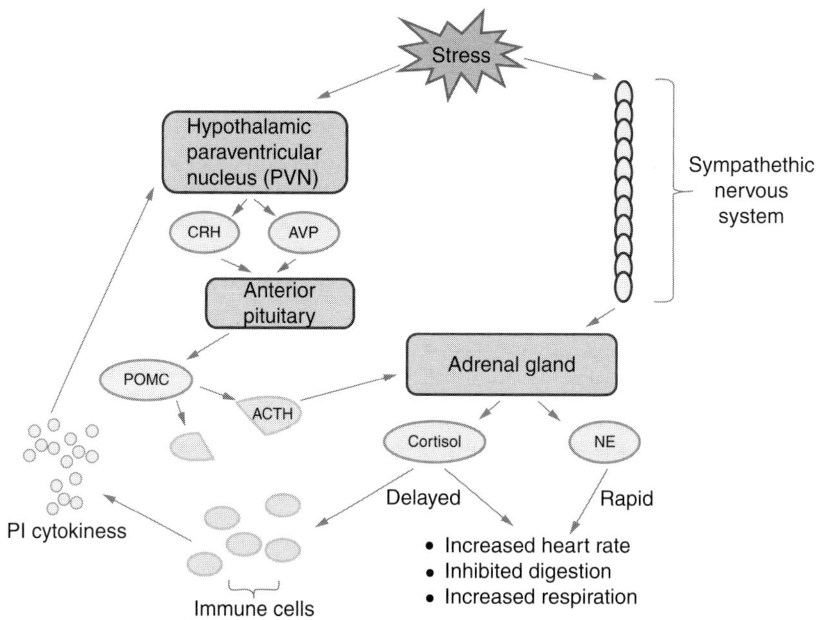

Fig. 15.1. Schematic of the effects of stress on the hypothalamic-pituitary axis and sympathetic nervous system. ACTH, adrenocorticotropin-releasing hormone; AVP, arginine-vasopressin; CRH, corticotrophin-releasing hormone; POMC, pro-opiomelanocortin. NE, norepinephrine.

sympathetic neurons in the intermediolateral cell column of the thoracolumbar spinal cord. In turn, these neurons connect with either cells of the adrenal medulla or those of the pre- or paravertebral ganglia that project to specific tissues. Activation of the SNS elicits what is referred to as the classic 'fight or flight' response, with catecholamines acting to drive a variety of relevant biological outcomes, including an increase in heart rate, increased force of heart contractions, increased peripheral vasoconstriction, increased blood pressure and increased energy mobilization (Ulrich-Lai and Herman, 2009).

Under normal 'unstressed' circumstances, the adrenal cortex releases CORT in a pulsatile and circadian-dependent manner with peak levels occurring just prior to waking. In contrast, exposure to a stressor dramatically alters this normal rhythm, increasing CORT release by an order of magnitude (Sorrells *et al.*, 2009). This massive surge is controlled via a number of brain regions, foremost amongst these the hypothalamic paraventricular nucleus (PVN). When activated, the PVN neurosecretory cells secrete corticotrophin-releasing hormone (CRH) and arginine-vasopressin (AVP) into the portal vessels of the median eminence. Together, these hormones traffic to the anterior pituitary to induce the production of a large precursor molecule known as pro-opiomelanocortin (POMC) (Vale *et al.*, 1981; Gillies *et al.*, 1982; Turnbull and Rivier, 1997). POMC, when cleaved, produces several peptides, one of which is adrenocorticotropin-releasing hormone (ACTH) (Buckingham *et al.*, 1992). Once in the peripheral circulation, ACTH travels to the adrenal cortex, where it initiates a sequence of reactions in which available stores of cholesterol are converted into circulating CORT that rapidly diffuses into the blood stream. Its physiological effects, however, are not immediate; first, these lipophilic molecules must diffuse passively across a cell's surface membrane and bind to either the high-affinity mineralocorticoid (MR) or low-affinity glucocorticoid receptor (GR) located within the cytoplasm, before translocating into the nucleus to influence gene transcription (Sorrells and Sapolsky, 2007). In broad terms, CORT release in response to stressful events is known to be capable of modulating multiple immune functions, including cytokine expression, immune cell trafficking, immune cell maturation, and the production of chemoattractants. Additionally, CORT can influence glucose metabolism, blood pressure, lipid metabolism, deposition of glycogen, neurotransmission, renal activity and muscle function. In most instances, the actions of stress-induced CORT are catabolic in nature, releasing energy from stored reserves, the ultimate purpose of which is hypothesized to be the provision of sufficient resources to deal with a perceived stressor.

Impact of stress response on inflammatory events

Inflammation is a complex multicellular process that is usually initiated by functional or structural disruption of body tissues. The ultimate endpoint of the inflammatory response is restoration of function. Typically, inflammatory responses in the periphery, whether localized or systemic in nature, involve the generation and release of acute-phase proteins, and pro-inflammatory (PI) cytokines such as interleukin (IL)-1, IL-6 and tumour necrosis factor-α (TNF-α). Additionally, peripheral inflammation involves recruitment and activation of leucocytes (cells of the immune system) such as neutrophils, macrophages and leucocytes (Benjamini *et al.*, 2000).

It was more than 70 years ago that the first evidence suggesting that stress influences immune function was reported (Chrousos and Gold, 1992). In the following decades the canonical view became that psychological stress, and by extension CORT, was unequivocally anti-inflammatory in nature. This view was supported by an extensive body of literature showing that high, stress-like levels of CORT (or synthetic versions of CORT) down-regulate the release of a large number of cytokines (Goujon *et al.*, 1997; Webster *et al.*, 2002), inhibit the expression of cellular adhesion molecules, which can disrupt the migration of leucocytes to the site of bacterial invasion (van de Stolpe *et al.*, 1993; Atsuta *et al.*, 1999), and suppress immunoglobulin production and leucocyte proliferation (Fleshner *et al.*, 1989; Cheng *et al.*, 1990). Although this view dominated for some time, it was at odds with the presumed biological purpose of stress, i.e. dealing with an immediate challenge. That is to say, it was not clear how suppressing immune function provided an adaptive benefit to the organism in the short term. In commenting on this issue, Sorrells and colleagues (Sorrells and Sapolsky, 2007; Sorrells *et al.*, 2009) highlighted that there seemed to be little reproductive benefit in an injured animal escaping predation only to subsequently succumb to infection. With the advent of improved sampling procedures, and biological assays with enhanced detection limits, this paradox has been largely resolved. The improvement in technology revealed that the early phase of the stress response is actually associated with an enhancement of immune function, rather than suppression, and that the suppressive effects of stress represent a form of negative feedback (Black, 2002; Black and Garbutt, 2002).

Peripheral pro-inflammatory effects of stress

It is now well established that high stress levels elevate peripheral levels of pro-inflammatory (PI) cytokines in humans (Miller *et al.*, 2009). These clinical findings are also completely consistent with the picture that has emerged from preclinical animal studies, where it has been possible to further probe the underlying mechanisms. Specifically, exposure to acute psychological stress prior to an inflammatory challenge can enhance immune function. Perhaps the best-known example of this comes from the group of Firdaus Dhabhar, involving an experimental procedure in which mice are exposed to an acute stressor prior to inducing a delayed type hypersensitivity (DTH) reaction via the cutaneous application of 2,4-dinitro-1-flurobenzene (DFNF). Specifically, Dbabhar's work demonstrated that acute stress administered before the introduction of DNFB significantly enhanced the magnitude of the DTH response, an effect that seems to be mediated by CORT-induced changes in leucocyte trafficking (Dhabhar and McEwen, 1997, 1999; Dhabhar, 1998, 2002; Dhabhar *et al.*, 2000). Similar stress-induced enhancements have also been found to occur with immunoglobulin production by B lymphocytes (Wood *et al.*, 1993; Shanks and Kusnecov, 1998). Even in the absence of any immunological challenge, acute stress can provoke the release of PI cytokines and acute-phase proteins in both rodents and humans as well as promote the activity of nuclear factor kappa-light-chain-enhancer of activated B cells (NFκB), a transcription factor intimately involved in the generation of pro-inflammatory responses (De Bosscher *et al.*, 2003; O'Connor *et al.*, 2003).

Central pro-inflammatory effects of stress

In the periphery, inflammatory processes are handled by a variety of innate immune cells. In the brain, however, inflammatory processes are primarily handled by highly specialized neural tissue support cells known as microglia (Fig. 15.2). Microglial cells normally represent 12–15% of all cells in the brain (Pessac *et al.*, 2001) and exist predominantly in a 'resting state' characterized by a ramified (highly branched) morphology (Streit *et al.*, 2004). Their role is to monitor the environment for potential threats to central nervous system (CNS) integrity and to respond to activating signals that are not usually present (e.g. PI cytokines, high levels of glucocorticoids, intracellular constituents or microbial structures), or factors that suddenly appear in an unusual format (Hanisch and Kettenmann, 2007). When microglia detect these danger signals they become activated and produce a number of biologically active molecules that drive a local neuroinflammatory response. Depending on their phase of activation, microglia can produce an array of PI and cytotoxic molecules, and in some instances can become antigen-presenting cells with many macrophage-like properties, such as the ability to phagocytose pathogens and cellular debris (Chew *et al.*, 2006). When activated, microglial cells are also known to proliferate, primarily through mitosis of resident microglial cells (Streit, 2006). This inflammation of neural tissue (hence, neuroinflammation) is normally beneficial in the short term (Neumann *et al.*, 2009) but, if chronic, can become maladaptive, resulting in disturbances of cell function and even cell damage owing to the release of cytotoxic free radicals (see excellent reviews in Block *et al.*, 2007; Gao and Hong, 2008). Importantly, activated microglia release a variety of substances that can modulate local neuronal signalling.

Preclinical studies have shown that stress elevates PI cytokine levels in the brain as well as peripherally (O'Connor *et al.*, 2003), and that, PI cytokines such as IL-1β act on microglia to promote proliferation and activation (Ganter *et al.*, 1992; Yu *et al.*, 1998). Moreover, a number of studies have now shown that acute stress promotes the morphological transition of microglia from a ramified-resting state to an activated state (Sugama *et al.*, 2007; Sugama, 2009), and that this response can be regionally specific and can vary in magnitude

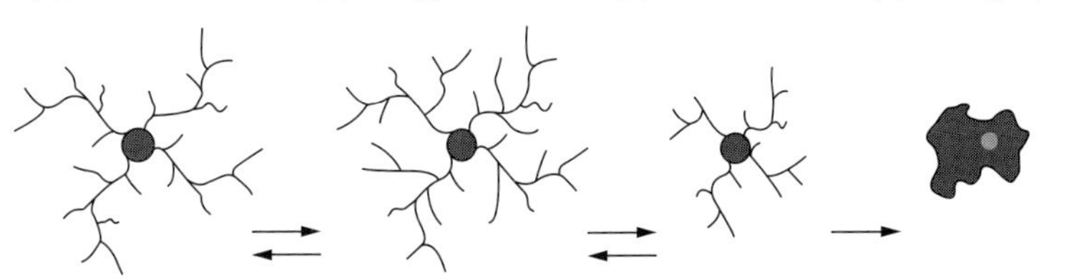

Fig. 15.2. Multistep schematic of microglial morphological remodelling. Microglial remodelling is known to occur in response to activating stimuli present in the cell's microenvironment. In their so-called 'resting' state, microglia exhibit a highly ramified appearance (a). On detection of an activating signal, microglia transform in a stimulus-dependent manner. Where an activating signal takes the form of neuronal damage or cell death, microglia may transform into hyper-ramified (b), then reactive (c) and finally phagocytic microglia (d). (From Hinwood *et al.*, 2011, with permission from Oxford University Press.)

over time (Frank *et al.*, 2007; Blandino *et al.*, 2009). In terms of chronic stress, Tynan and colleagues (Tynan *et al.*, 2010) have recently shown that stress selectively increases the number of microglia in certain stress-sensitive brain regions, and also causes a marked transition of microglia from a ramified-resting state to a non-resting state. These findings are consistent with the view that microglial activation could play an important role in controlling and/or adapting to stress. Hinwood and colleagues (2011) have subsequently extended this work by demonstrating chronic stress induced microglial activation is positively correlated with long-term neuronal activation in the prefrontal cortex, and that treating stressed animals with an inhibitor of microglial activation reduced the impact of stress on neuronal activation and microglial activation and improved stress induced cognitive impairments.

A crucial yet difficult question for researchers is whether the PI cytokines seen within the brain after exposure to stress are actually generated within the brain or traffic from the periphery into the brain. The difficulty associated with providing a firm answer to this question arises in part because of the cellular barrier that encases the brain, known as the blood brain barrier (BBB). The BBB is a vascular–endothelial barrier that restricts and regulates the movement of substances between the blood and the central nervous system. Initially, it was thought that peripherally generated cytokines were too large to passively diffuse through the barrier and that they could only gain access to the brain via specialized regions of the BBB known as the circumventricular organs (CVOs). The CVOs are essentially vascular windows in the BBB where the endothelial cells of the barrier are significantly more permeable. Entry of cytokines into the brain via the CVOs also meant that their effects were limited by diffusion. Evidence at the time, however, indicated that peripherally generated cytokines appeared to influence sites deep within the brain and distant to the CVOs. In the ensuing years several seminal studies by Banks and colleagues provided a compelling answer to why cytokines could exert actions at sites they apparently did not have access to. Specifically, Banks and colleagues demonstrated that the BBB does possess saturable transport systems that facilitate entry of a variety of PI cytokines, including IL-1β and TNF-α (Banks and Kastin, 1991, 1992; Banks *et al.*, 1994, 1995; Gutierrez *et al.*, 1993, Plotkin *et al.*, 1996). The existence of active transport mechanisms within the BBB provides a clear pathway through which peripherally generated PI cytokines can access deep tissue of the brain. It is also a finding that suggests strategies targeting peripherally generated cytokines should have central effects.

Importantly, several other pathways exist through which stress can trigger neuroinflammation. Firstly, stress can trigger the release of pro-inflammatory cytokines from microglia (Blandino *et al.*, 2006). The specific mechanisms through which this occurs are not completely characterized. It is recognized, however, that CORT can act on microglia to promote proliferation and activation (Sorrells *et al.*, 2009; Sorrells and Sapolsky, 2007) and of course CORT, which readily crosses the blood–brain barrier, is greatly elevated during stress. Secondly, it is recognized that PI cytokines can bind to receptors on the vagus nerve, altering neuronal signalling within the CNS (Bluthe *et al.*, 1994, 1996), which has the potential to activate microglia, triggering them to release PI cytokines. Moreover, circulating PI cytokines can bind to receptors present within the BBB to initiate the release of PI molecules within the brain (Schiltz and Sawchenko, 2002; Konsman *et al.*, 2004).

Pro-inflammatory cytokines and sickness behaviour

Although the behavioural consequences associated with stress-induced PI cytokines release are only now beginning to be investigated, research in this area is being heavily influenced by past research on the behavioural effects of infection. Specifically, it has long been known that viral and bacterial infection reliably elicit a cluster of behavioural changes collectively referred to as sickness behaviour (Dantzer *et al.*, 2008). Typically these behaviours include: fever, social withdrawal, loss of interest in activities normally considered to be pleasurable (anhedonia), reduced appetite, reduced thirst, disrupted sleep, irritability, fatigue, reduced attention, memory impairment and nausea (Dantzer *et al.*, 2008). It is now known that many of these behaviours are directly attributable to the increased levels of PI cytokines that accompany infection, because systemic or central infusion of PI cytokines induces the full repertoire of sickness behaviours (Kent *et al.*, 1992a,b). This is not true, however, for all PI cytokines; IL-6, despite its ability to produce fever, does not cause sickness behaviour (Dantzer *et al.*, 2008).

In the early 1990s a significant breakthrough was made when several research groups recognized that sickness behaviours were remarkably similar to the symptoms of depression. Indeed, the overlap was so striking that many started to investigate whether depression, a condition long thought to be caused by disturbed neurotransmission, was in fact driven by PI factors. The first to propose explicitly that depression was driven by PI molecules was Ronald Smith in a seminal paper published in 1991 (Smith, 1991). In support of this hypothesis Smith cited evidence demonstrating that non-depressed cancer patients administered PI cytokines developed symptoms sufficient to satisfy the diagnostic criteria for depression, and that these symptoms disappeared upon cessation of treatment. Smith reasoned that if depression was an inflammatory condition it would explain why there was such a high rate of co-morbidity between depression and other diseases with an inflammatory component, such as cardiovascular and autoimmune diseases. The hypothesis proposed by Smith was subsequently extended experimentally, most notably by Maes and colleagues, who demonstrated that patients with clinical depression exhibited higher levels of IL-6, IL-2 and TNF-α (Maes, 1993, 1995; Maes *et al.*, 1995; Mikova *et al.*, 2001).

Although the early reports indicating that depression was associated with enhanced peripheral inflammation were intriguing, it was clear to most researchers that the key issue to be determined was how this might relate to what was happening in the brain. Accordingly, it has been shown that IL-6 is elevated in the cerebrospinal fluid of patients with depression (Stubner *et al.*, 1999) and, even more recently, that the entire PI-cytokine network (at the mRNA level) is up-regulated, at post-mortem, in the brains of individuals with depression (Shelton *et al.*, 2010). Further, magnetic resonance imaging, positron emission tomography and post-mortem cell-counting studies have all demonstrated that the brains of patients with long-standing depression show significant cell loss (both glial and neuronal) (Rajkowska, 2002; Campbell and MacQueen, 2006; Koolschijn *et al.*, 2009), a known consequence of prolonged neuroinflammation. Finally, evidence that neuroinflammation may contribute to depression also comes from animal studies that have shown that central administration of PI cytokines induces depression-like behavioural changes that include impaired executive function, anhedonia, social withdrawal, anorexia and increased slow-wave sleep (Konsman *et al.*, 2002; Yirmiya *et al.*, 2002). Collectively, this body of evidence has contributed to the formulation of the neuroinflammatory theory of depression, which holds that depression arises as a result of disrupted neuronal signalling within mood regulatory nuclei.

Anti-inflammatory action of selective serotonin reuptake inhibitor antidepressants

For more than four decades the monoamine theory of depression has provided the primary theoretical justification for prescribing, to depressed patients, drugs that act by altering monoaminergic neurotransmission. In its original form, the theory proposed that depression arose as a result of a deficit in the level of noradrenaline and/or serotonin in the brain. Over time, the original theory has been revised. In its contemporary form it holds simply that monoamine systems seem to be able to modulate 'other brain neurobiologic systems which have a more primary role in depression' (Heninger *et al.*, 1996). Of the available antidepressants, the selective serotonin reuptake inhibitors (SSRIs) are the most widely prescribed in Australia, with more than 8 million prescriptions filled each year (Mant *et al.*, 2004). Driving their popularity is the fact that they are well tolerated and possess an excellent safety profile. Moreover, SSRI drug–drug interactions, side effects, and interactions with metabolic enzymes, are all well understood (Hemeryck and Belpaire, 2002; Helmeke *et al.*, 2008; Stahl, 2009; Fournier *et al.*, 2010).

SSRIs and serotonin and norepinephrine reuptake inhibitors (SNRIs) do, however, have one major drawback: they only provide complete and long-term control of symptoms in 50–60% of patients (Fava, 2003). Obviously, this is not ideal and has led a number of researchers to re-examine the putative mechanism of action through which these drugs exert their therapeutic effect; the hope being that, through improved knowledge, better use can be made of these important drugs. In this regard, perhaps the most significant development so far has been the realization that inflammation, and in particular inflammation of brain tissue (i.e. neuroinflammation), represents a major feature of depression (Maes *et al.*, 2008). The early evidence of a link between depression and inflammation (i.e. that depressed patients had elevated peripheral PI cytokine levels) resulted in studies that examined whether treatment with antidepressants altered circulating PI cytokine levels. As recently reported in a major review of the relevant literature, these studies showed that treatment of depressed patients with an SSRI or SNRI does indeed normalize serum levels of major inflammatory cytokines, including interleukin IL-1β, IL-6, TNF-α and interferon gamma (IFN-γ) (Janssen *et al.*, 2010). Complementing these clinical reports, there have been a considerable number of *in vitro* studies that have shown that SSRIs inhibit the responses of normal human and rodent peripheral immune system cells (particularly monocytes, macrophages and neutrophils) to agents that trigger inflammatory responses (Martensson and Nassberger, 1993; Sacerdote *et al.*, 1994; Xia *et al.*, 1996). The ability of SSRIs to reduce inflammation in the periphery is intriguing, but the obvious question is: does it translate through to an action in the brain that might be relevant to the treatment of depression? Evidence of an anti-inflammatory action in the periphery does not automatically constitute evidence of an anti-inflammatory action in the brain because the cells that are primary to inflammatory processes in the brain (the microglia) are distinct from the immune system cells that mediate the anti-inflammatory effects of SSRIs and SNRIs in the periphery (Wake *et al.*, 2009; Graeber, 2010). Recent studies have, however, provided evidence that at least some SSRIs can inhibit certain aspects of the microglial inflammatory response. For instance it has been reported that fluoxetine, paroxetine and sertraline can inhibit the ability of murine microglia to produce the PI cytokine TNF-α and the free radical nitric oxide (Hashioka *et al.*, 2007, 2009; Hwang *et al.*, 2008; Horikawa *et al.*, 2010). Collectively these results suggest that antidepressant medications, currently prescribed on the basis of their effectiveness rather than a complete theoretical understanding of their action might, in fact, owe at least some of their effectiveness as an antidepressant to their ability to alter the inflammatory status of the individual.

Does reducing inflammation improve mood?

Clearly, if inflammation is causally involved in producing depression it would stand to reason that inhibiting inflammation should reduce depressive symptoms. Unfortunately, there have been few experiments to directly address this issue. Some tantalizing evidence does, however, exist. For instance it has been shown that the cyclooxygenase-2 inhibitor celecoxib, when used in combination with the antidepressant reboxetine is more effective in improving symptoms than when reboxetine is combined with placebo (Muller *et al.*, 2006). In a similar vein, acetylsalicylic acid (i.e. aspirin) when given in combination with an antidepressant decreases the length of time taken for the antidepressant to show therapeutic effect. More recently, a phase III clinical trial examining the therapeutic effectiveness of entanercept, an anti-TNF-α agent in treating psoriasis, found that patients taking the drug reported improved symptoms of depression.

Importantly, the authors of the study found that this improvement seemed to be independent of changes in psoriatic symptoms (Tyring *et al.*, 2006). Finally, a meta-analysis of ten double-blind, placebo-controlled studies in which patients with mood disorders were treated with omega-3 polyunsaturated fatty acids found that omega-3 supplementation produced modest antidepressant effects (Song and Zhao, 2007). Studies examining the effects of omega-3 supplementation on mood disorders are reviewed in detail in Chapter 16. The role of regular exercise in ameliorating mood disorders is also discussed.

Summary and Conclusions

Psychological stress has long been identified as a major risk factor in the development of mood disorders such as depression. During the past several years it has been identified that stress may contribute to mood disturbance via the generation of PI molecules, including the PI cytokines and various acute-phase proteins. The evidence that PI molecules are responsible for changes in mood state is compelling, particularly evidence demonstrating that healthy individuals demonstrate enhanced negative mood following an immune challenge. The relationship between PI molecules and mood also aligns perfectly with the similarity observed between the symptoms of depression and those found to occur in individuals suffering from a viral or bacterial infection. Finally, after so many years of prescribing antidepressants while supposing that their effectiveness is derived from their ability to alter the level of monoamines, it is ironic to find that their mechanism of action might actually be attributable to their anti-inflammatory capacity. Given this, there is huge scope for research in this area, not least in how nutraceuticals and physical activity may be used as a stand-alone prophylactic treatment or complementary therapeutic intervention for stress-induced mood disorders.

References

Abdel-Salam, O.M. (2008) Drugs used to treat Parkinson's disease, present status and future directions. *CNS Neurological Disorders - Drug Targets* 7, 321–342.

Atsuta, J., Plitt, J., Bochner, B.S. and Schleimer, R.P. (1999) Inhibition of VCAM-1 expression in human bronchial epithelial cells by glucocorticoids. *American Journal of Respiratory Cell and Molecular Biology* 20, 643–650.

Banks, W.A. and Kastin, A.J. (1991) Blood to brain transport of interleukin links the immune and central nervous systems. *Life Sciences* 48, PL117–121.

Banks, W.A. and Kastin, A.J. (1992). The interleukins-1 alpha, -1 beta, and -2 do not acutely disrupt the murine blood-brain barrier. *International Journal of Immunopharmacology* 14, 629–636.

Banks, W.A., Kastin, A.J. and Gutierrez, E.G. (1994) Penetration of interleukin-6 across the murine blood-brain barrier. *Neuroscience Letters* 179, 53–56.

Banks, W.A., Kastin, A.J. and Broadwell, R.D. (1995) Passage of cytokines across the blood-brain barrier. *Neuroimmunomodulation* 2, 241–248.

Baune, B. (2009) Conceptual challenges of a tentative model of stress-induced depression. *PLoS ONE* 4, e4266.

Benjamini, E., Coico, R. and Sunshine, G. (2000) Immunology: a short course. Wiley-Liss, New York.

Black, P.H. (2002). Stress and the inflammatory response: a review of neurogenic inflammation. *Brain, Behavior, and Immunity* 16, 622–653.

Black, P.H. and Garbutt, L.D. (2002) Stress, inflammation and cardiovascular disease. *Journal of Psychosomatic Research* 52, 1–23.

Blandino, P., Jr, Barnum, C.J. and Deak, T. (2006) The involvement of norepinephrine and microglia in hypothalamic and splenic IL-1beta responses to stress. *Journal of Neuroimmunology* 173, 87–95.

Blandino, P., Jr, Barnum, C.J., Solomon, L.G., Larish, Y., Lankow, B.S., *et al.* (2009) Gene expression changes in the hypothalamus provide evidence for regionally-selective changes in IL-1 and microglial markers after acute stress. *Brain, Behavior, and Immunity* 23, 958–968.

Block, M.L., Zecca, L. and Hong, J.S. (2007) Microglia-mediated neurotoxicity: uncovering the molecular mechanisms. *Nature Reviews Neuroscience* 8, 57–69.

Bluthe, R.M., Walter, V., Parnet, P., Laye, S., Lestage, J., *et al.* (1994) Lipopolysaccharide induces sickness behaviour in rats by a vagal mediated mechanism. *Comptes Rendus de l Academie des Sciences. Serie III, Sciences de la Vie* 317, 499–503.

Bluthe, R.M., Michaud, B., Kelley, K.W. and Dantzer, R. (1996) Vagotomy attenuates behavioural effects of interleukin-1 injected peripherally but not centrally. *Neuroreport* 7, 1485–1488.

Buckingham, J., Smith, T., Loxley, H. and WD, O. (1992) The control of ACTH secretion. In: James, V.H.T. (ed) *The Adrenal Gland.* Raven Press, New York.

Campbell, S. and MacQueen, G. (2006) An update on regional brain volume differences associated with mood disorders. *Current Opinion in Psychiatry* 19, 25–33.

Checkley, S. (1996) The neuroendocrinology of depression and chronic stress. *British Medical Bulletin* 52, 597–617.

Cheng, G.J., Morrow-Tesch, J.L., Beller, D.I., Levy, E.M. and Black, P.H. (1990) Immunosuppression in mice induced by cold water stress. *Brain, Behavior, and Immunity* 4, 278–291.

Chew, L.J., Takanohashi, A. and Bell, M. (2006) Microglia and inflammation: impact on developmental brain injuries. *Mental Retardation and Developmental Disabilities Research* 12, 105–112.

Chrousos, G.P. and Gold, P.W. (1992) The concepts of stress and stress system disorders. Overview of physical and behavioral homeostasis. *Journal of the American Medical Association* 267, 1244–1252.

Dantzer, R., O'Connor, J.C., Freund, G.G., Johnson R.W. and Kelley, K.W. (2008) From inflammation to sickness and depression: when the immune system subjugates the brain. *Nature Reviews Neuroscience* 9, 46–56.

Day, T.A. (2005) Defining stress as a prelude to mapping its neurocircuitry: no help from allostasis. *Progress in Neuro-Psychopharmacology and Biological Psychiatry* 29, 1195–1200.

Day, T.A. and Walker, F.R. (2007). More appraisal please: a commentary on Pfaff *et al.* (2007) Relations between mechanisms of CNS arousal and mechanisms of stress. *Stress* 10, 311–313; discussion 314–315.

De Bosscher, K., Vanden Berghe, W. and Haegeman, G. (2003) The interplay between the glucocorticoid receptor and nuclear factor-kappaB or activator protein-1: molecular mechanisms for gene repression. *Endocrine Reviews* 24, 488–522.

Dhabhar, F.S. (1998) Stress-induced enhancement of cell-mediated immunity. *Annals of the New York Academy of Sciences* 840, 359–372.

Dhabhar, F.S. (2002) Stress-induced augmentation of immune function–the role of stress hormones, leukocyte trafficking, and cytokines. *Brain, Behavior, and Immunity* 16, 785–798.

Dhabhar, F.S. and McEwen, B.S. (1997) Acute stress enhances while chronic stress suppresses cell-mediated immunity in vivo: a potential role for leukocyte trafficking. *Brain, Behavior, and Immunity* 11, 286–306.

Dhabhar, F.S. and McEwen, B.S. (1999) Enhancing versus suppressive effects of stress hormones on skin immune function. *Proceedings of the National Academy of Sciences USA* 96, 1059–1064.

Dhabhar, F.S., Satoskar, A.R., Bluethmann, H., David, J.R. and McEwen, B.S. (2000) Stress-induced enhancement of skin immune function: A role for gamma interferon. *Proceedings of the National Academy of Sciences USA* 97, 2846–2851.

Fava, M. (2003) Diagnosis and definition of treatment-resistant depression. *Biological Psychiatry* 53, 649–659.

Fleshner, M., Laudenslager, M.L., Simons, L. and Maier, S.F. (1989) Reduced serum antibodies associated with social defeat in rats. *Physiology and Behavior* 45, 1183–1187.

Fournier, J.C., DeRubeis, R.J., Hollon, S.D., Dimidjian, S., Amsterdam, J.D., *et al.* (2010) Antidepressant drug effects and depression severity: a patient-level meta-analysis. *Journal of the American Medical Association* 303, 47–53.

Frank, M.G., Baratta, M.V., Sprunger, D.B., Watkins, L.R. and Maier, S.F. (2007) Microglia serve as a neuroimmune substrate for stress-induced potentiation of CNS pro-inflammatory cytokine responses. *Brain, Behavior, and Immunity* 21, 47–59.

Ganter, S., Northoff, H., Mannel, D. and Gebicke-Harter, P.J. (1992) Growth control of cultured microglia. *Journal of Neuroscience Research* 33, 218–230.

Gao, H.M. and Hong, J.S. (2008) Why neurodegenerative diseases are progressive: uncontrolled inflammation drives disease progression. *Trends in Immunology* 29, 357–365.

Gillies, G.E., Linton, E.A. and Lowry, P.J. (1982) Corticotropin releasing activity of the new CRF is potentiated several times by vasopressin. *Nature* 299, 355–357.

Goujon, E., Laye, S., Parnet, P. and Dantzer, R. (1997) Regulation of cytokine gene expression in the central nervous system by glucocorticoids: mechanisms and functional consequences. *Psychoneuroendocrinology* 22 Suppl 1, S75–S80.

Graeber, M.B. (2010) Changing face of microglia. *Science* 330, 783–788.
Gutierrez, E.G., Banks, W.A. and Kastin, A.J. (1993) Murine tumor necrosis factor alpha is transported from blood to brain in the mouse. *Journal of Neuroimmunology* 47, 169–176.
Hammen, C. (2005) Stress and depression. *Annual Review of Clinical Psychology* 1, 293–319.
Hanisch, U.K. and Kettenmann, H. (2007) Microglia: active sensor and versatile effector cells in the normal and pathologic brain. *Nature Neuroscience* 10, 1387–1394.
Hashioka, S., Klegeris, A., Monji, A., Kato, T., Sawada, M., *et al.* (2007) Antidepressants inhibit interferon-gamma-induced microglial production of IL-6 and nitric oxide. *Experimental Neurology* 206, 33–42.
Hashioka, S., McGeer, P.L., Monji, A. and Kanba, S. (2009) Anti-inflammatory effects of antidepressants: possibilities for preventives against Alzheimer's disease. *Central Nervous System Agents in Medicinal Chemistry* 9, 12–19.
Helmeke, C., Ovtscharoff, W., Jr., Poeggel, G. and Braun, K. (2008) Imbalance of immunohistochemically characterized interneuron populations in the adolescent and adult rodent medial prefrontal cortex after repeated exposure to neonatal separation stress. *Neuroscience* 152, 18–28.
Hemeryck, A. and Belpaire, F.M. (2002) Selective serotonin reuptake inhibitors and cytochrome P-450 mediated drug-drug interactions: an update. *Current Drug Metabolism* 3, 13–37.
Heninger, G.R., Delgado, P.L. and Charney, D.S. (1996) The revised monoamine theory of depression: a modulatory role for monoamines, based on new findings from monoamine depletion experiments in humans. *Pharmacopsychiatry* 29, 2–11.
Hinwood, M., Moranini, J., Day, T.A. and Walker, F.R. (2012) Evidence that microglia mediate the neurobiological effects of chronic psychological stress on the medial prefrontal cortex. *Cerebral Cortex* 22, 1442–1454.
Horikawa, H., Kato, T.A., Mizoguchi, Y., Monji, A., Seki, Y., *et al.* (2010). Inhibitory effects of SSRIs on IFN-gamma induced microglial activation through the regulation of intracellular calcium. *Progress in Neuro-Psychopharmacology and Biological Psychiatry* 34, 1306–1316.
Hwang, J., Zheng, L.T., Ock, J., Lee, M.G., Kim, S.H., *et al.* (2008). Inhibition of glial inflammatory activation and neurotoxicity by tricyclic antidepressants. *Neuropharmacology* 55, 826–834.
Janssen, D.G., Caniato, R.N., Verster, J.C. and Baune, B.T. (2010). A psychoneuroimmunological review on cytokines involved in antidepressant treatment response. *Human Psychopharmacology* 25, 201–-215.
Kent, S., Bluthe, R.M., Dantzer, R., Hardwick, A.J., Kelley, K.W., *et al.* (1992a) Different receptor mechanisms mediate the pyrogenic and behavioral effects of interleukin 1. *Proceedings of the National Academy of Sciences USA* 89, 9117–9120.
Kent, S., Bluthe, R.M., Kelley, K.W. and Dantzer, R. (1992b) Sickness behavior as a new target for drug development. *Trends in Pharmacological Sciences* 13, 24–28.
Konsman, J.P., Parnet, P. and Dantzer, R. (2002) Cytokine-induced sickness behaviour: mechanisms and implications. *Trends in Neurosciences* 25, 154–159.
Konsman, J.P., Vigues, S., Mackerlova, L., Bristow, A. and Blomqvist, A. (2004) Rat brain vascular distribution of interleukin-1 type-1 receptor immunoreactivity: relationship to patterns of inducible cyclooxygenase expression by peripheral inflammatory stimuli. *Journal of Comparative Neurology* 472, 113–129.
Koolhaas, J.M., Bartolomucci, A., Buwalda, B., de Boer, S.F., Flugge, G., *et al.* (2011) Stress revisited: a critical evaluation of the stress concept. *Neuroscience and Biobehavioral Reviews* 35, 1291–1301.
Koolschijn, P.C., van Haren, N.E., Lensvelt-Mulders, G.J., Hulshoff Pol, H.E. and Kahn, R.S. (2009) Brain volume abnormalities in major depressive disorder: a meta-analysis of magnetic resonance imaging studies. *Human Brain Mapping* 30, 3719–3735.
Maes, M. (1993) A review on the acute phase response in major depression. *Reviews in the Neurosciences* 4, 407–416.
Maes, M. (1995) Evidence for an immune response in major depression: a review and hypothesis. *Progress in Neuro-Psychopharmacology and Biological Psychiatry* 19, 11–38.
Maes, M., Meltzer, H.Y., Bosmans, E., Bergmans, R., Vandoolaeghe, E., *et al.* (1995) Increased plasma concentrations of interleukin-6, soluble interleukin-6, soluble interleukin-2 and transferrin receptor in major depression. *Journal of Affective Disorders* 34, 301–309.
Maes, M., Yirmyia, R., Noraberg, J., Brene, S., Hibbeln, J., *et al.* (2008) The inflammatory & neurodegenerative (I&ND) hypothesis of depression: leads for future research and new drug developments in depression. *Metabolic Brain Disease* 24, 27–53
Mant, A., Rondlo, V.A., Hall, W.D., Mitchell, P.B., Montgomery, W.S., *et al.* (2004) Making new choices about antidepressants in Australia: the long view 1975-2002. *Medical Journal of Australia* 181(7 Suppl), S21–S24.

Martensson, U. and Nassberger, L. (1993) Influence of antidepressants on mitogen stimulation of human lymphocytes. *Toxicology In Vitro* 7, 241–245.

Mikova, O., Yakimova, R., Bosmans, E., Kenis, G. and Maes, M. (2001) Increased serum tumor necrosis factor alpha concentrations in major depression and multiple sclerosis. *European Neuropsychopharmacology* 11, 203–208.

Miller, G.E., Rohleder, N. and Cole, S.W. (2009). Chronic interpersonal stress predicts activation of pro- and anti-inflammatory signaling pathways 6 months later. *Psychosomatic Medicine* 71, 57–62.

Muller, N., Schwarz, M.J., Dehning, S., Douhe, A., Cerovecki, A., *et al.* (2006) The cyclooxygenase-2 inhibitor celecoxib has therapeutic effects in major depression: results of a double-blind, randomized, placebo controlled, add-on pilot study to reboxetine. *Molecular Psychiatry* 11, 680–684.

Neumann, H., Kotter, M.R. and Franklin, R.J. (2009) Debris clearance by microglia: an essential link between degeneration and regeneration. *Brain* 132, 288–295.

O'Connor, K.A., Johnson, J.D., Hansen, M.K., Wieseler Frank, J.L., Maksimova, E., *et al.* (2003) Peripheral and central proinflammatory cytokine response to a severe acute stressor. *Brain Research* 991, 123–132.

Pessac, B., Godin, I. and Alliot, F. (2001) Microglia: origin and development. *Bulletin de l Academie Nationale de Medecine* 185, 337–346; discussion 346–337.

Plotkin, S.R., Banks, W.A. and Kastin, A.J. (1996) Comparison of saturable transport and extracellular pathways in the passage of interleukin-1 alpha across the blood-brain barrier. *Journal of Neuroimmunology* 67, 41–47.

Rajkowska, G. (2002) Cell pathology in mood disorders. *Seminars in Clinical Neuropsychiatry* 7, 281–292.

Sacerdote, P., Bianchi, M. and Panerai, A.E. (1994) Chlorimipramine and nortriptyline but not fluoxetine and fluvoxamine inhibit human polymorphonuclear cell chemotaxis in vitro. *General Pharmacology* 25, 409–412.

Schiltz, J.C. and Sawchenko, P.E. (2002) Distinct brain vascular cell types manifest inducible cyclooxygenase expression as a function of the strength and nature of immune insults. *Journal of Neuroscience* 22, 5606–5618.

Shanks, N. and Kusnecov, A.W. (1998) Differential immune reactivity to stress in BALB/cByJ and C57BL/6J mice: in vivo dependence on macrophages. *Physiology and Behavior* 65, 95–103.

Shelton, R.C., Claiborne, J., Sidoryk-Wegrzynowicz, M., Reddy, R., Aschner, M., *et al.* (2010) Altered expression of genes involved in inflammation and apoptosis in frontal cortex in major depression. *Molecular Psychiatry* 16, 751–762.

Smith, R.S. (1991) The macrophage theory of depression. *Medical Hypotheses* 35, 298–306.

Song, C. and Zhao, S. (2007) Omega-3 fatty acid eicosapentaenoic acid. A new treatment for psychiatric and neurodegenerative diseases: a review of clinical investigations. *Expert Opinion on Investigational Drugs* 16, 1627–1638.

Sorrells, S.F. and Sapolsky R.M. (2007) An inflammatory review of glucocorticoid actions in the CNS. *Brain, Behavior, and Immunity* 21, 259–272.

Sorrells, S.F., Caso, J.R., Munhoz, C.D. and Sapolsky, R.M. (2009) The stressed CNS: when glucocorticoids aggravate inflammation. *Neuron* 64, 33–39.

Stahl, S. (2009) *Stahl's Essential Psychopharmacology: Neuroscientific Basis and Practical Applications.* Cambridge University Press, New York.

Streit, W.J. (2006). Microglial senescence: does the brain's immune system have an expiration date? *Trends in Neuroscience* 29, 506–510.

Streit, W.J., Mrakm, R.E. and Griffin, W.S. (2004) Microglia and neuroinflammation: a pathological perspective. *Journal of Neuroinflammation* 1, 14.

Stubner, S., Schon, T., Padberg, F., Teipel, S.J., Schwarz, M.J., *et al.* (1999) Interleukin-6 and the soluble IL-6 receptor are decreased in cerebrospinal fluid of geriatric patients with major depression: no alteration of soluble gp130. *Neuroscience Letters* 259, 145–148.

Sugama, S. (2009) Stress-induced microglial activation may facilitate the progression of neurodegenerative disorders. *Medical Hypotheses* 73, 1031–1034.

Sugama, S., Fujita, M., Hashimoto, M. and Conti, B. (2007) Stress induced morphological microglial activation in the rodent brain: involvement of interleukin-18. *Neuroscience* 146, 1388–1399.

Turnbull, A.V. and Rivier, C. (1997) Corticotropin-releasing factor (CRF) and endocrine responses to stress: CRF receptors, binding protein, and related peptides. *Proceedings of the Society for Experimental Biology and Medicine* 215, 1–10.

Tynan, R.J., Naicker, S., Hinwood, M., Nalivaiko, E., Buller, K.M., *et al.* (2010) Chronic stress alters the density and morphology of microglia in a subset of stress-responsive brain regions. *Brain, Behavior, and Immunity* 24, 1058–1068.

Tyring, S., Gottlieb, A., Papp, K., Gordon, K., Leonardi, C., *et al.* (2006) Etanercept and clinical outcomes, fatigue, and depression in psoriasis: double-blind placebo-controlled randomised phase III trial. *Lancet* 367, 29–35.

Ulrich-Lai, Y.M. and Herman, J.P. (2009) Neural regulation of endocrine and autonomic stress responses. *Nature Reviews Neuroscience* 10, 397–409.

Vale, W., Spiess, J., Rivier, C. and Rivier, J. (1981) Characterization of a 41-residue ovine hypothalamic peptide that stimulates secretion of corticotropin and beta-endorphin. *Science* 213, 1394–1397.

van de Stolpe, A., Caldenhoven, E., Raaijmakers, J.A., van der Saag, P.T. and Koenderman, L. (1993) Glucocorticoid-mediated repression of intercellular adhesion molecule-1 expression in human monocytic and bronchial epithelial cell lines. *American Journal of Respiratory Cell and Molecular Biology* 8, 340–347.

Wake, H., Moorhouse, A.J., Jinno, S., Kohsaka, S. and Nabekura, J. (2009) Resting microglia directly monitor the functional state of synapses in vivo and determine the fate of ischemic terminals. *Journal of Neuroscience* 29, 3974–3980.

Webster, J.I., Tonelli, L. and Sternberg, E.M. (2002) Neuroendocrine regulation of immunity. *Annual Review of Immunology* 20, 125–163.

Wood, P.G., Karol, M.H., Kusnecov, A.W. and Rabin, B.S. (1993) Enhancement of antigen-specific humoral and cell-mediated immunity by electric footshock stress in rats. *Brain, Behavior, and Immunity* 7, 121–134.

Xia, Z., DePierre, J.W. and Nassberger, L. (1996) Tricyclic antidepressants inhibit IL-6, IL-1 beta and TNF-alpha release in human blood monocytes and IL-2 and interferon-gamma in T cells. *Immunopharmacology* 34, 27–37.

Yirmiya, R., Winocur, G. and Goshen, I. (2002) Brain interleukin-1 is involved in spatial memory and passive avoidance conditioning. *Neurobiology of Learning and Memory* 78, 379–389.

Yu, N., Zhang, X., Magistretti, P.J. and Bloom, F.E. (1998) IL-1-alpha and TNF-alpha differentially regulate CD4 and Mac-1 expression in mouse microglia. *Neuroimmunomodulation* 5, 42–52.

16 Depressive Disorders and Inflammation

R.K. McNamara*
Department of Psychiatry, University of Cincinnati College of Medicine, Ohio, USA

Introduction

Major psychiatric disorders including major depressive disorder (MDD) and bipolar disorder (BD) are characterized by recurrent severe depression, and depression frequently precedes the initial onset of mania and, by definition, bipolar I disorder (Conus *et al.*, 2008). In the USA, severe forms of MDD currently affect 2–7% of the population and up to 16–20% suffer from milder forms of the illness (Kessler *et al.*, 2007). The lifetime prevalence rate for BD is estimated at 1.0% for bipolar I disorder, 1.1% for bipolar II disorder and 2.4% for sub-threshold BD (4.4% total) (Kessler *et al.*, 2007). The initial onset of MDD and mania most frequently occurs during childhood and adolescence (Burke *et al.*, 1991;

* Author, robert.mcnamara@uc.edu

Chengappa *et al.*, 2003; Perlis *et al.*, 2009). Outcome data indicate that MDD and BD are associated with significant psychosocial morbidity and excess premature mortality attributable primarily to suicide and coronary heart disease (CHD) (Osby *et al.*, 2001; Angst *et al.*, 2002). In the year 2000, the World Health Organization identified MDD as the fourth ranked cause of disability and premature death in the world, and projected that by 2020 MDD will be the second most important cause of disability worldwide after cardiovascular disease (Murray and Lopez, 1997; WHO, 2000). Accordingly, developing a better understanding of pathogenic mechanisms and protective factors associated with the development of MDD and BD represents an urgent public health need.

Major advances in the treatment and prevention of mood disorders will be galvanized by the identification of pathogenic mechanisms conferring vulnerability. To this end, aggressive efforts have been devoted to identify susceptibility genes. A consistent pattern has yet to emerge, however, owing in part to the polygenic, heterogeneous and multifactorial nature of these disorders. Subtotal heritability estimates and monozygotic twin discordance rates indicate that environmental factors confer significant vulnerability (Merikangas *et al.*, 2002; Ehringer *et al.*, 2006). For example, a meta-analysis of community-based twin studies of MDD yielded a heritability estimate of 0.37, indicating that approximately two thirds of the liability is attributable to environmental factors (Sullivan *et al.*, 2000). Genetic factors play a greater, but not complete, etiological role in BD, with a heritability estimate of 0.59 (Tsuang and Faraone, 1990). Accordingly, aggressive efforts also need to be devoted to the identification of environmental risk factors, particularly in view of their amenability to modification and prevention.

There is a growing body of research aimed at identifying modifiable environmental risk factors for psychiatric disorders, and promising candidates include dietary deficiencies in micronutrients and regular physical activity (i.e. exercise). Of the different micronutrients implicated in the pathophysiology of mood disorders, which include Vitamin B9 (i.e. folate) and Vitamin E, a large body of evidence has implicated dietary long-chain omega-3 (LCn-3) fatty acid deficiency in the pathoetiology of MDD and BD (Hibbeln and Salem, 1995; Freeman *et al.*, 2006; Parker *et al.*, 2006a; Lin and Su, 2007; McNamara, 2009a; Appleton *et al.*, 2010). Additionally, evidence has also implicated dietary LCn-3 fatty acid deficiency as a risk factor for CHD in the general population (Harris, 2008) and in MDD patients (McNamara, 2009b). Importantly, the pathophysiology of mood disorders and CHD are associated with elevated pro-inflammatory signalling activity, which is down-regulated by increasing regular exercise and dietary LCn-3 fatty acid intake. The primary objective of this chapter is to review evidence implicating LCn-3 deficiency and exercise in the aetiology of pro-inflammatory signalling in mood disorders, and to evaluate their potential role as modifiable risk factors in the pathogenesis of MDD and BD.

LCn-3 Fatty Acid Deficiency in Mood Disorders

Background

Mammals require a dietary source of n-3 fatty acids to procure and maintain adequate concentrations of LCn-3 in peripheral and central tissues. Principal dietary sources of the vegetable shorter-chain n-3 fatty acid precursor α-linolenic acid (ALA, 18:3n-3) include flaxseed, linseed, canola, soy, chia seeds and perilla oils. The biosynthesis of LCn-3 fatty acids, including eicosapentaenoic acid (EPA, 20:5n-3) and docosahexaenoic acid (DHA, 22:6n-3), from ALA requires a series of microsomal desaturation and elongation reactions, and the final synthesis of DHA requires β-oxidation within peroxisomes. Enzymes mediating LCn-3 biosynthesis, including delta6- and delta5-desaturases, are regulated by multiple factors including gonadal hormones (Pawlosky *et al.*, 2003; Giltay *et al.*, 2004; McNamara *et al.*, 2009c; Childs *et al.*, 2010; Extier *et al.*, 2010), insulin (Brenner, 2003), dietary n-3 fatty acid intake (Igarashi *et al.*, 2007), as well as heritable polymorphisms in desaturase (Bokor *et al.*, 2010) and peroxisomal (Steinberg *et al.*, 2004) genes. In healthy adult humans residing in Western countries, ALA→EPA biosynthesis is limited and ALA→DHA and EPA→DHA biosynthesis is negligible (Brenna *et al.*, 2009). Preformed EPA and DHA can be obtained directly from the diet, particularly from fatty cold-water fish, including salmon, mackerel, herring, trout and tuna, as well as fish-oil and algal-derived supplements (Mozaffarian and Rim, 2006). Bypassing microsomal- and peroxisomal-mediated biosynthesis with preformed DHA is significantly more effective than ALA for increasing DHA composition in erythrocytes (Barceló-Coblijn *et al.*, 2008), breast milk (Francois *et al.*, 2003) and cortical grey matter (Su *et al.*, 1999).

An individual's LCn-3 'status' is determined by evaluating the fatty acid composition of blood (plasma phospholipids, erythrocytes and platelets), breast milk, peripheral (i.e. adipose and heart biopsies) and/or central (i.e. post-mortem brain) tissues by gas chromatography. Of these different options, erythrocyte membrane LCn-3 composition has emerged as a valid index of habitual (1–2 months) dietary LCn-3 fatty acid intake (Brown *et al.*, 1991; Katan *et al.*, 1997; Fekete *et al.*, 2009; Kuratko and Salem, 2009). Although different tissues exhibit differences in LCn-3 fatty acid turnover and composition, erythrocyte membrane LCn-3 fatty acid composition is positively correlated with plasma and platelet (Vidgren *et al.*, 1997), adipose (Leaf *et al.*, 1995; Hodson *et al.*, 2008; Ogura *et al.*, 2010), breast milk (Bergmann *et al.*, 2008) and myocardium (Harris *et al.*, 2004) LCn-3 composition. Erythrocyte membrane DHA composition is also positively correlated with brain grey matter DHA composition (Connor *et al.*, 1990; Carver *et al.*, 2001) as well as functional cortical activity (McNamara *et al.*, 2010a).

Mood disorders

Several independent studies have observed significant plasma phospholipid and/or erythrocyte membrane LCn-3 deficits in MDD patients with and without coronary syndromes relative to healthy controls (Maes *et al.*, 1996, 1999; Edwards *et al.*, 1998; Peet *et al.*, 1998; Frasure-Smith *et al.*, 2004; Parker *et al.*, 2006b; Amin *et al.*, 2008; Assies *et al.*, 2010; Baghai *et al.*, 2010; McNamara *et al.*, 2010b; Riemer *et al.*, 2010). A recent meta-analysis of 14 case-control fatty acid composition studies found significant deficits in EPA and DHA in MDD patients, whereas the principal LCn-6 fatty acid arachidonic acid was not different (Lin *et al.*, 2010). In BD patients, three independent studies have observed significant erythrocyte LCn-3 deficits compared with healthy controls (Chiu *et al.*, 2003; Ranjekar *et al.*, 2003; McNamara *et al.*, 2010b). Prospective longitudinal studies have found that low baseline plasma or erythrocyte DHA composition is associated with greater risk of developing postpartum depression (DeVriese *et al.*, 2003), depression following interferon-alpha (IFN-α) treatment (Su *et al.*, 2009), suicide in MDD patients (Sublette *et al.*, 2006), and CHD in the general population (Harris, 2008). Together, these studies provide strong evidence that both MDD and BD are associated with peripheral LCn-3 deficiency, and that these deficits may contribute to the aetiology of depressive symptoms as well as primary causes of premature excess mortality in MDD and BD patients.

The principle LCn-3 found in mammalian brain grey matter is DHA, which comprises approximately 15% of total fatty acid composition. The precursors of DHA, including ALA (18:3n-3), EPA (20:5n-3), and docosapentaenoic acid (22:5n-3), together comprise <1% of total brain fatty acid composition (McNamara *et al.*, 2008a; Carver *et al.*, 2001). A growing number of case-control studies have investigated the fatty acid composition of post-mortem brain grey matter from patients with MDD and BD, and some studies (McNamara *et al.*, 2007, 2008b; Conklin *et al.*, 2010) but not all (Lalovic *et al.*, 2007; Hamazaki *et al.*, 2010; Igarashi *et al.*, 2010), have observed significant DHA deficits. Although the reason for this discrepancy is not known, a number of important extraneous variables, including medications, diet, gender and methodological differences, may contribute (McNamara and Jandacek, 2011). Emerging evidence from human neuroimaging studies provide evidence for a role of dietary LCn-3 fatty acids in maintaining cortical metabolic and structural integrity (Hirashima *et al.*, 2004; Conklin *et al.*, 2007; Frangou *et al.*,

2007; Sublette *et al.*, 2009; McNamara *et al.*, 2010a). For example, a structural imaging study found that greater habitual LCn-3 fatty acid intake was associated with larger grey matter volumes in the anterior cingulate cortex, the right hippocampus and the right amygdala (Conklin *et al.*, 2007).

The aetiology of LCn-3 deficits observed in MDD and BD patients remains poorly understood, and may be attributable to several interacting variables including elevated lipid peroxidation secondary to impaired oxidative defence mechanisms (Peet *et al.*, 1998; Maes *et al.*, 2000; Sarandol *et al.*, 2007), folate deficiencies (Pita and Delgado, 2000; Umhau *et al.*, 2006), chronic alcohol exposure (Pawlosky and Salem, 1999; McNamara *et al.*, 2008b), and heritable polymorphisms in microsomal (Williard *et al.*, 2001; Schaeffer *et al.*, 2006; Martinelli *et al.*, 2008; Xie and Innis, 2008) and/or peroxisomal (Martinez, 1992; Steinberg *et al.*, 2004) biosynthesis genes. For example, recent studies have found that MDD patients exhibit reduced *FADS1* mRNA expression in post-mortem frontal cortex (Lalovic *et al.*, 2010; McNamara and Liu, 2011), and that patients with BD exhibit greater *FADS2* mRNA expression in post-mortem frontal cortex (Liu and McNamara, 2011). Moreover, a common polymorphism within the *FADS2* promoter is associated with greater transcription rates (Lattka *et al.*, 2010), and *FADS1* and *FADS2* are co-localized to chromosome 11q12-11q13.1, a locus found in a genome-wide linkage study to be associated with increased susceptibility to BD (Fallin *et al.*, 2004). Despite the potential multifactoral aetiology of LCn-3 deficits in MDD and BD patients, it is clear that dietary supplementation with preformed LCn-3 fatty acids (EPA+DHA) significantly increases erythrocyte and plasma EPA+DHA composition in MDD and BD patients to levels above those commonly observed in healthy controls (Marangell *et al.*, 2003; Su *et al.*, 2003; Silvers *et al.*, 2005; Grenyer *et al.*, 2007; Wozniak *et al.*, 2007; Mischoulon *et al.*, 2008; Clayton *et al.*, 2009). This finding suggests that dietary LCn-3 insufficiency is an important determinant of tissue LCn-3 deficits in MDD and BD patients. Furthermore, these data indicate that LCn-3 deficits in MDD and BD patients are preventable or reversible through dietary LCn-3 fatty acid supplementation. Therapeutic relevance is supported by controlled prospective intervention trials finding that chronic LCn-3 fatty acids (EPA+DHA) supplementation is associated with a significant advantage over placebo for the treatment of depressive symptoms in MDD patients (Freeman *et al.*, 2006; Lin and Su, 2007; Appleton *et al.*, 2010). Furthermore, cross-national and cross-sectional epidemiological studies have found that greater habitual dietary LCn-3 fatty acid (EPA+DHA) intake is associated with reduced lifetime prevalence rates of MDD and BD (Hibbeln, 1998, 2002; Noaghiul and Hibbeln, 2003; Peet, 2004).

LCn-3 Fatty Acids Negatively Regulate Inflammation

One consequence of chronic dietary n-3 fatty acid deficiency is a reciprocal increase in arachidonic acid (20:4n-6) biosynthesis from dietary linoleic acid (18:2n-6), and associated increases in peripheral and central membrane arachidonic acid composition (Moriguchi *et al.*, 2001; Igarashi *et al.*, 2007). Arachidonic acid is the principal substrate for cycloxygenase-2 (COX-2)-mediated biosynthesis of pro-inflammatory eicosanoids, including prostaglandin E_2 (PGE_2), and immune cell-membrane arachidonic acid composition is positively correlated with PGE_2 production (Calder, 2008). Feeding an arachidonic-acid-enriched diet significantly increases PGE_2 levels in rat brain (Song *et al.*, 2003, 2008), whereas a diet high in LCn-3 fatty acids significantly blunts elevations in brain PGE_2 levels following central infusions of IL-1β or systemic lipopolysaccharide (LPS) (Kozac *et al.*, 1997; Song *et al.*, 2003, 2004). Moreover, pharmacological inhibition of delta6-desaturase-mediated linoleic acid→arachidonic acid biosynthesis is associated with impaired eicosanoid synthesis (Obukowicz *et al.*, 1998). Importantly, PGE_2 stimulates biosynthesis of the cytokine interleukin-6 (IL-6) at the level of transcription via nuclear factor κB (NFκB) (Portanova *et al.*, 1996; Wang *et al.*, 2010). IL-6 in turn stimulates hepatic biosynthesis of acute phase proteins including C-reactive protein (CRP) (Castell *et al.*, 1989; Li *et al.*, 1990; Li and Goldmann, 1996; Pepys and Hirschfield, 2003). DHA and/or EPA blunts LPS- or IFN-γ-stimulated NFκB activation in macrophages (Komatsu *et al.*, 2003), COX-2-mediated PGE_2 synthesis (Strokin *et al.*, 2007), and TNF-α and/or IL-6 production in different cell lines (Khalfoun *et al.*, 1997; Hao *et al.*, 2010; Lu *et al.*, 2010). In rodent models, dietary-induced rat brain DHA deficits are associated with increased cytosolic phospholipase A_2 ($cPLA_2$) and COX-2 expression (Rao *et al.*, 2007), and greater IL-6 and/or TNF-α plasma concentrations (McNamara *et al.*, 2010c; Mingam *et al.*, 2008). Additional evidence suggests that the bioactive lipid metabolites of EPA and DHA have potent anti-inflammatory and inflammatory-resolving properties that are mediated in part by macrophage GPR120 receptors (Calder, 2008; Bazan *et al.*, 2010; Groeger *et al.*, 2010; Oh *et al.*, 2010; Serhan, 2010). Dietary LCn-3 fatty acid deficiency therefore might contribute to pro-inflammatory signalling by both direct and indirect interactions with inflammatory signalling pathways (Fig. 16.1).

In agreement with these basic science observations, clinical studies have found an inverse correlation between blood LCn-3 fatty acid levels and pro-inflammatory markers, including IL-6, TNF-α and the acute phase protein CRP, in healthy subjects (Ferrucci *et al.*, 2006; Micallef *et al.*, 2009) and CHD patients (Farzaneh-Far *et al.*, 2009). For example, in a cohort of 1123 human subjects, lower fasting plasma LCn-3 fatty acid composition was associated with significantly higher IL-6 and TNF-α concentrations (Ferrucci *et al.*, 2006). Other studies have found that greater habitual dietary LCn-3 fatty acid intake is inversely correlated with plasma IL-6 and CRP levels (Pischon *et al.*, 2003; Lopez-Garcia *et al.*, 2004). In addition, dietary supplementation with LCn-3 fatty acids (fish oil) decreases monocyte production of TNF-α in healthy subjects (Endres *et al.*, 1989; Meydani *et al.*, 1991; Caughey *et al.*, 1996). Furthermore, dietary LCn-3 fatty acid supplementation significantly reduced elevations in TNF-α, IL-6, CRP and PGE_2 following exercise compared with placebo (Phillips *et al.*, 2003; Tartibian *et al.*, 2011). Taken collectively, basic and clinical studies indicate that LCn-3 fatty acid status is an important determinant of constitutive pro-inflammatory signalling activity.

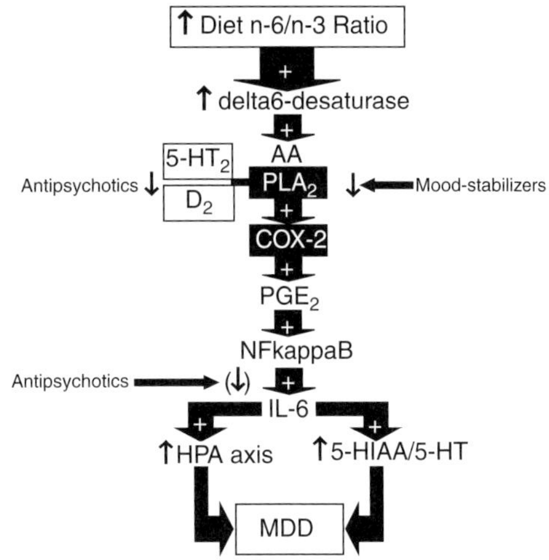

Fig. 16.1. Diagram illustrating the proposed pro-inflammatory signalling events resulting from dietary n-3 fatty acid deficiency. According to this model, dietary elevations in the n-6/n-3 ratio secondary to n-3 fatty acid deficiency up-regulate liver delta6-desaturase-mediated linoleic acid→arachidonic acid (AA) biosynthesis and immune cell membrane AA composition. Increased AA availability and mobilization via phospholipase A_2 (PLA_2) augments cycloxygenase-2 (COX-2)-mediated AA→prostaglandin E_2 (PGE_2) biosynthesis which in turn increases PGE_2→NFκB→IL-6 production. Elevated IL-6 concentrations increase hypothalamus–pituitary–adrenal (HPA) axis activity/reactivity and increase serotonin (5-HT) turnover, two prominent features associated with the pathophysiology of MDD. This pro-inflammatory signalling pathway may be down-regulated by atypical antipsychotics through blockade of dopamine D_2 and serotonin $5\text{-}HT_{2A/C}$ receptor-mediated PLA_2 activity and decreasing NFκB, and by mood-stabilizers by decreasing PLA_2 activity.

Inflammation in Major Mood Disorders

Animal studies

A body of preclinical research has found that stimulation of cytokine production increases behavioural indices of depression in rodents that are attenuated by antidepressant medications (Dantzer *et al.*, 2008). Conversely, TNF-α receptor (Simen *et al.*, 2006) and IL-6 (Chourbaji *et al.*, 2006) knockout mice exhibit reduced behavioural indices of depression. Moreover, the olfactory bulbectomized rat model of depression is associated with elevated central PLA_2 activity and pro-inflammatory PGE_2 production (Song *et al.*, 2009; Skelin *et al.*, 2011). Also, in rhesus monkeys, IFN-α administration, and associated increases in plasma IL-6 concentrations, led to a persistent increase in anxiety-like behaviour and depressive-like huddling in a subset of animals (Felger *et al.*, 2007). These preclinical studies support a link between elevations in pro-inflammatory signalling and depression-like behaviour that is responsive to antidepressant medications.

Clinical studies

Several case-control studies have investigated the inflammatory status of patients diagnosed with MDD. An early series of studies found that PGE_2 levels were significantly elevated in the plasma or saliva of MDD patients (Lieb *et al.*, 1983; Calabrese *et al.*, 1986; Ohishi *et al.*, 1988; Nishino *et al.*, 1989). More recently, studies have investigated cytokine levels in MDD patients. A meta-analysis of 24 of these case-control studies found that MDD patients exhibit significantly higher blood concentrations of IL-6 and TNF-α compared with healthy controls, whereas no significant differences were found for other pro-inflammatory (IL-1β, IL-2 and IFN-γ) or anti-inflammatory (IL-4, IL-8 and IL-10) cytokines (Dowlati *et al.*, 2010). Consistent with greater IL-6-induced CRP biosynthesis, case-control studies have also observed greater CRP levels in patients with depression (Lanquillon *et al.*, 2000; Kop *et al.*, 2002; Penninx *et al.*, 2003; Kling *et al.*, 2007). Epidemiological studies have found that higher CRP levels are associated with an increased adjusted risk for past and current depressive episodes in men but not women (Danner *et al.*, 2003; Ford and Erlinger 2004; Liukkonen *et al.*, 2006). Extensive evidence therefore suggests that elevations in pro-inflammatory signalling are a feature of MDD.

Case-control studies have also investigated peripheral cytokine levels in BD patients (Goldstein *et al.*, 2009). During depressive and acute manic episodes, BD patients exhibit greater IL-6, IL-6 receptor (IL-6R) and/or TNF-α levels compared with healthy controls (Maes *et al.*, 1995a; O'Brien *et al.*, 2006; Kim *et al.*, 2007; Ortiz-Dominguez *et al.*, 2007; Brietzke *et al.*, 2009). A subset of studies observed greater CRP levels during acute mania compared with BD patients during the depressive phase and healthy controls (Wadee *et al.*, 2002; Huang and Lin, 2007; Cunha *et al.*, 2008). Some studies (Dickerson *et al.*, 2007; Brietzke *et al.*, 2009), but not all (O'Brien *et al.*, 2006), found that IL-6 and CRP levels were positively correlated with manic symptom severity. In contrast, no differences were observed for TNF-α, IL-6 or CRP in euthymic BD patients compared with healthy controls (Cunha *et al.*, 2008; Brietzke *et al.*, 2009). These data suggest that elevated pro-inflammatory signalling is observed during both manic and depressive phases of BD, whereas elevations in CRP are unique to mania. Moreover, these data suggest that pro-inflammatory signalling resolves during euthymia, suggesting that this is a state (versus trait) feature of BD.

Additional evidence implicating inflammation in the pathoetiology of depression comes from prospective studies of non-depressed patients receiving chronic IFN-α therapy for the treatment of infectious disease. Approximately 20% to 50% of initially non-depressed patients receiving chronic IFN-α therapy develop clinically significant depression that responds to conventional antidepressant medications (Musselman *et al.*, 2001; Capuron *et al.*, 2002; Raison *et al.*, 2006). Subsequent studies have found that depression resulting from IFN-α is associated with elevations in peripheral (Prather *et al.*, 2009) and central (Raison *et al.*, 2008) IL-6 concentrations. It is also noteworthy that a significant percentage of hepatitis C patients receiving IFN-α therapy exhibit hypomanic and manic features, including irritability, sleep disturbances and hyperactivity (Constant *et al.*, 2005). Additionally, healthy subjects treated with endotoxin (*Salmonella abortus equi*) also exhibit symptoms of depression and anxiety that are correlated with increases in peripheral blood IL-6 and TNF-α concentrations (Reichenberg *et al.*, 2001). Moreover, elevations in IL-6 levels in response to influenza vaccination were amplified and prolonged in elderly patients with depressive symptoms (Glaser *et al.*, 2003). This body of evidence suggests that repeated activation of pro-inflammatory signalling networks can precipitate depression or mania in a subset of non-depressed patients, and that this response is associated with elevations in peripheral IL-6 concentrations.

A small number of case studies have investigated cytokine levels in the cerebrospinal fluid (CSF) of MDD and BD patients. One small study found that medication-free patients with acute severe depression had higher CSF concentrations of IL-1β, lower IL-6 and no change in TNF-α and there was a positive correlation between serum IL-1β and depression symptom severity (Levine *et al.*, 1999). Another study did not observe elevated CSF IL-6 concentrations in a small cohort of medication-free MDD patients (Carpenter *et al.*, 2004). A third study found CSF IL-6 concentrations was significantly higher in suicide attempters than in healthy control subjects and there was a significant positive correlation between CSF IL-6 levels, CSF levels of the serotonin metabolite 5-hydroxyindoleacetic acid (5-HIAA) and depression symptom severity (Lindqvist *et al.*, 2009). Another study found that euthymic BD patients exhibited greater CSF IL-1β levels, and lower CSF IL-6 levels, compared with in healthy controls (Söderlund *et al.*, 2011). Peripheral treatment with IFN-α increased CSF IL-6 concentrations in hepatitis C patients which were inversely correlated with CSF 5-HIAA concentrations (Raison *et al.*, 2008). The differential findings, particularly for IL-6, between CSF and plasma suggest that there may be dynamic mechanisms that regulate cytokine diffusion from peripheral to central compartments.

Case-control studies have also investigated the expression of inflammatory signalling markers in post-mortem brain tissue from MDD and BD patients. One study found that trans-membrane TNF protein expression was significantly greater in the frontal cortex (BA 46) of MDD patients compared with controls (Dean *et al.*, 2010). IL-4 mRNA expression was greater in frontal cortex (BA11) of female suicide victims and IL-13 mRNA expression was greater in male suicide victims (Tonelli *et al.*, 2008). This study also found a trend for greater TNF-α expression in female suicide victims, and no changes in IL-1β, IL-5 or IL-6 expression. Expression levels of enzymes involved in arachidonic acid metabolism, including $cPLA_2$ and COX-2, were elevated in the post-mortem frontal cortex of BD patients (Kim *et al.*, 2011). Moreover, higher protein and mRNA levels of IL-1β and IL-1R, but not TNF-α, were observed in the post-mortem frontal cortex of BD patients (Rao *et al.*, 2010). Another study did not observe changes in COX-2 expression in post-mortem frontal cortex of patients with MDD or BD, but did observe significant reductions in PGE_2 synthase (Maida *et al.*, 2006). Although these findings support central abnormalities in inflammatory signalling in MDD and BD patients, effects of prior chronic medication exposure on central cytokine levels complicate interpretation (see below). For example, it was found that elevated indices of arachidonic acid metabolism observed in the post-mortem frontal cortex (BA10) of drug-free BD patients were attenuated in patients treated with mood-stabilizer medications prior to death (McNamara *et al.*, 2008b).

Genetic association studies have begun to elucidate the potential contribution of single nucleotide polymorphisms (SNPs) in genes regulating inflammatory signalling pathways to the pathoetiology of MDD and BD. The PLA_2 BanI polymorphism was found to be associated with greater PLA_2 enzyme activity in platelets of schizophrenic patients (Barbosa *et al.*, 2007). In addition, a cross-sectional study found that serum PLA_2 activity was elevated in MDD and BD patients (Noponen *et al.*, 1993). A subsequent study found that calcium-independent PLA_2 activity was significantly greater in BD patients with a history of psychosis compared with those without history of psychosis and healthy controls (Ross *et al.*, 2006). The allele frequency of the PLA_2 BanI polymorphism was found to be greater in MDD, but not BD, patients compared with healthy controls

(Meira-Lima *et al.*, 2003; Papadimitiou *et al.*, 2003; Pae *et al.*, 2004; Dikeos *et al.*, 2006). Moreover, a recent prospective study found that the PLA_2 BanI polymorphism was associated with more somatic symptoms of depression in patients treated with IFN-α (Su *et al.*, 2010). Additionally, genetic studies have found that polymorphisms in delta6- (*FADS2*) and delta5-desaturase (*FADS1*) genes are associated with inflammation and CHD in the general population (Schaeffer *et al.*, 2006; Martinelli *et al.*, 2008). Together, these findings provide preliminary evidence for a potential genetic aetiology associated with elevated pro-inflammatory signalling in MDD.

Medication Effects

Antidepressants

A growing body of evidence suggests that antidepressant medications down-regulate pro-inflammatory signalling pathways (Castanon *et al.*, 2002). For example, *in vitro* studies have found that different antidepressants suppress LPS-induced production of pro-inflammatory cytokines including TNF-α and IL-6 (Kenis and Maes, 2002). Moreover, the development of cytokine-induced depressive-like behaviour in rodents is diminished by antidepressant medications (Yirmiya *et al.*, 2001). Rodent studies have also found, however, that chronic antidepressant treatments up-regulate PLA_2-mediated arachidonic acid turnover in rat brain, but do not alter COX-2 expression (Lee *et al.*, 2007, 2010) or arachidonic acid composition (McNamara *et al.*, 2010d). Although additional studies are required to clarify mechanisms, this preclinical evidence suggests that antidepressant medications interact with inflammatory signalling pathways.

Clinical studies have found that adjunctive treatment with celecoxib, which blocks COX-2-mediated arachidonic acid→PGE_2 production, augments the antidepressant effects of reboxetine in MDD patients (Muller *et al.*, 2006). Similarly, adjunctive treatment with acetylsalicylic acid (aspirin), also a COX-2 inhibitor, increased remission rates when added to fluoxetine in MDD patients previously nonresponsive to fluoxetine alone (Mendlewicz *et al.*, 2006). Other studies have found that significantly greater pre-treatment CRP levels in MDD patients were significantly reduced following a 6-week antidepressant treatment in both responders and non-responders (Lanquillon *et al.*, 2000), and that greater IL-6 and CRP levels are associated with reduced response to antidepressants (Maes *et al.*, 1997; Sluzewska *et al.*, 1997). Additionally, chronic treatment with the selective serotonin reuptake inhibitors did not significantly alter serum IL-6 concentrations in MDD patients (Maes *et al.*, 1995b; Jazayeri *et al.*, 2010). These preliminary clinical findings suggest that antidepressant medications may interact with different components of the inflammatory signalling pathway in a manner that is relevant to therapeutic effects.

Mood-stabilizers

Lithium chloride, and the anticonvulsants carbamazepine, sodium valproate and lamotrigine, are first-line treatments for acute mania and the prophylactic stabilization of mood oscillations in BD. A common mechanism of action of these medications is the down-regulation of $cPLA_2$-mediated arachidonic acid turnover and COX-2-mediated PGE_2 production (Rapoport and Bosetti, 2002; Rao *et al.*, 2008). The body of evidence supporting this mechanism has led to the 'arachidonic acid cascade' hypothesis of BD, which posits that elevated central COX-2-mediated arachidonic acid→PGE_2 production is a pathophysiological feature of BD that is suppressed by mood-stabilizer medications (Rapoport, 2008; Rao and Rapoport, 2009). Recent studies have also found that chronic neuroinflammation leading to elevated central PGE_2 production is significantly blunted in rats chronically treated with lithium (Basselin *et al.*, 2010). Chronic neuroinflammation is also associated with lateral ventricular enlargement and decreased hippocampal size in rodents (Hauss-Wegrzyniak *et al.*, 2000). It is therefore notable that lateral ventricular enlargement in BD (Kempton *et al.*, 2008) and reductions in hippocampal volume in MDD (Campbell *et al.*, 2004) are among the most robust and consistent neuroimaging features observed in case-control studies.

Consistent with these preclinical findings, clinical studies have found that chronic lithium treatment normalizes elevated IL-6R and IL-6, but not TNF-α levels in BD patients (Rapoport *et al.*, 1999; Kim *et al.*, 2007). *Ex vivo* studies have found that LPS-stimulated monocyte IL-6 production is greater in medication-free BD patients compared with healthy controls, and that this response is attenuated following lithium treatment (Knijff *et al.*, 2007). Another study found that lithium-treated BD patients exhibited fewer IL-6 secreting peripheral blood lymphocytes compared with healthy controls, and that the number of IL-6 secreting cells decreased significantly in medication-naïve BD patients following chronic lithium treatment (Boufidou *et al.*, 2004). In rapid cycling patients, serum IL-2R and IL-6R were increased compared with healthy controls, and were normalized following 30-day lithium treatment (Rapaport *et al.*, 1999). Another study did not observe significant alterations in elevated IL-6R in BD patients following semi-chronic treatment valproate (Maes *et al.*, 1995a). These clinical findings suggest that chronic lithium treatment has anti-inflammatory properties.

Antipsychotics

Atypical antipsychotic medications are efficacious in the treatment of acute mania, and are increasing being employed as the first-line treatment for acute mania in children and adolescents (Pfeifer *et al.*, 2010). Preclinical studies have found that atypical antipsychotic medications significantly attenuate IL-6 and TNF-α production in microglia cells following IFN-γ exposure (Kato *et al.*, 2007; Bian *et al.*, 2008), and in mice following peripheral LPS administration (Sugino *et al.*, 2009). Moreover, chronic risperidone treatment up-regulates delta-6 desaturase-mediated LCn-3 fatty acid biosynthesis and peripheral membrane LCn-3 fatty acid composition in rats (McNamara *et al.*, 2009d, 2011a) and normalizes constitutively elevated IL-6, TNF-α and CRP levels in n-3 fatty acid deficient rats (McNamara *et al.*, 2011b). It is also relevant that atypical antipsychotic medications are high-affinity antagonists at serotonin (5-HT) 5-$HT_{2A/C}$ and dopamine D_2 receptors (Richtand *et al.*, 2007), both of which are positively coupled to PLA_2-mediated arachidonic acid release (Piomelli *et al.*, 1991; Garcia and Kim, 1997; Nilsson *et al.*, 1998; Qu *et al.*, 2003). Some prior case-control studies have found that antipsychotic medications have immunosuppressive properties in schizophrenic patients (Drzyzga *et al.*, 2006) and adjunctive treatment with the COX-2 inhibitor celecoxib was found to be superior to risperidone alone in reducing symptom severity in schizophrenic patients (Akhondzadeh *et al.*, 2007). Together, these data suggest that atypical antipsychotic medications, like mood-stabilizers, suppress pro-inflammatory signalling activity and reactivity.

LCn-3 Fatty Acids and Inflammation in Mood Disorders

As discussed above, separate lines of evidence suggest that patients with MDD or BD exhibit both LCn-3 fatty acid deficiency and elevated pro-inflammatory signalling activity. Several animal studies have linked inflammation in mood disorders to brain fatty acid composition. For example, the Flinders Sensitive Line rat model of depression is associated with greater regional brain arachidonic acid composition (Green *et al.*, 2005). In addition, dietary-induced n-3 fatty acid deficiency is associated with elevated regional brain arachidonic acid composition, PLA_2 and COX-2 expression (Rao *et al.*, 2007) and elevated behavioural indices of depression (DeMar *et al.*, 2006). Remarkably, however, there have been few clinical studies that have directly investigated the link between LCn-3 fatty acid status and pro-inflammatory signalling in MDD and BD patients. One study found that greater plasma phospholipid n-6:n-3 ratios and depressive symptom severity were associated with greater TNF-α and IL-6 levels in elderly subjects (Kiecolt-Glaser *et al.*, 2007).

This finding is of particular interest in view of prior observations that a higher plasma LCn-6: LCn-3 ratio is positively correlated with manic (Sublette *et al.*, 2007) and depression (Adams *et al.*, 1996) symptom severity. In hepatitis C patients treated with IFN-α, baseline erythrocyte DHA composition (Su *et al.*, 2010) and plasma IL-6 concentrations (Prather *et al.*, 2009) were separately found to be significant predictors of treatment-emergent depression. The only intervention study to date found that chronic treatment with EPA (using 1 g/day) did not significantly alter serum IL-6 concentrations in MDD patients (Jazayeri *et al.*, 2010). Additional studies are clearly warranted to further elucidate the relationship between LCn-3 fatty acid status and pro-inflammatory signalling in MDD and BD.

Despite the paucity of evidence regarding the relationship between LCn-3 fatty acid deficiency and pro-inflammatory signalling in MDD and BD, parallel lines of preclinical and clinical evidence suggest that LCn-3 fatty acid deficiency and pro-inflammatory signalling similarly impact prominent pathophysiology features associated with mood dysregulation, including a dysregulation in central serotonin (5-HT) neurotransmission and hypothalamus–pituitary–adrenal (HPA) axis activity and reactivity.

Serotonin metabolism

Central serotonin neurotransmission has repeatedly been implicated in the pathophysiology (Arango *et al.*, 2002) and treatment (Vaswani *et al.*, 2003) of MDD, and to be modulated by LCn-3 fatty acids. For example, dietary n-3 fatty acid deficiency during perinatal development blunted fenfluramine-induced elevations in extracellular 5-HT content in the adult rat hippocampus (Kodas *et al.*, 2004). MDD patients also exhibited blunted fenfluramine-induced cerebral glucose metabolism in the prefrontal cortex (Anderson *et al.*, 2004). Moreover, plasma DHA concentrations were found to be positively correlated with the CSF levels of the principal metabolite of serotonin, 5-hydroxyindoleacetic acid (5-HIAA), in a cohort of healthy subjects (Hibbeln *et al.*, 1998). Furthermore, prospective studies have found that low plasma DHA composition (Sublette *et al.*, 2006) and low CSF 5-HIAA content (Placidi *et al.*, 2001) are both significant predictors of future suicidal behaviour in MDD patients. Perinatal n-3 fatty acid deficiency increases 5-HT_{2A} receptor binding in the adult rat prefrontal cortex (Delion *et al.*, 1996) and depressed suicide victims exhibit significant DHA deficits (McNamara *et al.*, 2007) and elevated 5-HT_{2A} receptor binding density (Arango *et al.*, 1990; Pandey *et al.*, 2002) in post-mortem prefrontal cortex. Chronic dietary n-3 fatty acid insufficiency is associated with reduced 5-HT synthesis and increased 5-HT metabolism in rat brain (McNamara *et al.*, 2009e) and depressive-like behaviour in the forced swim test (Demar *et al.*, 2006). Conversely, dietary-induced elevations in DHA composition increase 5-HT concentrations in rat frontal cortex (Chalon *et al.*, 1998; Vancassel *et al.*, 2008) and produce antidepressant-like effects in the forced swim test (Carlezon *et al.*, 2005; Huang *et al.*, 2008). Together, these associations support a link between LCn-3 fatty acid deficiency and pathophysiologically relevant alterations in central 5-HT metabolism.

Peripherally generated cytokines have also been found to interact with central 5-HT neurotransmission. For example, peripheral administration of IL-6 significantly increased 5-HIAA and the 5-HIAA/5-HT ratio in rat brain (Wang and Dunn, 1998), and significantly increased extracellular 5-HT concentrations in rat striatum (Zhang *et al.*, 2001). Furthermore, chronic dietary n-3 fatty acid deficiency increased constitutive peripheral (plasma) IL-6 concentrations, which were positively correlated with elevated 5-HIAA/5-HT ratios in different rat brain regions (McNamara *et al.*, 2010c) (Fig. 16.2). These findings are significant because medication-free MDD patients exhibit reduced indices of 5-HT synthesis (Rosa-Neto *et al.*, 2004), and significantly greater internal jugular venoarterial 5-HIAA plasma content relative to healthy controls (Barton *et al.*, 2008). Importantly, chronic treatment with fluoxetine significantly decreased 5-HIAA content and the 5-HIAA/5-HT ratio in rat frontal cortex (Unceta *et al.*, 2007; McNamara *et al.*,

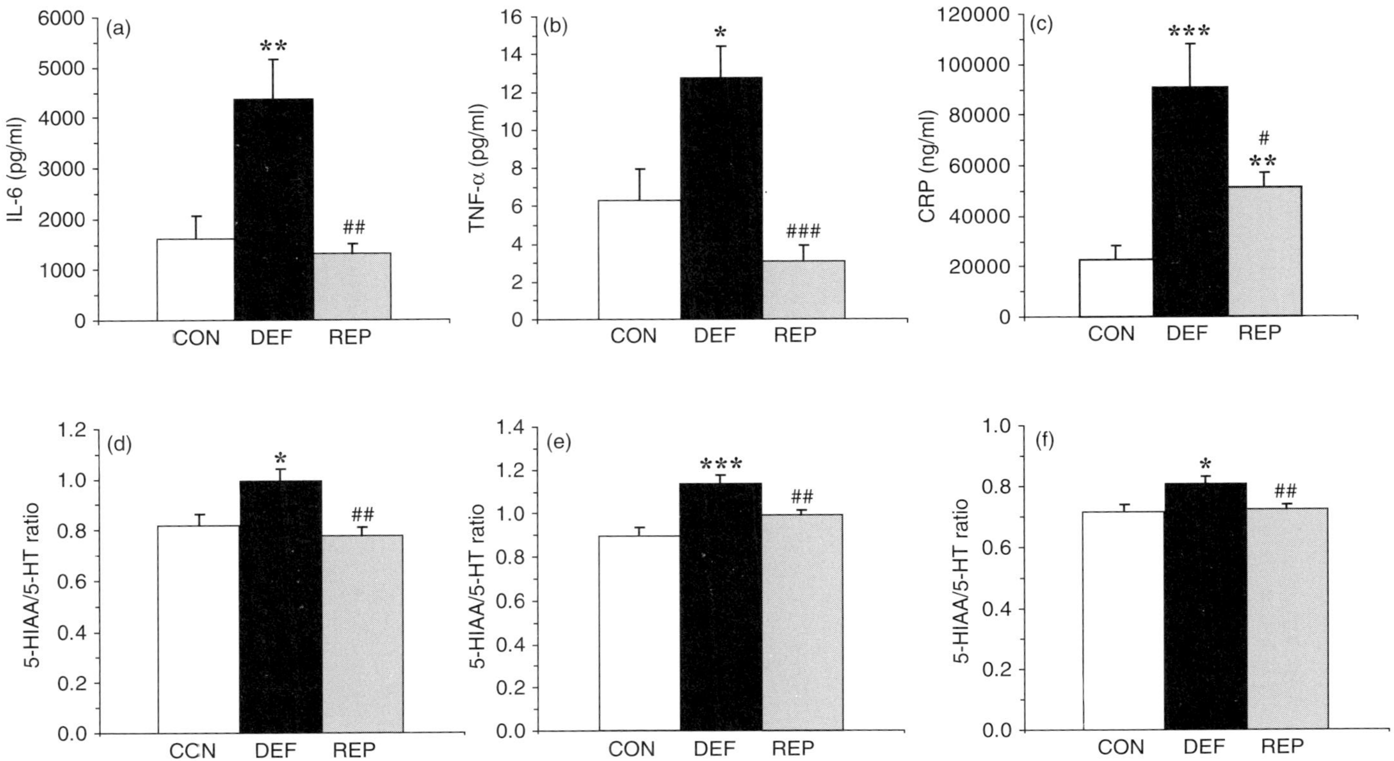

Fig. 16.2. Preclinical evidence linking LCn-3 fatty acid deficiency, elevated peripheral pro-inflammatory signalling activity and central alterations in 5-HT metabolism. Plasma concentrations of (a) interleukin-6 (IL-6, pg/ml), (b) tumour necrosis factor-alpha (TNF-α, pg/ml), (c) C-reactive protein (CRP, ng/ml); and serotonin turnover (5-HIAA/5-HT) in the (d) prefrontal cortex, (e) hypothalamus and (f) ventral striatum of control (CON, n = 10), n-3-deficient (DEF, n = 10) and n-3-repleted (REP, n = 10) rats. Among all rats (n = 30), plasma IL-6 levels were positively correlated with 5-HIAA/5-HT ratios in all brain regions. Values are group mean ± SEM. $^{*}p \leq 0.05$, $^{**}p \leq 0.01$, $^{***}p \leq 0.0001$ versus controls, $^{\#}p \leq 0.05$, $^{\#\#}p \leq 0.001$, $^{\#\#\#}p \leq 0.0001$ versus DEF rats. (From McNamara *et al.*, 2010c, with permission from Elsevier Science Inc.)

2010d) and CSF 5-HIAA content in MDD patients (Potter *et al.*, 1985; De Bellis *et al.*, 1993; Lundmark *et al.*, 1994; Sheline *et al.*, 1997; Barton *et al.*, 2008). Together, these data suggest that elevated peripheral IL-6 production in response to LCn-3 fatty acid deficiency may contribute to clinically relevant changes in central 5-HT metabolism that oppose the mechanism of action of antidepressant medications.

HPA axis

Several independent findings have implicated a dysregulation in HPA axis activity and reactivity in the pathophysiology of mood disorders (Pariante and Miller, 2001; Strohle and Holsboer, 2003). Emerging evidence suggests that pro-inflammatory cytokines alter HPA axis activity and reactivity. For example, acute cytokine administration induces the expression and release of corticotropin-releasing hormone (CRH), adrenocorticotropic hormone, and cortisol/corticosterone (Wang and Dunn, 1998; Beisuizen and Thijs, 2003). Pro-inflammatory cytokines have also been found to down-regulate glucocorticoid receptors, and may therefore impair glucocorticoid-receptor-mediated negative feedback on HPA activity (Pace and Miller, 2009). Stressful life events and psychosocial stressors have long been recognized as distal and proximal antecedents of affective episodes in MDD and BD (Post and Leverich, 2006). It is relevant, therefore, that childhood maltreatment or psychosocial stress were found to be associated with greater IL-6 and/or CRP production (McDade *et al.*, 2006; Danese *et al.*, 2007; Miller *et al.*, 2009). Furthermore, elevations in IL-6 in response to psychosocial stress were greater in MDD patients with early life stress (Pace *et al.*, 2006).

Preliminary evidence also suggests that LCn-3 fatty acids can modulate the activity and reactivity of the HPA axis. For example, LCn-3 fatty acid supplementation significantly blunted elevations in plasma cortisol elicited by psychosocial stress in healthy subjects (Delarue *et al.*, 2003) and significantly blunted elevated plasma cortisol in healthy subjects treated with LPS (Michaeli *et al.*, 2007). Moreover, chronic dietary supplementation with EPA significantly attenuated elevations in corticosterone levels elicited by central IL-1β administration in rats (Song *et al.*, 2004) and decreased serum cortisol levels in MDD patients (Jazayeri *et al.*, 2010). Finally, plasma DHA levels were found to be inversely correlated with CSF CRH levels in perpetrators of domestic violence (Hibbeln *et al.*, 2004). These findings suggest that LCn-3 fatty acids negatively regulate HPA axis activity and reactivity in response to psychosocial stress and pro-inflammatory signalling activity.

Physical Activity, Inflammation and Depression

Accumulating evidence from epidemiological studies (Kritz-Sliverstein *et al.*, 2001; Strawbridge *et al.*, 2002; Motl *et al.*, 2004) and a meta-analysis of intervention trials (Lawlor and Hopker, 2001) suggest that regular physical activity (i.e. exercise) may have antidepressant effects. A recent systematic review and meta-analysis of 23 intervention trials (907 participants) comparing the antidepressant effects of regular exercise with no treatment or a control intervention found support for an improvement in depressive symptoms in subjects diagnosed with MDD owing to regular exercise (Mead *et al.*, 2008). Although the mechanisms responsible for the therapeutic effect of exercise in MDD are not fully understood, regular exercise might diminish pro-inflammatory signalling pathways (Walsh *et al.*, 2011). Although acute and regular exercise are associated with increased skeletal muscle production of IL-6 in healthy human subjects (Pedersen *et al.*, 2001; Hiscock *et al.*, 2004; Nielsen and Pedersen, 2007), it has been proposed that this response may lead to a net anti-inflammatory effect through an up-regulation of anti-inflammatory molecules (Petersen and Pedersen, 2005; Mathur and Pedersen, 2008). Moreover, regular exercise was found to reduce skeletal muscle IL-6 and TNF-α production in rats under controlled dietary conditions (Lira *et al.*, 2009). This finding suggests that a progressive down-regulation in pro-inflammatory cytokine production in response to regular exercise might contribute to its antidepressant effects.

In contrast to the overall anti-inflammatory effects that seem to be induced by regular exercise, acute intense exercise may have different effects. Several studies have found that patients with chronic inflammatory diseases exhibit an augmented pro-inflammatory response to acute exercise that persists for a longer period after exercise cessation (Ploeger *et al.*, 2009). There have been few studies that have evaluated the effects of exercise on cytokine production in MDD patients. A preliminary study found that acute exercise was not associated with greater IL-6 levels in antidepressant-treated MDD patients compared with healthy controls after adjusting for baseline differences (Boettger *et al.*, 2010). In a second study of medication-free MDD patients, it was found that, although IL-6 and TNF-α progressively increased during acute exercise in patients and controls, the decrease in plasma IL-6 levels during the period following acute exercise were significantly greater in controls than patients (Hallberg *et al.*, 2010). Further studies are needed to determine whether regular exercise, found to have anti-inflammatory and antidepressant effects, results in a reduction in pro-inflammatory cytokine production in MDD patients. In view of evidence that LCn-3 fatty acid status is an important determinant of TNF-α, IL-6, CRP and PGE_2 production following exercise (Phillips *et al.*, 2003; Tartibian *et al.*, 2011), it will also be of interest to determine relationships between LCn-3 fatty acid status and pro-inflammatory cytokine production in response to acute and regular exercise in MDD patients.

Summary and Conclusions

A body of evidence from cross-sectional studies and associated meta-analyses have separately implicated LCn-3 fatty acid deficiency and elevated pro-inflammatory signalling activity in the pathoetiology of mood symptoms in MDD and BD. LCn-3 fatty acids negatively regulate pro-inflammatory signalling activity and increasing dietary LCn-3 fatty acid intake has both anti-inflammatory and antidepressant effects. Regular physical activity has anti-inflammatory effects that may contribute to the antidepressant role of exercise. Preclinical studies have found that LCn-3 fatty acid deficiency and elevated pro-inflammatory signalling impact central serotonin neurotransmission and HPA axis reactivity in MDD patients, which may oppose the mechanism of action of antidepressant medications. In general, medications that exhibit therapeutic efficacy in the treatment of acute and chronic mood symptoms in MDD or BD patients down-regulate different components of the pro-inflammatory signalling pathway. Taken collectively, these data implicate LCn-3 fatty acid deficiency and physical inactivity as modifiable risk factors for elevated pro-inflammatory signalling activity in MDD and BD. Additional research is warranted to investigate whether increasing LCn-3 fatty acid intake and/or physical activity can decrease inflammation and improve outcomes. Moreover, increasing LCn-3 fatty acid intake and/or physical activity may represent a feasible primary prevention strategy in youth that are at high risk for developing mood disorders. For example, LCn-3 fatty acid supplementation was found to prevent or delay the onset of psychosis in ultra-high-risk adolescents (Amminger *et al.*, 2010) and analogous trials in adolescents at high risk for developing MDD and BD are currently feasible (McNamara *et al.*, 2010e).

Acknowledgements and Disclosures

This work was supported in part by National Institute of Health grants MH083924 and AG03617, and a NARSAD Independent Investigator Award. The author has received research support from Martek Biosciences Inc, Inflammation Research Foundation, Ortho-McNeil Janssen, AstraZeneca, Eli Lilly, and is a member of the Inflammation Research Foundation scientific advisory board.

References

Adams, P.B., Lawson, S., Sanigorski, A. and Sinclair, A.J. (1996) Arachidonic acid to eicosapentaenoic acid ratio in blood correlates positively with clinical symptoms of depression. *Lipids* 31, S157–S161.

Akhondzadeh, S., Tabatabaee, M., Amini, H., Ahmadi, S.A., Abbasi, S.H., *et al.* (2007) Celecoxib as adjunctive therapy in schizophrenia: a double-blind, randomized and placebo-controlled trial. *Schizophrenia Research* 90, 179–185.

Amin, A.A., Menon, R.A., Reid, K.J., Harris, W.S. and Spertus, J.A. (2008) Acute coronary syndrome patients with depression have low blood cell membrane omega-3 fatty acid levels. *Psychosomatic Medicine* 70, 856–862.

Anderson, A.D., Oquendo, M.A., Parsey, R.V., Milak, M.S., Campbell, C., *et al.* (2004) Regional brain responses to serotonin in major depressive disorder. *Journal of Affective Disorders* 82, 411–417.

Angst, F., Stassen, H.H., Clayton, P.J. and Angst, J. (2002) Mortality of patients with mood disorders: follow-up over 34-38 years. *Journal of Affective Disorders* 68, 167–181.

Appleton, K.M., Rogers, P.J. and Ness, A.R. (2010) Updated systematic review and meta-analysis of the effects of n-3 long-chain polyunsaturated fatty acids on depressed mood. *American Journal of Clinical Nutrition* 91, 757–770.

Arango, V., Ernsberger, P., Marzuk, P.M., Chen, J.S., Tierney, H., *et al.* (1990) Autoradiographic demonstration of increased serotonin 5-HT2 and beta-adrenergic receptor binding sites in the brain of suicide victims. *Archives of General Psychiatry* 47, 1038–1047.

Arango, V., Underwood, M.D. and Mann, J.J. (2002) Serotonin brain circuits involved in major depression and suicide. *Progress in Brain Research* 136, 443–453.

Assies, J., Pouwer, F., Lok, A., Mocking, R.J., Bockting, C.L., *et al.* (2010) Plasma and erythrocyte fatty acid patterns in patients with recurrent depression: a matched case-control study. *Public Library of Science One* 5, e10635.

Baghai, T.C., Varallo-Bedarida, G., Born, C., Häfner, S., Schüle, C., *et al.* (2011) Major depressive disorder is associated with cardiovascular risk factors and low Omega-3 index. *Journal of Clinical Psychiatry* 72, 1242–1247.

Barbosa, N.R., Junqueira, R.M., Vallada, H.P. and Gattaz, W.F. (2007) Association between BanI genotype and increased phospholipase A2 activity in schizophrenia. *European Archives of Psychiatry and Clinical Neuroscience* 257, 340–343.

Barceló-Coblijn, G., Murphy, E.J., Othman, R., Moghadasian, M.H., Kashour, T., *et al.* (2008) Flaxseed oil and fish-oil capsule consumption alters human red blood cell n-3 fatty acid composition: a multiple-dosing trial comparing 2 sources of n-3 fatty acid. *American Journal of Clinical Nutrition* 88, 801–809.

Barton, D.A., Esler, M.D., Dawood, T., Lambert, E.A., Haikerwal, D., *et al.* (2008) Elevated brain serotonin turnover in patients with depression: effect of genotype and therapy. *Archives of General Psychiatry* 65, 38–46.

Basselin, M., Kim, H.W., Chen, M., Ma, K., Rapoport, S.I., *et al.* (2010) Lithium modifies brain arachidonic and docosahexaenoic metabolism in rat lipopolysaccharide model of neuroinflammation. *Journal of Lipid Research* 51, 1049–1056.

Bazan, N.G., Calandria, J.M. and Serhan, C.N. (2010) Rescue and repair during photoreceptor cell renewal mediated by docosahexaenoic acid-derived neuroprotectin D1. *Journal of Lipid Research* 51, 2018–2031.

Beishuizen, A. and Thijs, L.G. (2003) Endotoxin and the hypothalamo-pituitary-adrenal (HPA) axis. *Journal of Endotoxin Research,* 9, 3–24.

Bergmann, R.L., Haschke-Becher, E., Klassen-Wigger, P., Bergmann, K.E., Richter, R., *et al.* (2008) Supplementation with 200 mg/day docosahexaenoic acid from mid-pregnancy through lactation improves the docosahexaenoic acid status of mothers with a habitually low fish intake and of their infants. *Annals of Nutrition and Metabolism* 52, 157–166.

Bian, Q., Kato, T., Monji, A., Hashioka, S., Mizoguchi, Y., *et al.* (2008) The effect of atypical antipsychotics, perospirone, ziprasidone and quetiapine on microglial activation induced by interferon-gamma. *Progress in Neuropsychopharmacology and Biological Psychiatry* 32, 42–48.

Boettger, S., Müller, H.J., Oswald, K., Puta, C., Donath, L., *et al.* (2010) Inflammatory changes upon a single maximal exercise test in depressed patients and healthy controls. *Progress in Neuropsychopharmacology and Biological Psychiatry* 34, 475–478.

Bokor, S., Dumont, J., Spinneker, A., Gonzalez Gross, M., Nova, E., *et al.*, HELENA Study Group (2010) Single nucleotide polymorphisms in the FADS gene cluster are associated with delta-5 and delta-6 desaturase activities estimated by serum fatty acid ratios. *Journal of Lipid Research* 51, 2325–2333.

Boufidou, F., Nikolaou, C., Alevizos, B., Liappas, I.A. and Christodoulou, G.N. (2004) Cytokine production in bipolar affective disorder patients under lithium treatment. *Journal of Affective Disorders* 82, 309–313.

Brenna, J.T., Salem, N., Sinclair, A.J., Cunnane, S.C., International Society for the Study of Fatty Acids and Lipids, ISSFAL (2009) alpha-Linolenic acid supplementation and conversion to n-3 long-chain polyunsaturated fatty acids in humans. *Prostaglandins, Leukotrienes and Essential Fatty Acids* 80, 85–91.

Brenner, R.R. (2003) Hormonal modulation of delta6 and delta5 desaturases: case of diabetes. *Prostaglandins, Leukotrienes and Essential Fatty Acids* 68, 151–162.

Brietzke, E., Stertz, L., Fernandes, B.S., Kauer-Sant'anna, M., Mascarenhas, M., *et al.* (2009) Comparison of cytokine levels in depressed, manic and euthymic patients with bipolar disorder. *Journal of Affective Disorders* 116, 214–217.

Brown, A.J., Pang, E. and Roberts, D.C. (1991) Persistent changes in the fatty acid composition of erythrocyte membranes after moderate intake of n-3 polyunsaturated fatty acids: study design implications. *American Journal of Clinical Nutrition* 54, 668–673.

Burke, K.C., Burke, J.D., Rae, D.S. and Regier, D.A. (1991) Comparing age at onset of major depression and other psychiatric disorders by birth cohorts in five US community populations. *Archives of General Psychiatry* 48, 789-795.

Calabrese, J.R., Skwerer, R.G., Barna, B., Gulledge, A.D., Valenzuela, R., *et al.* (1986) Depression, immunocompetence, and prostaglandins of the E series. *Psychiatry Research* 17, 41-47.

Calder, P.C. (2008) The relationship between the fatty acid composition of immune cells and their function. *Prostaglandins, Leukotrienes and Essential Fatty Acids,* 79, pp. 101–108.

Campbell, S., Marriott, M., Nahmias, C. and MacQueen, G.M. (2004) Lower hippocampal volume in patients suffering from depression: a meta-analysis. *American Journal of Psychiatry* 161, 598–607.

Capuron, L., Hauser, P., Hinze-Selch, D., Miller, A.H. and Neveu, P.J. (2002) Treatment of cytokine-induced depression. *Brain, Behavior, and Immunity* 16, 575–580.

Carlezon, W.A., Mague, S.D., Parow, A.M., Stoll, A.L., Cohen, B.M., *et al.* (2005) Antidepressant-like effects of uridine and omega-3 fatty acids are potentiated by combined treatment in rats. *Biological Psychiatry* 57, 343–350.

Carpenter, L.L., Heninger, G.R., Malison, R.T., Tyrka, A.R. and Price, L.H. (2004) Cerebrospinal fluid interleukin (IL)-6 in unipolar major depression. *Journal of Affective Disorders* 79, 285–289.

Carver, J.D., Benford, V.J., Han, B. and Cantor, A.B. (2001) The relationship between age and the fatty acid composition of cerebral cortex and erythrocytes in human subjects. *Brain Research Bulletin* 56, 79–85.

Castanon, N., Leonard, B.E., Neveu, P.J. and Yirmiya, R. (2002) Effects of antidepressants on cytokine production and actions. *Brain, Behavior, and Immunity* 16, 569–574.

Castell, J.V., Andus, T., Kunz, D. and Heinrich, P.C. (1989) Interleukin-6. The major regulator of acute-phase protein synthesis in man and rat. *Annals of the New York Academy of Science* 557, 87–99.

Caughey, G.E., Mantzioris, E., Gibson, R.A., Cleland, L.G. and James, M.J. (1996) The effect on human tumor necrosis factor alpha and interleukin 1 beta production of diets enriched in n-3 fatty acids from vegetable oil or fish oil. *American Journal of Clinical Nutrition* 63, 116-122.

Chalon, S., Delion-Vancassel, S., Belzung, C., Guilloteau, D., Leguisquet, A.M., *et al.* (1998) Dietary fish oil affects monoaminergic neurotransmission and behavior in rats. *Journal of Nutrition* 128, 2512–2519.

Chengappa, K.N., Kupfer, D.J., Frank, E., Houck, P.R., Grochocinski, V.J., *et al.* (2003) Relationship of birth cohort and early age at onset of illness in a bipolar disorder case registry. *American Journal of Psychiatry* 160, 1636–1642.

Childs, C.E., Romeu-Nadal, M., Burdge, G.C. and Calder, P.C. (2010) The polyunsaturated fatty acid composition of hepatic and plasma lipids differ by both sex and dietary fat intake in rats. *Journal of Nutrition* 140, 245–250.

Chiu, C.C., Huang, S.Y., Su, K.P., Lu, M.L., Huang, M.C., *et al.* (2003) Polyunsaturated fatty acid deficit in patients with bipolar mania. *European Neuropsychopharmacology* 13, 99–103.

Chourbaji, S., Urani, A., Inta, I., Sanchis-Segura, C., Brandwein, C., *et al.* (006) IL-6 knockout mice exhibit resistance to stress-induced development of depression-like behaviors. *Neurobiology of Disease* 23, 587–594.

Clayton, E.H., Hanstock, T.L., Hirneth, S.J., Kable, C.J., Garg, M.L. *et al.* (2009) Reduced mania and depression in juvenile bipolar disorder associated with long-chain omega-3 polyunsaturated fatty acid supplementation. *European Journal of Clinical Nutrition* 63, 1037–1040.

Conklin, S.M., Gianaros, P.J., Brown, S.M., Yao, J.K., Hariri, A.R., *et al.* (2007) Long-chain omega-3 fatty acid intake is associated positively with corticolimbic gray matter volume in healthy adults. *Neuroscience Letters* 421, 209–212.

Conklin, S.M., Runyan, C.A., Leonard, S., Reddy, R.D., Muldoon, M.F., *et al.* (2010) Age-related changes of n-3 and n-6 polyunsaturated fatty acids in the anterior cingulate cortex of individuals with major depressive disorder. *Prostaglandins, Leukotrienes, and Essential Fatty Acids* 82, 111–119.

Connor, W.E., Neuringer, M. and Lin, D.S. (1990) Dietary effects on brain fatty acid composition: the reversibility of n-3 fatty acid deficiency and turnover of docosahexaenoic acid in the brain, erythrocytes, and plasma of rhesus monkeys. *Journal of Lipid Research* 31, 237–247.

Constant, A., Castera, L., Dantzer, R., Couzigou, P., de Ledinghen, V., *et al.* (2005) Mood alterations during interferon-alpha therapy in patients with chronic hepatitis C: evidence for an overlap between manic/hypomanic and depressive symptoms. *Journal of Clinical Psychiatry* 66, 1050–1057.

Conus, P., Ward, J., Hallam, K.T., Lucas, N., Macneil, C., *et al.* (2008) The proximal prodrome to first episode mania-a new target for early intervention. *Bipolar Disorders* 10, 555–565.

Cunha, A.B., Andreazza, A.C., Gomes, F.A., Frey, B.N., da Silveira, L.E., *et al.* (2008) Investigation of serum high-sensitive C-reactive protein levels across all mood states in bipolar disorder. *European Archives of Psychiatry and Clinical Neuroscience* 258, 300–304.

Danese, A., Pariante, C.M., Caspi, A., Taylor, A. and Poulton, R. (2007) Childhood maltreatment predicts adult inflammation in a life-course study. *Proceedings of the National Academy of Sciences USA* 104, 1319–1324.

Danner, M., Kasl, S.V., Abramson, J.L. and Vaccarino, V. (2003) Association between depression and elevated C-reactive protein. *Psychosomatic Medicine* 65, 347–356.

Dantzer, R., O'Connor, J.C., Freund, G.G., Johnson, R.W. and Kelley, K.W. (2008) From inflammation to sickness and depression: when the immune system subjugates the brain. *Nature Reviews Neuroscience* 9, 46–56.

De Bellis, M.D., Geracioti, T.D., Altemus, M. and Kling, M.A. (1993) Cerebrospinal fluid monoamine metabolites in fluoxetine-treated patients with major depression and in healthy volunteers. *Biological Psychiatry* 33, 636–641.

De Vriese, S.R., Christophe, A.B. and Maes, M. (2003) Lowered serum n-3 polyunsaturated fatty acid (PUFA) levels predict the occurrence of postpartum depression: further evidence that lowered n-PUFAs are related to major depression. *Life Sciences* 73, 3181–3187.

Dean, B., Tawadros, N., Scarr, E. and Gibbons, A.S. (2010) Regionally-specific changes in levels of tumour necrosis factor in the dorsolateral prefrontal cortex obtained postmortem from subjects with major depressive disorder. *Journal of Affective Disorders* 120, 245–248.

Delarue, J., Matzinger, O., Binnert, C., Schneiter, P., Chioléro, R., *et al.* (2003) Fish oil prevents the adrenal activation elicited by mental stress in healthy men. *Diabetes & Metabolism* 29, 289–295.

Delion, S., Chalon, S., Guilloteau, D., Besnard, J.C. and Durand, G. (1996) alpha-Linolenic acid dietary deficiency alters age-related changes of dopaminergic and serotoninergic neurotransmission in the rat frontal cortex. *Journal of Neurochemisty* 66, 1582–1591.

DeMar, J.C., Ma, K., Bell, J.M., Igarashi, M., Greenstein, D., *et al.* (2006) One generation of n-3 polyunsaturated fatty acid deprivation increases depression and aggression test scores in rats. *Journal of Lipid Research* 47, 172–180.

Dickerson, F., Stallings, C., Origoni, A., Boronow, J. and Yolken, R. (2007) Elevated serum levels of C-reactive protein are associated with mania symptoms in outpatients with bipolar disorder. *Progress in Neuropsychopharmacology and Biological Psychiatry* 31, 952–955.

Dikeos, D.G., Papadimitriou, G.N., Souery, D., Del-Favero, J., Massat, I., *et al.* (2006) Lack of genetic association between the phospholipase A2 gene and bipolar mood disorder in a European multicentre case-control study. *Psychiatric Genetics* 16, 169–171.

Dowlati, Y., Herrmann, N., Swardfager, W., Liu, H., Sham, L., *et al.* (2010) A meta-analysis of cytokines in major depression. *Biological Psychiatry* 67, 446–457.

Drzyzga, L., Obuchowicz, E., Marcinowska, A. and Herman, Z.S. (2006) Cytokines in schizophrenia and the effects of antipsychotic drugs. *Brain, Behavior, and Immunity* 20, 532–545.

Edwards, R., Peet, M., Shay, J. and Horrobin, D. (1998) Omega-3 polyunsaturated fatty acid levels in the diet and in red blood cell membranes of depressed patients. *Journal of Affective Disorders* 48, 149–155.

Ehringer, M.A., Rhee, S.H., Young, S., Corley, R. and Hewitt, J.K. (2006) Genetic and environmental contributions to common psychopathologies of childhood and adolescence: a study of twins and their siblings. *Journal of Abnormal Child Psychology* 34, 1–17.

Endres, S., Ghorbani, R., Kelley, V.E., Georgilis, K., Lonnemann, G., *et al.* (1989) The effect of dietary supplementation with n-3 polyunsaturated fatty acids on the synthesis of interleukin-1 and tumor necrosis factor by mononuclear cells. *New England Journal of Medicine* 320, 265–271.

Extier, A., Langelier, B., Perruchot, M.H., Guesnet, P., Van Veldhoven, P.P., *et al.* (2010) Gender affects liver desaturase expression in a rat model of n-3 fatty acid repletion. *Journal of Nutritional Biochemistry* 21, 180–187.

Fallin, M.D., Lasseter, V.K., Wolyniec, P.S., McGrath, J.A., Nestadt, G., *et al.* (2004) Genomewide linkage scan for bipolar-disorder susceptibility loci among Ashkenazi Jewish families. *American Journal of Human Genetics* 75, 204–219.

Farzaneh-Far, R., Harris, W.S., Garg, S., Na, B. and Whooley, M.A. (2009) Inverse association of erythrocyte n-3 fatty acid levels with inflammatory biomarkers in patients with stable coronary artery disease: The Heart and Soul Study. *Atherosclerosis* 205, 538–543.

Fekete, K., Marosvölgyi, T., Jakobik, V. and Decsi, T. (2009) Methods of assessment of n-3 long-chain polyunsaturated fatty acid status in humans: a systematic review. *American Journal of Clinical Nutrition* 89, 2070S–2084S.

Felger, J.C., Alagbe, O., Hu, F., Mook, D., Freeman, A.A., *et al.* (2007) Effects of interferon-alpha on rhesus monkeys: a nonhuman primate model of cytokine-induced depression. *Biological Psychiatry* 62, 1324–1333.

Ferrucci, L., Cherubini, A., Bandinelli, S., Bartali, B., Corsi, A., *et al.* (2006) Relationship of plasma polyunsaturated fatty acids to circulating inflammatory markers. *Journal of Clinical Endocrinology and Metabolism* 91, 439–446.

Ford, D.E. and Erlinger, T.P. (2004) Depression and C-reactive protein in US adults: data from the Third National Health and Nutrition Examination Survey. *Archive of Internal Medicine* 164, 1010–1014.

Francois, C.A., Connor, S.L., Bolewicz, L.C. and Connor, W.E. (2003) Supplementing lactating women with flaxseed oil does not increase docosahexaenoic acid in their milk. *American Journal of Clinical Nutrition* 77, 226–233.

Frangou, S., Lewis, M., Wollard, J. and Simmons, A. (2007) Preliminary in vivo evidence of increased N-acetyl-aspartate following eicosapentanoic acid treatment in patients with bipolar disorder. *Journal of Psychopharmacology* 21, 435–439.

Frasure-Smith, N., Lespérance, F. and Julien, P. (2004) Major depression is associated with lower omega-3 fatty acid levels in patients with recent acute coronary syndromes. *Biological Psychiatry* 55, 891–896.

Freeman, M.P., Hibbeln, J.R., Wisner, K.L., Davis, J.M., Mischoulon, D., *et al.* (2006) Omega-3 fatty acids: evidence basis for treatment and future research in psychiatry. *Journal of Clinical Psychiatry* 67, 1954–1967.

Garcia, M.C. and Kim, H.Y. (1997) Mobilization of arachidonate and docosahexaenoate by stimulation of the 5-HT2A receptor in rat C6 glioma cells. *Brain Research* 768, 43–48.

Giltay, E.J., Gooren, L.J., Toorians, A.W., Katan, M.B. and Zock, P.L. (2004) Docosahexaenoic acid concentrations are higher in women than in men because of estrogenic effects. *American Journal of Clinical Nutrition* 80, 1167–1174.

Glaser, R., Robles, T.F., Sheridan, J., Malarkey, W.B. and Kiecolt-Glaser, J.K. (2003) Mild depressive symptoms are associated with amplified and prolonged inflammatory responses after influenza virus vaccination in older adults. *Archives of General Psychiatry* 60, 1009–1014.

Goldstein, B.I., Kemp, D.E., Soczynska, J.K. and McIntyre, R.S. (2009) Inflammation and the phenomenology, pathophysiology, comorbidity, and treatment of bipolar disorder: a systematic review of the literature. *Journal of Clinical Psychiatry* 70, 1078–1090.

Green, P., Gispan-Herman, I. and Yadid, G. (2005) Increased arachidonic acid concentration in the brain of Flinders Sensitive Line rats, an animal model of depression. *Journal of Lipid Research* 46, 1093–1096.

Grenyer, B.F., Crowe, T., Meyer, B., Owen, A.J., Grigonis-Deane, E.M., *et al.* (2007) Fish oil supplementation in the treatment of major depression: a randomised double-blind placebo-controlled trial. *Progress in Neuropsychopharmacology and Biological Psychiatry* 31, 1393–1396.

Groeger, A.L., Cipollina, C., Cole, M.P., Woodcock, S.R., Bonacci, G., *et al.* (2010) Cyclooxygenase-2 generates anti-inflammatory mediators from omega-3 fatty acids. *Nature Chemical Biology* 6, 433–441.

Hallberg, L., Janelidze, S., Engstrom, G., Wisén, A.G., Westrin, A., *et al.* (2010) Exercise-induced release of cytokines in patients with major depressive disorder. *Journal of Affective Disorders* 126, 262–267.

Hamazaki, K., Choi, K.H. and Kim, H.Y. (2010) Phospholipid profile in the postmortem hippocampus of patients with schizophrenia and bipolar disorder: no changes in docosahexaenoic acid species. *Journal of Psychiatry Research* 44, 688–693.

Hao, W., Wong, O.Y., Liu, X., Lee, P., Chen, Y., *et al.* (2010) ω-3 fatty acids suppress inflammatory cytokine production by macrophages and hepatocytes. *Journal of Pediatric Surgery* 45, 2412–2418.

Harris, W.S. (2008) The omega-3 index as a risk factor for coronary heart disease. *American Journal of Clinical Nutrition* 87, 1997S–2002S.

Harris, W.S., Sands, S.A., Windsor, S.L., Ali, H.A., Stevens, T.L., *et al.* (2004) Omega-3 fatty acids in cardiac biopsies from heart transplantation patients: correlation with erythrocytes and response to supplementation. *Circulation* 110, 1645–1649.

Hauss-Wegrzyniak, B., Galons, J.P. and Wenk, G.L. (2000) Quantitative volumetric analyses of brain magnetic resonance imaging from rat with chronic neuroinflammation. *Experimental Neurology* 165, 347–354.

Hibbeln, J.R. (1998) Fish consumption and major depression. *Lancet* 351, 1213.

Hibbeln, J.R. (2002) Seafood consumption, the DHA content of mothers' milk and prevalence rates of postpartum depression: a cross-national, ecological analysis. *Journal of Affective Disorders* 69, 15–29.

Hibbeln, J.R. and Salem, N. (1995) Dietary polyunsaturated fatty acids and depression: when cholesterol does not satisfy. *American Journal of Clinical Nutrition* 62, 1–9.

Hibbeln, J.R., Linnoila, M., Umhau, J.C., Rawlings, R., George, D.T. *et al.* (1998) Essential fatty acids predict metabolites of serotonin and dopamine in cerebrospinal fluid among healthy control subjects, and early- and late-onset alcoholics. *Biological Psychiatry* 44, 235–242.

Hibbeln, J.R., Bissette, G., Umhau, J.C. and George, D.T. (2004) Omega-3 status and cerebrospinal fluid corticotrophin releasing hormone in perpetrators of domestic violence. *Biological Psychiatry* 56, 895–897.

Hirashima, F., Parow, A.M., Stoll, A.L., Demopulos, C.M., Damico, K.E., *et al.* (2004) Omega-3 fatty acid treatment and T(2) whole brain relaxation times in bipolar disorder. *American Journal of Psychiatry* 161, 1922–1924.

Hirschfield, G.M. and Pepys, M.B. (2003) C-reactive protein and cardiovascular disease: new insights from an old molecule. *Quarterly Journal of Medicine* 96, 793–807.

Hiscock, N., Chan, M.H., Bisucci, T., Darby, I.A. and Febbraio, M.A. (2004) Skeletal myocytes are a source of interleukin-6 mRNA expression and protein release during contraction: evidence of fiber type specificity. *Federation of American Societies for Experimental Biology* 18, 992–994.

Hodson, L., Skeaff, C.M. and Fielding, B.A. (2008) Fatty acid composition of adipose tissue and blood in humans and its use as a biomarker of dietary intake. *Progress in Lipid Research* 47, 348–380.

Huang, S.Y., Yang, H.T., Chiu, C.C., Pariante, C.M. and Su, K.P. (2008) Omega-3 fatty acids on the forced-swimming test. *Journal of Psychiatric Research* 42, 58–63.

Huang, T.L. and Lin, F.C. (2007) High-sensitivity C-reactive protein levels in patients with major depressive disorder and bipolar mania. *Progress in Neuropsychopharmacology and Biological Psychiatry* 31, 370–372.

Igarashi, M., Ma, K., Chang, L., Bell, J.M. and Rapoport, S.I. (2007) Dietary n-3 PUFA deprivation for 15 weeks upregulates elongase and desaturase expression in rat liver but not brain. *Journal of Lipid Research* 48, 2463–2470.

Igarashi, M., Ma, K., Gao, F., Kim, H.W., Greenstein, D., *et al.* (2010) Brain lipid concentrations in bipolar disorder. *Journal of Psychiatric Research,* 44, 177–182.

Jazayeri, S., Keshavarz, S.A., Tehrani-Doost, M., Djalali, M., Hosseini, M., *et al.* (2010) Effects of eicosapentaenoic acid and fluoxetine on plasma cortisol, serum interleukin-1beta and interleukin-6 concentrations in patients with major depressive disorder. *Psychiatry Resaerch* 178, 112–115.

Katan, M.B., Deslypere, J.P., van Birgelen, A.P., Penders, M. and Zegwaard, M. (1997) Kinetics of the incorporation of dietary fatty acids into serum cholesteryl esters, erythrocyte membranes, and adipose tissue: an 18-month controlled study. *Journal of Lipid Research* 38, 2012–2022.

Kato, T., Monji, A., Hashioka, S. and Kanba, S. (2007) Risperidone significantly inhibits interferon-gamma-induced microglial activation in vitro. *Schizophrenia Research* 92, 108–115.

Kempton, M.J., Geddes, J.R., Ettinger, U., Williams, S.C. and Grasby, P.M. (2008) Meta-analysis, database, and meta-regression of 98 structural imaging studies in bipolar disorder. *Archives of General Psychiatry* 65, 1017–1032.

Kenis, G. and Maes, M. (2002) Effects of antidepressants on the production of cytokines. *International Journal of Neuropsychopharmacology* 5, 401–412.

Kessler, R.C., Merikangas, K.R. and Wang, P.S. (2007) Prevalence, comorbidity, and service utilization for mood disorders in the United States at the beginning of the twenty-first century. *Annual Review in Clinical Psychology* 3, 137–158.

Khalfoun, B., Thibault, F., Watier, H., Bardos, P. and Lebranchu, Y. (1997) Docosahexaenoic and eisosapentaenoic acids inhibit in vitro human endothelial cell production of interleukin-6. In: Honn, K.V., Nigam,

S., Marnett, L.J. (eds) *Eicosanoids and Other Bioactive Lipids in Cancer, Inflammation, and Radiation Injury 2.* Plenum, New York.

Kiecolt-Glaser, J.K., Belury, M.A., Porter, K., Beversdorf, D.Q., Lemeshow, S., *et al.* (2007) Depressive symptoms, omega-6:omega-3 fatty acids, and inflammation in older adults. *Psychosomatic Medicine* 69, 217–224.

Kim, H.W., Rapoport, S.I. and Rao, J.S. (2011) Altered arachidonic acid cascade enzymes in postmortem brain from bipolar disorder patients. *Molecular Psychiatry* 16, 419–428.

Kim, Y.K., Jung, H.G., Myint, A.M., Kim, H. and Park, S.H. (2007) Imbalance between pro-inflammatory and anti-inflammatory cytokines in bipolar disorder. *Journal of Affective Disorders* 104, 91–95.

Kling, M.A., Alesci, S., Csako, G., Costello, R., Luckenbaugh, D.A., *et al.* (2007) Sustained low-grade pro-inflammatory state in unmedicated, remitted women with major depressive disorder as evidenced by elevated serum levels of the acute phase proteins C-reactive protein and serum amyloid A. *Biological Psychiatry* 62, 309–313.

Knijff, E.M., Breunis, M.N., Kupka, R.W., de Wit, H.J., Ruwhof, C., *et al.* (2007) An imbalance in the production of IL-1beta and IL-6 by monocytes of bipolar patients: restoration by lithium treatment. *Bipolar Disorders* 9, 743–753.

Kodas, E., Galineau, L., Bodard, S., Vancassel, S., Guilloteau, D., *et al.* (2004) Serotoninergic neurotransmission is affected by n-3 polyunsaturated fatty acids in the rat. *Journal of Neurochemistry* 89, 695–702.

Komatsu, W., Ishihara, K., Murata, M., Saito, H. and Shinohara, K. (2003) Docosahexaenoic acid suppresses nitric oxide production and inducible nitric oxide synthase expression in interferon-gamma plus lipopolysaccharide-stimulated murine macrophages by inhibiting the oxidative stress. *Free Radical Biology & Medicine* 34, 1006–1016.

Kop, W.J., Gottdiener, J.S., Tangen, C.M., Fried, L.P., McBurnie, M.A., *et al.* (2002) Inflammation and coagulation factors in persons > 65 years of age with symptoms of depression but without evidence of myocardial ischemia. *American Journal of Cardiology* 89, 419–424.

Kozak, W., Soszynski, D., Rudolph, K., Conn, C.A. and Kluger, M.J. (1997) Dietary n-3 fatty acids differentially affect sickness behavior in mice during local and systemic inflammation. *American Journal of Physiology* 272, 1298–1307.

Kritz-Silverstein, D., Barrett-Connor, E. and Corbeau, C. (2001) Cross-sectional and prospective study of exercise and depressed mood in the elderly: the Rancho Bernardo study. *American Journal of Epidemiology* 153, 596–603.

Kuratko, C.N. and Salem, N. (2009) Biomarkers of DHA status. *Prostaglandins, Leukotrienes, and Essential Fatty Acids* 81, 111–118.

Lalovic, A., Levy, E., Canetti, L., Sequeira, A., Montoudis, A., *et al.* (2007) Fatty acid composition in postmortem brains of people who completed suicide. *Journal of Psychiatry and Neuroscience* 32, 363–370.

Lalovic, A., Klempan, T., Sequeira, A., Luheshi, G. and Turecki, G. (2010) Altered expression of lipid metabolism and immune response genes in the frontal cortex of suicide completers. *Journal of Affective Disorders* 120, 24–31.

Lanquillon, S., Krieg, J.C., Bening-Abu-Shach, U. and Vedder, H. (2000) Cytokine production and treatment response in major depressive disorder. *Neuropsychopharmacology* 22, 370–379.

Lattka, E., Eggers, S., Moeller, G., Heim, K., Weber, M., *et al.* (2010) A common FADS2 promoter polymorphism increases promoter activity and facilitates binding of transcription factor ELK1. *Journal of Lipid Research* 51, 182–191.

Lawlor, D.A. and Hopker, S.W. (2001) The effectiveness of exercise as an intervention in the management of depression: systematic review and meta-regression analysis of randomised controlled trials. *British Medical Journal* 322, 763–767.

Leaf, D.A., Connor, W.E., Barstad, L. and Sexton, G. (1995) Incorporation of dietary n-3 fatty acids into the fatty acids of human adipose tissue and plasma lipid classes. *American Journal of Clinical Nutrition* 62, 68–73.

Lee, H.J., Rao, J.S., Ertley, R.N., Chang, L., Rapoport, S.I., *et al.* (2007) Chronic fluoxetine increases cytosolic phospholipase A(2) activity and arachidonic acid turnover in brain phospholipids of the unanesthetized rat. *Psychopharmacology* 190, 103–115.

Lee, H.J., Rao, J.S., Chang, L., Rapoport, S.I. and Kim, H.W. (2010) Chronic imipramine but not bupropion increases arachidonic acid signaling in rat brain: is this related to ‘switching’ in bipolar disorder? *Molecular Psychiatry* 15, 602–614.

Levine, J., Barak, Y., Chengappa, K.N., Rapoport, A., Rebey, M. *et al.* (1999) Cerebrospinal cytokine levels in patients with acute depression. *Neuropsychobiology* 40, 171–176.

Li, S.P. and Goldmann, N.D. (1996) Regulation of human C-reactive protein gene expression by two synergistic IL-6 responsive elements. *Biochemistry* 35, 9060–9068

Li, S.P., Liu, T.Y. and Goldman, N.D. (1990) cis-acting elements responsible for interleukin-6 inducible C-reactive protein gene expression. *Journal of Biological Chemistry* 265, 4136–4142.

Lieb, J., Karmali, R. and Horrobin, D. (1983) Elevated levels of prostaglandin E2 and thromboxane B2 in depression. *Prostaglandins, Leukotrienes and Medicine* 10, 361–367.

Lin, P.Y. and Su, K.P. (2007) A meta-analytic review of double-blind, placebo-controlled trials of antidepressant efficacy of omega-3 fatty acids. *Journal of Clinical Psychiatry* 68, 1056–1061.

Lin, P.Y., Huang, S.Y. and Su, K.P. (2010) A meta-analytic review of polyunsaturated fatty acid compositions in patients with depression. *Biological Psychiatry* 68, 140–147.

Lindqvist, D., Janelidze, S., Hagell, P., Erhardt, S., Samuelsson, M., *et al.* (2009) Interleukin-6 is elevated in the cerebrospinal fluid of suicide attempters and related to symptom severity. *Biological Psychiatry* 66, 287–292.

Lira, F.S., Koyama, C.H., Yamashita, A.S., Rosa, J.C., Zanchi, N.E., *et al.* (2009) Chronic exercise decreases cytokine production in healthy rat skeletal muscle. *Cell Biochemistry and Function* 27, 458–461.

Liu, Y. and McNamara, R.K. (2011) Elevated delta-6 desaturase (*FADS2*) gene expression in the prefrontal cortex of patients with bipolar disorder. *Journal of Psychiatry Research* 45, 269–272.

Liukkonen, T., Silvennoinen-Kassinen, S., Jokelainen, J., Räsänen, P., Leinonen, M., *et al.* (2006) The association between C-reactive protein levels and depression: Results from the northern Finland 1966 birth cohort study. *Biological Psychiatry* 60, 825–830.

Lopez-Garcia, E., Schulze, M.B., Manson, J.E., Meigs, J.B., Albert, C.M., *et al.* (2004) Consumption of (n-3) fatty acids is related to plasma biomarkers of inflammation and endothelial activation in women. *Journal of Nutrition* 134, 1806–1811.

Lu, D.Y., Tsao, Y.Y., Leung, Y.M. and Su, K.P. (2010) Docosahexaenoic acid suppresses neuroinflammatory responses and induces heme oxygenase-1 expression in BV-2 microglia: implications of antidepressant effects for omega-3 fatty acids. *Neuropsychopharmacology* 35, 2238–2248.

Lundmark, J., Wålinder, J., Alling, C., Manniche, P.M. and Dalgaard, L. (1994) The effect of paroxetine on cerebrospinal fluid concentrations of neurotransmitter metabolites in depressed patients. *European Neuropsychopharmacology* 4, 1–6.

Maes, M., Bosmans, E., Calabrese, J., Smith, R. and Meltzer, H.Y. (1995a) Interleukin-2 and interleukin-6 in schizophrenia and mania: effects of neuroleptics and mood stabilizers. *Journal of Psychiatry Research* 29, 141–152.

Maes, M., Meltzer, H.Y., Bosmans, E., Bergmans, R., Vandoolaeghe, E., *et al.* (1995b) Increased plasma concentrations of interleukin-6, soluble interleukin-6, soluble interleukin-2 and transferrin receptor in major depression. *Journal of Affective Disorders* 34, 301–309.

Maes, M., Smith, R., Christophe, A., Cosyns, P., Desnyder, R., *et al.* (1996) Fatty acid composition in major depression: decreased omega 3 fractions in cholesteryl esters and increased C20:4 omega 6/C20:5 omega 3 ratio in cholesteryl esters and phospholipids. *Journal of Affective Disorders* 38, 35–46.

Maes, M., Bosmans, E., De Jongh, R., Kenis, G., Vandoolaeghe, E. *et al.* (1997) Increased serum IL-6 and IL-1 receptor antagonist concentrations in major depression and treatment resistant depression. *Cytokine* 9, 853–858.

Maes, M., Christophe, A., Delanghe, J., Altamura, C., Neels, H., *et al.* (1999) Lowered omega3 polyunsaturated fatty acids in serum phospholipids and cholesteryl esters of depressed patients. *Psychiatry Research,* 85, 275–291.

Maes, M., De Vos, N., Pioli, R., Demedts, P., Wauters, A., *et al.* (2000) Lower serum vitamin E concentrations in major depression. Another marker of lowered antioxidant defenses in that illness. *Journal of Affective Disorders* 58, 241–246.

Maida, M.E., Hurley, S.D., Daeschner, J.A., Moore, A.H. and O'Banion, M.K. (2006) Cytosolic prostaglandin E2 synthase (cPGES) expression is decreased in discrete cortical regions in psychiatric disease. *Brain Research* 1103, 164–172.

Marangell, L.B., Martinez, J.M., Zboyan, H.A., Kertz, B., Kim, H.F., *et al.* (2003) A double-blind, placebo-controlled study of the omega-3 fatty acid docosahexaenoic acid in the treatment of major depression. *American Journal of Psychiatry* 160, 996–998.

Martinelli, N., Girelli, D., Malerba, G., Guarini, P., Illig, T., *et al.* (2008) FADS genotypes and desaturase activity estimated by the ratio of arachidonic acid to linoleic acid are associated with inflammation and coronary artery disease. *American Journal of Clinical Nutrition* 88, 941–949.

Martinez, M. (1992) Abnormal profiles of polyunsaturated fatty acids in the brain, liver, kidney and retina of patients with peroxisomal disorders. *Brain Research* 583, 171–182.

Mathur, N. and Pedersen, B.K. (2008) Exercise as a mean to control low-grade systemic inflammation. *Mediators of Inflammation* doi:10.1155/2008/109502.

McDade, T.W., Hawkley, L.C. and Cacioppo, J.T. (2006) Psychosocial and behavioral predictors of inflammation in middle-aged and older adults: the Chicago health, aging, and social relations study. *Psychosomatic Medicine* 68, 376–381.

McNamara, R.K. (2009a) Evaluation of docosahexaenoic acid deficiency as a preventable risk factor for recurrent affective disorders: Current status, future directions, and dietary recommendations. *Prostoglandins, Leukotrienes, and Essential Fatty Acids* 81, 223–231.

McNamara, R.K. (2009b) Membrane omega-3 fatty acid deficiency as a preventable risk factor for comorbid coronary heart disease in major depressive disorder. *Cardiovascular Psychiatry and Neurology* 9, 1–13.

McNamara, R.K. and Jandacek, R. (2011) Investigation of postmortem brain polyunsaturated fatty acid composition in psychiatric disorders: Limitations, challenges, and future directions. *Journal of Psychiatry Research* 45, 44–46.

McNamara, R.K. and Liu, Y. (2011) Reduced fatty acid biosynthesis gene expression in the prefrontal cortex of patients with major depressive disorder. *Journal of Affective Disorders* 129, 359–363.

McNamara, R.K., Hahn, C.-G., Jandacek, R., Rider, T., Tso, P., *et al.* (2007) Selective deficits in the omega-3 fatty acid docosahexaenoic acid in the postmortem orbitofrontal cortex of patients with major depressive disorder. *Biological Psychiatry* 62, 17–24.

McNamara, R.K., Liu, Y., Jandacek, R., Rider, T. and Tso, P. (2008a) The aging human orbitofrontal cortex: Decreasing polyunsaturated fatty acid composition and associated increases in lipogenic gene expression and stearoyl-CoA desaturase activity. *Prostoglandins, Leukotrienes, and Essential Fatty Acids* 78, 293–304.

McNamara, R.K., Jandacek, R., Rider, T., Tso, P., Stanford, K., *et al.* (2008b) Deficits in docosahexaenoic acid and associated elevations in the metabolism of arachidonic acid and saturated fatty acids in the postmortem orbitofrontal cortex of patients with bipolar disorder. *Psychiatric Research* 160, 285–299.

McNamara, R.K., Able, J.A., Liu, Y., Jandacek, R., Rider, T. *et al.* (2009a) Gender differences in rat erythrocyte and brain docosahexaenoic acid composition: Role of ovarian hormones and dietary omega-3 fatty acid composition. *Psychoneuroendocrinology* 34, 532–539.

McNamara, R.K., Able, J.A., Jandacek, R., Rider, T. and Tso, P. (2009b) Chronic risperidone treatment preferentially increases rat erythrocyte and prefrontal cortex omega-3 fatty acid composition: Evidence for augmented biosynthesis. *Schizophrenia Research* 107, 150–157.

McNamara, R.K., Able, J., Liu, Y., Jandacek, R., Rider, T., *et al.* (2009c) Omega-3 fatty acid deficiency during perinatal development increases serotonin turnover in the prefrontal cortex and decreases midbrain tryptophan hydroxylase-2 expression in adult female rats: dissociation from estrogenic effects. *Journal of Psychiatry Research* 43, 656–663.

McNamara, R.K., Able, J.A., Jandacek, R., Rider, T., Tso, P., *et al.* (2010a) Docosahexaenoic acid supplementation increases prefrontal cortex activation during sustained attention in healthy boys: A placebo-controlled, dose-ranging, functional magnetic resonance imaging study. *American Journal of Clinical Nutrition* 91, 1060–1067.

McNamara, R.K., Jandacek, R., Rider, T., Tso, P., Dwivedi, Y., *et al.* (2010b) Selective deficits in erythrocyte docosahexaenoic acid composition in adult patients with bipolar disorder and major depressive disorder. *Journal of Affective Disorders* 126, 303–311.

McNamara, R.K., Jandacek, R., Rider, T., Tso, P., Cole-Strauss, A., *et al.* (2010c) Omega-3 fatty acid deficiency increases constitutive pro-inflammatory cytokine production in rats: relationship with central serotonin turnover. *Prostaglandins, Leukotrienes, and Essential Fatty Acids* 83, 185–191.

McNamara, R.K., Able, J.A., Rider, T., Tso, P. and Jandacek, R. (2010d) Effect of chronic fluoxetine treatment on male and female rat erythrocyte and prefrontal cortex fatty acid composition. *Progress in Neuropsychopharmacology and Biological Psychiatry* 34, 1317–1321.

McNamara, R.K., Nandagopal, J.J., Strakowski, S.M., DelBello, M.P. (2010e) Preventative strategies for early-onset bipolar disorder: Towards a clinical staging model. *CNS Drugs* 24, 983–996.

McNamara, R.K., Rider, T., Jandacek, R., Tso, P., Cole-Strauss, A., *et al.* (2011a) Differential effects of antipsychotic medications on polyunsaturated fatty acid biosynthesis in rats: Relationship with liver delta6-desaturase expression. *Schizophrenia Research* 129, 57–65.

McNamara, R.K., Jandacek, R., Rider, T. and Tso, P. (2011b) Chronic risperidone normalizes elevated pro-inflammatory cytokine and C-reactive protein production in omega-3 fatty acid deficient rats. *European Journal of Pharmacology* 652, 152–156.

Mead, G.E., Morley, W., Campbell, P., Greig, C.A., McMurdo, M., *et al.* (2009) Exercise for depression. *Cochrane Database of Systematic Reviews* 3, CD004366.

Meira-Lima, I., Jardim, D., Junqueira, R., Ikenaga, E. and Vallada, H. (2003) Allelic association study between phospholipase A2 genes and bipolar affective disorder. *Bipolar Disorders* 5, 295–299.

Mendlewicz, J., Kriwin, P., Oswald, P., Souery, D., Alboni, S., *et al.* (2006) Shortened onset of action of antidepressants in major depression using acetylsalicylic acid augmentation: a pilot open-label study. *International Journal of Clinical Psychopharmacology* 21, 227–231.

Merikangas, K.R., Chakravarti, A., Moldin, S.O., Araj, H., Blangero, J.C., *et al.* (2002) Future of genetics of mood disorders research. *Biological Psychiatry* 52, 457–477.

Meydani, S.N., Endres, S., Woods, M.M., Goldin, B.R., Soo, C., *et al.* (1991) Oral (n-3) fatty acid supplementation suppresses cytokine production and lymphocyte proliferation: comparison between young and older women. *Journal of Nutrition* 121, 547–555.

Micallef, M.A., Munro, I.A. and Garg, M.L. (2009) An inverse relationship between plasma n-3 fatty acids and C-reactive protein in healthy individuals. *European Journal of Clinical Nutrition* 63, 1154–1156.

Michaeli, B., Berger, M.M., Revelly, J.P., Tappy, L. and Chioléro, R. (2007) Effects of fish oil on the neuroendocrine responses to an endotoxin challenge in healthy volunteers. *Clinical Nutrition* 26, 70–77.

Miller, G.E., Rohleder, N. and Cole, S.W. (2009) Chronic interpersonal stress predicts activation of pro- and anti-inflammatory signaling pathways 6 months later. *Psychosomatic Medicine* 71, 57–62.

Mingam, R., Moranis, A., Bluthé, R.M., De Smedt-Peyrusse, V., Kelley, K.W., *et al.* (2008) Uncoupling of interleukin-6 from its signalling pathway by dietary n-3-polyunsaturated fatty acid deprivation alters sickness behaviour in mice. *European Journal of Neuroscience* 28, 1877–1886.

Mischoulon, D., Best-Popescu, C., Laposata, M., Merens, W., Murakami, J.L., *et al.* (2008) A double-blind dose-finding pilot study of docosahexaenoic acid (DHA) for major depressive disorder. *European Neuropsychopharmacology* 18, 639–645.

Moriguchi, T., Loewke, J., Garrison, M., Catalan, J.N. and Salem, N. (2001) Reversal of docosahexaenoic acid deficiency in the rat brain, retina, liver, and serum. *Journal of Lipid Research* 42, 419–427.

Motl, R.W., Birnbaum, A.S., Kubik, M.Y. and Dishman, R.K. (2004) Naturally occurring changes in physical activity are inversely related to depressive symptoms during early adolescence. *Psychosomatic Medicine* 66, 336–342.

Mozaffarian, D. and Rimm, E.B. (2006) Fish intake, contaminants, and human health: evaluating the risks and the benefits. *Journal of the American Medical Association* 296, 1885–1899.

Müller, N., Schwarz, M.J., Dehning, S., Douhe, A., Cerovecki, A., *et al.* (2006) The cyclooxygenase-2 inhibitor celecoxib has therapeutic effects in major depression: results of a double-blind, randomized, placebo controlled, add-on pilot study to reboxetine. *Molecular Psychiatry* 11, 680–684.

Murray, C.J. and Lopez, A.D. (1997) Global mortality, disability, and the contribution of risk factors: Global Burden of Disease Study. *Lancet* 349, 1436–1442.

Musselman, D.L., Lawson, D.H., Gumnick, J.F., Manatunga, A.K., Penna, S., *et al.* (2001) Paroxetine for the prevention of depression induced by high-dose interferon alfa. *New England Journal of Medicine* 344, 961–966.

Nielsen, A.R. and Pedersen, B.K. (2007) The biological roles of exercise-induced cytokines: IL-6, IL-8, and IL-15. *Applied Physiology, Nutrition, and Metabolism* 32, 833–839.

Nilsson, C.L., Hellstrand, M., Ekman, A. and Eriksson, E. (1998) Direct dopamine D2-receptor-mediated modulation of arachidonic acid release in transfected CHO cells without the concomitant administration of a Ca2+-mobilizing agent. *British Journal of Pharmacology* 124, 1651–1658.

Nishino, S., Ueno, R., Ohishi, K., Sakai, T. and Hayaishi, O. (1989) Salivary prostaglandin concentrations: possible state indicators for major depression. *American Journal of Psychiatry* 146, 365–368.

Noaghiul, S. and Hibbeln, J.R. (2003) Cross-national comparisons of seafood consumption and rates of bipolar disorders. *American Journal of Psychiatry* 160, 2222–2227.

Noponen, M., Sanfilipo, M., Samanich, K., Ryer, H., Ko, G., *et al.* (1993) Elevated PLA2 activity in schizophrenics and other psychiatric patients. *Biological Psychiatry* 34, 641–649.

O'Brien, S.M., Scully, P., Scott, L.V. and Dinan, T.G. (2006) Cytokine profiles in bipolar affective disorder: focus on acutely ill patients. *Journal of Affective Disorders* 90, 263–267.

Obukowicz, M.G., Welsch, D.J., Salsgiver, W.J., Martin-Berger, C.L., Chinn, K.S., *et al.* (1998) Novel, selective delta6 or delta5 fatty acid desaturase inhibitors as antiinflammatory agents in mice. *Journal of Pharmacology and Experimental Therapeutics* 287, 157–166.

Ogura, T., Takada, H., Okuno, M., Kitade, H., Matsuura, T., *et al.* (2010) Fatty acid composition of plasma, erythrocytes and adipose: their correlations and effects of age and sex. *Lipids* 45, 137–144.

Oh, D.Y., Talukdar, S., Bae, E.J., Imamura, T., Morinaga, H., *et al.* (2010) GPR120 is an omega-3 fatty acid receptor mediating potent anti-inflammatory and insulin-sensitizing effects. *Cell* 142, 687–698.

Ohishi, K., Ueno, R., Nishino, S., Sakai, T. and Hayaishi, O. (1988) Increased level of salivary prostaglandins in patients with major depression. *Biological Psychiatry* 23, 326–334.

Ortiz-Domínguez, A., Hernández, M.E., Berlanga, C., Gutiérrez-Mora, D., Moreno, J., *et al.* (2007) Immune variations in bipolar disorder: phasic differences. *Bipolar Disorders* 9, 596–602.

Osby, U., Brandt, L., Correia, N., Ekbom, A. and Sparén, P. (2001) Excess mortality in bipolar and unipolar disorder in Sweden. *Archives of General Psychiatry* 58, 844–850.

Pace, T.W. and Miller, A.H. (2009) Cytokines and glucocorticoid receptor signaling. Relevance to major depression. *Annals of the New York Academy of Science* 1179, 86–105.

Pace, T.W., Mletzko, T.C., Alagbe, O., Musselman, D.L., Nemeroff, C.B., *et al.* (2006) Increased stress-induced inflammatory responses in male patients with major depression and increased early life stress. *American Journal of Psychiatry* 163, 1630–1633.

Pae, C.U., Yu, H.S., Kim, J.J., Lee, C.U., Lee, S.J., *et al.* (2004) BanI polymorphism of the cytosolic phospholipase A2 gene and mood disorders in the Korean population. *Neuropsychobiology* 49, 185–188.

Pandey, G.N., Dwivedi, Y., Rizavi, H.S., Ren, X., Pandey, S.C., *et al.* (2002) Higher expression of serotonin 5-HT(2A) receptors in the postmortem brains of teenage suicide victims. *American Journal of Psychiatry* 159, 419–429.

Papadimitriou, G.N., Dikeos, D.G., Souery, D., Del-Favero, J., Massat, I., *et al.* (2003) Genetic association between the phospholipase A2 gene and unipolar affective disorder: a multicentre case-control study. *Psychiatric Genetics* 13, 211–220.

Pariante, C.M. and Miller, A.H. (2001) Glucocorticoid receptors in major depression: relevance to pathophysiology and treatment. *Biological Psychiatry* 49, 391–404.

Parker, G.B., Gibson, N.A., Brotchie, H., Heruc, G., Rees, A.M. *et al.* (2006a) Omega-3 fatty acids and mood disorders. *American Journal of Psychiatry* 163, 969–978.

Parker, G.B., Heruc, G.A., Hilton, T.M., Olley, A., Brotchie, H., *et al.* (2006b) Low levels of docosahexaenoic acid identified in acute coronary syndrome patients with depression. *Psychiatry Research* 141, 279–286.

Pawlosky, R.J. and Salem, N. (1999) Alcohol consumption in rhesus monkeys depletes tissues of polyunsaturated fatty acids and alters essential fatty acid metabolism. *Alcoholism: Clinical and Experimental Research* 23, 311–317.

Pawlosky, R.J., Hibbeln, J., Lin, Y. and Salem, N. (2003) n-3 fatty acid metabolism in women. *British Journal of Nutrition* 90, 993–994.

Pedersen, B.K., Steensberg, A., Fischer, C., Keller, C., Ostrowski, K., *et al.* (2001) Exercise and cytokines with particular focus on muscle-derived IL-6. *Exercise Immunology Review* 7, 18–31.

Peet, M. (2004) International variations in the outcome of schizophrenia and the prevalence of depression in relation to national dietary practices: an ecological analysis. *British Journal of Psychiatry* 184, 404–408.

Peet, M., Murphy, B., Shay, J. and Horrobin, D. (1998) Depletion of omega-3 fatty acid levels in red blood cell membranes of depressive patients. *Biological Psychiatry* 43, 315–319.

Penninx, B.W., Kritchevsky, S.B., Yaffe, K., Newman, A.B., Simonsick, E.M., *et al.* (2003) Inflammatory markers and depressed mood in older persons: results from the Health, Aging and Body Composition study. *Biological Psychiatry* 54, 566–572.

Perlis, R.H., Miyahara, S., Marangell, L.B., STEP-BD Investigators (2004) Long-Term implications of early onset in bipolar disorder: data from the first 1000 participants in the systematic treatment enhancement program for bipolar disorder (STEP-BD). *Biological Psychiatry* 55, 875–881.

Petersen, A.M. and Pedersen, B.K. (2005) The anti-inflammatory effect of exercise. *Journal of Applied Physiology* 98, 1154–1162.

Pfeifer, J.C., Kowatch, R.A. and DelBello, M.P. (2010) Pharmacotherapy of bipolar disorder in children and adolescents: recent progress. *CNS Drugs* 24, 575–593.

Phillips, T., Childs, A.C., Dreon, D.M., Phinney, S. and Leeuwenburgh, C. (2003) A dietary supplement attenuates IL-6 and CRP after eccentric exercise in untrained males. *Medicine & Science in Sports & Exercise* 35, 2032–2037.

Piomelli, D., Pilon, C., Giros, B., Sokoloff, P., Martres, M.P., *et al.* (1991) Dopamine activation of the arachidonic acid cascade as a basis for D1/D2 receptor synergism. *Nature* 353, 164–167.

Pischon, T., Hankinson, S.E., Hotamisligil, G.S., Rifai, N., Willett, W.C. and Rimm, E.B. (2003) Habitual dietary intake of n-3 and n-6 fatty acids in relation to inflammatory markers among US men and women. *Circulation* 108, 155–160.

Pita, M.L. and Delgado, M.J. (2000) Folate administration increases n-3 polyunsaturated fatty acids in rat plasma and tissue lipids. *Thrombosis and Haemostasis* 84, 420–423.

Placidi, G.P., Oquendo, M.A., Malone, K.M., Huang, Y.Y., Ellis, S.P., *et al.* (2001) Aggressivity, suicide attempts, and depression: relationship to cerebrospinal fluid monoamine metabolite levels. *Biological Psychiatry* 50, 783–791.

Ploeger, H.E., Takken, T., de Greef, M.H. and Timmons, B.W. (2009) The effects of acute and chronic exercise on inflammatory markers in children and adults with a chronic inflammatory disease: a systematic review. *Exercise Immunology Review* 15, 6–41.

Portanova, J.P., Zhang, Y., Anderson, G.D., Hauser, S.D., Masferrer, J.L., *et al.* (1996) Selective neutralization of prostaglandin E2 blocks inflammation, hyperalgesia, and interleukin 6 production in vivo. *Journal of Experimental Medicine* 18, 4883–4891.

Post, R.M. and Leverich, G.S. (2006) The role of psychosocial stress in the onset and progression of bipolar disorder and its comorbidities: the need for earlier and alternative modes of therapeutic intervention. *Development and Psychopathology* 18, 1181–1211.

Potter, W.Z., Scheinin, M., Golden, R.N., Rudorfer, M.V., Cowdry, R.W., *et al.* (1985) Selective antidepressants and cerebrospinal fluid. Lack of specificity on norepinephrine and serotonin metabolites. *Archives of General Psychiatry* 42, 1171–1177.

Prather, A.A., Rabinovitz, M., Pollock, B.G. and Lotrich, F.E. (2009) Cytokine-induced depression during IFN-alpha treatment: the role of IL-6 and sleep quality. *Brain, Behavior and Immunity* 23, 1109–1116.

Qu, Y., Chang, L., Klaff, J., Balbo, A. and Rapoport, S.I. (2003) Imaging brain phospholipase A2 activation in awake rats in response to the 5-HT2A/2C agonist (+/–)2,5-dimethoxy-4-iodophenyl-2-aminopropane (DOI). *Neuropsychopharmacology* 28, 244–252.

Raison, C.L., Capuron, L. and Miller, A.H. (2006) Cytokines sing the blues: inflammation and the pathogenesis of depression. *Trends in Immunology* 27, 24–31.

Raison, C.L., Borisov, A.S., Majer, M., Drake, D.F., Pagnoni, G., *et al.* (2009) Activation of central nervous system inflammatory pathways by interferon-alpha: relationship to monoamines and depression. *Biological Psychiatry* 65, 296–303.

Ranjekar, P.K., Hinge, A., Hegde, M.V., Ghate, M., Kale, A., *et al.* (2003) Decreased antioxidant enzymes and membrane essential polyunsaturated fatty acids in schizophrenic and bipolar mood disorder patients. *Psychiatry Research,* 121, 109–122.

Rao, J.S. and Rapoport, S.I. (2009) Mood-stabilizers target the brain arachidonic acid cascade. *Current Molecular Pharmacology* 2, 207–214.

Rao, J.S., Ertley, R.N., DeMar, J.C., Rapoport, S.I., Bazinet, R.P., *et al.* (2007) Dietary n-3 PUFA deprivation alters expression of enzymes of the arachidonic and docosahexaenoic acid cascades in rat frontal cortex. *Molecular Psychiatry* 12, 151–157.

Rao, J.S., Lee, H.J., Rapoport, S.I. and Bazinet, R.P. (2008) Mode of action of mood stabilizers: is the arachidonic acid cascade a common target? *Molecular Psychiatry* 13, 585–596.

Rao, J.S., Harry, G.J., Rapoport, S.I. and Kim, H.W. (2010) Increased excitotoxicity and neuroinflammatory markers in postmortem frontal cortex from bipolar disorder patients. *Molecular Psychiatry* 15, 384–392.

Rapaport, M.H., Guylai, L. and Whybrow, P. (1999) Immune parameters in rapid cycling bipolar patients before and after lithium treatment. *Journal of Psychiatric Research* 33, 335–340.

Rapoport, S.I. (2008) Brain arachidonic and docosahexaenoic acid cascades are selectively altered by drugs, diet and disease. *Prostaglandins, Leukotrienes, and Essential Fatty Acids* 79, 153–156.

Rapoport, S.I. and Bosetti, F. (2002) Do lithium and anticonvulsants target the brain arachidonic acid cascade in bipolar disorder? *Archives of General Psychiatry* 59, 592–596.

Reichenberg, A., Yirmiya, R., Schuld, A., Kraus, T., Haack, M., *et al.* (2001) Cytokine-associated emotional and cognitive disturbances in humans. *Archives of General Psychiatry* 58, 445–452.

Richtand, N.M., Welge, J.A., Logue, A.D., Keck, P.E., Strakowski, S.M. *et al.* (2007) Dopamine and serotonin receptor binding and antipsychotic efficacy. *Neuropsychopharmacology* 32, 1715–1726.

Riemer, S., Maes, M., Christophe, A. and Rief, W. (2010) Lowered omega-3 PUFAs are related to major depression, but not to somatization syndrome. *Journal of Affective Disorders* 123, 173–180.

Rosa-Neto, P., Diksic, M., Okazawa, H., Leyton, M., Ghadirian, N., *et al.* (2004) Measurement of brain regional alpha-[11C]methyl-L-tryptophan trapping as a measure of serotonin synthesis in medication-free patients with major depression. *Archives of General Psychiatry* 61, 556–563.

Ross, B.M., Hughes, B., Kish, S.J. and Warsh, J.J. (2006) Serum calcium-independent phospholipase A2 activity in bipolar affective disorder. *Bipolar Disorders* 8, 265–270.

Sarandol, A., Sarandol, E., Eker, S.S., Erdinc, S., Vatansever, E., *et al.* (2007) Major depressive disorder is accompanied with oxidative stress: short-term antidepressant treatment does not alter oxidative-antioxidative systems. *Human Psychopharmacology* 22, 67–73.

Serhan, C.N. (2010) Novel lipid mediators and resolution mechanisms in acute inflammation: to resolve or not? *American Journal of Pathology* 177, 1576–1591.

Sheline, Y., Bardgett, M.E. and Csernansky, J.G. (1997) Correlated reductions in cerebrospinal fluid 5-HIAA and MHPG concentrations after treatment with selective serotonin reuptake inhibitors. *Journal of Clinical Psychopharmacology* 17, 11–14.

Silvers, K.M., Woolley, C.C., Hamilton, F.C., Watts, P.M. and Watson, R.A. (2005) Randomised double-blind placebo-controlled trial of fish oil in the treatment of depression. *Prostaglandins, Leukotrienes, and Essential Fatty Acids* 72, 211–218.

Simen, B.B., Duman, C.H., Simen, A.A. and Duman, R.S. (2006) TNFalpha signaling in depression and anxiety: behavioral consequences of individual receptor targeting. *Biological Psychiatry* 59, 775–785.

Skelin, I., Kovačević, T., Sato, H. and Diksic, M. (2011) Upregulated arachidonic acid signalling in the olfactory bulbectomized rat model of depression. *Neurochemistry International* 58, 483–488.

Sluzewska, A., Sobieska, M. and Rybakowski, J.K. (1997) Changes in acute-phase proteins during lithium potentiation of antidepressants in refractory depression. *Neuropsychobiology* 35, 123–127.

Söderlund, J., Olsson, S.K., Samuelsson, M., Walther-Jallow, L., Johansson, C., *et al.* (2011) Elevation of cerebrospinal fluid interleukin-1ß in bipolar disorder. *Journal of Psychiatry & Neuroscience* 36, 114–118.

Song, C., Li, X., Leonard, B.E. and Horrobin, D.F. (2003) Effects of dietary n-3 or n-6 fatty acids on interleukin-1beta-induced anxiety, stress, and inflammatory responses in rats. *Journal of Lipid Research* 44, 1984–1991.

Song, C., Phillips, A.G., Leonard, B.E. and Horrobin, D.F. (2004) Ethyl-eicosapentaenoic acid ingestion prevents corticosterone-mediated memory impairment induced by central administration of interleukin-1beta in rats. *Molecular Psychiatry* 9, 630–638.

Song, C., Manku, M.S. and Horrobin, D.F. (2008) Long-chain polyunsaturated fatty acids modulate interleukin-1beta-induced changes in behavior, monoaminergic neurotransmitters, and brain inflammation in rats. *Journal of Nutrition* 138, 954–963.

Song, C., Zhang, X.Y. and Manku, M. (2009) Increased phospholipase A2 activity and inflammatory response but decreased nerve growth factor expression in the olfactory bulbectomized rat model of depression: effects of chronic ethyl-eicosapentaenoate treatment. *Journal of Neuroscience* 29, 14–22.

Steinberg, S., Chen, L., Wei, L., Moser, A., Moser, H., *et al.* (2004) The PEX Gene Screen: molecular diagnosis of peroxisome biogenesis disorders in the Zellweger syndrome spectrum. *Molecular Genetics and Metabolism* 83, 252–263.

Strawbridge, W.J., Deleger, S., Roberts, R.E. and Kaplan, G.A. (2002) Physical activity reduces the risk of subsequent depression for older adults. *American Journal of Epidemiology* 156, 328–334.

Ströhle, A. and Holsboer, F. (2003) Stress responsive neurohormones in depression and anxiety. *Pharmacopsychiatry* 36, S207–S214.

Strokin, M., Sergeeva, M. and Reiser, G. (2007) Prostaglandin synthesis in rat brain astrocytes is under the control of the n-3 docosahexaenoic acid, released by group VIB calcium-independent phospholipase A2. *Journal of Neurochemistry* 102, 1771–1782.

Su, H.M., Bernardo, L., Mirmiran, M., Ma, X.H., Corso, T.N., Nathanielsz, P.W. and Brenna, J.T. (1999) Bioequivalence of dietary alpha-linolenic and docosahexaenoic acids as sources of docosahexaenoate accretion in brain and associated organs of neonatal baboons. *Pediatric Research* 45, 87–93.

Su, K.P., Huang, S.Y., Chiu, C.C. and Shen, W.W. (2003) Omega-3 fatty acids in major depressive disorder. A preliminary double-blind, placebo-controlled trial. *European Neuropsychopharmacology* 13, 267–271.

Su, K.P., Huang, S.Y., Peng, C.Y., Lai, H.C., Huang, C.L., *et al.* (2010) Phospholipase A2 and cyclooxygenase 2 genes influence the risk of interferon-alpha-induced depression by regulating polyunsaturated fatty acids levels. *Biological Psychiatry* 67, 550–557.

Sublette, M.E., Hibbeln, J.R., Galfalvy, H., Oquendo, M.A. and Mann, J.J. (2006) Omega-3 polyunsaturated essential fatty acid status as a predictor of future suicide risk. *American Journal of Psychiatry* 163, 1100–1102.

Sublette, M.E., Bosetti, F., DeMar, J.C., Ma, K., Bell, J.M., *et al.* (2007) Plasma free polyunsaturated fatty acid levels are associated with symptom severity in acute mania. *Bipolar Disorders* 9, 759–765.

Sublette, M.E., Milak, M.S., Hibbeln, J.R., Freed, P.J., Oquendo, M.A., *et al.* (2009) Plasma polyunsaturated fatty acids and regional cerebral glucose metabolism in major depression. *Prostaglandins, Leukotrienes, and Essential Fatty Acids* 80, 57–64.

Sugino, H., Futamura, T., Mitsumoto, Y., Maeda, K. and Marunaka, Y. (2009) Atypical antipsychotics suppress production of proinflammatory cytokines and up-regulate interleukin-10 in lipopolysaccharide-treated mice. *Progress in Neuropsychopharmacology and Biological Psychiatry* 33, 303–307.
Sullivan, P.F., Neale, M.C. and Kendler, K.S. (2000) Genetic epidemiology of major depression: review and meta-analysis. *American Journal of Psychiatry* 157, 1552–1562.
Tartibian, B., Maleki, B.H. and Abbasi, A. (2011) Omega-3 fatty acids supplementation attenuates inflammatory markers after eccentric exercise in untrained men. *Clinical Journal of Sport Medicine* 21, 131–137.
Tonelli, L.H., Stiller, J., Rujescu, D., Giegling, I., Schneider, B., *et al.* (2008) Elevated cytokine expression in the orbitofrontal cortex of victims of suicide. *Acta Psychiatrica Scandinavica* 117, 198–206.
Tsuang, M.T. and Faraone, S.V. (1990) *The Genetics of Mood Disorders*. Johns Hopkins University Press, Baltimore, Maryland.
Umhau, J.C., Dauphinais, K.M., Patel, S.H., Nahrwold, D.A., Hibbeln, J.R., *et al.* (2006) The relationship between folate and docosahexaenoic acid in men. *European Journal of Clinical Nutrition* 60, 352–357.
Unceta, N., Barrondo, S., Ruiz de Azúa, I., Gómez-Caballero, A., Goicolea, M.A., *et al.* (2007) Determination of fluoxetine, norfluoxetine and their enantiomers in rat plasma and brain samples by liquid chromatography with fluorescence detection. *Journal of Chromatography. B Analytical Technologies in the Biomedical and Life Sciences* 852, 519–528.
Vancassel, S., Leman, S., Hanonick, L., Denis, S., Roger, J., *et al.* (2008) n-3 polyunsaturated fatty acid supplementation reverses stress-induced modifications on brain monoamine levels in mice. *Journal of Lipid Research* 49, 340–348.
Vaswani, M., Linda, F.K. and Ramesh, S. (2003) Role of selective serotonin reuptake inhibitors in psychiatric disorders: a comprehensive review. *Progress in Neuropsychopharmacology and Biological Psychiatry* 27, 85–102.
Vidgren, H.M., Agren, J.J., Schwab, U., Rissanen, T., Hänninen, O., *et al.* (1997) Incorporation of n-3 fatty acids into plasma lipid fractions, and erythrocyte membranes and platelets during dietary supplementation with fish, fish oil, and docosahexaenoic acid-rich oil among healthy young men. *Lipids* 32, 697–705.
Wadee, A.A., Kuschke, R.H., Wood, L.A., Berk, M., Ichim, L., *et al.* (2002) Serological observations in patients suffering from acute manic episodes. *Human Psychopharmacology* 17, 175–179.
Walsh, N.P., Gleeson, M., Shephard, R.J., Gleeson, M., Woods, J.A., *et al.* (2011) Position statement. Part one: Immune function and exercise. *Exercise Immunology Review* 17, 6–63.
Wang, J. and Dunn, A.J. (1998) Mouse interleukin-6 stimulates the HPA axis and increases brain tryptophan and serotonin metabolism. *Neurochemistry International* 33, 143–154.
Wang, P., Zhu, F. and Konstantopoulos, K. (2010) Prostaglandin E2 induces interleukin-6 expression in human chondrocytes via cAMP/protein kinase A- and phosphatidylinositol 3-kinase-dependent NF-kappaB activation. *American Journal of Physiology - Cell Physiology* 298, 1445–1456.
Williard, D.E., Nwankwo, J.O., Kaduce, T.L., Harmon, S.D., Irons, M., *et al.* (2001) Identification of a fatty acid delta6-desaturase deficiency in human skin fibroblasts. *Journal of Lipid Research* 42, 501–508.
World Health Organization (2000) Cross-national comparisons of the prevalences and correlates of mental disorders. WHO International Consortium in Psychiatric Epidemiology. *Bulletin of the World Health Organization* 78, 413–426.
Wozniak, J., Biederman, J., Mick, E., Waxmonsky, J., Hantsoo, L., *et al.* (2007) Omega-3 fatty acid monotherapy for pediatric bipolar disorder: a prospective open-label trial. *European Neuropsychopharmacology* 17, 440–447.
Xie, L. and Innis, S.M. (2008) Genetic variants of the FADS1 FADS2 gene cluster are associated with altered (n-6) and (n-3) essential fatty acids in plasma and erythrocyte phospholipids in women during pregnancy and in breast milk during lactation. *Journal of Nutrition* 138, 2222–2228.
Yirmiya, R., Pollak, Y., Barak, O., Avitsur, R., Ovadia, H., *et al.* (2001) Effects of antidepressant drugs on the behavioral and physiological responses to lipopolysaccharide (LPS) in rodents. *Neuropsychopharmacology* 24, 531–544.
Zhang, J., Terreni, L., De Simoni, M.G. and Dunn, A.J. (2001) Peripheral interleukin-6 administration increases extracellular concentrations of serotonin and the evoked release of serotonin in the rat striatum. *Neurochemistry International* 38, 303–308.

17 Asthma and Inflammation

H.A. Scott,*[,1,2] M.L. Garg,[3] P.G. Gibson[1,2] and L.G. Wood[1,2,3]
[1]*Centre for Asthma and Respiratory Disease;* [2]*Respiratory and Sleep Medicine, John Hunter Hospital, Newcastle and* [3]*School of Biomedical Sciences & Pharmacy, University of Newcastle, Australia*

Introduction

Asthma is a respiratory disease characterized by airway inflammation, airway hyperresponsiveness and variable airflow obstruction that is often reversible (Jeukendrup *et al.*, 2000; Busse and Lemanske Jr, 2001; GINA Executive Committee, 2010). These characteristics lead to symptoms of asthma such as wheezing, shortness of breath, chest tightness, cough and sputum production. The severity of these symptoms may range from transient to persistent and may be exacerbated by various exposures, such as allergens and environmental pollutants (Wark and Gibson, 2006). It is estimated that asthma affects 300 million people globally (GINA Executive Committee) and accounts for 1 in every 250 deaths, many of which are preventable (Masoli *et al.*, 2004). Asthma is responsible for 1% of disability-adjusted life years (DALYs) worldwide, which is equivalent to that of diabetes and schizophrenia (Masoli *et al.*, 2004). The clinical signs of asthma are manageable with appropriate treatment, with inhaled glucocorticoids currently the most effective means of reducing airway inflammation. Their use is associated with improved lung function and quality of life, and reduced airways hyperresponsiveness and exacerbation severity (GINA Executive Committee, 2010).

* Corresponding author, hayley.scott@newcastle.edu.au

Asthma is considered an allergic disease, involving activation of the acquired immune response resulting in interleukin (IL)-5-mediated eosinophilic airway inflammation (Douwes *et al.*, 2002). Eosinophilic airway inflammation results when inhaled allergens activate Th2 helper T cells and mast cells via immunoglobulin (Ig)E, which induces inflammation by causing the release of histamine, leukotrienes and Th2 cytokines including IL-4, IL-5 and IL-13 (Teran, 1999; Busse and Lemanske Jr, 2001; Fahy, 2009). Once released, IL-5 travels to the bone marrow promoting the release of eosinophils into the circulation, which then migrate to lung tissue causing respiratory epithelial damage (Busse and Lemanske Jr, 2001). Eosinophils release inflammatory mediators such as leukotrienes (which causes injury to airway tissues) and granulocyte-macrophage colony-stimulating factor (which prolongs eosinophil survival) (Busse and Lemanske Jr, 2001). Inhaled allergens therefore activate the allergic pathway in asthma and lead to an eosinophilic pattern of airway inflammation, tissue damage, bronchial responsiveness and airway obstruction.

A non-eosinophilic pattern of inflammation has also been described in asthma, with a subgroup of asthmatics demonstrating IL-8-driven neutrophilic airway inflammation. This asthma phenotype involves a persistence of asthma symptoms and airways hyperresponsiveness in the absence of airway eosinophilia (Simpson *et al.*, 2006). Neutrophilic airway inflammation is being increasingly recognized as having an important role in asthma, because less than 50% of asthma cases are attributable to allergy (Pearce *et al.*, 1999). Those with neutrophilic asthma tend to be older, non-atopic and have a later onset of disease compared with those with an eosinophilic pattern of airway inflammation (Green *et al.*, 2002; Simpson *et al.*, 2006). Environmental exposures such as ozone, pollutants, viruses and bacterial endotoxins induce neutrophilic airway inflammation and airway obstruction in susceptible individuals with asthma (Douwes *et al.*, 2002). This inflammation involves the innate immune response, with increased levels of Toll-like receptor (TLR)-4 and TLR-2 observed in the airways of individuals with neutrophilic asthma (Simpson *et al.*, 2007).

Systemic inflammation is also evident in asthma, with the pro-inflammatory mediators IL-6 (Ström *et al.*,1996; Paeratakul *et al.*, 1998; Huang and Pan, 2001) and C-reactive protein (CRP) (Miyamoto *et al.*, 2007) elevated in the serum of asthmatics compared with healthy subjects. We have recently demonstrated that systemic inflammation is specific to the subgroup of asthmatics with a neutrophilic inflammatory phenotype. We also reported that systemic inflammation, specifically circulating IL-6, is associated with reduced lung function and worse asthma control (Wood *et al.*, 2011a). IL-6 has previously been shown to be important to airway responses. Genetically IL-6-deficient O_3-exposed mice have reduced airway neutrophils (Kaser *et al.*, 2008). Furthermore, systemic administration of IL-6 antibodies reduces innate airway hyperresponsiveness in an obese murine model (Patel *et al.*, 2004).

Anti-inflammatory treatments in asthma

As described above, the inflammatory response is central to asthma aetiology and symptomatology. Pharmacological treatment includes glucocorticoids, which controls airway inflammation. Although glucocorticoids are very effective in reducing eosinophilic airway inflammation, those with a neutrophilic pattern of airway inflammation are resistant to this medication and, in fact, glucocorticoids may enhance airway neutrophilia (Cox, 1995). Alternative treatments that manage neutrophilic airway inflammation in asthma are therefore needed. This highlights the potential for nutrition/physical activity interventions to be utilized in asthma. This chapter summarizes the scientific and epidemiological evidence supporting the use of such interventions to modulate the clinical and inflammatory manifestations of asthma.

Dietary Modulation of Inflammation in Asthma

The recent dramatic increase in asthma incidence in Westernized countries (Masoli *et al.*, 2004) and in those migrating from a developing to a Western country (Gibson *et al.*, 2003; Pereg *et al.*, 2008; Wang *et al.*, 2008) suggests that features of a Western lifestyle, such as dietary intake, promote asthma onset and development. This may be due to various components of a Western diet that promote inflammation. A high fat intake, low antioxidant intake and obesity, resulting from chronic metabolic surplus, all cause innate immune activation, which contributes to asthma. The discordance between evolutionary genetic traits and the comparatively recent emergence of a Westernized dietary pattern might underlie the recent increase in asthma incidence and worsening of asthma symptoms in susceptible individuals (Cordain *et al.*, 2005).

Dietary fat

The role of fatty acids in modifying the inflammatory environment in asthma is particularly important; however, only a limited number of observational and intervention studies have examined its association with asthma incidence and symptoms. These studies demonstrate variable results, which is possibly due to the populations being studied and the type of dietary measure performed. Most epidemiological research has estimated dietary fat intake by self-administered questionnaire, which has limitations.

An excessive dietary fat intake leads to increased levels of circulating lipids, which activate innate immune pathways leading to increased levels of pro-inflammatory mediators. The type of fatty acid consumed has varying effects on cellular membranes and thus the inflammatory pattern exhibited. Saturated fatty acids (SFAs) activate innate immune responses via TLR4 and TLR2, leading to activation of nuclear factor κB (NFκB) and the up-regulation of pro-inflammatory cytokines such as TNF-α, IL-6 and IL-8 (Lee *et al.*, 2004; Lee and Hwang, 2006). Conversely, omega-3 polyunsaturated fatty acids (PUFAs) and monounsaturated fatty acids (MUFAs) inhibit this pathway (Lee and Hwang, 2006).

The omega-6 polyunsaturated fatty acid linoleic acid is converted to arachidonic acid in the body, which is then enzymatically converted to the pro-inflammatory eicosanoids prostaglandin (PG)E_2 and leukotriene (LT) B_4 (Field *et al.*, 2002). LTB_4 enhances the Th1 response, thereby increasing the production of pro-inflammatory cytokines such as TNF-α and IL-6, and stimulating neutrophil infiltration (Calder, 1998; Field *et al.*, 2002). Because this fatty acid predominates in a Western diet, a high proportion of linoleic acid is present in cellular membranes (Calder, 1998). Conversely, the incorporation of the omega-3 PUFAs eicosapentaenoic (EPA) and docosahexaenoic acid (DHA) into cellular membranes reduces levels of these pro-inflammatory eicosanoids and increases production of the far less biologically active eicosanoids PGE_3 and LTB_5 (Calder, 1998). As such, omega-3 fatty acids are considered anti-inflammatory fatty acids.

Observational studies

A number of large epidemiological studies indicate that dietary fat intake affects respiratory health. A high dietary fat intake seems to be associated with asthma incidence (Ström *et al.*, 1996), airway hyperresponsiveness (Wanger *et al.*, 2005) and asthma severity (Misso *et al.*, 2005). Furthermore, an association between plasma triglyceride levels and adult-onset wheeze has been observed (Bodner *et al.*, 1999).

In recent decades, the relative proportions of dietary fatty acids have changed. Consumption of polyunsaturated fats has increased owing to an increase in margarine and vegetable oil consumption and a decreased intake of butter and lard (Black and Sharpe, 1997). It has been hypothesized that this higher consumption of omega-6 and reduction in omega-3 has led to an increased prevalence of allergic sensitization and might account for the recent increase in asthma development (Black and Sharpe, 1997).

One recent study examined the relationship between fatty acids and airway inflammation in asthma, and observed that the proportion of plasma SFAs was positively associated with neutrophilic airway inflammation, whereas the level of plasma MUFA was inversely associated with neutrophilic airway inflammation, in males (Scott *et al.*, 2011). Interestingly, this relationship was not evident in females; possibly owing to sex differences in the storage and release of fatty acids (Scott *et al.*, 2011). Males have a significantly higher fatty acid uptake and rate of lipolysis in the visceral abdominal depot compared with age- and body mass index (BMI)-matched females (Shi and Clegg, 2009). These fatty acids are mostly transported directly to the liver, where SFAs potently activate the TLR4 pathway leading to the release of pro-inflammatory cytokines (de Luca and Olefsky, 2008). This larger flux of fatty acids in males may result in greater sensitivity to fatty-acid-induced inflammation, therefore providing a possible explanation for this sexually dimorphic association.

OMEGA-3 FATTY ACIDS. Omega-3 fatty acids suppress neutrophil function (Turner *et al.*, 2008) and a higher intake is associated with better lung function (Jia *et al.*, 2004; Lago *et al.*, 2007; McKeever *et al.*, 2008a) (Table 17.1). Woods *et al.* (2004) found plasma omega-3 fatty acids were associated with fewer asthma attacks in the preceding 3 months, fewer nocturnal asthma symptoms in the preceding 12 months and reduced bronchial reactivity, in a sample of 1601 young adults with and without asthma. Numerous cross-sectional studies have reported an association between oily fish consumption and a reduced odds of current asthma (Hodge *et al.*, 1996; Kris-Etherton *et al.*, 1999; Murray *et al.*, 2006; Tabak *et al.*, 2006; National Heart Foundation of Australia, 2009) (Table 17.1). In terms of circulating concentration (Woods *et al.*, 2004; Bolte *et al.*, 2006) or estimated dietary intake (Hodge *et al.*, 1996; Broadfield *et al.*, 2004; Miyamoto *et al.*, 2007; McKeever *et al.*, 2008a; Miyake *et al.*, 2008; Rodríguez-Rodríguez *et al.*, 2010) of omega-3 fatty acids the evidence remains inconsistent (Table 17.1).

OMEGA-6 FATTY ACIDS. The association between omega-6 fatty acids and asthma outcomes has been examined extensively, with several authors finding that dietary intake of omega-6 fatty acids (estimated via questionnaire) is not significantly associated with current asthma (Hodge *et al.*, 1996; Huang and Pan, 2001; McKeever *et al.*, 2008a; Miyake *et al.*, 2008). The measurement of circulating fatty acids seems, however, to demonstrate a more significant effect. For example, a cross-sectional study of 526 children aged 8–11 years found that plasma arachidonic acid was associated with increased odds of asthma, whereas plasma linoleic acid was associated with decreased odds (Bolte *et al.*, 2006) (Table 17.1). Another epidemiological study examined plasma fatty acids and found that, although there was no association with odds of current asthma, a higher circulating omega-6 level was associated with increased airway hyperresponsiveness (Woods *et al.*, 2004) (Table 17.1). Furthermore, a higher omega-6 fatty acid intake has been associated with poorer lung function (McKeever *et al.*, 2008a) and increased odds of wheeze (Miyake *et al.*, 2008) (Table 17.1).

SATURATED FATTY ACIDS. A cross-sectional study of 1166 adolescents showed that a 1 standard deviation increase in saturated fat intake doubled the risk of current asthma (Huang and Pan, 2001), whereas another study in young adults found an increased SFA intake was associated with increased odds of airway hyperresponsiveness (Soutar *et al.*, 1997) (Table 17.1). Some studies, however, have found no association between saturated fat intake and current asthma (Hodge *et al.*, 1996; Woods *et al.*, 2004; Murray *et al.*, 2006; Miyamoto *et al.*, 2007; Miyake *et al.*, 2008; National Heart Foundation of Australia, 2009) or atopy (Woods *et al.*, 2004), and therefore large epidemiological studies utilizing quality measures of dietary intake are required to determine the strength of this association.

MONOUNSATURATED FATTY ACIDS. MUFA seem to have either a neutral (Hodge *et al.*, 1996; Simopoulos, 2002; Woods *et al.*, 2004; Bolte *et al.*, 2006; Murray *et al.*, 2006; Miyamoto *et al.*, 2007; Miyake *et al.*, 2008; Rodríguez-Rodríguez *et al.*, 2010) or protective effect (Von Schacky, 2010) on asthma risk (Table 17.1). Additional studies are required to determine the inflammatory and clinical effects of this fatty acid on asthma status.

SUMMARY. The epidemiological evidence examining the effect of dietary fat on inflammation in asthma is weak. Most studies have

Table 17.1. Cross-sectional studies examining the association of fatty acids with inflammation, current asthma, lung function, asthma symptoms.

	Population	FA measure	Outcome measure	Omega-6	Omega-3	SFA	MUFA
Bolte *et al.*, 2005	n = 7124 18–79 years	FFQ	Current asthma	↑			
Bolte *et al.*, 2006	r = 526 7–11 years	Serum cholesterol esters	Current asthma	↓ LA; ↑ AA	–		–
			FEV_1	↑ LA; ↓ AA	–		–
Broadfield *et al.*, 2004	n = 178 Mean age 43 years	Erythrocyte cell membranes	Current asthma	↓	–		
Chatzi *et al.*, 2007	n = 460 6.5 years	Fish intake (FFQ)	Atopy		↓ (Fish)		
			Current wheeze		– (Fish)		
de Luis *et al.*, 2005	n = 108 Mean age 24–27 years	3-day food diary	FEV_1		↑		
Fluge *et al.*, 1998	n = 4300 20–44 years	Fish intake FFQ	Wheeze		– (Fish)		
			Chest tightness		– (Fish)		
			Asthma attack		– (Fish)		
Hodge *et al.*, 1996	n = 574 8–11 years	Fish intake	Current asthma		↓ (Fish)		
		FFQ		–	–	–	–
Huang and Pan, 2001	n = 1166 13–17 years	24-h food recall	Current asthma	–	–	↑	↓
Laerum *et al.*, 2007	n = 16187 23–54 years	Fish intake FFQ	Current asthma		↓ (Fish)		
McKeever *et al.*, 2008	n = 13820 20–59 years	FFQ	Current asthma	–	–		
			FEV_1	↓	–		
			Wheeze	–	↑		
Miyake *et al.*, 2008	n = 25033 6–15 years	Brief diet history questionnaire	Current asthma	–	–	–	–
			Wheeze	↑	↑	–	–
Miyamoto *et al.*, 2007	n = 1002 pregnant females	Diet history questionnaire	Current asthma	–	–	–	–
Murray *et al.*, 2006	n = 74 3–5 years	FFQ	Current asthma	↑ (total PUFA) – (omega-6 and omega-3)		–	–

Continued

Table 17.1. Continued.

	Population	FA measure	Outcome measure	Omega-6	Omega-3	SFA	MUFA
Nagel and Linseisen, 2005	n = 525 35–65 years	FFQ	Current asthma	–	–	–	–
Rodriguez-Rodriguez *et al.*, 2010	n = 638 8–13 years	3-day food diary	Current asthma	–	–	↑	–
Schwartz and Weiss, 1994	n = 2526 30+ years	FFQ	FEV_1		↑ (Fish intake)		
Soutar *et al.*, 1997	n = 116 Mean age 37–38 years	7-day FFQ	AHR	– (Total PUFA)		↑	↑
Tabak *et al.*, 2006	n = 598 8–13 years	FFQ	Current asthma		↓ (Fish intake)		
			Wheeze		↓ (Fish intake)		
Woods *et al.*, 2004	n = 1601 20–44 years	FFQ	Current asthma	–	–	–	–
			Atopy	–	–	–	–
			Asthma attack past 3 months	–	↓	–	–
			Nocturnal symptoms	–	↓	–	–
			DRS	↑	↓	–	–

↑, increased risk; ↓, decreased risk; –, no effect observed; AA, arachidonic acid; AHR, airway hyperresponsiveness; DRS, dose response slope calculated as the provocation fall (%) ÷ provocation dose of methacholine; FFQ, food frequency questionnaire; FA, fatty acid; FEV_1, forced expiratory volume in 1 s; LA, linoleic acid.

utilized dietary questionnaires rather than conducting plasma fatty acid measures. Further cross-sectional studies performing direct measures of fatty acids are warranted to elucidate their role in asthma aetiology and the clinical course of the disease.

Interventional studies

Although cross-sectional studies have examined asthma from a clinical perspective, interventional studies provide stronger evidence in terms of mechanisms driving an association between fatty acids and asthma. Two recent studies have examined the effect of a high fat intake on inflammation in asthma. Wood *et al.* (2011b) demonstrated that a high-fat meal, containing 49 g mixed fat (SFA, PUFA, MUFA), modified innate immune responses, with significantly increased sputum neutrophilia and TLR4 mRNA expression, and suppressed bronchodilator recovery in subjects with asthma. Another study by de Vries *et al.* (2009) found a significant reduction in lung eosinophils and IL-5 in allergic mice fed a high-fat diet. This suggests that dietary fat may modulate innate and allergic pathways differentially. Another study examined the potential anti-inflammatory effects of omega-3 fatty acids on the eosinophilic asthma pathway. There was no reported effect of 5 weeks supplementation with 0.69 g omega-3 PUFA on sputum eosinophils, exhaled nitric oxide (eNO) or bronchial reactivity in 12 subjects with asthma (Schubert *et al.*, 2009).

The ratio of omega-6:omega-3 PUFA has been examined in children from infanthood until 5 years of age. No effect was seen on asthma risk (Marks *et al.*, 2006). Another study supplemented children with omega-3 PUFA before birth (via the supplementation of mother). Although this had no effect on risk of asthma development, other asthma measures, including wheeze, bronchodilator use and nocturnal coughing, were significantly reduced in those children with a higher plasma concentration of omega-3 (Mihrshahi *et al.*, 2004). Bitalgi *et al.* (2009) found 1000 mg/day omega-3 supplementation for 6 weeks in children with asthma resulted in improved asthma control and lung function, and a reduction in sputum eosinophils.

SUMMARY. Few interventional trials have examined the role of dietary fat in asthma. Taken together, these studies suggest that fatty acids have the potential to modulate inflammatory pathways in asthma. Further work is needed, however, to elucidate how this could be relevant to asthma management.

Obesity

Both obesity and asthma have concurrently increased in prevalence and incidence in recent decades (Australian Centre for Asthma Monitoring 2007). Obesity and asthma are associated conditions, with obesity conferring twice the risk of asthma development (Beuther and Sutherland, 2007). Obese asthmatics experience more severe asthma symptoms, a poorer quality of life, reduced lung function, increased dyspnoea, and increased hospitalizations and emergency room visits compared with asthmatics of a healthy weight (Camargo Jr *et al.*, 1999; Sin *et al.*, 2002; Thomson *et al.*, 2003; Dixon *et al.*, 2006; Vortmann and Eisner, 2008). The effect of obesity on airway hyperresponsiveness is uncertain, with a positive association between BMI and airway hyperresponsiveness observed in some (Celedon *et al.*, 2001; Chinn *et al.*, 2002; Litonjua *et al.*, 2002) but not all studies (Soutar *et al.*, 1997). Because both obesity and asthma are chronic inflammatory states, it has been suggested that inflammation might be the common link.

Observational studies

Studies suggest that the association between obesity and asthma is stronger in non-atopic (Kronander *et al.*, 2004; Appleton *et al.*, 2006) females (Shaheen *et al.*, 1999; Beckett *et al.*, 2001, Celedon *et al.*, 2001; Chen *et al.*, 2002; Guerra *et al.*, 2002; Loebroks *et al.*, 2008). Although this is not a universal observation (Huovinen *et al.*, 2003; Ford *et al.*, 2004b), it is supported by Haldar *et al.* (2008) who conducted a cluster analysis and found a clinical asthma phenotype that was predominantly female with an absence of sputum eosinophils despite a high symptom expression.

Various cytokines and adipokines released by adipose tissue, such as IL-6 and CRP, may contribute to asthma progression and development. Indeed, asthma severity is worse in subjects with a higher concentration of circulating IL-6 independent of BMI (Dixon *et al.*, 2006), whereas airflow limitation is more severe in an elderly population with elevated CRP (Melbye *et al.*, 2007). Adipokines, such as leptin and adiponectin, may contribute to the link between obesity and asthma. Leptin levels are elevated in subjects who are both obese and asthmatic, with an increased circulating leptin concentration associated with increased odds of current asthma (Gurkan *et al.*, 2004; Sood *et al.*, 2006; Nagel *et al.*, 2009). Interestingly, Sood *et al.* (2006) found a significant association between leptin and asthma risk for pre-menopausal females, but not for males or post-menopausal females. It is plausible that the association of leptin with increased asthma risk is being driven by neutrophilic airway inflammation. Leptin increases neutrophil function and activation via TNF-α (Zarkesh-Esfahani *et al.*, 2004) and inhibits neutrophil apoptosis (Bruno *et al.*, 2005). This inflammation may extend to the airways of asthmatic individuals, leading to increased neutrophilic airway inflammation. Indeed in a mouse pneumococcal pneumonia model, exogenous leptin stimulated the innate immune response leading to increased neutrophils and IL-6 in bronchoalveolar fluid (MacDougald and Burant, 2007). Adiponectin may also play a role in asthma. Sood *et al.* (2008) found adiponectin concentrations to be lower in females with asthma compared with those without asthma; however, the concentration in males does not differ by asthma status. Furthermore, a lower circulating adiponectin concentration seems to be associated with increased odds of current asthma in pre-menopausal females, but not males, after adjustment for BMI (Sood *et al.*, 2008). Shore *et al.* (2006) has demonstrated that adiponectin infusion suppresses eosinophilic and neutrophilic airway inflammation and attenuates airway hyperresponsiveness in ovalbumin (OVA)-sensitized mice. Similarly, Medoff *et al.* (2009) found that OVA-sensitized adiponectin-deficient mice have enhanced eosinophilic airway inflammation and pulmonary vascular remodelling compared with wild-type mice. These studies suggest that adiponectin deficiency may worsen asthma and augment airway inflammation. Evidence is, however, currently limited and further investigation is therefore warranted.

Several researchers have examined the association between obesity and airway inflammation and have found no association between obesity and sputum eosinophilia (Todd *et al.*, 2007; Lessard *et al.*, 2008; Sutherland *et al.*, 2008b) or exhaled nitric oxide (eNO) (Sutherland *et al.*, 2008b). Indeed, sputum eosinophils (van Veen *et al.*, 2008) and eNO (Komakula *et al.*, 2007; van Veen *et al.*, 2008; Berg *et al.*, 2011) may in fact be inversely associated with obesity, suggesting a shift from the Th2 response. It is therefore evident that eosinophilic airway inflammation is not driving the association between asthma and obesity. Neutrophilic airway inflammation has been examined as a driver of the obese–asthma phenotype in only a small number of studies. We recently reported a positive association between BMI and sputum neutrophilia (Scott *et al.*, 2011). Interestingly, when stratified by sex this association was only statistically significant in females. Three recent studies report no association between obesity and neutrophilic airway inflammation (Todd *et al.*, 2007; Lessard *et al.*, 2008; Sutherland *et al.*, 2008b). Interestingly, however, all three studies show a clear non-significant trend towards increased sputum neutrophils as BMI classification increased (Todd *et al.*, 2007; Lessard *et al.*, 2008; Sutherland *et al.*, 2008b). The lack of statistical significance in these studies is possibly due to the small sample size in two studies (Lessard *et al.*, 2008; Sutherland *et al.*, 2008b), sex differences not being considered in two instances (Todd *et al.*, 2007; Lessard *et al.*, 2008) and the large variation generally observed in the measurement of sputum cells (Table 17.2).

Interventional studies

Obesity increases the risk of asthma development and worsens asthma symptoms, so reversibility with weight loss would be expected. Indeed, weight loss does seem to improve asthma symptoms, lung function and quality of life, and reduce

Table 17.2. Summary of studies examining the relationship between obesity and airway inflammation in subjects with asthma.

	Normal weight (BMI <25 kg/m^2)	Obese (BMI ≥30 kg/m^2)	*P*-value
Lessard *et al.* (2008)			
% Neutrophils[a]	31.6 ± 21.8	48.6 ± 21.3	>0.05
% Eosinophils[a]	2.6 ± 3.7	4.6 ± 12.9	>0.05
Scott *et al.* (2011)			
% Neutrophils[a]	37.8 ± 21.9	50.8 ± 23.0	0.01
% Eosinophils	1.3 (0.5, 5.3)	1.4 (0.3, 3.0)	0.32
Sutherland *et al.* (2008)			
% Neutrophils	22.4 (9.7, 27.4)	28.9 (17.2, 43.8)	0.27[b]
% Eosinophils	10.7 (5.6, 35.5)	11.3 (7.5, 25.9)	0.98[b]
Todd *et al.* (2007)			
% Neutrophils[a]	52.1 ± 29.2	60.5 ± 27.4	>0.05
% Eosinophils	0.7 (0, 53.0)	0.5 (0, 34.3)	>0.05

Data presented as median (IQR) or [a]mean ± SD. [b]*P*-value is calculated from the interaction between obesity and asthma in subjects with and without asthma.

asthma medication usage (Dixon *et al.*, 1999; Stenius-Aarniala *et al.*, 2000; Aaron *et al.*, 2004; Eneli *et al.*, 2008). Weight loss therefore provides an alternate treatment route to increasing inhaled corticosteroid medication, which has limited effectiveness in obese individuals (Peters-Golden *et al.*, 2006; Boulet and Franssen, 2007; Sutherland *et al.*, 2008a). Surprisingly, the majority of studies have been conducted in individuals undergoing bariatric surgery, with asthma not measured objectively and/or as the primary outcome (Macgregor and Greenberg, 1993; Dixon *et al.*, 1999; Simard *et al.*, 2004; Ahroni *et al.*, 2005; Nelson *et al.*, 2006; Sultan *et al.*, 2009).

Dietary restriction has been examined in several studies; however, only one randomized controlled trial has been conducted. This study employed a 14-week dietary restriction, resulting in a weight loss of 14.5% and corresponding improvements to forced expiratory volume in 1 s (FEV_1) of 7.2% and forced vital capacity (FVC) of 8.6% (Stenius-Aarniala *et al.*, 2000). Subjects in the weight-loss group had significantly reduced dyspnoea and rescue medication usage compared with controls, and in the year following the intervention had significantly fewer asthma exacerbations (Stenius-Aarniala *et al.*, 2000). Non-randomized trials also demonstrate that dietary restriction improves clinical asthma outcomes such as FEV_1 (Hakala *et al.*, 2000; Aaron *et al.*, 2004), FVC (Hakala *et al.*, 2000), quality of life (Aaron *et al.*, 2004), dyspnoea (Hakala *et al.*, 2000) and asthma control (Johnson *et al.*, 2007). Few studies have examined inflammatory outcomes after weight loss; however, Johnson *et al.* (2007) found an 8-week caloric restriction resulted in a significant reduction in TNF-α, whereas CRP was unchanged. This was only a very small study, however (n = 10), so it is likely that it was not powered to detect change in this marker. A number of surgical trials has been conducted solely in asthmatic subjects and these trials suggest that bariatric surgery does indeed reduce asthma symptoms and asthma medication usage, and improve lung function (Macgregor and Greenberg, 1993; Maniscalco *et al.*, 2008; Dixon *et al.*, 2011), despite no change to eNO (Maniscalco *et al.*, 2008) or sputum eosinophils (Dixon *et al.*, 2011). Interestingly, the effect of weight loss on airway inflammation, measured using sputum cell counts, has only been examined by Dixon *et al.* (2011) in a small study of asthmatic adults. Bariatric surgery resulted in no change to sputum neutrophils or eosinophils, despite improvements to lung function and asthma symptoms, and a trend towards reduced airway hyperresponsiveness (Dixon *et al.*, 2011).

Summary

In summary, research into the obese–asthma phenotype has largely focused on modifying clinical asthma outcomes rather than mechanisms driving this association. Gaining a better understanding of the mechanisms involved in the reversibility of the obese–asthma phenotype with weight loss is therefore paramount to ensuring optimal management of this population. A limited amount of evidence suggests that airway neutrophilia may be a feature of obese asthma, particularly in females. The ability of weight loss to reduce neutrophilic inflammation in asthma requires further exploration.

Antioxidants

A low antioxidant intake can contribute to inflammation by reducing host defences against reactive oxygen species (ROS). ROS are produced during normal cellular activities, such as during respiration. Antioxidants, including the enzymatic antioxidants superoxide dismutase (SOD) and glutathione peroxidise (GSH-Px), and the non-enzymatic antioxidants ascorbic acid and α-tocopherol, prevent ROS from reaching a concentration that may cause damage within the cell of a healthy host. In certain diseases, however, ROS production overwhelms antioxidant defences causing oxidative stress. (Slade *et al.*, 1993; Nadeem *et al.*, 2008). Asthma, a disease with an underlying inflammatory pathology, depletes antioxidants. For example, subjects with asthma have low levels of ascorbic acid, α-tocopherol and carotenoids in the lungs despite adequate dietary intake (Kelly *et al.*, 1999; Wood *et al.*, 2005). Indeed, poor antioxidant status has been linked to an increased risk of asthma development and deterioration of asthma control (Wood *et al.*, 2003; Nadeem *et al.*, 2008) owing to oxidative stress. A low dietary antioxidant intake can exacerbate oxidative stress by further reducing antioxidant protection. The role of exogenous antioxidants in relation to asthma risk, inflammation and asthma outcomes has been investigated in a number of epidemiological and interventional studies, which are discussed below.

Observational studies

Large-scale epidemiological studies show that antioxidants may be protective against asthma (Shaheen *et al.*, 2001; Rubin *et al.*, 2004). Indeed, nutrient deficiencies of ascorbic acid, vitamin E and β-carotene have been linked with asthma exacerbation and poorer lung function, with asthmatic subjects having reduced levels of antioxidants in the lungs compared with healthy subjects (Kelly *et al.*, 1999; Wood *et al.*, 2005). Trolox equivalent antioxidant capacity (TEAC) is an indicator of overall oxidant stress and has been found to be significantly reduced in plasma during an acute asthma exacerbation when compared with stable asthmatics (Rahman *et al.*, 1996). Further, TEAC was significantly reduced in stable asthma compared with healthy controls (Rahman *et al.*, 1996). This is supported by Katsoulis *et al.* (2003) who observed a significantly lower total antioxidant status (TAS) at time of admission to hospital for a severe asthma exacerbation compared with discharge, which is probably due to increased oxidative stress during exacerbation. Furthermore, improvement to TAS during the hospital admission correlated with an improvement to FEV_1. Fabian *et al.* (2011) found that children with asthma had a significantly lower total antioxidant capacity, whereas malondialdehyde (MDA), a marker of lipid peroxidation, correlated with eNO, suggesting that this increased airway inflammation and oxidative stress modifies antioxidant activity in asthma. Other authors have reported a positive association between oxidative stress and airway hyperresponsiveness (Katsumata *et al.*, 1990; Saleh *et al.*, 1998). These studies suggest that oxidant–antioxidant imbalance may contribute to the development and progression of asthma.

FRUIT AND VEGETABLES. The intake of fruit and vegetables has decreased considerably in Western societies causing reduced lung antioxidant defences. This is hypothesized to have contributed to the increased prevalence of asthma in recent decades due to shifting oxidant–antioxidant balance (Seaton *et al.*, 1994). Observational studies consistently report beneficial associations of fruit and vegetable intake on lung function. For example, Cook *et al.* (1997) found FEV_1 was 79 ml higher in children who reported eating fruit more than once a day compared with children who reported never eating fruit. This is supported by longitudinal data from an adult population that shows that over a 7-year period those who had the greatest reduction in fresh fruit intake had a 107-ml reduction in their FEV_1 compared with those who did not change fresh fruit intake (Carey *et al.*, 1998). Fruit consumption also modifies risk of asthma development. For example, apple consumption was inversely associated with odds of asthma in a population aged 16–50 years (Shaheen *et al.*, 2001), whereas apple juice concentrate and banana consumption was inversely associated with wheeze in children (Okoko *et al.*, 2007). Low fruit consumption has also been associated with increased risk of cough (Antova *et al.*, 2003), wheeze (Chatzi *et al.*, 2007a,b) and rhinitis (Chatzi *et al.*, 2007a) in children. In addition to whole foods, numerous observational studies have examined the impact of specific antioxidants on asthma outcomes and these are discussed below.

VITAMIN A. Vitamin A is a fat-soluble vitamin and there are also a number of provitamin A compounds including β-carotene, lycopene and β-cryptoxanthin. These compounds exert antioxidant activity, with large epidemiological studies suggesting favourable effects in terms of asthma risk. For example, NHANES III data show that both serum α-carotene and β-carotene levels are associated with a reduced risk of asthma in children, whereby an increase of 1 standard deviation corresponded to 10% and 15% reduced odds of asthma, respectively (Harik-Khan *et al.*, 2004; Rubin *et al.*, 2004). Conversely, Okuda *et al.* (2010) found no association between α-carotene, β-carotene, lycopene or β-cryptoxanthin and asthma risk in a smaller sample of 396 Japanese children. In terms of asthma outcomes, dietary carotenoids seem to benefit respiratory function cross-sectionally in both adults and children (Grievink *et al.*, 1998; Bodner *et al.*, 1999; Hu and Cassano, 2000; Schünemann *et al.*, 2001; McKeever *et al.*, 2008b); however, they do not seem to modify symptom expression such as wheeze (Grievink *et al.*, 1998). Carotenoid intake has also been shown to be protective against lung function decline in young adults in two large epidemiological trials (Guénégou *et al.*, 2006; Thyagarajan *et al.*, 2011).

Vitamin A itself has also been examined, although somewhat less extensively. Lung function is positively associated with serum vitamin A levels in adults and a higher dietary vitamin A intake in children (Morabia *et al.*, 1990; Gilliland *et al.*, 2003; McKeever *et al.*, 2008b). One large well-characterized epidemiological study, however, cited no association between estimated dietary intake of vitamin A and lung function (Shahar *et al.*, 1994) and therefore conclusions regarding this antioxidant are limited.

VITAMIN C. Vitamin C is a water-soluble antioxidant that acts as an electron donor to a number of compounds including ROS, and is the most abundant antioxidant on the airway surface of the lung (Slade *et al.*, 1993). Studies generally support a beneficial role for vitamin C in terms of asthma risk (Ford *et al.*, 2004a; Harik-Khan *et al.*, 2004; Rubin *et al.*, 2004) and lung function (Grievink *et al.*, 1998; Hu *et al.*, 1998; Hu and Cassano, 2000; Gilliland *et al.*, 2003). For example, the NHANES III data shows a 10% reduction in asthma risk for every 1 SD increase in serum vitamin C in children aged 4–16 years (Rubin *et al.*, 2004). In those exposed to passive smoking, this was a 40% reduction in asthma risk for every 1 standard deviation increase in serum vitamin C (Rubin *et al.*, 2004). Hu *et al.* (1998) examined 3085 Chinese adults aged 35–64 years and found that for every 100 mg increase in daily vitamin C intake, FEV_1 was increased by 21.6 ml and FVC by 24.9 ml. Examination of 2566 children aged 11–19 years showed that girls with a low intake of vitamin C had a poorer FEV_1 and FVC, whereas boys with a low intake had a poorer FVC compared with those with a higher vitamin C intake (Gilliland *et al.*, 2003). A case-control study found an inverse association between dietary intake of vitamin C and bronchial reactivity, whereby those with the lowest intake of vitamin C had a fivefold increased risk of airway hyperresponsiveness to methacholine (Soutar *et al.*, 1997).

VITAMIN E. Vitamin E is a lipid-soluble antioxidant that protects against membrane injury by preventing autoxidation of lipids and converts ROS to less active forms (Wood and Gibson, 2009). Vitamin E describes a group of compounds including four tocopherols and four tocotrienols. Observational studies report a beneficial effect of vitamin E on lung function (Hu and Cassano, 2000; Schünemann *et al.*, 2001; Gilliland *et al.*, 2003), asthma control (Bakkeheim *et al.*, 2011), wheeze (Bodner *et al.*, 1999; Devereux *et al.*, 2006) and IgE sensitization (Fogarty *et al.*, 2000). These findings are supported by large epidemiological trials, which show that a higher maternal intake of vitamin A reduces offspring wheeze at 2 years (Litonjua *et al.*, 2006) and asthma risk at 5 years (Devereux *et al.*, 2006).

Interventional studies

Numerous interventional studies also indicate that dietary antioxidants are important to respiratory health, in terms of both asthma outcomes and inducing changes in inflammation. The inflammatory consequences of oxidant–antioxidant imbalance in asthma have been examined in both murine and human interventional studies. Oxidative stress causes the infiltration of inflammatory cells into the airways including eosinophils, neutrophils and lymphocytes (Sagai *et al.*, 1996; Saleh *et al.*, 1998). These inflammatory cells produce oxidants, leading to increased airway hyperresponsiveness and poorer lung function (Schünemann *et al.*, 1997; Horváth *et al.*, 1998; Saleh *et al.*, 1998).

Dietary or supplemental antioxidants assist in maintaining oxidant–antioxidant balance in the airways and modulates the infiltration of inflammatory cells. This was demonstrated in a study in which 10 days of a low antioxidant diet increased sputum neutrophilia in adults with asthma, whereas subsequent 7-day supplementation with a lycopene-rich treatment, provided as either tomato juice or tomato extract, reduced airway neutrophil concentrations (Wood *et al.*, 2008). Similarly, Blackwell *et al.* (1996), using a rat model, found that treatment of the lung with N-acetylcysteine significantly reduced airway neutrophilia after exposure to endotoxin. Antioxidant supplementation also seems to modify Th2 responses in asthma. In a murine model, supplementation of OVA-sensitized mice with tomato extract led to significantly reduced airway concentrations of IL-4, IL-5 and eosinophils (Hazlewood *et al.*, 2011). Guinea pigs treated with vitamin C for 26 days had a significant reduction in both BAL eosinophils and neutrophils after OVA challenge (Haines *et al.*, 2011). Further, rats supplemented with γ-tocopherol for 4 days had a 74% reduction in airway eosinophils after OVA challenge compared with rats not treated with γ-tocopherol, while there was a trend towards reduced neutrophils (non-significant reduction of 48%) (Wagner *et al.*, 2007). There was also a significant reduction in IL-5 and IL-13 concentrations in the lung (Wagner *et al.*, 2007).

Only a small number of intervention trials have examined the effect of antioxidant supplementation or restriction on clinical asthma outcomes. For example, the study by Wood *et al.* (2008) found that not only did a low antioxidant diet increase airway neutrophils but subjects experienced a deterioration in their lung function and asthma control. Several interventional studies have shown beneficial effects on lung function of supplementing cyclists (Grievink *et al.*, 1999), street workers (Romieu *et al.*, 1998) and children (Romieu *et al.*, 2002) with vitamins C and E. Maternal supplementation with vitamin A, but not β-carotene, in a chronically undernourished population resulted in significant improvements in lung function of offspring at ages 9–13 years (Checkley *et al.*, 2010). Others have, however, failed to observe a benefit. For example, supplementation of 35 asthmatics with 500 mg vitamin E for 6 weeks had no effect on lung function or asthma symptoms in adults with asthma (Pearson *et al.*, 2004). In another trial, maternal antioxidant supplementation with high-dose vitamin C and E during pregnancy had no effect on respiratory outcomes of infants at 2 years of age (Greenough *et al.*, 2010). Further, a recent Cochrane review does not support an association between vitamin C supplementation and lung function or symptoms in those with asthma (Kaur *et al.*, 2009). However, this review of nine studies included only 330 participants and therefore the current evidence is limited. These discrepancies of antioxidant supplementation on clinical asthma outcomes may be due to the differing populations being examined, with at-risk populations seeming to receive greater benefit from such supplementation. Further, it seems that combined antioxidant supplements, or whole foods, might exert greater benefit than isolated antioxidant nutrients alone.

Summary

Taken together, the experimental and epidemiological evidence suggests that a low intake of exogenous antioxidants augments inflammatory processes and in turn leads to increased risk of asthma development. Asthma itself induces an oxidant–antioxidant imbalance, which is associated with poorer asthma outcomes including increased airway inflammation and airway hyperresponsiveness, and poorer lung function. Although additional high-quality interventional trials are required, the current epidemiological evidence and existing interventional evidence suggest an important role of dietary antioxidants in both reducing inflammatory processes in asthma and decreasing the risk of asthma development.

Physical Activity and Modulation of Inflammation in Asthma

Exercise may cause increased airway resistance in individuals with asthma, leading to exercise-induced bronchoconstriction (EIB); however, pre-treatment with medications such as inhaled beta-agonists can prevent or reduce risk of EIB (McFadden Jr and Gilbert, 1994). None the less, fear of inducing asthma symptoms may deter those with asthma from participating in physical activity. Indeed, a number of studies indicate that those with asthma seem to have a lower fitness level than those without asthma (Clark and Cochrane, 1988; Wong *et al.*, 2001), suggesting that this is the case. Participation in regular exercise is recommended for both adults and children with asthma to reduce asthma-related physical impairment (National Heart Lung and Blood Institute, 2007). Indeed, studies suggest that regular participation in exercise may reduce the risk of asthma exacerbation (Garcia-Aymerich *et al.*, 2009), improve asthma symptoms (Ford *et al.*, 2003) and reduce airway hyperresponsiveness (Shaaban *et al.*, 2007). The mechanisms by which these benefits occur are uncertain; however, the anti-inflammatory role of regular exercise is implicated.

Observational studies

Several observational studies support an association between physical activity level and risk of asthma. For example, Cheng *et al.* (2010) examined 123 children aged 7–14 years and found asthmatic children were significantly less likely to participate in exercise. The asthmatic children with a lower exercise level were more likely to believe that exercise would make their asthma worse, had a poorer lung function and poorer asthma-related quality of life, compared with asthmatic children with a higher exercise participation (Cheng *et al.*, 2010). Similarly, in a cohort of 155 children aged 3–5 years, a history of asthma and wheezing was associated with a lower level of exercise (Firrincieli *et al.*, 2005). In a longitudinal cohort, children with a lower fitness level at baseline were more likely to have developed asthma within 10 years (Rasmussen *et al.*, 2000). Similarly in adults, observational studies report an increased physical activity level is associated with reduced odds of current asthma (Ford *et al.*, 2003; Teramoto and Moonie, 2011) and asthma exacerbation (Garcia-Aymerich *et al.*, 2009), and improved health (Dogra and Baker, 2006). Others report no effect of exercise on asthma development, however (Chen *et al.*, 2001; Berntsen *et al.*, 2009; Benet *et al.*, 2011), with some reporting an increased risk of asthma (Ownby *et al.*, 2007), wheeze (Nystad *et al.*, 2001) and airway hyperresponsiveness (Shaaban *et al.*, 2007) in those who are more active. This equivocal evidence is possibly due to differences in the populations studied and the effect of exercise intensity not being assessed in most instances.

Interventional studies

Changes to clinical asthma outcomes have been investigated after exercise training.

A Cochrane review found no effect of physical training on lung function; however, there was a non-significant reduction in wheeze (Ram *et al.*, 2005). Of the 355 subjects included in the review, only 129 had lung function measures recorded and, with the considerable variation in the exercise interventions prescribed, differing exercise intensities and durations, further quality studies measuring lung function and other objective clinical measures such as asthma-related quality of life, symptoms and medication usage are needed. A more recent study found that a 9-week swimming or golf programme in 45 children aged 7–14 years resulted in significant improvements to asthma symptoms, quality of life and a reduction in urgent physician visits for asthma (Weisgerber *et al.*, 2008). A 10-week high-intensity exercise training programme in asthmatic adults significantly improved lung function, whereas there was a reduction in the proportion of subjects experiencing EIA (Emtner *et al.*, 1996). Two months of aerobic training in asthmatic children aged 8–16 years resulted in a significant reduction in the use of both inhaled and oral corticosteroids (Neder *et al.*, 1999). These studies indicate the need to investigate further the clinical effects of exercise training in asthma in order to provide a strong level of evidence.

Interventional studies examining the mechanisms by which physical activity may improve asthma outcomes are lacking. The available evidence suggests, however, that exercise may reduce airway inflammation. Mendes *et al.* (2011) found 3 months of aerobic training significantly reduced sputum eosinophils and eNO in subjects with asthma, with these reductions being greater in asthmatics with more severe eosinophilia at baseline. This intervention also resulted in significantly more symptom-free days and fewer asthma exacerbations during the 3-month follow-up period compared with control subjects (Mendes *et al.*, 2011). The mechanism by which physical activity reduces airway eosinophilia has been explored in several murine models. OVA-sensitized mice exercised on a treadmill at a moderate intensity for 45 min had a significant reduction in bronchoalveolar lavage (BAL) eosinophils compared with sedentary control mice (Hewitt *et al.*, 2009). This corresponded with an increased expression of IL-10 and IL-1ra, and reduced expression of the Th2-derived cytokines IL-5 and IL-4 (Hewitt *et al.*, 2009; Vieira *et al.*, 2007, 2008). These inflammatory changes may be driving the observed reduction in airway eosinophils.

Summary

Despite the fact that guidelines recommend regular physical activity to minimize asthma-related impairment, those with asthma are less likely to exercise. Fear of deteriorating asthma control might be a contributing factor. There seems to be a role of moderate-intensity exercise in reducing asthma-associated airway inflammation. Further investigation of asthma outcomes and the mechanisms driving a reduction in airway inflammation after moderate-intensity exercise are needed to better inform our understanding of exercise as a potential treatment strategy in asthma.

Summary and Conclusions

Both innate and acquired immune pathways are important in asthma, with the activation of each leading to a different pattern of airway inflammation. Evidence from available mechanistic studies suggests that physical activity, antioxidant intake and dietary fat intake can modulate the acquired immune response (Fig. 17.1). Obesity, dietary fat intake and antioxidant intake have been shown to influence the innate immune system. Data describing the effect of dietary fat, adiposity, antioxidants and exercise on clinical asthma outcomes are limited. It is plausible, however, that these factors may each provide useful adjunct asthma therapies. Our understanding of the inflammatory and clinical role of diet and exercise in asthma is improving, but there remains a need for further high-quality trials in order to strengthen the existing evidence base. This will better inform the clinical management of this population.

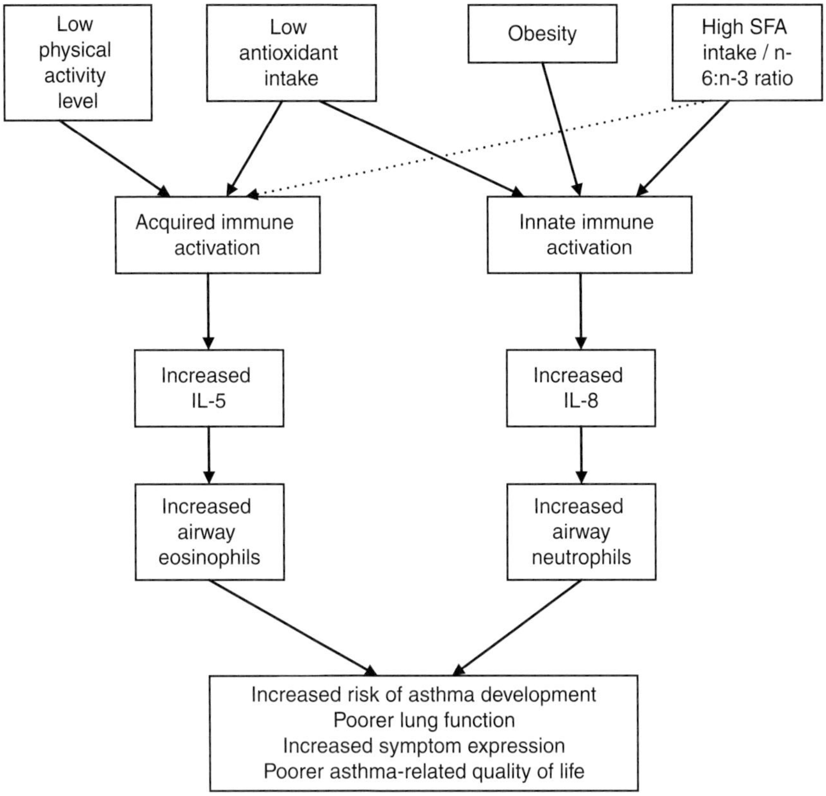

Fig. 17.1. Summary of the hypothesized inflammatory effects of physical activity, antioxidants, obesity and dietary fat intake on inflammation and clinical outcomes in asthma. IL, interleukin; SFA, saturated fatty acid.

References

Aaron, S.D., Fergusson, D., Dent, R., Chen, Y., Vandemheen, K.L. and Dales, R.E. (2004) Effect of Weight Reduction on Respiratory Function and Airway Reactivity in Obese Women. *Chest* 125, 2046–2052.

Ahroni, J.H., Montgomery, K.F. and Watkins, B.M. (2005). Laparoscopic adjustable gastric banding: weight loss, co-morbidities, medication usage and quality of life at one year. *Obesity Surgery* 15, 641–647.

Antova, T., Pattenden, S., Nikiforov, B., Leonardi, G.S., Boeva, B., *et al.* (2003) Nutrition and respiratory health in children in six Central and Eastern European countries. *Thorax* 58, 231–236.

Appleton, S.L., Adams, R.J., Wilson, D.H., Taylor, A.W. and Ruffin, R.E. (2006) Central obesity is associated with nonatopic but not atopic asthma in a representative population sample. *Journal of Allergy and Clinical Immunology* 118, 1284–1291.

Australian Centre for Asthma Monitoring (2007) Asthma in Australia: findings from the 2004–05 National Health Survey. Cat. no. ACM 10. Canberra: Australian Institute of Health and Welfare.

Bakkeheim, E., Mowinckel, P., Carlsen, K.H., Burney, P. and Carlsen, K.C.L. (2011) Altered oxidative state in schoolchildren with asthma and allergic rhinitis. *Pediatric Allergy and Immunology* 22, 178–185.

Beckett, W.S., Jacobs Jr, D.R., Yu, X., Iribarren, C. and Williams, O.D. (2001) Asthma is associated with weight gain in females but not males, independent of physical activity. *American Journal of Respiratory and Critical Care Medicine* 164, 2045–2050.

Benet, M., Varraso, R., Kauffmann, F., Romieu, I., Antó, J.M., *et al.* (2011) The effects of regular physical activity on adult-onset asthma incidence in women. *Respiratory Medicine* 105, 1104–1107.

Berg, C.M., Thelle, D.S., Rosengren, A., Lissner, L., Torén, K., *et al.* (2011) Decreased fraction of exhaled nitric oxide in obese subjects with asthma symptoms. *Chest* 139, 1109–1116.

Berntsen, S., Carlsen, K.C.L., Anderssen, S.A., Mowinckel, P., Hageberg, R., *et al.* (2009) Norwegian adolescents with asthma are physical active and fit. *Allergy* 64, 421–426.

Beuther, D.A. and Sutherland, E.R. (2007) Overweight, obesity, and incident asthma: a meta-analysis of prospective epidemiologic studies. *American Journal of Respiratory and Critical Care Medicine* 175, 661–666.

Biltagi, M.A., Baset, A.A., Bassiouny, M., Kasrawi, M.A. and Attia, M. (2009) Omega-3 fatty acids, vitamin C and Zn supplementation in asthmatic children: a randomized self-controlled study. *Acta Paediatrica* 98, 737–742.

Black, P.N. and Sharpe, S. (1997) Dietary fat and asthma: is there a connection? *European Respiratory Journal* 10, 6–12.

Blackwell, T.S., Blackwell, T.R., Holden, E.P., Christman, B.W. and Christman, J.W. (1996) In Vivo Antioxidant Treatment Suppresses Nuclear Factor-κB Activation and Neutrophilic Lung Inflammation. *The Journal of Immunology* 157, 1630–1637.

Bodner, C., Godden, D., Brown, K., Little, J., Ross, S. *et al.* (1999) Antioxidant intake and adult-onset wheeze: a case±control study. *European Respiratory Journal* 13, 22–30.

Bolte, G., Kompauer, I., Fobker, M., Cullenz, P., Keilk, U., *et al.* (2006) Fatty acids in serum cholesteryl esters in relation to asthma and lung function in children. *Clinical and Experimental Allergy* 36, 293–302.

Boulet, L.-P. and Franssen, E. (2007) Influence of obesity on response to fluticasone with or without salmeterol in moderate asthma. *Respiratory Medicine* 101, 2240–2247.

Broadfield, E.C., Mckeever, T.M., Whitehurst, A., Lewis, S.A., Lawson, N., *et al.* (2004) A case–control study of dietary and erythrocyte membrane fatty acids in asthma. *Clinical and Experimental Allergy* 34, 1232–1236.

Bruno, A., Conus, S., Schmid, I. and Simon, H.-U. (2005) Apoptotic pathways are inhibited by leptin receptor activation in neutrophils. *The Journal of Immunology* 174, 8090–8096.

Busse, W.W. and Lemanske Jr, R.F. (2001) Asthma. *New England Journal of Medicine* 344, 350–362.

Calder, P.C. (1998) Fat chance of immunomodulation. *Immunology Today* 19, 244–247.

Camargo Jr, C.A., Weiss, S.T., Zhang, S., Willett, W.C. and Speizer, F.E. (1999) Prospective study of body mass index, weight change, and risk of adult-onset asthma in women. *Archives of Internal Medicine* 159, 2582–2588.

Carey, I.M., Strachan, D.P. and Cook, D.G. (1998) Effects of changes in fresh fruit consumption on ventilatory function in healthy British adults. *American Journal of Respiratory and Critical Care Medicine* 158, 728–733.

Celedon, J.C., Palmer, L.J., Litonjua, A.A., Weiss, S.T., Wang, B., *et al.* (2001) Body mass index and asthma in adults in families of subjects with asthma in Anqing, China. *American Journal of Respiratory and Critical Care Medicine* 164, 1835–1840.

Chatzi, L., Apostolaki, G., Bibakis, I., Skypala, I., Bibaki-Liakou, V., Tzanakis, N., Kogevinas, M. & Cullinan, P. (2007a) Protective effect of fruits, vegetables and the Mediterranean diet on asthma and allergies among children in Crete. *Thorax,* 62, 677–683.

Chatzi, L., Torrent, M., Romieu, I., Garcia-Esteban, R., Ferrer, C., *et al.* (2007b) Diet, wheeze, and atopy in school children in Menorca, Spain. *Pediatric Allergy and Immunology* 18, 480–485.

Checkley, W., West Jr, K.P., Wise, R.A., Baldwin, M.R., Wu, L., *et al.* (2010) Maternal vitamin A supplementation and lung function in offspring. *New England Journal of Medicine* 362, 1784–1894.

Chen, Y., Dales, R. and Krewski, D. (2001) Leisure-time energy expenditure in asthmatics and non-asthmatics. *Respiratory Medicine,* 95, 13–18.

Chen, Y., Dales, R., Tang, M. and Krewski, D. (2002) Obesity may increase the incidence of asthma in women but not in men: longitudinal observations from the Canadian National Population Health Surveys. *American Journal of Epidemiology* 155, 191–197.

Cheng, B.-L., Huang, Y., Shu, C., Lou, X.-L., Fu, Z. *et al.* (2010) A cross-sectional survey of participation of asthmatic children in physical activity. *World Journal of Pediatrics* 6, 238–243.

Chinn, S., Jarvis, D. and Burney, P. (2002) Relation of bronchial responsiveness to body mass index in the ECRHS. *Thorax* 57, 1028–1033.

Clark, C.J. and Cochrane, L.M. (1988) Assessment of work performance in asthma for determination of cardiorespiratory fitness and training capacity. *Thorax* 43, 745–749.

Cook, D.G., Carey, I.M., Whincup, P.H., Papacosta, O., Chirico, S., *et al.* (1997) Effect of fresh fruit consumption on lung function and wheeze in children. *Thorax* 52, 628–633.

Cordain, L., Eaton, S.B., Sebastian, A., Mann, N., Lindeberg, S., *et al.* (2005) Origins and evolution of the Western diet: health implications for the 21st century. *American Journal of Clinical Nutrition* 81, 341–354.

Cox, G. (1995) Glucocorticoid treatment inhibits apoptosis in human neutrophils. *The Journal of Immunology* 154, 4719–4725.

De Luca, C. and Olefsky, J.M. (2008) Inflammation and insulin resistance. *FEBS Letters* 582, 97–105.

De Vries, A., Hazlewood, L., Fitch, P.M., Seckl, J.R., Foster, P., *et al.* (2009) High-fat feeding redirects cytokine responses and decreases allergic airway eosinophilia. *Clinical and Experimental Allergy* 39, 731–739.

Devereux, G., Turner, S.W., Craig, L.C.A., Mcneill, G., Martindale, S., *et al.* (2006) Low maternal vitamin E intake during pregnancy is associated with asthma in 5-year-old children. *American Journal of Respiratory and Critical Care Medicine* 174, 499–507.

Dixon, A.E., Shade, D.M., Cohen, R.I., Skloot, G.S., Holbrook, J.T., *et al.* (2006) Effect of obesity on clinical presentation and response to treatment in asthma. *Journal of Asthma* 43, 553–558.

Dixon, A.E., Pratley, R.E., Forgione, P.M., Kaminsky, D.A., Whittaker-Leclair, L.A., *et al.* (2011) Effects of obesity and bariatric surgery on airway hyperresponsiveness, asthma control, and inflammation. *Journal of Allergy and Clinical Immunology* 128, 508–515.

Dixon, J.B., Chapman, L. and O'Brien, P. (1999) Marked Improvement in Asthma after Lap-Band® Surgery for Morbid Obesity. *Obesity Surgery* 9, 385–389.

Dogra, S. and Baker, J. (2006) Physical activity and health in Canadian asthmatics. *Journal of Asthma* 43, 795–799.

Douwes, J., Gibson, P., Pekkanen, J. and Pearce, N. (2002) Non-eosinophilic asthma: importance and possible mechanisms. *Thorax* 57, 643–648.

Emtner, M., Herala, M. and Stålenheim, G. (1996) High-intensity physical training in adults with asthma: a 10-week rehabilitation program. *Chest* 109, 323–330.

Eneli, I.U., Skybo, T. and Camargo Jr, C.A. (2008) Weight loss and asthma: a systematic review. *Thorax* 63, 671–676.

Fabian, E., Pölöskey, P., Kósa, L., Elmadfa, I. and Réthy, L.A. (2011) Activities of antioxidant enzymes in relation to oxidative and nitrosative challenges in childhood asthma. *Journal of Asthma* 48, 351–357.

Fahy, J.V. (2009) Eosinophilic and neutrophilic inflammation in asthma. *Proceedings of the American Thoracic Society* 6, 256–259.

Field, C.J., Johnson, I.R. and Schley, P.D. (2002) Nutrients and their role in host resistance to infection. *Journal of Leukocyte Biology* 71, 16–32.

Firrincieli, V., Keller, A., Ehrensberger, R., Platts-Mills, J., Shufflebarger, C., *et al.* (2005) Decreased physical activity among head start children with a history of wheezing: use of an accelerometer to measure activity. *Pediatric Pulmonology* 40, 57–63.

Fogarty, A., Lewis, S., Weiss, S. and Britton, J. (2000) Dietary vitamin E, IgE concentrations, and atopy. *The Lancet* 356, 1573–1574.

Ford, E.S., Heath, G.W., Mannino, D.M. and Redd, S.C. (2003) Leisure-time physical activity patterns among US adults with asthma. *Chest* 124, 432–437.

Ford, E.S., Mannino, D.M. and Redd, S.C. (2004a) Serum antioxidant concentrations among U.S. adults with self-reported asthma. *Journal of Asthma* 41, 179–187.

Ford, E.S., Mannino, D.M., Redd, S.C., Mokdad, A.H. and Mott, J.A. (2004b) Body mass index and asthma incidence among USA adults. *European Respiratory Journal,* 24, 740–744.

Garcia-Aymerich, J., Varraso, R., Antó, J.M. and Camargo Jr, C.A. (2009) Prospective study of physical activity and risk of asthma exacerbations in older women. *American Journal of Respiratory and Critical Care Medicine* 179, 999–1003.

Gibson, P.G., Henry, R.L., Shah, S., Powell, H. and Wang, H. (2003) Migration to a Western country increases asthma symptoms but not eosinophilic airway inflammation. *Pediatric Pulmonology* 36, 209–215.

Gilliland, F.D., Berhane, K.T., Li, Y.-F., Gauderman, W.J., Mcconnell, R., *et al.* (2003) Children's lung function and antioxidant vitamin, fruit, juice, and vegetable intake. *American Journal of Epidemiology* 158, 576–584.

GINA Executive Committee Global Initiative for Asthma: Global strategy for asthma management and prevention, Updated 2010. http://www.ginasthma.com (Accessed July 2011).

Green, R.H., Brightling, C.E., Woltmann, G., Parker, D., Wardlaw, A.J., *et al.* (2002) Analysis of induced sputum in adults with asthma: identification of subgroup with isolated sputum neutrophilia and poor response to inhaled corticosteroids. *Thorax* 57, 875–879.

Greenough, A., Shaheen, S.O., Shennan, A., Seed, P.T. and Poston, L. (2010) Respiratory outcomes in early childhood following antenatal vitamin C and E supplementation. *Thorax* 65, 998–1003.

Grievink, L., Smit, H.A., Ocké, M.C., Van 'T Veer, P. and Kromhout, D. (1998) Dietary intake of antioxidant (pro)-vitamins, respiratory symptoms and pulmonary function: the MORGEN study. *Thorax* 53, 166–171.

Grievink, L., Zijlstra, A.G., Ke, X. and Brunekreef, B. (1999) Double-blind intervention trial on modulation of ozone effects on pulmonary function by antioxidant supplements. *American Journal of Epidemiology* 149, 306–314.

Guénégou, A., Leynaert, B., Pin, I., Le Moël, G., Zureik, M., *et al.* (2006) Serum carotenoids, vitamins A and E, and 8 year lung function decline in a general population. *Thorax* 61, 320–326.

Guerra, S., Sherrill, D.L., Bobadilla, A., Martinez, F.D. and Barbee, R.A. (2002) The relation of body mass index to asthma, chronic bronchitis, and emphysema. *Chest* 122, 1256–1263.

Gurkan, F., Atamer, Y., Ece, A., Kocyigit, Y., Tuzun, H., *et al.* (2004) Serum leptin levels in asthmatic children treated with an inhaled corticosteroid. *Annals of Allergy, Asthma and Immunology* 93, 277–280.

Haines, D.D., Varga, B., Bak, I., Juhasz, B., Mahmoud, F.F., *et al.* (2011) Summative interaction between astaxanthin, Ginkgo biloba Extract (EGb761) and Vitamin C in suppression of respiratory inflammation: A comparison with ibuprofen. *Phytotherapy Research* 25, 128–136.

Hakala, K., Stenius-Aarniala, B. and Sovijärvi, A. (2000) Effects of weight loss on peak flow variability, airways obstruction, and lung volumes in obese patients with asthma. *Chest* 118, 1315–1321.

Haldar, P., Pavord, I.D., Shaw, D.E., Berry, M.A., Thomas, M., *et al.* (2008) Cluster analysis and clinical asthma phenotypes. *American Journal of Respiratory and Critical Care Medicine* 178, 218–224.

Harik-Khan, R.I., Muller, D.C. and Wise, R.A. (2004) Serum vitamin levels and the risk of asthma in children. *American Journal of Epidemiology* 159, 351–357.

Hazlewood, L.C., Wood, L.G., Hansbro, P.M. and Foster, P.S. (2011) Dietary lycopene supplementation suppresses Th2 responses and lung eosinophilia in a mouse model of allergic asthma. *The Journal of Nutritional Biochemistry* 22, 95–100.

Hewitt, M., Creel, A., Estell, K., Davis, I.C. and Schwiebert, L.M. (2009) Acute exercise decreases airway inflammation, but not responsiveness, in an allergic asthma model. *American Journal of Respiratory Cell and Molecular Biology* 40, 83–89.

Hodge, L., Salome, C.M., Peat, J.K., Haby, M.M., Xuan, W., *et al.* (1996) Consumption of oily fish and childhood asthma risk. *The Medical Journal of Australia* 164, 137–140.

Horváth, I., Donnelly, L.E., Kiss, A., Kharitonov, S.A., Lim, S., *et al.* (1998) Combined use of exhaled hydrogen peroxide and nitric oxide in monitoring asthma. *American Journal of Respiratory and Critical Care Medicine* 158, 1042–1046.

Hu, G. and Cassano, P.A. (2000) Antioxidant nutrients and pulmonary function: The Third National Health and Nutrition Examination Survey (NHANES III). *American Journal of Epidemiology* 151, 975–981.

Hu, G., Zhang, X., Chen, J., Peto, R., Campbell, T.C., *et al.* (1998) Dietary vitamin C intake and lung function in rural China. *American Journal of Epidemiology* 148, 594–599.

Huang, S. and Pan, W. (2001) Dietary fats and asthma in teenagers: analyses of the first Nutrition and Health Survey in Taiwan (NAHSIT). *Clinical and Experimental Allergy* 31, 1875–1880.

Huovinen, E., Kaprio, J. and Koskenvuo, M. (2003) Factors associated to lifestyle and risk of adult onset asthma. *Respiratory Medicine* 97, 273–280.

Jeukendrup, A.E., Vet-Joop, K., Sturk, A., Stegen, J., Senden, J., *et al.* (2000) Relationship between gastrointestinal complaints and endotoxaemia, cytokine release and the acute-phase reaction during and after a long-distance triathlon in highly trained men. *Clinical Science* 98, 47–55.

Jia, S.H., Li, Y., Parodo, J., Kapus, A., Fan, L., *et al.* (2004) Pre-B cell colony-enhancing factor inhibits neutrophil apoptosis in experimental inflammation and clinical sepsis. *The Journal of Clinical Investigation* 113, 1318–1327.

Johnson, J.B., Summer, W., Cutler, R.G., Martin, B., Hyun, D.-H., *et al.* (2007) Alternate day calorie restriction improves clinical findings and reduces markers of oxidative stress and inflammation in overweight adults with moderate asthma. *Free Radical Biology and Medicine* 42, 665–674.

Kaser, S., Tatarczyk, T., Stadlmayr, A., Ciardi, C., Ress, C., *et al.* (2008) Effect of obesity and insulin sensitivity on adiponectin isoform distribution. *European Journal of Clinical Investigation* 38, 827–834.

Katsoulis, K., Kontakiotis, T., Leonardopoulos, I., Kotsovili, A., Legakis, I.N., *et al.* (2003) Serum total antioxidant status in severe exacerbation of asthma: correlation with the severity of the disease. *Journal of Asthma* 40, 847–854.

Katsumata, U., Miura, M., Ichinose, M., Kimura, K., Takahashi, T., *et al.* (1990) Oxygen radicals produce airway constriction and hyperresponsiveness in anesthetized cats. *American Review of Respiratory Disease* 141, 1158–1161.

Kaur, B., Rowe, B. and Arnold, E. (2009) Vitamin C supplementation for asthma. Cochrane Database of Systematic Reviews 2009, Issue 1. Art. No.: CD000993. DOI: 10.1002/14651858.CD000993.pub3.

Kelly, F.J., Mudway, I., Blomberg, A., Frew, A. and Sandström, T. (1999) Altered lung antioxidant status in patients with mild asthma. *The Lancet* 354, 482–483.

Komakula, S., Khatri, S., Mermis, J., Savill, S., Haque, S., *et al.* (2007) Body mass index is associated with reduced exhaled nitric oxide and higher exhaled 8-isoprostanes in asthmatics. *Respiratory Research* 8, 32.

Kris-Etherton, P.M., Pearson, T.A., Wan, Y., Hargrove, R.L., Moriarty, K., *et al.* (1999) High-monounsaturated fatty acid diets lower both plasma cholesterol and triacylglycerol concentrations. *The American Journal of Clinical Nutrition* 70, 1009–1015.

Kronander, U.N., Falkenberg, M. and Zetterström, O. (2004) Prevalence and incidence of asthma related to waist circumference and BMI in a Swedish community sample. *Respiratory Medicine* 98, 1108–1116.

Lago, F., Dieguez, C., Gómez-Reino, J. and Gualillo, O. (2007) Adipokines as emerging mediators of immune response and inflammation. *Nature Clinical Practice Rheumatology* 3, 716–724.

Lee, J.Y. and Hwang, D.A. (2006) The modulation of inflammatory gene expression by lipids: mediation through Toll-like receptors. *Molecules and Cells* 21, 174–185.

Lee, J.Y., Zhao, L., Youn, H.S., Weatherill, A.R., Tapping, R., *et al.* (2004) Saturated fatty acid activates but polyunsaturated fatty acid inhibits Toll-like receptor 2 dimerized with Toll-like receptor 6 or 1. *The Journal of Biological Chemistry* 279, 16971–16979.

Lessard, A., Turcotte, H., Cormier, Y. and Boulet, L.-P. (2008) Obesity and asthma: A specific phenotype? *Chest* 134, 317–323.

Litonjua, A.A., Sparrow, D., Celedon, J.C., Demolles, D. and Weiss, S.T. (2002) Association of body mass index with the development of methacholine airway hyperresponsiveness in men: the Normative Aging Study. *Thorax* 57, 581–585.

Litonjua, A.A., Rifas-Shiman, S.L., Ly, N.P., Tantisira, K.G., Rich-Edwards, J.W., *et al.* (2006) Maternal antioxidant intake in pregnancy and wheezing illnesses in children at 2 y of age. *The American Journal of Clinical Nutrition* 84, 903–911.

Loebroks, A., Apfelbacher, C.J., Amelang, M. and Stürmer, T. (2008) Obesity and Adult Asthma: Potential Effect Modification by Gender, But Not by Hay Fever. *Annals of Epidemiology* 18, 283–289.

Macdougald, O.A. and Burant, C.F. (2007) The rapidly expanding family of adipokines. *Cell Metabolism* 6, 159–161.

Macgregor, A.M.C. and Greenberg, R.A. (1993) Effect of surgically induced weight loss on asthma in the morbidly obese. *Obesity Surgery* 3, 15–21.

Maniscalco, M., Zeddaa, A., Faraonea, S., Cerbonec, M.R., Cristianoc, S., *et al.* (2008) Weight loss and asthma control in severely obese asthmatic females. *Respiratory Medicine* 102, 102–108.

Marks, G.B., Mihrshahi, S., Kemp, A.S., Tovey, E.R., Webb, K., *et al.* & For the Childhood Asthma Prevention Study Team (2006) Prevention of asthma during the first 5 years of life: A randomized controlled trial. *Journal of Allergy and Clinical Immunology* 118, 53–61.

Masoli, M., Fabian, D., Holt, S., Beasley, R. & For the Global Initiative for Asthma (GINA) Program (2004) The global burden of asthma: executive summary of the GINA Dissemination Committee Report. *Allergy* 59, 469–478.

Mcfadden Jr, E.R. & Gilbert, I.A. (1994) Exercise-Induced Asthma. *The New England Journal of Medicine,* 330, 1362-1367.

Mckeever, T.M., Lewis, S.A., Cassano, P.A., Ocké, M., Burney, P., *et al.* (2008a) The relation between dietary intake of individual fatty acids, FEV1 and respiratory disease in Dutch adults. *Thorax* 63, 208–214.

Mckeever, T.M., Lewis, S.A., Smit, H.A., Burney, P., Cassano, P.A., *et al.* (2008b) A multivariate analysis of serum nutrient levels and lung function. *Respiratory Research* 9, 67.

Medoff, B.D., Okamoto, Y., Leyton, P., Meiqian, Sandall, B.P., Raher, M.J., *et al.* (2009) Adiponectin deficiency increases allergic airway inflammation and pulmonary vascular remodelling. *American Journal of Respiratory Cell and Molecular Biology* 41, 397–406.

Melbye, H., Halvorsen, D.S., Hartz, I., Medbø, A., Brox, J., *et al.* (2007) Bronchial airflow limitation, smoking, body mass index, and statin use are strongly associated with the C-reactive protein level in the elderly. The Tromsø Study 2001. *Respiratory Medicine* 101, 2541–2549.

Mendes, F.a.R., Almeida, F.A., Cukier, A., Stelmach, R., Jacob-Filho, W., *et al.* (2011) Effects of aerobic training on airway inflammation in asthmatic patients. *Medicine and Science in Sports and Exercise* 43, 197–203.

Mihrshahi, S., Peat, J.K., Webb, K., Oddy, W., Marks, G.B., *et al.* & For the Caps Team (2004) Effect of omega-3 fatty acid concentrations in plasma on symptoms of asthma at 18 months of age. *Pediatric Allergy and Immunology* 15, 517–522.

Misso, N.L.A., Brooks-Wildhaber, J., Ray, S., Vally, H. and Thompson, P.J. (2005) Plasma concentrations of dietary and nondietary antioxidants are low in severe asthma. *European Respiratory Journal* 26, 257–264.

Miyake, Y., Sasakiw, S., Arakawaz, M., Tanaka, K., Murakami, K., *et al.* (2008) Fatty acid intake and asthma symptoms in Japanese children: The Ryukyus Child Health Study. *Clinical and Experimental Allergy* 38, 1644–1650.

Miyamoto, S., Miyake, Y., Sasaki, S., Tanaka, K., Ohya, Y., *et al.* Osaka Maternal and Child Health Study Group (2007) Fat and fish intake and asthma in Japanese women: baseline data from the Osaka Maternal and Child Health Study. *The International Journal of Tuberculosis and Lung Disease* 11, 103–109.

Morabia, A., Menkes, M.J.S., Comstock, G.W. and Tockman, M.S. (1990) Serum retinol and airway obstruction. *American Journal of Epidemiology* 132, 77–82.

Murray, C.S., Simpson, B., Kerry, G., Woodcock, A. and Custovic, A. (2006) Dietary intake in sensitized children with recurrent wheeze and healthy controls: a nested case–control study. *Allergy* 61, 438–442.

Nadeem, A., Masood, A. and Siddiqui, N. (2008) Oxidant-antioxidant imbalance in asthma: scientific evidence, epidemiological data and possible therapeutic options. *Therapeutic Advances in Respiratory Disease* 2, 215–235.

Nagel, G., Koenig, W., Rapp, K., Wabitsch, M., Zoellner, I. *et al.* (2009) Associations of adipokines with asthma, rhinoconjunctivitis, and eczema in German schoolchidren. *Pediatric Allergy and Immunology* 20, 81–88.

National Heart Foundation of Australia (2009) *Summary of Evidence: Dietary Fats and Dietary Cholesterol for Cardiovascular Health.* National Heart Foundation of Australia.

National Heart Lung and Blood Institute (2007) National Asthma Education and Prevention Program Expert Panel Report 3: guidelines for the diagnosis and management of asthma. National Heart, Lung, and Blood Institute, Bethesda.

Neder, J.A., Nery, L.E., Silva, A.C., Cabral, A.L.B. and Fernandes, A.L.G. (1999) Short term effects of aerobic training in the clinical management of moderate to severe asthma in children. *Thorax* 54, 202–206.

Nelson, W.K., Fatima, J., Houghton, S.G., Thompson, G.B., Kendrick, M.L., *et al.* (2006) The malabsorptive very, very long limb Roux-en-Y gastric bypass for super obesity: Results in 257 patients. *Surgery* 140, 517–523.

Nystad, W., Nafstad, P. and Harris, J.R. (2001) Physical activity affects the prevalence of reported wheeze. *European Journal of Epidemiology* 17, 209–212.

Okoko, B.J., Burney, P.G., Newson, R.B., Potts, J.F. and Shaheen, S.O. (2007) Childhood asthma and fruit consumption. *European Respiratory Journal* 29, 1161–1168.

Okuda, M., Bando, N., Terao, J., Sasaki, S., Sugiyama, S., *et al.* (2010) Association of serum carotenoids and tocopherols with atopic diseases in Japanese children and adolescents. *Pediatric Allergy and Immunology* 21, e705–e710.

Ownby, D.R., Peterson, E.L., Nelson, D., Joseph, C.C.L., *et al.* (2007) The relationship of physical activity and percentage of body fat to the risk of asthma in 8- to 10-year-old children. *Journal of Asthma* 44, 885–889.

Paeratakul, S., Popkin, B.M., Keyou, G., Adair, L.S. and Stevens, J. (1998) Changes in diet and physical activity affect the body mass index of Chinese adults. *International Journal of Obesity* 22, 424–431.

Patel, S.D., Rajala, M.W., Rossetti, L., Scherer, P.E. and Shapiro, L. (2004) Disulfide-dependent multimeric assembly of resistin family hormones. *Science* 304, 1154–1158.

Pearce, N., Pekkanen, J. and Beasley, R. (1999) How much asthma is really attributable to atopy? *Thorax* 54, 268–272.

Pearson, P.J.K., Lewis, S.A., Britton, J. and Fogarty, A. (2004) Vitamin E supplements in asthma: a parallel group randomised placebo controlled trial. *Thorax* 59, 652–656.

Pereg, D., Tirosh, A., Lishner, M., Goldberg, A., Shochat, T., *et al.* (2008) Prevalence of asthma in a large group of Israeli adolescents: influence of country of birth and age at migration. *Allergy* 63, 1040–1045.

Peters-Golden, M., Swern, A., Bird, S.S., Hustad, C.M., Grant, E., *et al.* (2006) Influence of body mass index on the response to asthma controller agents. *European Respiratory Journal* 27, 495–503.
Rahman, I., Morrison, D., Donaldson, K. and Macnee, W. (1996) Systemic oxidative stress in asthma, COPD, and smokers. *American Journal of Respiratory and Critical Care Medicine* 154, 1055–1060.
Ram, F.S.F., Robinson, S., Black, P.N. and Picot, J. (2005) Physical training for asthma. *Cochrane Database of Systematic Reviews* 2005, Issue 4. Art. No.: CD001116. DOI: 10.1002/14651858.CD001116.pub2.
Rasmussen, F., Lambrechtsen, J., Siersted, H.C., Hansen, H.S. and Hansen, N.C.G. (2000) Low physical fitness in childhood is associated with the development of asthma in young adulthood: the Odense schoolchild study. *European Respiratory Journal* 16, 866–870.
Rodríguez-Rodríguez, E., Perea, J.M., Jiménez, A.I., Rodríguez-Rodríguez, P., López-Sobaler, A.M., *et al.* (2010) Fat intake and asthma in Spanish schoolchildren. *European Journal of Clinical Nutrition* 64, 1065–1071.
Romieu, I., Meneses, F., Ramirez, M., Ruiz, S., Perez Padilla, R., *et al.* (1998) Antioxidant supplementation and respiratory functions among workers exposed to high levels of ozone. *American Journal of Respiratory and Critical Care Medicine* 158, 226–232.
Romieu, I., Sienra-Monge, J.J., Ramirez-Aguilar, M., Tellez-Rojo, M.M., Moreno-Macias, H., *et al.* (2002) Antioxidant supplementation and lung functions among children with asthma exposed to high levels of air pollutants. *American Journal of Respiratory and Critical Care Medicine* 166, 703–709.
Rubin, R.N., Navon, L. and Cassano, P.A. (2004) Relationship of serum antioxidants to asthma prevalence in youth. *American Journal of Respiratory and Critical Care Medicine* 169, 393–398.
Sagai, M., Furuyama, A. and Ichinose, T. (1996) Biological effects of diesel exhaust particles (DEP). III. Pathogenesis of asthma like symptoms in mice. *Free Radical Biology and Medicine* 21, 199–209.
Saleh, D., Ernst, P., Lim, S., Barnes, P.J. and Giad, A. (1998) Increased formation of the potent oxidant peroxynitrite in the airways of asthmatic patients is associated with induction of nitric oxide synthase: effect of inhaled glucocorticoid. *The Journal of the Federation of American Societies for Experimental Biology* 12, 929–937.
Schubert, R., Kitz, R., Beermann, C., Rose, M.A., Lieb, A., *et al.* (2009) Effect of n-3 polyunsaturated fatty acids in asthma after low-dose allergen challenge. *International Archives of Allergy and Immunology* 148, 321–329.
Schünemann, H.J., Muti, P., Freudenheim, J.L., Armstrong, D., Browne, R., *et al.* (1997) Oxidative stress and lung function. *American Journal of Epidemiology* 146, 939–948.
Schünemann, H.J., Brydon, J.B., Freudenheim, J.L., Muti, P., Browne, R.W., *et al.* (2001) The relation of serum levels of antioxidant vitamins C and E, retinol and carotenoids with pulmonary function in the general population. *American Journal of Respiratory and Critical Care Medicine* 163, 1246–1255.
Scott, H.A., Gibson, P.G., Garg, M.L. and Wood, L.G. (2011) Airway inflammation is augmented by obesity and fatty acids in asthma. *European Respiratory Journal* 38, 594–602.
Seaton, A., Godden, D.J. and Brown, K. (1994) Increase in asthma: a more toxic environment or a more susceptible population? *Thorax* 49, 171–174.
Shaaban, R., Leynaert, B., Soussan, D., Antó, J.M., Chinn, S., *et al.* (2007) Physical activity and bronchial hyperresponsiveness: European Community Respiratory Health Survey II. *Thorax* 62, 403–410.
Shahar, E., Folsom, A.R., Melnick, S.L., Tockman, M.S., Comstock, G.W., *et al.* (1994) Does dietary vitamin A protect against airway obstruction? *American Journal of Respiratory and Critical Care Medicine* 150, 978–982.
Shaheen, S.O., Sterne, J.a.C., Montgomery, S.M. and Azima, H. (1999) Birth weight, body mass index and asthma in young adults. *Thorax* 54, 396–402.
Shaheen, S.O., Sterne, J.a.C., Thompson, R.L., Songhurst, C.A., Margetts, B.M., *et al.* (2001) Dietary antioxidants and asthma in adults: population-based case–control study. *American Journal of Respiratory and Critical Care Medicine* 164, 1823–1828.
Shi, H. and Clegg, D.J. (2009) Sex differences in the regulation of body weight. *Physiology and Behavior* 97, 199–204.
Shore, S.A., Terry, R.D., Flynt, L., Xu, A. and Hug, C. (2006) Adiponectin attenuates allergen-induced airway inflammation and hyperresponsiveness in mice. *Journal of Allergy and Clinical Immunology* 118, 389–395.
Simard, B., Turcotte, H., Marceau, P., Biron, S., Hould, F.S., *et al.* (2004) Asthma and sleep apnea in patients with morbid obesity: outcome after bariatric surgery. *Obesity Surgery* 14, 1381–1388.
Simopoulos, A.P. (2002) The importance of the ratio of omega-6/omega-3 essential fatty acids. *Biomedicine and Pharmacotherapy* 56, 365–379.

Simpson, J.L., Scott, R.J., Boyle, M.J. and Gibson, P.G. (2006) Inflammatory subtypes in asthma: assessment and identification using induced sputum. *Respirology* 11, 54–61.
Simpson, J.L., Grissell, T.V., Douwes, J., Scott, R.J., Boyle, M.J., *et al.* (2007) Innate immune activation in neutrophilic asthma and bronchiectasis. *Thorax* 62, 211–218.
Sin, D.D., Jones, R.L. and Man, S.F.P. (2002) Obesity is a risk factor for dyspnea but not for airflow obstruction. *Archives of Internal Medicine* 162, 1477–1481.
Slade, R., Crissman, K., Norwood, J. and Hatch, G. (1993) Comparison of antioxidant substances in bronchoalveolar lavage cells and fluid from humans, guinea pigs, and rats. *Experimental Lung Research* 19, 469–484.
Sood, A., Cui, X., Qualls, C., Beckett, W.S., Gross, M.D., *et al.* (2008) Association between asthma and serum adiponectin concentration in women. *Thorax* 63, 877–882.
Sood, A., Ford, E.S. and Camargo Jr, C.A. (2006) Association between leptin and asthma in adults. *Thorax* 61, 300–305.
Soutar, A., Seaton, A. and Brown, K. (1997) Bronchial reactivity and dietary antioxidants. *Thorax* 52, 166–170.
Spivak, H., Hewitt, M.F., Onn, A. and Half, E.E. (2005) Weight loss and improvement of obesity-related illness in 500 U.S. patients following laparoscopic adjustable gastric banding procedure. *The American Journal of Surgery* 189, 27–32.
Stenius-Aarniala, B., Poussa, T., Kvarnström, J., Grönlund, E.-L., Ylikahri, M., *et al.* (2000) Immediate and long term effects of weight reduction in obese people with asthma: randomised controlled study. *BMJ* 320, 827–832.
Ström, K., Janzon, L., Mattisson, I., Rosberg, H.E. and Arborelius, M. (1996) Asthma but not smoking-related airflow limitation is associated with a high fat diet in men: results from the population study "Men born in 1914", Malmö, Sweden. *Monaldi Archives for Chest Disease* 51, 16–21.
Sultan, S., Parikh, M., Youn, H., Kurian, M., Fielding, G., *et al.* (2009) Early U.S. outcomes after laparoscopic adjustable gastric banding in patients with a body mass index less than 35 kg/m^2. *Surgical Endoscopy* 23, 1569–1573.
Sutherland, E.R., Goleva, E., Strand, M., Beuther, D.A. and Leung, D.Y.M. (2008a) Body mass and glucocorticoid response in asthma. *American Journal of Respiratory and Critical Care Medicine* 178, 682–687.
Sutherland, T.J.T., Cowan, J.O., Young, S., Goulding, A., Grant, A.M., *et al.* (2008b) The association between obesity and asthma: interactions between systemic and airway inflammation. *American Journal of Respiratory and Critical Care Medicine,* 178, 469–475.
Tabak, C., Wijga, A.H., De Meer, G., Janssen, N.a.H., Brunekreef, B., *et al.* (2006) Diet and asthma in Dutch school children (ISAAC-2). *Thorax* 61, 1048–1053.
Teramoto, M. and Moonie, S. (2011) Physical activity participation among adult Nevadans with self-reported asthma. *Journal of Asthma* 48, 517–522.
Teran, L.M. (1999) Chemokines and IL-5: major players of eosinophil recruitment in asthma. *Clinical and Experimental Allergy* 29, 287–290.
Thomson, C.C., Clark, S., Camargo Jr, C.A. and On Behalf of the Marc Investigators (2003) Body mass index and asthma severity among adults presenting to the emergency department. *Chest* 124, 795–802.
Thyagarajan, B., Meyer, K.A., Smith, L.J., Beckett, W.S., Williams, O.D., *et al.* (2011) Serum carotenoid concentrations predict lung function evolution in young adults: the coronary artery risk development in young adults (CARDIA) Study. *American Journal of Clinical Nutrition* 94, 1211–1218.
Todd, D.C., Armstrong, S., D'silva, L., Allen, C.J., Hargreave, F.E., *et al.* (2007) Effect of obesity on airway inflammation: a cross-sectional analysis of body mass index and sputum cell counts. *Clinical and Experimental Allergy* 37, 1049–1054.
Turner, D., Steinhart, A.H. and Griffiths, A.M. (2008) Omega 3 fatty acids (fish oil) for maintenance of remission in ulcerative colitis. *Cochrane Database of Systematic Reviews* 2007, Issue 3. Art. No.: CD006443. DOI: 10.1002/14651858.CD006443.pub2.
Van Veen, I.H., Ten Brinke, A., Sterk, P.J., Rabe, K.F. and Bel, E.H. (2008) Airway inflammation in obese and nonobese patients with difficult-to-treat asthma. *Allergy* 63, 570–574.
Vieira, R.P., Claudino, R.C., Duarte, A.C.L.S., Santos, A.N.B.G., Perini, A., *et al.* (2007) Aerobic exercise decreases chronic allergic lung inflammation and airway remodeling in mice. *American Journal of Respiratory and Critical Care Medicine* 176, 871–877.
Vieira, R.P., De Andrade, V.F., Duarte, A.C.S., Dos Santos, Â.B.G., Mauad, T., *et al.* (2008) Aerobic conditioning and allergic pulmonary inflammation in mice. II. Effects on lung vascular and parenchymal

inflammation and remodeling. *American Journal of Physiology - Lung Cellular and Molecular Physiology* 295, L670–L679.

Von Schacky, C. (2010) Omega-3 fatty acids vs. cardiac disease-the contribution of the omega-3 index. *Cell and Molecular Biology* 56, 93–101.

Vortmann, M. and Eisner, M.D. (2008) BMI and health status among adults with asthma. *Obesity* 16, 146–152.

Wagner, J.G., Jiang, Q., Harkema, J.R., Ames, B.N., Illek, B., *et al.* (2007) γ-Tocopherol prevents airway eosinophilia and mucous cell hyperplasia in experimentally induced allergic rhinitis and asthma. *Clinical and Experimental Allergy* 38, 501–511.

Wang, H.-Y., Wong, G.W.K., Chen, Y.-Z., Ferguson, A.C., Greene, J.M., *et al.* (2008) Prevalence of asthma among Chinese adolescents living in Canada and in China. *Canadian Medical Association Journal* 179, 1133–1142.

Wanger, J., Clausen, J.L., Coates, A., Pedersen, O.F., Brusasco, V., *et al.* (2005) Standardisation of the measurement of lung volumes. *European Respiratory Journal* 26, 511–522.

Wark, P.a.B. and Gibson, P.G. (2006) Asthma exacerbations · 3: Pathogenesis *Thorax* 61, 909–915.

Weisgerber, M., Webber, K., Meurer, J., Danduran, M., Berger, S., *et al.* (2008) Moderate and vigorous exercise programs in children with asthma: safety, parental satisfaction, and asthma outcomes. *Pediatric Pulmonology* 43, 1175–1182.

Wong, T.W., Yu, T.S., Wang, X.R. and Robinson, P. (2001) Predicted maximal oxygen uptake in normal Hong Kong Chinese schoolchildren and those with respiratory diseases. *Pediatric Pulmonology* 31, 126–132.

Wood, L.G. and Gibson, P.G. (2009) Dietary factors lead to innate immune activation in asthma. *Pharmacology and Therapeutics,* 123, 37–53.

Wood, L.G., Gibson, P.G. and Garg, M.L. (2003) Biomarkers of lipid peroxidation, airway inflammation and asthma. *European Respiratory Journal* 21, 177–186.

Wood, L.G., Garg, M.L., Blake, R.J., Garcia-Caraballo, S. and Gibson, P.G. (2005) Airway and circulating levels of carotenoids in asthma and healthy controls. *Journal of the American College of Nutrition* 24, 448–455.

Wood, L.G., Garg, M.L., Powell, H. and Gibson, P.G. (2008) Lycopene-rich treatments modify noneosinophilic airway inflammation in asthma: Proof of concept. *Free Radical Research* 42, 94–102.

Wood, L.G., Baines, K.J., Fu, J., Scott, H.A. and Gibson, P.G. (2011a) The neutrophilic inflammatory phenotype is associated with systemic inflammation in asthma. *Chest,* in press.

Wood, L.G., Garg, M.L. and Gibson, P.G. (2011b) A high-fat challenge increases airway inflammation and impairs bronchodilator recovery in asthma. *Journal of Allergy and Clinical Immunology* 127, 1133–1140.

Woods, R.K., Raven, J.M., Walters, E.H., Abramson, M J. and Thien, F.C.K. (2004) Fatty acid levels and risk of asthma in young adults. *Thorax* 59, 105–110.

Zarkesh-Esfahani, H., Pockley, A.G., Wu, Z., Hellewell, P.G., Weetman, A.P., *et al.* (2004) Leptin indirectly activates human neutrophils *via* induction of TNF-α. *The Journal of Immunology* 172, 1809–1814.

18 Inflammatory Bowel Disease and Inflammation

L.R. Ferguson*
Discipline of Nutrition, The University of Auckland, New Zealand; Nutrigenomics, New Zealand

Introduction

Crohn's disease (CD) and ulcerative colitis (UC) are two forms of inflammatory bowel diseases (IBD), a group of chronic, episodic inflammatory conditions of the large and small intestines. The two forms of the disease differ primarily in their location and severity. CD is more severe and can affect any part of the gastrointestinal tract, whereas UC is restricted to the colon and the rectum. Both forms of the disease have profound effects on quality of life, and their incidence and prevalence has been increasing in recent years. For

* Author, l.ferguson@auckland.ac.nz

example, whereas paediatric IBD was considered to be relatively rare in New Zealand in the 1960s, it is now much more common, particularly in parts of the South Island (Yap *et al.*, 2008). Both innate and adaptive immune responses are thought to play a role in inflammation in IBD. A particular type of T helper cells, known as Th17, seem critical to this response (Abraham and Cho, 2009).

Nutrition plays a complex role in both forms of IBD. It might play a causal role, interacting with various other factors in contributing to disease susceptibility (Amre *et al.*, 2007; D'Souza *et al.*, 2008). Around 100 susceptibility genes have been identified to date, some common across both diseases and others specific to one or other form (Anderson *et al.*, 2010; Franke *et al.*, 2010). It seems that either the presence or absence of certain dietary components, together with components of the gut-associated microbial ecosystem (microbiome) (Goodman *et al.*, 2009; Turnbaugh *et al.*, 2009; Goodman and Gordon, 2010) provide environmental triggers for the development, and also affect the course, of the disease (Persson *et al.*, 1993; Kugathasan *et al.*, 2007; Bernstein *et al.*, 2008; D'Souza *et al.*, 2008; Yamamoto *et al.*, 2009; Haller *et al.*, 2010; Triggs *et al.*, 2010) (Fig. 18.1). Nutrition may provide a primary therapy for active disease, and maintenance of remission (Akobeng, 2008; Buchanan *et al.*, 2009; Gassull, 2009; Kuriyama *et al.*, 2009; Coeffier *et al.*, 2010). Conversely, certain dietary items in certain patients may lead to a flare-up of symptoms (Triggs *et al.*, 2010). Because many patients become malnourished during the course of the disease, other nutritional support may also be required (Valentini *et al.*, 2008; Conklin and Oliva-Hemker, 2010).

Physical activity may also play a role in IBD susceptibility, although data are not extensive or consistent (Sonnenberg, 1990; Narula and Fedorak, 2008). There has been a general belief that the health of IBD patients will benefit from regular exercise, potentially reducing stress and some disease symptoms (Ball, 1998; Ng *et al.*, 2006; Moreno *et al.*, 2007; Narula and Fedorak, 2008; Packer *et al.*, 2010). An ongoing programme of physical activity (PA) has been suggested to improve bone mineral density, immunological response and psychological health. Some IBD patients might, however, be restricted as to the nature of exercise they are able to perform (Brevinge *et al.*, 1995).

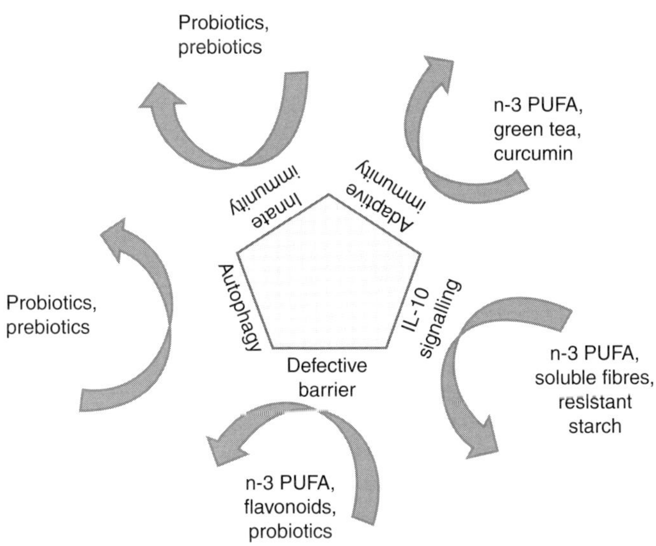

Fig. 18.1. Potential gene–diet interactions in IBD. The five main gene pathways associated with IBD, and examples of various nutrients, identified in the text, that may interact with these. IL, interleukin; PUFA, polyunsaturated fatty acid.

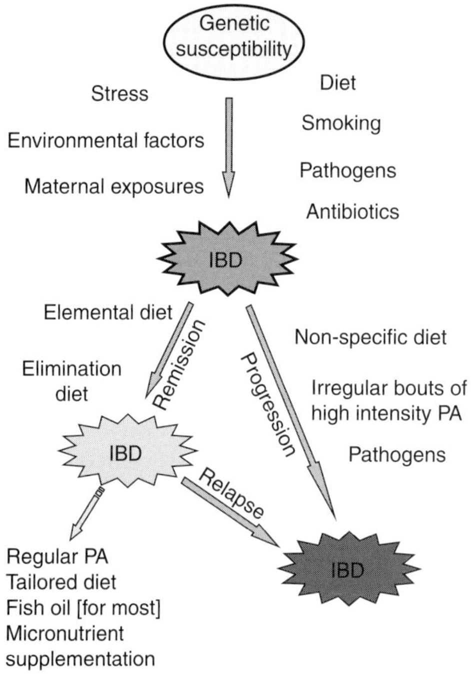

Fig. 18.2. Points at which nutrition and physical activity may impact on IBD risk and disease progression. PA, physical activity.

This chapter will consider the role of both diet and exercise in the development and progression of the disease. An illustration of potential interactions is provided in Fig. 18.2. Several recent area-specific reviews are already available and examples are highlighted in Table 18.1.

The Nature of Inflammation in IBD

Inflammation is a normal cellular response to some sort of exogenous stimulus, such as a chemical insult or bacterial pathogen, working through the immune system (Ferguson and Laing, 2010). Immune responses can be divided into innate immunity and adaptive immunity, which interact at different levels to modify immune response. There are two types of adaptive immunity. Humoral immunity involves the production of antibodies by B cells, whereas in cell-mediated immunity, $CD8^+$ cytotoxic T (Tc) cells and $CD4^+$ helper T cells (Th) are the main cell types. Th cells, depending on the signals they receive, can differentiate into Th1, Th2, Th17, Treg cells and other cell types with specific actions. Th cells can become activated when they come into contact with a molecule attached to the surface of antigen-presenting cells. Early studies on Th cells focussed on Th1 and Th2. A subset of Th cells, known as Th17, have emerged, however, as critical players in inflammation in IBD (Abraham and Cho, 2009; Dambacher *et al.*, 2009; Koenders and Van Den Berg, 2010).

Th17 cells are distinct from other subsets of Th cells as they specifically express the cytokine IL-17, thereby differentiating them from interferon gamma (IFN-γ) producing Th1 cells, or IL-4 producing Th2 cells. Th17 cells also produce IL-6, IL-21, IL-22, IL-23, IL-26 and various chemokines (Liang *et al.*, 2006; Nurieva *et al.*, 2007; Wilson *et al.*, 2007). It seems that Th17 cells are positively regulated by the expression of IL-23 from antigen-presenting cells (Langrish *et al.*, 2005; Kobayashi *et al.*, 2008). Expression of the gene encoding IL-23 is particularly affected in IBD (Ferguson *et al.*, 2010a).

Nutritional Aspects of IBD

Nutrition in the epidemiology of IBD

Data from several case-control studies are available. For example, Bernstein and co-workers (Bernstein *et al.*, 2006) performed an age, gender and geographic residence matched case-control study on IBD risk factors, on the basis of cases drawn from the population-based University of Manitoba IBD Research Registry and controls from the population-based Manitoba Health Registry. They reported that dietary risk factors for either form of the disease included having drunk unpasteurized milk or having eaten pork. D'Sousa *et al.* (2008) also did a case-control study across three tertiary hospitals in Canada. They sought to assess pre-disease diet and to determine gender-specific dietary patterns and assess associated risks for CD. They established several risk patterns. In

Table 18.1. Examples of recent systematic reviews relevant to nutrition and physical activity in IBD.

Year of publication	Topic	Scope	Endpoint	Reference
2009	Epidemiology of causes	Dietary risk factors and the therapeutic efficacy of nutritional interventions	IBD	Yamamoto *et al.*, 2009
2010	Epidemiology of causes	Microbial ecology, human genetics, and immune responses. Also exogenous infections, use of antibiotics and diet	IBD	Bernstein, 2010
2010	Epidemiology of causes	Dietary causes	IBD	Chapman-Kiddell *et al.*, 2010
2010	Gene–diet interactions	Nutrigenomics in disease susceptibility and progression	IBD	Ferguson, 2010
2010	Host–microbe interactions	Necessity of homeostasis to reduce or resolve gut inflammation	Inflammation	Garrett *et al.*, 2010
2010	Host gene–diet–microbe interactions	Functional role of diet and gut bacteria in causing and modulating IBD	IBD	Sartor, Baker *et al.*, 2009; Haller, 2010; Hansen *et al.*, 2010
2010	Omega-3 polyunsaturated fatty acids	Critique of variability of sources used in clinical trials to date	IBD	Ferguson *et al.*, 2010
2010	Probiotics and prebiotics	Infant formulae supplemented with probiotics and/or prebiotics compared with unsupplemented formulae	Growth and adverse effects	Braegger *et al.*, 2010
2008	Probiotics	Clinical studies before and after 2005; mechanism of action	IBD	Fedorak and Dieleman, 2008
2010	Prebiotics	Mechanism of action and level of clinical evidence for efficacy	Health and wellness	Roberfroid *et al.*, 2010
2010	Diet therapy in treatment	Why self-assessment is important, and development of a methodology	CD	Brown and Roy, 2010
2010	Diet therapy in treatment	Effects on growth and malnutrition	IBD	Hartman *et al.*, 2009; Mijac *et al.*, 2010
2010	Diet therapy in treatment	Similarities and differences with regard to the nutritional complications and the approach to nutritional management in both children and adults	IBD	Conklin and Oliva-Hemker, 2010
2010	Malnutrition	Malnutrition and impaired muscle strength	IBD	Valentini *et al.*, 2008
2008	Physical activity	Role of exercise in aetiology, disease remission and progression	IBD	Narula and Fedorak, 2008
2009	Physical activity	Comparison of effects of acute and chronic exercise on inflammation	Inflammatory markers in IBD and related diseases	Ploeger *et al.*, 2009
2010	Physical activity	Effects of exercise on quality of life and immune status	IBD	Packer *et al.*, 2010

girls, a high intake of meats, fatty foods and desserts was positively associated with CD. A second dietary pattern was characterized by high levels of vegetables, fruits, olive oil, fish, grains and nuts and was inversely associated with CD in both genders. A common criticism of such studies is, however, that they depend upon accurate recording of pre-illness diet and are subject to inaccuracies.

More definitive data may be possible from prospective studies, such as one seeking to determine the relationship between the intake of nutrients and the development of UC in 260,686 men and women aged 20–80 years, as part of the large European prospective cohort study (EPIC) (Hart *et al.*, 2008). Only 139 subjects with incident UC were identified, and no dietary associations detected, apart from a marginally significant positive association with the highest quartile of intake of linoleic acid and an increased risk of UC.

Nutrition and the IBD patient

Nutrition not only affects the probability of IBD, but also profoundly affects its course. Aghdassi *et al.* (2007) considered dietary intake in 74 Canadian patients with CD, with a mean age of 35.7 ± 1.4 years and body mass index (BMI) of 23.05 ± 0.45. All patients completed a 7-day food record and a diary for CD Activity Index. Although energy and protein intakes were within the recommended levels, the intake of total carbohydrates, total fat and saturated fat intake exceeded the recommended levels in a significant number of the patients, whereas their intakes of certain micronutrients were sub-optimal.

In general, there is a very high prevalence of food sensitivities in these patients, and enteral nutrition is considered a first-line therapy that will place the majority of CD patients into remission (Akobeng, 2008; Buchanan *et al.*, 2009; Gassull, 2009; Hebuterne *et al.*, 2009; Heuschkel, 2009; Kuriyama *et al.*, 2009; Yamamoto *et al.*, 2010). The basic problem is that it is not possible to establish general dietary guidelines that will maintain remission in all patients (Hartman *et al.*, 2009; Shamir, 2009; Conklin and Oliva-Hemker, 2010; Triggs *et al.*, 2010). Certain foods may trigger symptoms in one group of individuals but suppress symptoms in others. There are very few foods that most IBD patients can safely eat in unlimited amounts and, in consequence, their diets tend to be restricted. Consequently, malnutrition can become a serious problem (Filippi *et al.*, 2006; Valentini *et al.*, 2008; Hartman *et al.*, 2009; Mijac *et al.*, 2010).

Detrimental foods in IBD

Foods known to lead to adverse symptoms include dairy products, wheat, corn and certain fruits and vegetables. In our own studies, highly spiced foods, including Indian or Thai curries of various types, high-energy drinks and beer also gave a high number of adverse symptoms (Triggs *et al.*, 2010). However, there is no 'one size fits all'. A food-symptom diary may be helpful in establishing which particular foods cause the adverse symptoms, followed by a customized elimination diet.

Beneficial foods in IBD

In our Auckland studies (Triggs *et al.*, 2010), we identified fresh white fish, salmon, tuna, yoghurt, gluten-free products, porridge oats, boiled potatoes, banana, soya milk and goats milk as the ten foods most likely to be considered beneficial by our IBD patients. There are, however, a number of other foods that also seem beneficial by certain groups in certain circumstances, and might help to regulate disease symptoms. Examples of these would include pumpkin and kumara (depending upon the cooking methods) and drinks such as ginger ale, providing this is allowed to go flat before consumption.

Malnutrition in IBD

Paediatric patients with IBD commonly have impaired nutritional status and growth (Kugathasan *et al.*, 2007; Pfefferkorn *et al.*, 2009; Shamir, 2009). Nutritional deficiencies in such patients result from a combination of inadequate nutrient intake, malabsorption and protein-losing enteropathy (Hartman *et al.*, 2009). They might also be a consequence of the metabolic disturbances directly induced by the diseases and/or their common treatments, especially corticosteroids. Surgical procedures will also play a role.

Protein-energy malnutrition (PEM) is defined as a 'state of nutrition in which a deficiency or excess (or imbalance) of energy, protein, and other nutrients causes measurable adverse effects on tissue/body form (body shape, size and composition) and function, and clinical outcome' (Valentini *et al.*, 2008). Approximately 75% of patients with active IBD show evidence for PEM.

It is very common to find multiple vitamin and mineral deficiencies in IBD patients. Identifying and correcting such micronutrient deficiencies can improve growth and also reduce the possibility of co-morbid conditions such as osteopenia and anaemia (Filippi *et al.*, 2006; Hartman *et al.*, 2009; Shamir, 2009; Shamir *et al.*, 2010). IBD patients have high prevalence of decreased BMD and vitamin K and D deficiency, probably caused by malabsorption of these vitamins (Kuwabara *et al.*, 2009). For example, CD patients with terminal ileal resections are at increased risk for vitamin B12 malabsorption (Duerksen *et al.*, 2006). These authors suggested that the length of terminal ileum resected correlated with the degree of abnormality in test results.

Micronutrient deficiencies can have important consequences, including hyperhomocysteinemia, which is associated with a higher risk of cardiovascular disease. Iron-deficiency anaemia is an especially important problem for both adults and children with IBD. Intravenous iron administration may be superior to oral iron supplementation to rectify this (Shamir, 2009). Ensuring adequate bone health is also important to the nutritional management of IBD, although guidelines for screening and therapeutic interventions for low bone-mineral density are lacking in children (Conklin and Oliva-Hemker, 2010). Screening for nutritional deficiencies in chronic disease patients is warranted and should be mandatory. Managing the deficiencies involves simple nutritional guidelines, micronutrient supplements and nutritional support.

Although the exact figures have varied according to the population, there have been previous reports that a high proportion of CD patients have a BMI below 20 (Kugathasan *et al.*, 2007). However, a recent report from two North American multicentre cohorts found the situation, at least in that country, may be changing (Kugathasan *et al.*, 2007). Kugathasan and co-workers studied clinical, demographic and BMI data from 783 patients with newly diagnosed IBD in comparison with similar figures from 2748 healthy children. Low BMI (<5%) was seen in 22–24% of children with CD and 7–9% of children with UC; however, 10% of children with CD and 20–30% of children with UC had a BMI at diagnosis that would be classed as overweight or obese.

Gene–diet or epigene–diet interactions in IBD

The fields of nutrigenetics and nutrigenomics consider gene–diet interactions in relation to both the impact of genetic variation on nutrient requirements and also of nutrient regulation of the expression of genes (Ferguson, 2010). It is now apparent that there are a substantial number of genes involved in IBD susceptibility, some distinct to the individual diseases and others overlapping between the two (Anderson *et al.*, 2010; Franke *et al.*, 2010). The nature of the pathways involved may suggest distinct nutritional approaches, depending on the affected gene pathways (Fig. 18.2). Nutrigenetic approaches may be the most viable approach to maintaining disease remission at present, and preventing disease development in the future.

Haller (2010) recognized nutrigenomics as 'a transdisciplinary approach to understand the impact of nutrition and/or microbes as prime environmental triggers in shaping the dynamic range between health and diseases'. He suggested that the application of the various -omics technologies, including transcriptomics, proteomics and metabolomics will be the way forwards in defining the functional role of diet on the gut microbiota in modulating chronic degenerative diseases including IBD.

Epigenetic effects are also apparent in IBD, and might be affected by dietary items, especially the status of certain micronutrients (Barnett *et al.*, 2010). The epigenome is regulated via DNA methylation, histone modification and non-coding RNA. Barnett and co-workers (Barnett *et al.*, 2010) have described the plasticity of epigenetic modifications that occur owing to low selenium and folate levels in the diet during gestation and lactation.

Dietary Modulation of Inflammation in IBD

Recent reviews on this topic (Cosnes *et al.*, 2010) have concluded that a Western diet was associated with increased risk of IBD. The major constituents of such a diet may affect intestinal inflammation via several mechanisms (Chapman-Kiddell *et al.*, 2010). These include the effects of insulin resistance, modification of intestinal permeability, the pro- or anti-inflammatory role of various types of polyunsaturated fatty acids, and the effect of various nutrients on host microbiota. Amre and co-workers (2007) concluded that imbalances in the consumption of polyunsaturated fatty acids, vegetables and fruits are associated with an increased risk for CD in children.

Root vegetables and gourds

Root vegetables are plant roots (any underground part of a plant) used as a vegetable. They are generally storage organs, which act as carbohydrate stores. They differ in the balance between sugars, starches and other types of carbohydrate, and the levels of these. True roots include *Beta vulgaris* (beetroot), certain *Brassica* spp. (rutabaga and turnip), *Daucus carota* subsp. *sativus* (carrot) and *Apium graveolens rapaceum* (celeriac). The sweet potato or kumara (*Ipomoea batatas*) is more formally a tuberous root. Another good carbohydrate source is the pumpkin, which is actually a gourd, and can be a cultivar of any of the species *Cucurbita pepo, Cucurbita mixta, Cucurbita maxima* and *Cucurbita moschata*.

Considering the range of effects seen in response to different vegetables, the various root vegetables identified above may be more likely than other types of vegetable to be neutral or beneficial to IBD patients (Triggs *et al.*, 2010). This is also generally true for pumpkins. We have suggested that a common characteristic of all these foods is that they have high starch and are somewhat bland. They may help maintain homeostasis in the gastrointestinal system, rather than direct effects on inflammation.

The effect of these vegetables may, however, be modified according to cooking method. Plain boiled root vegetables such as potatoes or carrots, or high-starch vegetables such as pumpkin may generally be unlikely to lead to a flare up of symptoms, whereas high-fat and/or high-sugar preparation methods can generally change an otherwise beneficial root vegetable to become detrimental.

Green vegetables

There is some confusion in the literature at present in relation to the consumption of green leafy vegetables. There are some recommendations being given to minimize the consumption of fermentable oligo-, di- and monosaccharides, and polyols (FODMAPS). These dietary practices have been shown to have short-term effects on some of the bloating and wind sometimes associated with the diseases (Gearry *et al.*, 2009). In particular, these dietary practices are leading to a very substantial reduction in the intake of brassicaceous vegetables in IBD patients. Although there may be some (variable) short-term symptoms that seem beneficial, there is a concern that the long-term effect is likely to be one of malnutrition, given the range of important nutrients in this group of plants (Barrett and Gibson, 2010). Additionally, regular broccoli consumption has been repeatedly shown to reduce oxidative stress and inflammation, using several different biomarkers (Cho *et al.*, 2006; Traka *et al.*, 2008; Vasanthi *et al.*, 2009). This effect is dependent upon having an intact glutathione S-transferase Mu gene (GSTM1), and is thought to act through modulating nuclear factor-erythroid factor 2 (Nrf2)-mediated stress responses (Kim *et al.*, 2010).

Fruits

Although some fairly bland fruits such as banana seem to show beneficial symptoms, a range of fruits tend to be avoided by IBD patients, possibly because of their slightly acid properties (Triggs *et al.*, 2010).

Fats

Although high-fat diets seem generally detrimental in IBD, the nature of the fat makes a large difference, and this may interact with genotype. Ferreira and co-workers (Ferreira *et al.*, 2010) showed that high intakes of saturated and monounsaturated fats, with low intake of long-chain omega-3 polyunsaturated acids (n-3 PUFAs), and a high n-3:n-6 PUFA ratio are associated with active CD. This effect was particularly strong in individuals carrying variants of certain cytokine and apoptotic genes. The desirability of high n-3 PUFA intake would be consistent with the tendency found in our dietary studies for high fish or high oily fish diets to be desirable (Triggs *et al.*, 2010).

Dietary conjugated linoleic acid and long-chain n-3 PUFAs such as docosahexaenoic acid (DHA) or eicosapentaenoic acid (EPA) have been proposed as pharmaceutical agents for use in active IBD. Although EPA has shown anti-inflammatory efficacy in animal models of IBD, such as the IL-10 (-/-) mouse model (Knoch *et al.*, 2009), their use in the clinic has been controversial (Bassaganya-Riera and Hontecillas, 2010).

In our own review of the available literature on n-3 PUFAs in clinical trials, we have raised a number of concerns about data interpretation (Ferguson *et al.*, 2010). There has been a lack of consistency in the formulations tested, the method of presentation and the storage of the supplements (where this was the method of administration). It is generally recognized that it is the long-chain n-3 PUFAs that are most likely to be beneficial. Because they are typically produced from marine sources, however, accumulation of pollutants may lead to adverse contaminants. Also, these products can be oxidized, and the way in which they are purified and stored is essential to their likely efficacy. In the context of variable endpoints, the available data do not argue against the use of n-3 PUFAs in general.

Even otherwise desirable, well-balanced, appropriately stored and administered long-chain n-3 PUFA may have adverse effects in certain genotypes. Woodworth *et al.* (2010) studied the effects of dietary fish oil enriched with DHA on experimentally induced colitis in a mouse model. When genetically susceptible mice were exposed to *Helicobacter hepaticus*, mild colitis was observed within 4 weeks. Contrary to expectations, feeding these mice diets enriched in fish oils induced severe colitis, and led to signs of impaired immune response.

Curcumin

Curcumin (diferulolylmethane) is the active ingredient of turmeric and a major constituent of curry powder, to which it imparts the characteristic yellow colour. Curcumin has been used in traditional Asian and African medicine to treat a wide range of conditions, albeit with varying levels of evidence. It shows preclinical and clinical potential in reducing relapse rate in UC, but has not been adequately tested in CD to date (Epstein *et al.*, 2010a,b). For example, Larmonier and co-workers (Larmonier *et al.*, 2008) investigated the effects of dietary curcumin at a range of doses on the development of colitis, immune activation, and *in vivo* nuclear factor κB (NFκB) activity in germ-free IL-10(-/-) or mice colonized with specific pathogen-free microflora. They demonstrated that curcumin was moderately effective against the development of colitis in these animals, with moderately improved colonic morphology. In human studies, Epstein and co-workers (Epstein *et al.*, 2010b) studied curcumin-treated mucosal biopsies from both children and adults with IBD. They showed reduced p38 MAPK activation, enhanced IL-10 and reduced IL-1β, as well as dose-dependent suppression of matrix metalloproteases in the curcumin-treated group. The authors suggest that these data would be consistent with a primary mechanism of action via inhibition of NFκB.

MDR1 is a candidate gene for UC that is significantly associated with risk of this disease in certain population groups such as New Zealand (Huebner *et al.*, 2009). Nones and co-workers (Nones *et al.*, 2009) studied the effects of curcumin in multidrug resistance gene-deficient (mdr1a-/-) mice. These mice spontaneously develop intestinal inflammation, with pathology similar to IBD. Curcumin (at 0.2% in the diet) significantly reduced the histological signs of colonic inflammation in these mice.

Prebiotics and probiotics

It seems that changing public health practices are leading to altered microbial exposures over time, in New Zealand as well as many other Westernized societies (Green *et al.*, 2006; Han *et al.* 2010). The hygiene hypothesis suggests that lack of early exposure to a range of microbes may negatively impact on appropriate development of the adaptive immune response, and enhance sensitivity to certain diseases (Bernstein *et al.*, 2006; Bernstein, 2010). In common with other autoimmune diseases, it seems that poor hygiene at an early stage of life may be a protective factor against CD (Han *et al.*, 2010). It is well recognized that the human colonic microbiota is central to the induction of disordered immune function and inflammation (Baker *et al.*, 2009; Garrett *et al.*, 2010; Haller, 2010). The 'pathogenic community' describes a condition in which the stability of the microbial ecosystem of the healthy human gut is disrupted in response to host genetics and destabilized immunity (Garrett *et al.*, 2010). Where they have been studied, most individuals with IBD are characterized by 'dysbiosis', in which one or a few potentially harmful microorganisms are dominant, creating a disease-prone situation (Baker *et al.*, 2009; Frank *et al.*, 2010; Hansen *et al.*, 2010). The probability of this condition may be modulated according to genotype (Frank *et al.*, 2010). It may also be affected by exposure to antibiotics and by diet.

Both prebiotics and probiotics have the potential to modulate the gut microbiome, and both have been suggested to have a potentially beneficial role in IBD. Roberfroid *et al.* (2010) defined the action of a prebiotic as: 'the selective stimulation of growth and/ or activity(ies) of one or a limited number of microbial genus(era)/species in the gut microbiota that confer(s) health benefits to the host'. They cite human intervention studies that have unequivocally demonstrated that consumption of certain food products can result in statistically significant changes in the composition of the gut microbiota. Of considerable relevance to IBD is that this modification of the microbiome associates with apparently beneficial changes in the activity of the immune system. In parallel, it improves stool quality (pH, frequency and consistency), reduces the risk of gastroenteritis and infections, and improves general well-being.

Probiotics are living commensal microorganisms of the intestinal tract that are commonly sold through the health-food market under the claim that, 'if ingested regularly, they are capable of modulating the gut microbiota'. There is evidence that they affect the gastrointestinal tract and associated immune system, and have numerous effects on intestinal function and immune responses (Fedorak, 2008). There is also evidence to suggest that certain probiotics may have a potentially beneficial role in IBD, especially in paediatric disease (Braegger *et al.*, 2010). In particular, the evidence would seem clear that probiotics are effective for the treatment as well as for primary and secondary prevention of pouchitis (Floch *et al.*, 2008; Braegger *et al.*, 2010). Pouchitis describes a condition whereby a neo-rectum, created in patients after total proctocolectomy, becomes chronically inflamed. Various literature analyses would agree that mixtures are more effective than single strains, which have been the subject of most previous studies (Ewaschuk *et al.*, 2006; Akobeng, 2008; Fedorak, 2008; Fedorak and Dieleman, 2008; Gerasimidis *et al.*, 2008;

Braegger *et al.*, 2010; Shamir, 2010) Fedorak and co-workers (Floch *et al.*, 2008) critically evaluated the probiotic clinical studies, especially those involving the well-characterized mixture VSL#3. This mixture contains eight specially selected strains of bacteria: *Streptococcus thermophilus*, *Bifidobacterium breve*, *Bifidobacterium longum*, *Bifidobacterium infantis*, *Lactobacillus acidophilus*, *Lactobacillus plantarum*, *Lactobacillus paracasei* and *Lactobacillus delbrueckii* subsp. *bulgaricus*. The current evidence base would seem to support but not prove the possibility that probiotic mixtures are beneficial for immune function, gut microbiota modulation and at least some forms of IBD.

There is, at present, a considerable research effort seeking to expand the range of food vehicles that can be used for human consumption of probiotics and prebiotics. Both may be consumed as a component of yoghurts, be drunk as a 'shot', be incorporated into a capsule, into baby foods, etc. From their reviews of the current literature, Braegger and co-workers (Braegger *et al.*, 2010) suggested that the administration of probiotic- and/or prebiotic-supplemented formula to healthy infants does not raise safety concerns with regard to growth and adverse effects. They do not consider, however, that there are sufficient data to recommend the routine use of probiotic- and/or prebiotic-supplemented formulae. Instead, they suggest further studies, using validated clinical outcome measures to assess the effects of probiotic and/or prebiotic supplementation of formulae.

Physical Activity in the Aetiology of IBD

Several sets of epidemiological data have related regular PA to reduced risk of IBD (Sonnenberg, 1990; Persson *et al.*, 1993; D'Inca *et al.*, 1999, 2000). For example, a case-control study in Sweden concluded that daily and weekly exercise over a significant time period, e.g. 5 years, significantly reduced the risk for CD but not UC, as compared with randomly selected, healthy controls. Prospective studies, however, have revealed only small and rather inconsistent associations between sedentary occupations and IBD risk. There is evidence that short-term high-intensity exercise may adversely affect immune response, and this could be a factor in the emergence of the disease (Narula and Fedorak, 2008; Tuan *et al.*, 2008).

Effects of moderate and regular exercise

There is some evidence that moderate and regular PA significantly increases the quality of life for IBD patients, and may also be associated with decreased disease activity (Narula and Fedorak, 2008; Ploeger *et al.*, 2009; Cosnes, 2010; Packer *et al.*, 2010). It may also contribute to increased muscle mass and the prevention of osteoporosis.

A systematic review of the human IBD literature to December 2008 (Packer *et al.*, 2010) considered outcome measures of health-related quality of life, clinical disease indicators or immune function where PA was used as a primary intervention for symptom control. In total, seven studies were included in this systematic review: five were on PA and quality-of-life measures and inflammatory disease markers, and two on PA and immune measures. Four studies out of five showed that regular PA significantly increased quality of life and decreased disease activity, as assessed by questionnaires. They found no evidence, however, that PA affected immune outcomes in patients with IBD.

There seems reason to advocate a programme of moderate and regular PA for patients with quiescent IBD as well as other chronic diseases such as rheumatoid arthritis, while caution is still needed for patients with active disease (D'Incà *et al.*, 1999, 2000; Loudon *et al.*, 1999; Crumbock *et al.*, 2009; Packer *et al.*, 2010). Given the increased measures of overweight and obesity now being seen in IBD (Kugathasan *et al.*, 2007), it is of interest that regular and moderate PA leads to a reduction in BMI (Loudon *et al.*, 1999). It is also a potentially effective method of increasing BMD in CD, and may slow the rate of bone loss and reduce the risk of orthotic fractures in later life (Robinson *et al.*, 1998).

Effects of heavy endurance exercise

Heavy endurance exercise may lead to an acute, albeit transient, inflammatory response that is likely to enhance rather than reduce the symptoms of IBD (D'Incà *et al.*, 2000).

Reduction in exercise ability associated with IBD symptoms

Patients with IBD, especially CD, often show symptoms of general fatigue and decreased muscle function that may affect their quality of life, and also their ability to cope with regular PA. This is especially true for patients who have had extensive resections (Peters *et al.*, 2001). Brevinge and co-workers (Brevinge *et al.*, 1995) showed that maximal exercise load was reduced marginally (by 9%) in IBD patients without small bowel resection, by 22% in patients with moderate small bowel resection (15–30% resection) and by 40% in patients with extensive bowel resection (more than 50%). The effect was greater than predicted by reduction in muscle mass, and the authors suggested that malabsorption played a causal role. Similar studies in paediatric patients led to similar conclusions (Ploeger *et al.*, 2010).

Summary and Conclusions

CD and UC are forms of IBD, a group of chronic recurrent inflammatory conditions of the large and small intestines, whose incidence is increasing in some countries. There is strong evidence for genetic susceptibility to both forms of the disease, but the probability of disease development will be modified by diet and lifestyle factors (Fig. 18.1). The gut microbiota also plays a key role, the nature of which will be modulated by diet and lifestyle factors. Nutrition and PA play a complex role in the aetiology of IBD (Fig. 18.2). At present, however, it is difficult to establish the relative roles of genetics, nutrition, PA, stress and infections, and the way in which these interact, in increased risk of the disease.

For those patients with IBD, nutrition and PA will profoundly affect both the control of disease symptoms and rate of disease progression. Each IBD patient has a distinctive genetic profile and nature of disease presentation. It will become increasingly important to recognize a need for personalized dietary and PA regimes for symptom control. Dietary factors that may reduce symptoms are few in nature, whereas there is an extensive list of potentially adverse items. In consequence, malnutrition is common in this group of patients, and may be part of the reason for decreased general health and strength that may impact their ability to cope with regular PA programmes. There is a strong need for better co-ordinated studies that combine groups internationally, with similar protocols, in order to strengthen the currently available databases on these important topics.

Acknowledgements

Nutrigenomics New Zealand is a collaboration among The University of Auckland, Plant and Food Research Ltd and AgResearch Ltd. It is funded by the New Zealand Ministry of Science and Innovation.

References

Abraham, C. and Cho, J. (2009) Interleukin-23/Th17 pathways and inflammatory bowel disease. *Inflammatory Bowel Diseases* 15, 1090–1100.

Aghdassi, E., Wendland, B.E., Stapleton, M., Raman, M. and Allard, J.P. (2007) Adequacy of nutritional intake in a Canadian population of patients with Crohn's disease. *Journal of the American Dietetic Association* 107, 1575–1580.

Akobeng, A.K. (2008) Review article: the evidence base for interventions used to maintain remission in Crohn's disease. *Alimentary Pharmacology and Therapeutics* 27, 11–18.

Amre, D.K., D'Souza, S., Morgan, K., Seidman, G., Lambrette, P., *et al.* (2007) Imbalances in dietary consumption of fatty acids, vegetables, and fruits are associated with risk for Crohn's disease in children. [Erratum appears in *American Journal of Gastroenterology* (2007) 102, 2614]. *American Journal of Gastroenterology* 102, 2016–2025.

Anderson, C.A., Boucher, G., Lees, C.W., Franke, A., *et al.* (2010) Meta-analysis identifies 29 additional ulcerative colitis risk loci, increasing the number of confirmed associations to 47. *Nature Genetics* 43, 246–252.

Baker, P.I., Love, D.R. and Ferguson, L.R. (2009) Role of gut microbiota in Crohn's disease. *Expert Review of Gastroenterology and Hepatology* 3, 535–546.

Ball, E. (1998) Exercise guidelines for patients with inflammatory bowel disease. *Gastroenterology Nursing* 21, 108–111.

Barnett, M., Bermingham, E., Mcnabb, W., Bassett, S., Armstrong, K., *et al.* (2010) Investigating micronutrients and epigenetic mechanisms in relation to inflammatory bowel disease. *Mutation Research* 690, 71–80.

Barrett, J.S. and Gibson, P.R. (2010) Development and validation of a comprehensive semi-quantitative food frequency questionnaire that includes FODMAP intake and glycemic index. *Journal of the American Dietetic Association* 110, 1469–1476.

Bassaganya-Riera, J. and Hontecillas, R. (2010) Dietary conjugated linoleic acid and n-3 polyunsaturated fatty acids in inflammatory bowel disease. *Current Opinion in Clinical Nutrition and Metabolic Care* 13, 569–573.

Bernstein, C.N. (2010) Epidemiologic clues to inflammatory bowel disease. *Current Gastroenterology Reports* 12, 495–501.

Bernstein, C.N. and Shanahan, F. (2008) Disorders of a modern lifestyle: reconciling the epidemiology of inflammatory bowel diseases. *Gut* 57, 1185–1191.

Bernstein, C.N., Rawsthorne, P., Cheang, M. and Blanchard, J.F. (2006) A population-based case control study of potential risk factors for IBD. *American Journal of Gastroenterology* 101, 993–1002.

Braegger, C., Chmielewska, A., Decsi, T., Kolacek, S., Mihatsch, W., *et al.* (2010) Supplementation of infant formula with probiotics and/or prebiotics: a systematic review and comment by the ESPGHAN committee on nutrition. *Journal of Pediatric Gastroenterology and Nutrition* 52, 238–250.

Brevinge, H., Berglund, B., Bosaeus, I., Tolli, J., Nordgren, S., *et al.* (1995) Exercise capacity in patients undergoing proctocolectomy and small bowel resection for Crohn's disease. *British Journal of Surgery* 82, 1040–1045.

Brown, A.C. and Roy, M. (2010) Does evidence exist to include dietary therapy in the treatment of Crohn's disease? *Expert Review of Gastroenterology and Hepatology* 4, 191–215.

Buchanan, E., Gaunt, W.W., Cardigan, T., Garrick, V., Mcgrogan, P., *et al.* (2009) The use of exclusive enteral nutrition for induction of remission in children with Crohn's disease demonstrates that disease phenotype does not influence clinical remission. *Alimentary Pharmacology and Therapeutics* 30, 501–507.

Chapman-Kiddell, C.A., Davies, P.S.W., Gillen, L. and Radford-Smith, G.L. (2010) Role of diet in the development of inflammatory bowel disease. *Inflammatory Bowel Diseases* 16, 137–151.

Cho, E.J., Lee, Y.A., Yoo, H.H. and Yokozawa, T. (2006) Protective effects of broccoli (*Brassica oleracea*) against oxidative damage in vitro and in vivo. *Journal of Nutritional Science and Vitaminology* 52, 437–444.

Coeffier, M., Marion-Letellier, R. and Dechelotte, P. (2010) Potential for amino acids supplementation during inflammatory bowel diseases. *Inflammatory Bowel Diseases* 16, 518–524.

Conklin, L.S. and Oliva-Hemker, M. (2010) Nutritional considerations in pediatric inflammatory bowel disease. *Expert Review of Gastroenterology and Hepatology* 4, 305–317.

Cosnes, J. (2010) Smoking, physical activity, nutrition and lifestyle: environmental factors and their impact on IBD. *Digestive Diseases* 28, 411–417.

Crumbock, S.C., Loeb, S.J. and Fick, D.M. (2009) Physical activity, stress, disease activity, and quality of life in adults with Crohn disease. *Gastroenterology Nursing* 32, 188–195.

D'Inca, R., Varnier, M., Mestriner, C., Martines, D., D'odorico, A. *et al.* (1999) Effect of moderate exercise on Crohn's disease patients in remission. *Italian Journal of Gastroenterology and Hepatology,* 31, 205–10.

D'Inca, R., Varnier, M., D'Odorico, A. and Sturniolo, G.C. (2000) Exercise and inflammatory bowel disease: immunological aspects. *Exercise Immunology Review* 6, 43–53.

D'Souza, S., Levy, E., Mack, D., Israel, D., Lambrette, P., *et al.* (2008) Dietary patterns and risk for Crohn's disease in children. *Inflammatory Bowel Diseases* 14, 367–373.

Dambacher, J., Beigel, F., Zitzmann, K., De Toni, E.N., Goke, B., *et al.* (2009) The role of the novel Th17 cytokine IL-26 in intestinal inflammation. *Gut* 58, 1207–1217.

Duerksen, D.R., Fallows, G. and Bernstein, C.N. (2006) Vitamin B12 malabsorption in patients with limited ileal resection. *Nutrition* 22, 1210–1213.

Epstein, J., Sanderson, I.R. and Macdonald, T.T. (2010a) Curcumin as a therapeutic agent: the evidence from in vitro, animal and human studies. *British Journal of Nutrition* 103, 1545–1557.

Epstein, J., Docena, G., Macdonald, T.T. and Sanderson, I.R. (2010b) Curcumin suppresses p38 mitogen-activated protein kinase activation, reduces IL-1beta and matrix metalloproteinase-3 and enhances IL-10 in the mucosa of children and adults with inflammatory bowel disease. *British Journal of Nutrition* 103, 824–832.

Ewaschuk, J.B., Tejpar, Q.Z., Soo, I., Madsen, K. and Fedorak, R.N. (2006) The role of antibiotic and probiotic therapies in current and future management of inflammatory bowel disease. *Current Gastroenterology Reports* 8, 486–498.

Fedorak, R.N. (2008) Understanding why probiotic therapies can be effective in treating IBD. *Journal of Clinical Gastroenterology* 42 Suppl 3, S111–S115.

Fedorak, R.N. (2010) Probiotics in the management of ulcerative colitis. *Gastroenterology and Hepatology* 6, 688–690.

Fedorak, R.N. and Dieleman, L.A. (2008) Probiotics in the treatment of human inflammatory bowel diseases: update 2008. *Journal of Clinical Gastroenterology* 42 Suppl 2, S97–S103.

Ferguson, L.R. (2010) Nutrigenomics and inflammatory bowel diseases. *Expert Review of Clinical Immunology* 6, 573–583.

Ferguson, L.R. and Laing, W.A. (2010) Chronic inflammation, mutation and human disease. *Mutation Research* 690, 1–2.

Ferguson, L.R., Smith, B.G. and James, B.J. (2010) Combining nutrition, food science and engineering in developing solutions to Inflammatory bowel diseases – omega-3 polyunsaturated fatty acids as example. *Food and Function* 1, 60–72.

Ferreira, P., Cravo, M., Guerreiro, C.S., Tavares, L., Santos, P.M., *et al.* (2010) Fat intake interacts with polymorphisms of Caspase9, FasLigand and PPARgamma apoptotic genes in modulating Crohn's disease activity. *Clinical Nutrition* 29, 819–23.

Filippi, J., Al-Jaouni, R., Wiroth, J.-B., Hebuterne, X. and Schneider, S.M. (2006) Nutritional deficiencies in patients with Crohn's disease in remission. *Inflammatory Bowel Diseases* 12, 185–191.

Floch, M.H., Walker, W.A., Guandalini, S., Hibberd, P., Gorbach, S., *et al.* (2008) Recommendations for probiotic use–2008. *Journal of Clinical Gastroenterology* 42 Suppl 2, S104–S108.

Frank, D.N., Robertson, C.E., Hamm, C.M., Kpadeh, Z., Zhang, T., *et al.* (2010) Disease phenotype and genotype are associated with shifts in intestinal-associated microbiota in inflammatory bowel diseases. *Inflammatory Bowel Diseases* 17, 179–184.

Franke, A., Mcgovern, D.P.B., Barrett, J.C., Wang, K., *et al.* (2010) Genome-wide meta-analysis increases to 71 the number of confirmed Crohn's disease susceptibility loci. *Nature Genetics* 42, 1118–1125.

Garrett, W.S., Gordon, J.I. and Glimcher, L.H. (2010) Homeostasis and inflammation in the intestine. *Cell* 140, 859–870.

Gassull, M.A. (2009) Can nutritional therapy replace pharmacologic therapy in pediatric Crohn's disease? *Nature Clinical Practice Gastroenterology and Hepatology* 6, 80–81.

Gearry, R.B., Irving, P.M., Barrett, J.S., Nathan, D.M., Shepherd, S.J. and Gibson, P.R. (2009) Reduction of dietary poorly absorbed short-chain carbohydrates (FODMAPs) improves abdominal symptoms in patients with inflammatory bowel disease-a pilot study. *Journal of Crohn's and Colitis* 3, 8–14.

Gerasimidis, K., Mcgrogan, P., Hassan, K. and Edwards, C.A. (2008) Dietary modifications, nutritional supplements and alternative medicine in paediatric patients with inflammatory bowel disease. *Alimentary Pharmacology and Therapeutics* 27, 155–165.

Goodman, A.L. and Gordon, J.I. (2010) Our unindicted coconspirators: human metabolism from a microbial perspective. *Cell Metabolism* 12, 111–116.

Goodman, A.L., Mcnulty, N.P., Zhao, Y., Leip, D., Mitra, R.D., *et al.* (2009) Identifying genetic determinants needed to establish a human gut symbiont in its habitat. *Cell Host and Microbe* 6, 279–289.

Green, C., Elliott, L., Beaudoin, C. and Bernstein, C.N. (2006) A population-based ecologic study of inflammatory bowel disease: searching for etiologic clues. *American Journal of Epidemiology* 164, 615–623; discussion 624–628.

Haller, D. (2010) Nutrigenomics and IBD: the intestinal microbiota at the cross-road between inflammation and metabolism. *Journal of Clinical Gastroenterolog,* 44 Suppl 1, S6–S9.

Han, D.Y., Fraser, A.G., Dryland, P. and Ferguson, L.R. (2010) Environmental factors in the development of chronic inflammation: a case-control study on risk factors for Crohn's disease within New Zealand. *Mutation Research,* 690, 116–22.

Hansen, J., Gulati, A. and Sartor, R.B. (2010) The role of mucosal immunity and host genetics in defining intestinal commensal bacteria. *Current Opinion in Gastroenterology* 26, 564–571.

Hart, A.R., Luben, R., Olsen, A., Tjonneland, A., Linseisen, J., *et al.* (2008) Diet in the aetiology of ulcerative colitis: a European prospective cohort study. *Digestion* 77, 57–64.

Hartman, C., Eliakim, R. and Shamir, R. (2009) Nutritional status and nutritional therapy in inflammatory bowel diseases. *World Journal of Gastroenterology* 15, 2570–2578.

Hebuterne, X., Filippi, J., Al-Jaouni, R. and Schneider, S. (2009) Nutritional consequences and nutrition therapy in Crohn's disease. *Gastroenterologie Clinique et Biologique* 33 Suppl 3, S235–S244.

Heuschkel, R. (2009) Enteral nutrition should be used to induce remission in childhood Crohn's disease. *Digestive Diseases* 27, 297–305.

Huebner, C., Browning, B.L., Petermann, I., Han, D.Y., Philpott, M., *et al.* (2009) Genetic analysis of MDR1 and inflammatory bowel disease reveals protective effect of heterozygous variants for ulcerative colitis. *Inflammatory Bowel Diseases* 15, 1784–1793.

Kim, J., Cha, Y.-N. and Surh, Y.-J. (2010) A protective role of nuclear factor-erythroid 2-related factor-2 (Nrf2) in inflammatory disorders. *Mutation Research* 690, 12–23.

Knoch, B., Barnett, M.P.G., Zhu, S., Park, Z.A., Nones, K., *et al.* (2009) Genome-wide analysis of dietary eicosapentaenoic acid- and oleic acid-induced modulation of colon inflammation in interleukin-10 gene-deficient mice. *Journal of Nutrigenetics and Nutrigenomics* 2, 9–28.

Kobayashi, T., Okamoto, S., Hisamatsu, T., Kamada, N., Chinen, H., *et al.* (2008) IL23 differentially regulates the Th1/Th17 balance in ulcerative colitis and Crohn's disease. *Gut,* 57, 1682–1689.

Koenders, M.I. and Van Den Berg, W.B. (2010) Translational mini-review series on Th17 cells: are T helper 17 cells really pathogenic in autoimmunity? *Clinical and Experimental Immunology* 159, 131–136.

Kugathasan, S., Nebel, J., Skelton, J.A., Markowitz, J., Keljo, D., *et al.* and Wisconsin Pediatric Inflammatory Bowel Disease, A. and Pediatric Inflammatory Bowel Disease Collaborative Research, G. (2007) Body mass index in children with newly diagnosed inflammatory bowel disease: observations from two multi-center North American inception cohorts. *Journal of Pediatrics* 151, 523–527.

Kuriyama, M., Kato, J., Morimoto, N., Fujimoto, T., Kono, H., *et al.* and Japan West Crohn's Disease Study, G. (2009) Enteral nutrition improves health-related quality of life in Crohn's disease patients with long disease duration. *Hepato-Gastroenterology* 56, 321–327.

Kuwabara, A., Tanaka, K., Tsugawa, N., Nakase, H., Tsuji, H., *et al.* (2009) High prevalence of vitamin K and D deficiency and decreased BMD in inflammatory bowel disease. *Osteoporosis International* 20, 935–942.

Langrish, C.L., Chen, Y., Blumenschein, W.M., Mattson, J., Basham, B., *et al.* (2005) IL-23 drives a pathogenic T cell population that induces autoimmune inflammation. *The Journal of Experimental Medicine* 201, 233–240.

Larmonier, C.B., Uno, J.K., Lee, K.-M., Karrasch, T., Laubitz, D., *et al.* (2008) Limited effects of dietary curcumin on Th-1 driven colitis in IL-10 deficient mice suggest an IL-10-dependent mechanism of protection. *American Journal of Physiology - Gastrointestinal and Liver Physiology* 295, G1079–G1091.

Liang, S.C., Tan, X.Y., Luxenberg, D.P., Karim, R., Dunussi-Joannopoulos, K., *et al.* (2006) Interleukin (IL)-22 and IL-17 are coexpressed by Th17 cells and cooperatively enhance expression of antimicrobial peptides. *Journal of Experimental Medicine* 203, 2271–2279.

Loudon, C.P., Corroll, V., Butcher, J., Rawsthorne, P. and Bernstein, C.N. (1999) The effects of physical exercise on patients with Crohn's disease. *American Journal of Gastroenterology* 94, 697–703.

Mallon, D.P. and Suskind, D.L. (2010) Nutrition in pediatric inflammatory bowel disease. *Nutrition in Clinical Practice* 25, 335–339.

Mijac, D.D., Jankovic, G.L.J., Jorga, J. and Krstic, M.N. 2010. Nutritional status in patients with active inflammatory bowel disease: prevalence of malnutrition and methods for routine nutritional assessment. *European Journal of Internal Medicine,* 21, 315–9.

Moreno, D.A., Lopez-Berenguer, C. and Garcia-Viguera, C. (2007) Effects of stir-fry cooking with different edible oils on the phytochemical composition of broccoli. *Journal of Food Science* 72, S064–S068.

Narula, N. and Fedorak, R.N. (2008) Exercise and inflammatory bowel disease. *Canadian Journal of Gastroenterology* 22, 497–504.

Ng, V., Millard, W., Lebrun, C. and Howard, J. (2006) Exercise and Crohn's disease: speculations on potential benefits. *Canadian Journal of Gastroenterology* 20, 657–660.

Nones, K., Dommels, Y.E.M., Martell, S., Butts, C., Mcnabb, W.C., *et al.* (2009) The effects of dietary curcumin and rutin on colonic inflammation and gene expression in multidrug resistance gene-deficient (mdr1a-/-) mice, a model of inflammatory bowel diseases. *British Journal of Nutrition* 101, 169–181.

Nurieva, R., Yang, X.O., Martinez, G., Zhang, Y., Panopoulos, A.D., *et al.* (2007) Essential autocrine regulation by IL-21 in the generation of inflammatory T cells. *Nature* 448, 480–483.

Packer, N., Hoffman-Goetz, L. and Ward, G. (2010) Does physical activity affect quality of life, disease symptoms and immune measures in patients with inflammatory bowel disease? A systematic review. *Journal of Sports Medicine and Physical Fitness* 50, 1–18.

Persson, P.G., Leijonmarck, C.E., Bernell, O., Hellers, G. and Ahlbom, A. (1993) Risk indicators for inflammatory bowel disease. *International Journal of Epidemiology* 22, 268–272.

Peters, H.P., De Vries, W.R., Vanberge-Henegouwen, G.P. and Akkermans, L.M. (2001) Potential benefits and hazards of physical activity and exercise on the gastrointestinal tract. *Gut* 48, 435–439.

Pfefferkorn, M., Burke, G., Griffiths, A., Markowitz, J., Rosh, J., *et al.* (2009) Growth abnormalities persist in newly diagnosed children with crohn disease despite current treatment paradigms. *Journal of Pediatric Gastroenterology and Nutrition* 48, 168–174.

Ploeger, H.E., Takken, T., De Greef, M.H.G. and Timmons, B.W. (2009) The effects of acute and chronic exercise on inflammatory markers in children and adults with a chronic inflammatory disease: a systematic review. *Exercise Immunology Review* 15, 6–41.

Ploeger, H.E., Takken, T., Wilk, B., Issenman, R.M., Sears, R., *et al.* (2010) Exercise capacity in pediatric patients with inflammatory bowel disease. *Journal of Pediatrics* 158, 814–819.

Roberfroid, M., Gibson, G.R., Hoyles, L., Mccartney, A.L., Rastall, R., *et al.* (2010) Prebiotic effects: metabolic and health benefits. *British Journal of Nutrition* 104 Suppl 2, S1–S63.

Robinson, R.J., Krzywicki, T., Almond, L., Al-Azzawi, F., Abrams, K., *et al.* (1998) Effect of a low-impact exercise program on bone mineral density in Crohn's disease: a randomized controlled trial. *Gastroenterology* 115, 36–41.

Sartor, R.B. (2010) Genetics and environmental interactions shape the intestinal microbiome to promote inflammatory bowel disease versus mucosal homeostasis. *Gastroenterology* 139, 1816–1819.

Shamir, R. (2009) Nutritional aspects in inflammatory bowel disease. *Journal of Pediatric Gastroenterology and Nutrition* 48 Suppl 2, S86–S88.

Shamir, R. (2010) Nutrition and growth in inflammatory bowel disease. *Journal of Pediatric Gastroenterology and Nutrition* 51 Suppl 3, S131–S132.

Sonnenberg, A. (1990) Occupational distribution of inflammatory bowel disease among German employees. *Gut* 31, 1037–1040.

Traka, M., Gasper, A.V., Melchini, A., Bacon, J.R., Needs, P.W., *et al.* (2008) Broccoli consumption interacts with GSTM1 to perturb oncogenic signalling pathways in the prostate. *PLoS ONE* 3, e2568.

Triggs, C.M., Munday, K., Hu, R., Fraser, A.G., Gearry, R.B., *et al.* (2010) Dietary factors in chronic inflammation: food tolerances and intolerances of a New Zealand Caucasian Crohn's disease population. *Mutation Research* 690, 123–138.

Tuan, T.C., Hsu, T.G., Fong, M.C., Hsu, C.F., Tsai, K.K.C., *et al.* (2008) Deleterious effects of short-term, high-intensity exercise on immune function: evidence from leucocyte mitochondrial alterations and apoptosis. *British Journal of Sports Medicine* 42, 11–15.

Turnbaugh, P.J., Ridaura, V.K., Faith, J.J., Rey, F.E., Knight, R. *et al.* (2009) The effect of diet on the human gut microbiome: a metagenomic analysis in humanized gnotobiotic mice. *Science Translational Medicine* 1, 6ra14.

Valentini, L., Schaper, L., Buning, C., Hengstermann, S., Koernicke, T., *et al.* (2008) Malnutrition and impaired muscle strength in patients with Crohn's disease and ulcerative colitis in remission. *Nutrition* 24, 694–702.

Vasanthi, H.R., Mukherjee, S. and Das, D.K. (2009) Potential health benefits of broccoli- a chemico-biological overview. *Mini-Reviews in Medicinal Chemistry* 9, 749–759.

Wilson, N.J., Boniface, K., Chan, J.R., Mckenzie, B.S., Blumenschein, W.M., *et al.* (2007) Development, cytokine profile and function of human interleukin 17-producing helper T cells. *Nature immunology* 8, 950–957.

Woodworth, H.L., Mccaskey, S.J., Duriancik, D.M., Clinthorne, J.F., Langohr, I.M., *et al.* (2010) Dietary fish oil alters T lymphocyte cell populations and exacerbates disease in a mouse model of inflammatory colitis. *Cancer Research* 70, 7960–7969.

Yamamoto, T., Nakahigashi, M. and Saniabadi, A.R. (2009) Review article: diet and inflammatory bowel disease–epidemiology and treatment. *Alimentary Pharmacology and Therapeutics* 30, 99–112.

Yamamoto, T., Nakahigashi, M., Umegae, S. and Matsumoto, K. (2010) Enteral nutrition for the maintenance of remission in Crohn's disease: a systematic review. *European Journal of Gastroenterology and Hepatology* 22, 1–8.

Yap, J., Wesley, A., Mouat, S. and Chin, S. (2008) Paediatric inflammatory bowel disease in New Zealand. *New Zealand Medical Journal* 121, 19–34.

19 Ageing and Inflammation

C. Nowson,*,[1] J.A. Grieger,[2] D. Cameron-Smith[1,3]
[1]Deakin University Centre for Physical Activity and Nutrition Research, Burwood, Australia; [2]Flinders University Nutrition and Dietetics, Bedford Park, Australia; [3]Liggins Institute, University of Auckland, New Zealand

Introduction

The number of older people worldwide is rapidly increasing. During ageing, a number of physiological changes occur. Cross-sectional studies have identified that the prevalence of high body weight or obesity (i.e body mass index (BMI) >30 kg/m^2) increases with age up to about 60 years, and then declines (Seidell and Visscher, 2000); with gradual reductions in fat free mass, height and bone mass (Going *et al.*, 1995,) Ageing is also associated with alterations in the immune system. Immunosenescence is the term used to describe the deterioration and dysregulation of the immune system. Although there is a view that immunosenescence is a generalized, age-related, unidirectional decline in immune responses, there is evidence that there are changes to the immune system that may enhance as well as diminish function. Nearly every component of the immune system undergoes dramatic age-associated restructuring, leading to complex remodelling with compensatory mechanisms and qualitative alterations in function. Furthermore, ageing is

* Corresponding author, nowson@deakin.edu.au

associated with declining levels of both spontaneous and recreational physical activity. Whether these habitual changes in muscular function contribute to the inflammatory burden of ageing has yet to be fully elucidated.

The inflammatory response may either be 'acute' or 'chronic'. The acute inflammatory response lasts 2–3 days, is initiated by several chemical mediators and is down-regulated once the stimulus has been removed. Chronic inflammation is persistent inflammation, with continual recruitment of monocytes, and later lymphocytes, to the site of injury. Chronic inflammation is of particular interest as it has been implicated in the aetiology of several diseases including cardiovascular disease (CVD), diabetes, rheumatoid arthritis, cancer and neurodegenerative diseases such as Alzheimer's disease (AD), which are associated with ageing. This chronic, low-grade inflammation has been termed 'inflammaging' (Franceschi *et al.*, 2000), and is initiated by internal and environmental stimuli (De Martinis *et al.*, 2005). It has been proposed that 'inflammaging' can be accompanied by anti-inflammatory processes, which are also major determinants not only of immunosenescence but eventually of global ageing and longevity (Franceschi *et al.*, 2007).

Conversely, a number of observational studies have demonstrated reduced circulatory concentrations of inflammatory biomarkers in aged individuals. These large population studies include the Third National Health and Nutrition Examination survey (NHANES III) (Abramson and Vaccarino, 2002), the British Regional Heart Study (Wannamethee *et al.*, 2002), the Cardiovascular Health Study (Geffken *et al.*, 2001) and the Health ABC Study (Schaap *et al.*, 2009). In these studies, an independent and inverse relationship with plasma C-reactive protein (CRP) has been established. Furthermore, this relationship is influenced by the intensity and frequency of exercise in older populations.

Inflammation and ageing

All components of the immune system succumb to ageing. Increased activity of natural killer (NK) cells has been associated with healthier ageing (Mariani *et al.*, 1999), whereas low activity of NK cells has been associated with less healthy ageing (Kmiec *et al.*, 2001). During ageing, the immune system is compromised owing to persistent increases in pro-inflammatory markers, particularly interleukin-6 (IL-6), tumour necrosis factor alpha (TNF-α), and interleukin one beta (IL-1β) (Fagiolo *et al.*, 1993; Shurin *et al.*, 2007); and the limited evidence available seems to indicate that levels of anti-inflammatory cytokines, particularly IL-10, tend to be reduced (Shurin *et al.*, 2007; Saurwein-Teissl *et al.*, 2000). There is a reduction in T and B lymphocytes (Paganelli *et al.*, 1992; Sansoni *et al.*, 1993) with ageing, but an increase in effector CD8+ CD28– T cells (Fagnoni *et al.*, 1996), which may be the result of persistent viruses.

Compared with those from younger subjects, peripheral blood mononuclear cells from older people produce higher amounts of pro-inflammatory cytokines (Fagiolo *et al.*, 1993). One hypothesis (Fig. 19.1) proposes that the beneficial effects of inflammation that are activated to defend against infections early in life and in adulthood become detrimental later in life. Therefore, those who age well have a life-long lower immune response to stimuli and those who mounted a robust inflammatory response to fight infections early in life may be disadvantaged later in life and vice versa (Franceschi *et al.*, 2000). This would assume that centenarians, at young age, were more susceptible and prone to infectious diseases. Genetic factors also are thought to influence the capacity to mount an immune response; this varies between individuals, as does the rate of reaching the threshold of pro-inflammatory status at which disease/disability occurs. In centenarians, the time needed to reach the pathologically high inflammatory state threshold is extremely long. Generally centenarians live without disability until very old age, despite the fact that most of them have raised inflammatory markers (Bruunsgaard *et al.*, 1999). Therefore there is no clear link between measured inflammatory markers and disability in old age.

To answer key questions, more ageing studies on humans need to be conducted. Laboratory animals are raised and kept in relatively sterile environments with minimal

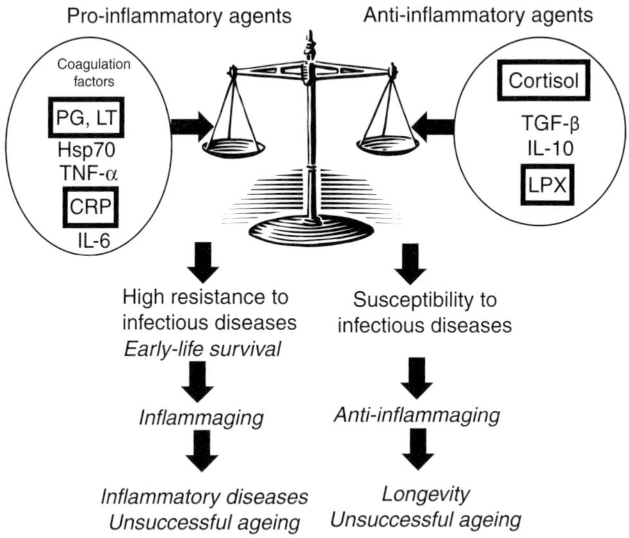

Fig. 19.1. The balancing between pro- and anti-inflammatory agents. Efficient inflammatory responses can confer high resistance to infectious diseases, but also an increased susceptibility to inflammation-based diseases later in life. On the other side, low inflammatory responses, while rendering increased susceptibility to infectious diseases, can confer a survival advantage in old age. CRP, C-reactive protein; Hsp70, 70 kDa heat shock proteins (ubiquitously expressed heat shock proteins that help to protect cells from stress); IL, interleukin; LPX, lipoxins; LT, leukotrienes; PG, prostaglandins; TGF-β, transforming growth factor beta; TNF-α, tumour necrosis factor alpha. Bold boxes indicate factors for which their contribution to longevity has not been studied yet. (From Franceschi *et al.*, 2007, with permission from Elsevier Ltd.)

exposure to antigenic stimuli. In contrast, humans are exposed to an enormous range of microbes and challenges to the immune system. Humans have evolved a complex lymphocyte-based immune system with an enormous variety of bacterial species present in the intestinal flora (Pancer and Cooper, 2006). There is evidence that alterations in the microflora seen in frail elderly people contribute to increases in inflammatory status and that alterations in gut flora have been related to multi-system organ failure, colon cancer and inflammatory bowel diseases (Guarner, 2006). It has been proposed that nutritional interventions that modify the intestinal microbiota could reduce the pro-inflammatory effects of age-related changes in the microflora and reinforce the mucosal barrier or modulate the cellular activation pathways that drive and/or inhibit pro-inflammatory processes (Schiffrin *et al.*, 2010). A complex remodelling of the immune system during ageing occurs that might be a sign of decreased immune competence. Interventions that reduce inflammation may therefore be an effective strategy to combat a number of age-related diseases.

Obesity and energy (calorie) restriction

In animal models there is good evidence to show that restricting energy intake, known as 'calorie restriction' (CR), improves health and slows ageing in mammals. The reasons for this are still under investigation. Sir2-like proteins (sirtuins) are a family of NAD$^+$-dependent deacetylases that play important roles in gene silencing, DNA repair, DNA recombination and ageing in model organisms. When diet is restricted through caloric restriction, lifespan is extended in diverse species, suggesting that there is a conserved mechanism for nutrient regulation of ageing (Wood *et al.*, 2004).

It seems that CR, in the absence of malnutrition, delays ageing and prevents ageing-related diseases through multiple mechanisms including a reduction in chronic inflammation in older people. It has been proposed that energy accumulation is involved in the generation of the chronic inflammatory state seen in old age. There is also emerging evidence that the inflammatory response induces energy expenditure in a feedback manner to protect against energy surplus in obesity (Ye and Keller, 2010). Therefore, under 'normal' circumstances the inflammatory response helps to protect against obesity. This feedback system can, however, become deficient (inflammation resistance), and energy expenditure is actually reduced, leading to the development of obesity. In addition, it has been suggested that in the peripheral tissues, inflammation induces fat mobilization and oxidation to promote energy expenditure and is thus useful to prevent obesity, which also may induce energy disposal through glucose excretion in urine as a result of insulin resistance and hyperglycemia (Bastard *et al.*, 2006). In the brain, inflammation may inhibit food intake and activate neurons for energy expenditure. This is ideal to prevent obesity, but would be detrimental in the very old, where frailty and weight loss is of greatest concern.

Nutrition, Inflammation and Ageing

Diet may play a key role in ameliorating inflammation and reducing the burden of a number of diseases (Pitsavos *et al.*, 2007; Panagiotakos *et al.*, 2009). Although cross-sectional and longitudinal studies have shown some associations between dietary intakes of nutrients or nutritional status with inflammatory markers, limited intervention studies have been conducted in the older population. The burden of chronic disease is largely borne by older people owing to age-related increases in the incidence of CVD, cancer, dementia and osteoporosis, yet much of the research has not included the elderly but has focused on middle-aged adults. Thus, it can be difficult to extrapolate these research findings to old age because the elderly group are more likely to have a number of co-morbidities that are associated with inflammation.

A number of organ-specific age-related diseases have been found to have an inflammatory pathogenesis, including cancer, type 2 diabetes mellitus (T2DM), atherosclerosis, AD, osteoporosis, as well as obesity, depression and dementia. There are some epidemiological data and randomized controlled trials assessing diet and inflammation in common diseases of older adults, and the role of physical activity.

Cardiovascular disease

Atherosclerosis, leading to CVD, is characterized by a generalized cellular inflammatory response and inflammation, known to play a central role in mediating all phases of atherosclerosis, from the initiation of the atherosclerotic lesion to the eventual rupture of the unstable plaque (Blake and Ridker, 2002). During ageing, oxidative stress is also increased (Jira *et al.*, 1996; Napoli *et al.*, 1997), which may be a consequence of decreased nitric oxide bioavailability and endothelium-dependent vasodilatation, an increase in pro-inflammatory cytokines (Donato *et al.*, 2007, 2008) or a decrease in the presence of antioxidants (Napoli *et al.*, 1997). The oxidation of LDL cholesterol, which plays a key role in the development of atherogenesis, has been shown to be increased in the elderly. The inflammation that ensues stimulates pro-inflammatory signalling pathways leading to an inflammatory response, ultimately leading to the formation of atherosclerotic plaques. Reactive oxygen species (ROS) (superoxide anions, hydroxyl radicals and hydrogen peroxide) may be generated exogenously or produced intracellularly. Normally, cells defend themselves against ROS damage through antioxidants (e.g. vitamin E, vitamin C, selenium) (Herrera and Barbas, 2001; Padayatty *et al.*, 2003). However, an imbalance between oxidants and antioxidants results in oxidative stress, and increases in ROS can activate a number of signalling pathways that have been linked to atherosclerosis (Steinberg *et al.*, 1989; Witztum, 1994). Key participants in this process, which can be measured in serum, are the pro-inflammatory cytokines and acute phase reactants such as CRP. During acute inflammation, CRP and some acute-phase reactants can increase up to 10,000-fold. CRP has recently been used as a marker of sub-clinical atherosclerosis in identifying at-risk individuals: in middle-aged populations, high-sensitivity CRP (hs-CRP) was found to add prognostic information beyond that conveyed by all lipid measures (Ridker *et al.*, 2005). There is a graded, dose–response association between hs-CRP and CVD that remains after adjustment for other risk factors such as blood lipids. Lipids seem to add predictive value above that of currently established risk factors (Pearson *et al.*, 2003), although their prognostic value in the very old may be limited (Kritchevsky *et al.*, 2005).

Dietary patterns, inflammatory markers

A number of studies, conducted predominantly in healthy middle-aged men and women, have demonstrated inverse associations between a prudent dietary pattern and biomarkers of inflammation, specifically CRP and E-selectin, and a positive association between a 'Western' diet and CRP concentrations (Lopez-Garcia *et al.*, 2004a). A dietary pattern that included whole grains, fruit, nuts and green leafy vegetables was inversely associated with CRP, IL-6, homocysteine and soluble intercellular adhesion molecule-1 (Nettleton *et al.*, 2006); whereas a 'Mediterranean-style' has been found to be associated with reduced serum concentrations of hs-CRP, IL-6 and homocysteine (Chrysohoou *et al.*, 2004; Esposito *et al.*, 2004). Both fruit and vegetable intakes have been found to be inversely associated with plasma CRP concentrations in a study conducted in middle-aged women (Esmaillzadeh *et al.*, 2006); and in a cross-sectional study in older men free of CVD, fruit and dietary vitamin C intakes were negatively associated with CRP concentrations (Wannamethee *et al.*, 2006). Similar results were found in cross-sectional studies in Hispanic white elders (Gao *et al.*, 2004). In a 10-year cohort study, among those aged between 45 and 75 years, variety but not quantity of fruit and vegetables was associated with a lower serum CRP concentration (Bhupathiraju and Tucker, 2011).

There have been few randomized controlled trials (RCTs) investigating the role of dietary factors on markers of inflammation in older people. One RCT, in persons aged 55–80 years of age at high cardiovascular risk, found that a Mediterranean diet that included olive oil, down-regulated cellular and humoral inflammatory pathways related to atherosclerosis, through a reduction in CRP, IL-6 and endothelial and monocyte adhesion molecules and chemokines, whereas a low-fat diet did not show these effects (Estruch, 2010). This is not, however, a consistent finding in all studies. One trial found no effect of a Mediterranean diet on CRP, but baseline levels of CRP were low in participants of whom 80% were taking a statin drug, possibly explaining the negative finding (Michalsen *et al.*, 2006).

Dietary fat, inflammatory markers

Trans fatty acid (TFA) intake in women has been positively associated with markers of systemic inflammation: specifically, to soluble TNF-α receptors 1 and 2, IL-6 and CRP in the Nurses' Health Study I and II (Mozaffarian *et al.*, 2004). Adjusting for serum lipid concentrations partly attenuated these associations, suggesting that they might be partly mediated by effects of TFAs on serum lipids. Perhaps inflammatory markers such as CRP are useful predictors of response to dietary intervention. For example, in a study among generally healthy adults, those with higher CRP concentrations had a smaller and non-significant reduction in total and low-density lipoprotein (LDL) cholesterol, but a significant and greater increase in triglycerides, on a reduced-fat/low-cholesterol diet (Erlinger *et al.*, 2003).

In agreement with epidemiological studies, a carefully controlled dietary intervention study showed that consumption of *trans* and saturated fatty acids might be associated with increased risk of coronary artery disease in humans, mediated through pro-inflammatory cytokines, acute-phase proteins and adhesion molecules. Consumption of a diet rich in TFA (8% TFA for 8 weeks) led to significant increases in plasma CRP and IL-6 in healthy men (mean age 42 years) (Baer *et al.*, 2004). A similar study, however, conducted in older men and women (range 52–73 years), failed to show any changes in CRP levels with increased TFA consumption (6% substitution) over a shorter time period of 35 days (Lichtenstein *et al.*, 2003).

Although plant sterols reduce blood lipids (Gagliardi *et al.*, 2010), they seem to have little or no effect on inflammatory markers (Houweling *et al.*, 2009). In contrast to saturated and *trans* fatty acids, polyunsaturated fats, specifically the long-chain omega-3 PUFAs eicosapentanoic acid (EPA) and docosahexanoic acid (DHA), have well documented anti-inflammatory properties (Galli and Calder, 2009) and also effectively reduce serum triglycerides. Long-chain omega-3 PUFAs are mainly found in fish, particularly oily fish like salmon. Evidence from three cohort studies showed that dietary long-chain omega-3 PUFAs (Lopez-Garcia *et al.*, 2004b; Niu *et al.*, 2006; He *et al.*, 2008) and consumption of non-fried fish (He *et al.*, 2008) were associated with lower levels of inflammation (Table 19.1).

Of the nine reported RCTs in healthy elderly or in patients at high risk for CVD or with hyperlipidemia, five were found to reduce some markers of inflammation in response to fish oil (Thies *et al.*, 2001a,b,c; Bechoua *et al.*, 2003; Wu *et al.*, 2004). One study utilizing whole fish found a reduction in CRP (Tsitouras *et al.*, 2008) and two studies reported non-significant results (Berstad *et al.*, 2003; Pot *et al.*, 2010a) (Table 19.2). The applicability of these studies to the general population of older people is not clear because the amount of fish and/or fish oil consumed was extremely high and would not be achievable by most older people.

Other foods/nutrients, inflammation

There is inconsistent evidence for other foods, particularly those containing polyphenols, on markers of inflammation in patients at risk for CVD. Polyphenolic compounds are known for their antioxidant properties. They include resveratrol, curcumin, quercetin and (–)-epigallocatechin-3-gallate (EGCG), and are found in red wine/grapes, curry powder, fruits/vegetables and green tea, respectively. Polyphenols have the capacity to modulate the associated biological states of oxidative stress and chronic inflammation that are found to contribute to the aetiology of various diseases, and limited intervention studies have been conducted.

In a randomized crossover feeding trial of men and women ~70 years of age (n = 42) and at high risk of CVD (either had diabetes or ≥3 of the following cardiovascular disease risk factors: tobacco smoking, hypertension, elevated blood lipids or obesity), consumption of 40 g cocoa powder with 500 ml skimmed milk/day for 4 weeks significantly decreased P-selectin and ICAM-1 concentrations, whilst consumption of skimmed milk only had no significant effect for hsCRP, IL-6 or the expression of adhesion molecules on T lymphocyte surfaces (Monagas *et al.*, 2009). In another RCT, in a younger age group who were at high risk for CVD (elevated blood pressure, elevated blood lipids and elevated hematocrit or smoking), supplementation with bilberry juice significantly decreased plasma concentrations of CRP, IL-6 and IL-15 over a 4-week period (Karlsen *et al.*, 2010). There is evidence in those at greatest risk of CVD that foods containing polyphenols may modulate the inflammation processes and could result in health benefits, and the benefits of such foods should be explored further in older adults.

Diabetes

Type II diabetes (T2DM) is highly prevalent in the older population (International Diabetes Federation and World Health Organisation Diabetes Uni, 2007), brought about by the age-related impairment of pancreatic β cells leading to decreasing insulin production. The link between inflammation and T2DM may be through insulin resistance (IR), perhaps the result of TNF-α (Hotamisligil *et al.*, 1993; Aljada *et al.*, 2002) or IL-6 (Senn *et al.*, 2002) inhibiting insulin signalling. High levels of

Table 19.1. Summary of evidence of dietary associations with markers of inflammation in older people: cross-sectional studies.

Study description	Sample and characteristics	Intervention/methods	Main outcomes	Conclusions
He *et al.*, 2008 Location: USA Study design: Population based-study	Multi-Ethnic Study of Atherosclerosis n = 5677 Age: 45–84 years Population: Men and women free of CVD	Self administered Food Frequency Questionnaire (FFQ)	Long-chain PUFA was inversely associated with IL-6 concentrations Non-fried fish was inversely associated with IL-6, CRP, ICAM-1 and fibrinogen Fried fish consumption associated with increased CRP and IL-6	Some association Long-chain n-3 PUFAs and fish were associated with improved levels of inflammation and endothelial activation
Lopez-Garcia *et al.*, 2004 Location: USA Study design: Cross-sectional	Subgroup of women from the Nurses Health Study n = 727 Age: ~56 years Population: Healthy women	Self-administered FFQ	Highest quintile of total dietary n-3 PUFA (ALA+EPA+DHA) had a significantly lower concentration of CRP, IL-6 E-selectin, soluble vascular adhesion molecule (VCAM-1) and soluble intracellular adhesion molecule (sICAM-1) compared with the highest quintile	Some association Dietary n-3 PUFA intake (at least 60 g fish/week) was associated with decreased levels of inflammatory markers
Niu *et al.*, 2006 Location: Japan Study design: Cross-sectional	n = 971 Age: ~76 years Population: Healthy men and women	Self-administered diet-history questionnaire	Increasing total n-3 PUFA intakes was associated with decreased CRP Increasing intakes of long-chain n-3 PUFA (EPA+DHA) across quartiles was associated with a decreased odds of high CRP	Some association Higher intake of n-3 PUFAs from fish products was independently associated with a lower prevalence of CRP concentrations ≥1 mg/l

ALA, alpha linolenic acid; CRP, C-reactive protein; CVD, cardiovascular disease; DHA, docosahexanoic acid; EPA, eicosapentanoic acid; IL-6, interleukin 6; ICAM-1, intercellular adhesion molecule 1; n-3 PUFA, omega-3 polyunsaturated fatty acids; VCAM-1, vascular adhesion molecule.

Table 19.2. Summary of evidence of dietary factors with markers of inflammation in older people: randomized controlled studies.

Study description	Sample and characteristics	Intervention/methods	Main outcomes	Conclusions
Pot *et al.*, 2010a; Geelen *et al.*, 2004 Location: Netherlands Study design: Parallel, double-blind, placebo-controlled trial	n = 77 Age: 50–70 years Population: Healthy men and women	Fish oil (700 mg EPA + 560 mg DHA) versus placebo (high oleic sunflower oil) Duration: 12 weeks	Fish oil supplementation had no effect on serum IL-6, IL-1β or TNF-α versus placebo Fish oil supplementation had no effect on CRP concentrations vs placebo	No evidence of effect Healthy middle-aged population may not benefit from fish oil as an anti-inflammatory agent
Berstad *et al.*, 2003 Location: Norway Study design: Placebo-controlled double-blind, randomized study, with 2×2 factorial	n = 171 Age: 65–71 years Population: Men at high risk for CHD	Group 1: 2.4 g of esterified n-3 PUFA, no dietary advice; Group 2: Dietary advice (to increase fruit, vegetable, fish and vegetable oil intakes, and decrease use of fat from meat and animal sources) + placebo capsules; Group 3: 2.4 g of n-3 PUFA + dietary advice, Group 4: Placebo capsules, no dietary advice Fish oil groups also consumed 12 mg α-tocopherol/day Duration: 18 months	Both n-3 PUFA supplementation groups increased serum EPA and DHA 18 months of fish oil supplementation did not affect serum E-selectin, VCAM-1, ICAM-1, or endothelial markers A decrease in E-selectin was reported in the dietary intervention group	Some selective effect No dose-response association between the increases in serum EPA and DHA and changes in inflammatory markers
Thies *et al.*, 2001a,b Location: UK Study design: Randomized, placebo-controlled, double-blind parallel study	n = 46 Age: 55–75 years Population: Healthy men and women	2 g ALA versus 770 mg GLA versus 680 mg AA versus 720 mg DHA versus 720 mg EPA + 280 mg DHA/day Duration: 12 weeks	720 mg EPA + 280 mg DHA decreased Natural Killer cell activity This decrease was fully reversed by 4 weeks after supplementation had ceased DHA supplementation alone (720 mg/day) had no effect GLA and FO caused a significant decrease in lymphocyte proliferation	Negative effect Moderate supplementation with EPA (but not other n-6 or n-3 PUFA) decreased NK cell activity in healthy subjects Some selective effect Moderate level GLA or EPA but not other n-6 or n-3 PUFA can decrease lymphocyte proliferation but not production of interleukin-2 or IFN-γ

Continued

Table 19.2. Continued.

Study description	Sample and characteristics	Intervention/methods	Main outcomes	Conclusions
			No effect on the production of IL-2 or IFN-γ by PBMC	
Thies *et al.*, 2001c Location: UK Study design: Randomized, placebo-controlled, double-blind, parallel study	n = 46 Age: 55–75 years Population: Healthy men and women	720 mg EPA + 280 mg DHA/day Duration: 12 weeks	Supplementation decreased VCAM-1 by 28% and decreased E-selectin by 17% Fish oil supplementation did not affect ICAM-1 or inflammatory cell numbers or neutrophil and monocyte responses	Some selective effect Fish oil supplementation containing moderate levels of EPA+DHA can decrease some markers of endothelial activation
Tsitouras *et al.*, 2008 Location: USA Study design: Single intervention study	n = 12 Age: ~66 years Population: Healthy older men and women	Control: 720 g of lean fish/week Intervention: 720 g of fatty fish/ week + 15 ml of sardine oil/day Duration: 6-week control period, 8-week intervention	After the intervention period, serum CRP concentrations decreased with a trend towards a reduction in IL-6	Some selective effect Regular consumption of fatty fish may beneficially affect endothelial inflammatory markers such as CRP
Bechoua, 2003 Location: France Study design: Double-blind, randomized controlled trial	n = 20 Age: 70–83 years (mean 75.6 years) Population: Healthy, non-institutionalized elderly	Fish oil (150 mg DHA + 30 mg EPA) Placebo Both groups received vitamin E (0.17 mg α-tocopherol for the placebo and 0.54 mg for the marine oil Duration: 6 weeks	The proliferative responses of PBMCs to various mitogens decreased in the fish oil group versus placebo	Some selective effect A low dose of EPA+DHA was sufficient to markedly decrease the proliferative response of lymphocytes to mitogenic lectins and antigens
Wu *et al.*, 2004 Location: USA Study design: Randomized, double blind placebo-controlled study	n = 40 Age: > 65 years Population: Healthy elderly men and women	300 mg EPA + 200 mg DHA was given to all subjects PLUS varying doses of vitamin E (100 mg, 200 mg or 40 mg Placebo Duration: 3 months	LPS stimulated production of IL-1β decreased with the 200 mg vitamin E No change following the other doses No significant reduction in the production of concanalvin A stimulated IL-6 or TNF-α	Some selective effect Vitamin E in combination with fish oil may contribute to the reduction in inflammatory cytokines observed

ALA, alpha linolenic acid; AA, arachidonic acid; CHD, coronary heart disease; CRP, C-reactive protein; DHA, docosahexanoic acid; EPA, eicosapentanoic acid; FO, fish oil; GLA, gamma linolenic acid; ICAM-1, intercellular adhesion molecule 1; IL-6, interleukin 6; IL-1β, interleukin 1-beta; IL-2, interleukin 2; IFN-γ, interferon gamma; LPS, lipopolysaccharide; NK, natural killer; PBMC, peripheral blood mononuclear cells; n-3 PUFA, omega-3 polyunsaturated fatty acids; TNF-α, tumour necrosis factor alpha; VCAM-1, vascular adhesion molecule.

CRP and IL-6 have been shown to be independent predictors for the development of T2DM (Pradhan *et al.*, 2001; Dandona *et al.*, 2004). Despite these emerging links, there are few randomized controlled studies in older patients with T2DM evaluating the impact on inflammation through dietary strategies.

Cancer

Similarly, for cancer, the prevalence in older adults is high (World Cancer Research Fund / American Institute for Cancer Research, 2007). Studies in rats have identified that chronic inflammation accelerates tumour formation in mice lacking the ability to repair DNA damage (Meira *et al.*, 2008). In humans, there is increasing evidence that chronic inflammatory states in the gastrointestinal tract are associated with increased incidence of *Helicobacter pylori* infection, gastric cancer and coeliac disease. Coeliac disease is associated with intestinal lymphoma and other forms of cancer, especially adenocarcinoma in the gastrointestinal tract (Catassi *et al.*, 2005). The age-associated changes in the immune system, with reduction in function of the thymus, is marked (Wang *et al.*, 2010), with inflammatory infiltrates predominantly represented by CD3(+) T lymphocytes and macrophages. It is difficult, however, to ascribe the inflammatory response, particularly the change in T-cell distribution to the age-related increased incidence of cancer in older people. Despite positive associations identifying higher intakes of some fruits and vegetables, cereal products, dairy products and fibre-rich foods with reduced risk of inflammation and potential reduction in colorectal cancer (Lund *et al.*, 2011), limited RCTs have been carried out assessing a reduction in cancer cells or inflammation with dietary strategies (Cheng *et al.*, 2003; Courtney *et al.*, 2007; Pot *et al.*, 2010a,b).

Alzheimer's disease, dementia and impaired cognition

Alzheimer's disease (AD) is the most common cause of dementia and is characterized by a progressive decline in memory function (Blennow *et al.*, 2006). Old age is the predominant risk factor for AD, and the prevalence of AD increases almost exponentially from 1% at 60–64 years of age to 25% or more at 85 years old and older (Blennow *et al.*, 2006).

One of the key drivers of dementia is reduced blood flow to the brain. There is evidence that stroke and a number of cardiovascular risk factors, especially raised blood pressure, are important in the development of both vascular and degenerative forms of dementia (i.e. AD) and cognitive impairment (Gorelick, 2004). There is evidence that fish oils, which contain n-3 PUFA, reduce blood pressure, especially in older and hypertensive subjects (Geleijnse *et al.*, 2002), and reduce plasma triglycerides (Robinson and Stone, 2006). The inflammatory pathways are a key component for the development of thrombosis and endothelial dysfunction, which are linked in the development of atherosclerosis. Western diets tend to be high in n-6 fatty acids, notably linoleic acid, which is a precursor of arachidonic acid (AA), and comparatively low in the n-3 PUFAs, alpha-linolenic acid and the long-chain marine fatty acids DHA and EPA. It is thought that diets high in n-6 and low in n-3 PUFA lead to more AA in brain phospholipids, which leads to a pro-inflammatory environment that contributes to the development of AD (Cole *et al.*, 2010). The large prospective Framingham Heart Study among 899 men and women (median age of 76 years) who were followed up for 9.1 years, found that those in the upper quartile of plasma phosphatidylcholine DHA levels, with a mean fish intake of 3.0 servings/week, had a 47% reduction in risk of developing all-cause dementia (Schaefer *et al.*, 2006). A recent review using data from cross-sectional and longitudinal population-based studies concluded that there is an indication that higher intakes of saturated fatty acids could have negative effects on cognitive function and contribute to mild cognitive impairment, whilst in creased fish consumption and high intake of monounsaturated fatty acids and PUFAs, particularly n-3 PUFA, reduces risk for cognitive decline (Solfrizzi *et al.*, 2010). Another review also supported that low fish and DHA intakes contribute significantly to the risk of AD, with lower blood DHA levels also linked to a higher risk of cognitive decline and AD (Cunnane *et al.*, 2009). Currently there is no evidence from RCTs to support these findings, however.

Depression

The cause of depression associated with ageing is unclear. Although depression often occurs in combination with other disorders (Alexopoulos, 2005), it tends to worsen the outcomes of these illnesses and increases mortality. Studies have found that, with ageing, there is an increase in immune cells of the brain, mediators of inflammation and brain atrophy (Lucin and Wyss-Coray, 2009). Both human and animal studies have found that genes related to cellular stress and inflammation are up-regulated with age, whereas genes related to synaptic function, growth factors and trophic support are down-regulated (Lucin and Wyss-Coray, 2009).

There is also a growing body of research indicating a link between depression and increased levels of pro-inflammatory cytokines. Increased concentrations of CRP and pro-inflammatory cytokines have been observed in depressed, but otherwise healthy, patients (Schlatter *et al.*, 2004). Stressors activate the hypothalamo–pituitary–adrenal (HPA) axis and the sympathetic nervous system, and the products of these systems then alter the function of immune organs and cells elevating pro-inflammatory cytokines. These cytokines may pass through the blood–brain barrier and alter pathways involved in depression such as neurotransmitter metabolism (Maier and Watkins, 1998). Hyper-secretion of corticotropin-releasing hormone (CRH) under these conditions may provide the substrate linking stress and depression. Thus, the relationship between depression and inflammation appears bi-directional, and each may be stimulated by the other.

In a recent analysis of the NHANES data, the risk of moderate to severe depression was significantly greater in the highest quartiles of CRP (ordinal regression; OR = 1.84), white blood cell count (OR = 1.70) and platelet counts (OR = 1.41) (Kobrosly and van Wijngaarden, 2010). In an Australian retrospective cohort study, serum CRP was found to be an independent risk marker for *de novo* major depressive disorder in women (Pasco *et al.*, 2010). Additionally, there is growing, albeit inconsistent, evidence of a link between various nutritional components, such as n-3 PUFAs found in fish, and depression. The brain and central nervous system (CNS) contain high concentrations of n-3 PUFAs, and it has been suggested that n-3 PUFAs may be involved in neurotransmitter synthesis, degradation, release, reuptake and binding, resulting in neurotransmitter activity that has been associated with reduced levels of depression and low mood (Liperoti *et al.*, 2009).

A few RCTs have been performed to assess the effect of fish oils on depression in the elderly and have found no effect. Two studies, one in mild to moderately depressed elderly (mean age 85 years) receiving 12 weeks of daily consumption of fish oil (1480 mg EPA + DHA) and another in independently living elderly (n = 302, mean age 70 years) receiving daily fish oil supplementation with 1800 mg or 400 mg EPA + DHA for 13 or 26 weeks, found no effect of the supplements on cognitive function (Rogers *et al.*, 2008), depression scores or anxiety (van de Rest *et al.*, 2008b) or quality of life. Another study found that n-3 PUFA supplementation improved depressive symptoms but only in non-apolipoprotein E4 carriers (van de Rest *et al.*, 2008a), indicating that some people may be more responsive to specific dietary interventions. A meta-analysis evaluating the effect of n-3 PUFAs on depressed mood concluded that there was considerable heterogeneity in the outcome, with some support of a benefit of n-3 PUFAs in those with a clinically diagnosed depressive illness, but no evidence of any benefit in individuals without a diagnosis of depressive illness (Appleton *et al.*, 2010). Again, the link between reducing inflammation through dietary strategies and reducing depression has not been evaluated in RCT. The high prevalence of depression associated with cancer, diabetes and coronary heart disease, all conditions that increase with increasing age (Jackson *et al.*, 2004) and are characterized by inflammation, should provide the impetus to evaluate the efficacy of dietary interventions in preventing depression by reducing inflammation.

Physical Activity, Inflammation and Ageing

Physical activity itself is involved in the recruitment and activation of skeletal muscle (Fig. 19.2). Within the muscle, intense exercise is associated with the generation of an inflammatory response (Nieman *et al.*, 1995). Cytokines and other peptides that are produced, expressed and released by muscle fibres and exert either paracrine or endocrine effects are classified as 'myokines' (Febbraio and Pedersen, 2005). These myokines include both pro- and anti-inflammatory cytokine species (Pedersen and Febbraio, 2008). It is hypothesized that the profile of secreted myokines reflects the severity of muscular damage, with more severe traumatic muscular damage eliciting a cytokine profile necessary for the recruitment, invasion and activation of inflammatory cells, including macrophages and neutrophils, necessary for degradation and ultimately repair of the damaged tissues (Tidball, 2005). Although differences in the production of myokines is evident in studies that have focused on the expression within myofibres, the overall differences in pro- versus anti-inflammatory responses between young and older individuals remains unknown. Indeed, it has yet to be established how regular exercise (or exercise training) is able to lower the inflammatory load of ageing (Mathur and Pedersen, 2008). There are two plausible mechanisms. The first is that inactivity itself is associated with increased muscular inflammation. This is demonstrated in disuse models, where restricting or preventing muscle activity results in the activation of stress-signalling pathways within the muscle (Evans *et al.*, 2010). Whether this results in greater secretion of pro-inflammatory cytokines into the circulation is not understood. The second theory is that in response to the pro-inflammatory stimuli imposed by exercise itself, the muscle elicits an increased compensatory or buffering response. This is characterized by hormesis, which is a dose–response phenomenon characterized by a low-dose stimulation, high-dose inhibition, resulting in either a J-shaped or an inverted U-shaped dose–response (Nunn *et al.*, 2010). Accordingly it is thought

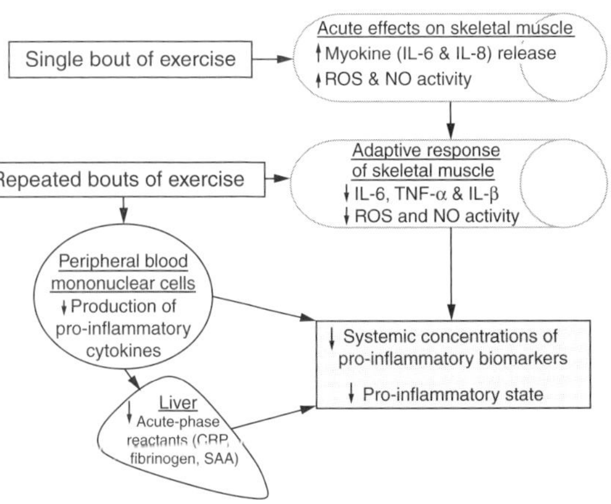

Fig. 19.2. Schematic of adaptations to exercise training potentially underlying improvements in chronic inflammation. Adaptive responses in inflammatory and redox-sensitive pathways in skeletal muscle, as well as potential adaptive responses in innate immune cells, may serve to protect against chronic systemic low-grade inflammation. CRP, C-reactive protein; IL, interleukin; NO, nitric oxide; ROS, reactive oxygen species; SAA, serum amyloid a; TGF-β, transforming growth factor beta; TNF-α, tumour necrosis factor alpha. (From Nicklas *et al.*, 2009, with permission from Lippincott Williams & Wilkins.)

that periodic and short-term exposure to a pro-inflammatory load will elicit a greater and compensatory rise in protective and anti-inflammatory defences, such that an overall reduction in inflammatory load is present. Although neither mechanism has been examined *in vivo*, clear and consistent intervention data are providing evidence that exercise is an important defence against age-related inflammation (Mathur and Pedersen, 2008).

Physical activity: observational studies

A number of observational studies have demonstrated reduced circulatory concentrations of inflammatory biomarkers in aged individuals. The large population studies that have correlated the impact of exercise participation and circulating inflammatory variables include the Third National Health and Nutrition Examination Survey (NHANES III) (Abramson and Vaccarino, 2002), the British Regional Heart Study (Wannamethee *et al.*, 2002), the Cardiovascular Health Study (Geffken *et al.*, 2001) and the Health ABC Study (Schaap *et al.*, 2009). In these studies an independent and inverse relationship with plasma CRP and other markers, including TNF-α and IL-6, has been established. Furthermore, this relationship is influenced by the intensity and frequency of exercise in older populations. Indeed in the NHANES III cohort, an increased self-reported physical activity frequency from 4 to 21 times/month to almost daily activity (>22 times/month) resulted in a decrease in the percentage of the population with elevated CRP from 9.7% to 6.5% (Abramson *et al.*, 2002). Comparing these results with those of the sedentary individuals, in whom 15.1% had elevated CRP, physical activity with increasing frequency is beneficial.

Physical activity: randomized controlled trials

Intervention studies with either structured supervised or unsupervised community exercise participation in older cohorts overwhelmingly support the benefits of greater exercise in ameliorating chronic inflammation in the elderly. Of the studies completed to date, structured studies in high-risk populations should be noted. Such studies have examined the benefits of exercise training in older people with coronary heart disease (Walther *et al.*, 2008) and T2DM (Brooks *et al.*, 2007). The studies demonstrated reductions in circulating CRP and IL-6 in these populations. In an otherwise healthy population of older men and women, The Lifestyle Interventions and Independence for Elders (LIFE) trial provides RCT evidence of an improvement in inflammatory load in a community-dwelling population (Nicklas *et al.*, 2008). Over a 12-month intervention period, 424 elderly people (70–89 years) engaged in a physical activity programme consisting of aerobic, strength and flexibility exercises. Both IL-6 and CRP concentrations were reduced, although, importantly, those with the greatest pre-intervention inflammatory load had the greatest reductions.

Summary and Conclusions

Ageing can generally be viewed as a pro-inflammatory state and the chronic diseases that manifest in older people, such as CVD, cancer, T2DM and dementia, are characterized by increased levels of inflammation. As such, it is difficult to separate the effects of ageing from disease states because these occur concurrently. Many nutrients, foods and dietary patterns have been associated with inflammation. Cross-sectionally and longitudinally, these relationships in general mirror those seen for blood lipids and cardiovascular risk. To date there have only been short-term dietary intervention studies evaluating markers of inflammation, with conflicting results. Currently it is not possible to make any firm recommendations as there are many unknowns. For example, it is possible that diet influences the metabolism of pro-inflammatory cytokines, without a concomitant change in the overall inflammatory process. Furthermore, the significance in terms of health and progression of disease, of small reductions in inflammatory markers, is not known. We do not know if these small, short-term reductions in inflammatory markers actually translate to equivalent positive health benefits demonstrated in cross-sectional or prospective studies. In addition, it may be that inflammatory markers such as CRP are useful to predict risk, or respond to dietary intervention, whilst remaining resistant to significant long-term reductions. None the less, it is feasible that dietary factors will be found to have an impact on the overall inflammatory response and could reduce some of the disease burden associated with ageing or even assist in extending the lifespan. Hence, more randomized trials conducted in older people are needed to demonstrate the long-term efficacy of dietary interventions.

Despite the initial pro-inflammatory response to exercise, longer-term improvements in inflammation are evident in older individuals. Further studies are required to provide both mechanistic insights to understand the biological basis for these improvements, but also to ascertain the dose, frequency and types of exercise that are required.

References

Abramson, J.L. and Vaccarino, V. (2002) Relationship between physical activity and inflammation among apparently healthy middle-aged and older US adults. *Archives of Internal Medicine* 162, 1286–1292.

Alexopoulos, G.S. (2005) Depression in the elderly. *Lancet* 365, 1961–1970.

Aljada, A., Ghanim, H., Assian, E. and Dandona, P. (2002) Tumor necrosis factor-alpha inhibits insulin-induced increase in endothelial nitric oxide synthase and reduces insulin receptor content and phosphorylation in human aortic endothelial cells. *Metabolism* 51, 487–491.

Appleton, K.M., Rogers, P.J. and Ness, A.R. (2010) Updated systematic review and meta-analysis of the effects of n-3 long-chain polyunsaturated fatty acids on depressed mood. *American Journal of Clinical Nutrition* 91, 757–770.

Baer, D.J., Judd, J.T., Clevidence, B.A. and Tracy, R.P. (2004) Dietary fatty acids affect plasma markers of inflammation in healthy men fed controlled diets: a randomized crossover study. *American Journal of Clinical Nutrition* 79, 969–973.

Bastard, J.P., Maachi, M., Lagathu, C., Kim, M.J., Caron, M., *et al.* (2006) Recent advances in the relationship between obesity, inflammation, and insulin resistance. *European Cytokine Network* 17, 4–12.

Bechoua, S., Dubois, M., Vericel, E., Chapuy, P., Lagarde, M., *et al.* (2003) Influence of very low dietary intake of marine oil on some functional aspects of immune cells in healthy elderly people. *British Journal of Nutrition* 89, 523–531.

Berstad, P., Seljeflot, I., Veierod, M.B., Hjerkinn, E.M., Arnesen, H., *et al.* (2003) Supplementation with fish oil affects the association between very long-chain n-3 polyunsaturated fatty acids in serum non-esterified fatty acids and soluble vascular cell adhesion molecule-1. *Clinical Science (London)* 105, 13–20.

Bhupathiraju, S.N. and Tucker, K.L. (2011) Greater variety in fruit and vegetable intake is associated with lower inflammation in Puerto Rican adults. *American Journal of Clinical Nutrition* 93, 37–46.

Blake, G.J. and Ridker, P.M. (2002) Inflammatory bio-markers and cardiovascular risk prediction. *Journal of Internal Medicine* 252, 283–294.

Blennow, K., De Leon, M.J. and Zetterberg, H. (2006) Alzheimer's disease. *Lancet* 368, 387–403.

Brooks, N., Layne, J.E., Gordon, P.L., Roubenoff, R., Nelson, M.E., *et al.* (2007) Strength training improves muscle quality and insulin sensitivity in Hispanic older adults with type 2 diabetes. *International Journal of Medical Sciences* 4, 19–27.

Bruunsgaard, H., Andersen-Ranberg, K., Jeune, B., Pedersen, A.N., Skinhoj, P., *et al.* (1999) A high plasma concentration of TNF-alpha is associated with dementia in centenarians. *Journals of Gerontology. Series A, Biological Sciences and Medical Sciences* 54, M357–M364.

Catassi, C., Bearzi, I. and Holmes, G.K. (2005) Association of celiac disease and intestinal lymphomas and other cancers. *Gastroenterology* 128, S79–S86.

Cheng, J., Ogawa, K., Kuriki, K., Yokoyama, Y., Kamiya, T., *et al.* (2003) Increased intake of n-3 polyunsaturated fatty acids elevates the level of apoptosis in the normal sigmoid colon of patients polypectomized for adenomas/tumors. *Cancer Letters* 193, 17–24.

Chrysohoou, C., Panagiotakos, D.B., Pitsavos, C., Das, U.N. and Stefanadis, C. (2004) Adherence to the Mediterranean diet attenuates inflammation and coagulation process in healthy adults: The ATTICA Study. *Journal of American College of Cardiology* 44, 152–158.

Cole, G.M., Ma, Q.L. and Frautschy, S.A. (2010) Dietary fatty acids and the aging brain. *Nutrition Reviews* 68 Suppl 2, S102–S111.

Courtney, E.D., Matthews, S., Finlayson, C., Di Pierro, D., Belluzzi, A., *et al.* (2007) Eicosapentaenoic acid (EPA) reduces crypt cell proliferation and increases apoptosis in normal colonic mucosa in subjects with a history of colorectal adenomas. *International Journal of Colorectal Disease* 22, 765–776.

Cunnane, S.C., Plourde, M., Pifferi, F., Begin, M., Feart, C. *et al.* (2009) Fish, docosahexaenoic acid and Alzheimer's disease. *Progress in Lipid Research* 48, 239–256.

Dandona, P., Aljada, A. and Bandyopadhyay, A. (2004) Inflammation: the link between insulin resistance, obesity and diabetes. *Trends in Immunology* 25, 4–7.

De Martinis, M., Franceschi, C., Monti, D. and Ginaldi, L. (2005) Inflamm-ageing and lifelong antigenic load as major determinants of ageing rate and longevity. *Federation of European Biochemical Societies* 579, 2035–2039.

Donato, A.J., Black, A.D., Jablonski, K.L., Gano, L.B. and Seals, D.R. (2008) Aging is associated with greater nuclear NF kappa B, reduced I kappa B alpha, and increased expression of proinflammatory cytokines in vascular endothelial cells of healthy humans. *Aging Cell* 7, 805–812.

Donato, A.J., Eskurza, I., Silver, A.E., Levy, A.S., Pierce, G.L., *et al.* (2007) Direct evidence of endothelial oxidative stress with aging in humans: relation to impaired endothelium-dependent dilation and upregulation of nuclear factor-kappaB. *Circulation Research* 100, 1659–1666.

Erlinger, T.P., Miller, E.R., 3rd, Charleston, J. and Appel, L.J. (2003) Inflammation modifies the effects of a reduced-fat low-cholesterol diet on lipids: results from the DASH-sodium trial. *Circulation* 108, 150–154.

Esmaillzadeh, A., Kimiagar, M., Mehrabi, Y., Azadbakht, L., Hu, F.B., *et al.* (2006) Fruit and vegetable intakes, C-reactive protein, and the metabolic syndrome. *American Journal of Clinical Nutrition* 84, 1489–1497.

Esposito, K., Marfella, R., Ciotola, M., Di Palo, C., Giugliano, F., *et al.* (2004) Effect of a mediterranean-style diet on endothelial dysfunction and markers of vascular inflammation in the metabolic syndrome: a randomized trial. *Journal of the American Medical Association* 292, 1440–1446.

Estruch, R. (2010) Anti-inflammatory effects of the Mediterranean diet: the experience of the PREDIMED study. *Proceedings of the Nutrition Society* 69, 333–340.

Evans, W.J., Paolisso, G., Abbatecola, A.M., Corsonello, A., Bustacchini, S., *et al.* (2010) Frailty and muscle metabolism dysregulation in the elderly. *Biogerontology* 11, 527–536.

Fagiolo, U., Cossarizza, A., Scala, E., Fanales-Belasio, E., Ortolani, C., *et al.* (1993) Increased cytokine production in mononuclear cells of healthy elderly people. *European Journal of Immunology* 23, 2375–2378.

Fagnoni, F.F., Vescovini, R., Mazzola, M., Bologna, G., Nigro, E., Lavagetto, G., Franceschi, C., Passeri, M. and Sansoni, P. (1996) Expansion of cytotoxic CD8+ CD28– T cells in healthy ageing people, including centenarians. *Immunology* 88, 501–507.

Febbraio, M.A. and Pedersen, B.K. (2005) Contraction-induced myokine production and release: is skeletal muscle an endocrine organ? *Exercise and Sport Sciences Review* 33, 114–119.

Franceschi, C., Bonafe, M., Valensin, S., Olivieri, F., De Luca, M., *et al.* (2000) Inflamm-aging. An evolutionary perspective on immunosenescence. *Annals of the New York Academy of Sciences* 908, 244–254.

Franceschi, C., Capri, M., Monti, D., Giunta, S., Olivieri, F., *et al.* (2007) Inflammaging and anti-inflammaging: a systemic perspective on aging and longevity emerged from studies in humans. *Mechanisms of Ageing and Development* 128, 92–105.

Gagliardi, A.C., Maranhao, R.C., De Sousa, H.P., Schaefer, E.J. and Santos, R.D. (2010) Effects of margarines and butter consumption on lipid profiles, inflammation markers and lipid transfer to HDL particles in free-living subjects with the metabolic syndrome. *European Journal of Clinical Nutrition* 64, 1141–1149.

Galli, C. and Calder, P.C. (2009) Effects of fat and fatty acid intake on inflammatory and immune responses: a critical review. *Annals of Nutrition and Metabolism* 55, 123–139.

Gao, X., Bermudez, O.I. and Tucker, K.L. (2004) Plasma C-reactive protein and homocysteine concentrations are related to frequent fruit and vegetable intake in Hispanic and non-Hispanic white elders. *Journal of Nutrition* 134, 913–918.

Geffken, D.F., Cushman, M., Burke, G.L., Polak, J.F., Sakkinen, P.A., *et al.* (2001) Association between physical activity and markers of inflammation in a healthy elderly population. *American Journal of Epidemiology* 153, 242–250.

Geleijnse, J.M., Giltay, E.J., Grobbee, D.E., Donders, A.R. and Kok, F.J. (2002) Blood pressure response to fish oil supplementation: metaregression analysis of randomized trials. *Journal of Hypertension* 20, 1493–1499.

Going, S., Williams, D. and Lohman, T. (1995) Aging and body composition: biological changes and methodological issues. *Exercise and Sport Sciences Reviews* 23, 411–458.

Gorelick, P.B. (2004) Risk factors for vascular dementia and Alzheimer disease. *Stroke* 35, 2620–2622.

Guarner, F. (2006) Enteric flora in health and disease. *Digestion* 73 Suppl 1, 5–12.

He, K., Liu, K., Daviglus, M.L., Mayer-Davis, E., Jenny, N.S., *et al.* (2008) Intakes of long-chain n-3 polyunsaturated fatty acids and fish in relation to measurements of subclinical atherosclerosis. *American Journal of Clinical Nutrition* 88, 1111–1118.

Herrera, E. and Barbas, C. (2001) Vitamin E: action, metabolism and perspectives. *Journal of Physiology and Biochemistry* 57, 43–56.

Hotamisligil, G.S., Shargill, N.S. and Spiegelman, B.M. (1993) Adipose expression of tumor necrosis factor-alpha: direct role in obesity-linked insulin resistance. *Science* 259, 87–91.

Houweling, A.H., Vanstone, C.A., Trautwein, E.A., Duchateau, G.S. and Jones, P.J. (2009) Baseline plasma plant sterol concentrations do not predict changes in serum lipids, C-reactive protein (CRP) and plasma plant sterols following intake of a plant sterol-enriched food. *European Journal of Clinical Nutrition* 63, 543–551.

International Diabetes Federation and World Health Organisation Diabetes Uni (2007) Diabetes Atlas, third edition, International Diabetes Federation, 2007. Diabetes and Cardiovascular Disease: Time to Act, International Diabetes Federation, 2001. World Health Organisation Diabetes Uni. Available at: http://www.diabetesaustralia.com.au/en/Understanding-Diabetes/Diabetes-Globally/.

Jackson, J.L., Dezee, K. and Berbano, E. (2004) Can treating depression improve disease outcomes? *Annals of Internal Medicine* 140, 1054–1056.

Jira, W., Spiteller, G. and Schramm, A. (1996) Increase in hydroxy fatty acids in human low density lipoproteins with age. *Chemistry and Physics of Lipids* 84, 165–173.

Karlsen, A., Paur, I., Bohn, S.K., Sakhi, A.K., Borge, G.I., *et al.* (2010) Bilberry juice modulates plasma concentration of NF-kappaB related inflammatory markers in subjects at increased risk of CVD. *European Journal of Nutrition* 49, 345–355.

Kmiec, Z., Mysliwska, J., Rachon, D., Kotlarz, G., Sworczak, K., *et al.* (2001) Natural killer activity and thyroid hormone levels in young and elderly persons. *Gerontology* 47, 282–288.

Kobrosly, R. and Van Wijngaarden, E. (2010) Associations between immunologic, inflammatory, and oxidative stress markers with severity of depressive symptoms: an analysis of the 2005–2006 National Health and Nutrition Examination Survey. *Neurotoxicology* 31, 126–133.

Kritchevsky, S.B., Cesari, M. and Pahor, M. (2005) Inflammatory markers and cardiovascular health in older adults. *Cardiovascular Research* 66, 265–75.

Lichtenstein, A.H., Erkkila, A.T., Lamarche, B., Schwab, U.S., Jalbert, S.M., *et al.* (2003) Influence of hydrogenated fat and butter on CVD risk factors: remnant-like particles, glucose and insulin, blood pressure and C-reactive protein. *Atherosclerosis* 171, 97–107.

Liperoti, R., Landi, F., Fusco, O., Bernabei, R. and Onder, G. (2009) Omega-3 polyunsaturated fatty acids and depression: a review of the evidence. *Current Pharmaceutical Design* 15, 4165–4172.

Lopez-Garcia, E., Schulze, M.B., Fung, T.T., Meigs, J.B., Rifai, N., *et al.* (2004a) Major dietary patterns are related to plasma concentrations of markers of inflammation and endothelial dysfunction. *American Journal of Clinical Nutrition* 80, 1029–35.

Lopez-Garcia, E., Schulze, M.B., Manson, J.E., Meigs, J.B., Albert, C.M., *et al.* (2004b) Consumption of (n-3) fatty acids is related to plasma biomarkers of inflammation and endothelial activation in women. *Journal of Nutrition* 134, 1806–1811.

Lucin, K.M. and Wyss-Coray, T. (2009) Immune activation in brain aging and neurodegeneration: too much or too little? *Neuron* 64, 110–122.

Lund, E.K., Belshaw, N.J., Elliott, G.O. and Johnson, I.T. (2011) Recent advances in understanding the role of diet and obesity in the development of colorectal cancer. *Proceedings of the Nutrition Society* 1–11.

Maier, S.F. and Watkins, L.R. (1998) Cytokines for psychologists: implications of bidirectional immune-to-brain communication for understanding behavior, mood, and cognition. *Psychological Review* 105, 83–107.

Mariani, E., Ravaglia, G., Forti, P., Meneghetti, A., Tarozzi, A., *et al.* (1999) Vitamin D, thyroid hormones and muscle mass influence natural killer (NK) innate immunity in healthy nonagenarians and centenarians. *Clinical and Experimental Immunology* 116, 19–27.

Mathur, N. and Pedersen, B.K. (2008) Exercise as a mean to control low-grade systemic inflammation. *Mediators of Inflammation* 2008, 109502.

Meira, L.B., Bugni, J.M., Green, S.L., Lee, C.W., Pang, B., *et al.* (2008) DNA damage induced by chronic inflammation contributes to colon carcinogenesis in mice. *Journal of Clinical Investigation* 118, 2516–2525.

Michalsen, A., Lehmann, N., Pithan, C., Knoblauch, N.T., Moebus, S., *et al.* (2006) Mediterranean diet has no effect on markers of inflammation and metabolic risk factors in patients with coronary artery disease. *European Journal of Clinical Nutrition* 60, 478–485.

Monagas, M., Khan, N., Andres-Lacueva, C., Casas, R., Urpi-Sarda, M., *et al.* (2009) Effect of cocoa powder on the modulation of inflammatory biomarkers in patients at high risk of cardiovascular disease. *American Journal of Clinical Nutrition* 90, 1144–1150.

Mozaffarian, D., Pischon, T., Hankinson, S.E., Rifai, N., Joshipura, K., *et al.* (2004) Dietary intake of trans fatty acids and systemic inflammation in women. *American Journal of Clinical Nutrition* 79, 606–612.

Napoli, C., Abete, P., Corso, G., Malorni, A., Postiglione, A., *et al.* (1997) Increased low-density lipoprotein peroxidation in elderly men. *Coronary Artery Disease* 8, 129–136.

Nettleton, J.A., Steffen, L.M., Mayer-Davis, E.J., Jenny, N.S., Jiang, R., *et al.* (2006) Dietary patterns are associated with biochemical markers of inflammation and endothelial activation in the Multi-Ethnic Study of Atherosclerosis (MESA). *American Journal of Clinical Nutrition* 83, 1369–1379.

Nicklas, B.J., Hsu, F.C., Brinkley, T.J., Church, T., Goodpaster, B.H., *et al.* (2008) Exercise training and plasma C-reactive protein and interleukin-6 in elderly people. *Journal of the American Geriatrics Society* 56, 2045–2052.

Nicklas, B.J., Brinkley, T.E., Nicklas, B.J. and Brinkley, T.E. (2009) Exercise training as a treatment for chronic inflammation in the elderly. *Exercise and Sport Sciences Reviews* 37, 165–170.

Nieman, D.C., Henson, D.A., Sampson, C.S., Herring, J.L., Suttles, J., *et al.* (1995) The acute immune response to exhaustive resistance exercise. *International Journal of Sports Medicine* 16, 322–328.

Niu, K., Hozawa, A., Kuriyama, S., Ohmori-Matsuda, K., Shimazu, T., *et al.* (2006) Dietary long-chain n-3 fatty acids of marine origin and serum C-reactive protein concentrations are associated in a population with a diet rich in marine products. *American Journal of Clinical Nutrition* 84, 223–229.

Nunn, A.V., Guy, G.W., Brodie, J.S. and Bell, J.D. (2010) Inflammatory modulation of exercise salience: using hormesis to return to a healthy lifestyle. *Nutrition and Metabolism (London)* 7, 87.

Padayatty, S.J., Katz, A., Wang, Y., Eck, P., Kwon, O., *et al.* (2003)Vitamin C as an antioxidant: evaluation of its role in disease prevention. *Journal of the American College of Nutrition* 22, 18–35.

Paganelli, R., Quinti, I., Fagiolo, U., Cossarizza, A., Ortolani, C., *et al.* (1992) Changes in circulating B cells and immunoglobulin classes and subclasses in a healthy aged population. *Clinical and Experimental Immunology* 90, 351–354.

Panagiotakos, D.B., Dimakopoulou, K., Katsouyanni, K., Bellander, T., Grau, M., *et al.* (2009) Mediterranean diet and inflammatory response in myocardial infarction survivors. *International Journal of Epidemiology* 38, 856–866.

Pancer, Z. and Cooper, M.D. (2006) The evolution of adaptive immunity. *Annual Review of Immunology* 24, 497–518.

Pasco, J.A., Nicholson, G.C., Williams, L.J., Jacka, F.N., Henry, M.J., *et al.* (2010) Association of high-sensitivity C-reactive protein with de novo major depression. *British Journal of Psychiatry* 197, 372–377.

Pearson, T.A., Mensah, G.A., Alexander, R.W., Anderson, J.L., Cannon, R.O., 3rd, *et al.* (2003) Markers of inflammation and cardiovascular disease: application to clinical and public health practice: A statement for healthcare professionals from the Centers for Disease Control and Prevention and the American Heart Association. *Circulation* 107, 499–511.

Pedersen, B.K. and Febbraio, M.A. (2008) Muscle as an endocrine organ: focus on muscle-derived interleukin-6. *Physiological Reviews* 88, 1379–1406.

Pitsavos, C., Panagiotakos, D.B., Tzima, N., Lentzas, Y., Chrysohoou, C., *et al.* (2007) Diet, exercise, and C-reactive protein levels in people with abdominal obesity: the ATTICA epidemiological study. *Angiology* 58, 225–233.

Pot, G.K., Geelen, A., Majsak-Newman, G., Harvey, L.J., Nagengast, F.M., *et al.* (2010a) Increased consumption of fatty and lean fish reduces serum C-reactive protein concentrations but not inflammation markers in feces and in colonic biopsies. *Journal of Nutrition* 140, 371–376.

Pot, G.K., Habermann, N., Majsak-Newman, G., Harvey, L.J., Geelen, A., *et al.* (2010b) Increasing fish consumption does not affect genotoxicity markers in the colon in an intervention study. *Carcinogenesis* 31, 087–91.

Pradhan, A.D., Manson, J.E., Rifai, N., Buring, J.E. and Ridker, P.M. (2001) C-reactive protein, interleukin 6, and risk of developing type 2 diabetes mellitus. *Journal of the American Medical Association* 286, 327–334.

Ridker, P.M., Rifai, N., Cook, N.R., Bradwin, G. and Buring, J.E. (2005) Non-HDL cholesterol, apolipoproteins A-I and B100, standard lipid measures, lipid ratios, and CRP as risk factors for cardiovascular disease in women. *Journal of the American Medical Association* 294, 326–333.

Robinson, J.G. and Stone, N.J. (2006) Antiatherosclerotic and antithrombotic effects of omega-3 fatty acids. *American Journal of Cardiology* 98, 39i–49i.

Rogers, P.J., Appleton, K.M., Kessler, D., Peters, T.J., Gunnell, D., *et al.* (2008) No effect of n-3 long-chain polyunsaturated fatty acid (EPA and DHA) supplementation on depressed mood and cognitive function: a randomised controlled trial. *British Journal of Nutrition* 99, 421–431.

Sansoni, P., Cossarizza, A., Brianti, V., Fagnoni, F., Snelli, G., *et al.* (1993) Lymphocyte subsets and natural killer cell activity in healthy old people and centenarians. *Blood,* 82, 2767–2773.

Saurwein-Teissl, M., Blasko, I., Zisterer, K., Neuman, B., Lang, B. *et al.* (2000) An imbalance between pro- and anti-inflammatory cytokines, a characteristic feature of old age. *Cytokine* 12, 1160–1161.

Schaap, L.A., Pluijm, S.M., Deeg, D.J., Harris, T.B., Kritchevsky, S.B., *et al.* (2009) Higher inflammatory marker levels in older persons: associations with 5-year change in muscle mass and muscle strength. *Journals of Gerontology. Series A, Biological Sciences and Medical Sciences* 64, 1183–1189.

Schaefer, E.J., Bongard, V., Beiser, A.S., Lamon-Fava, S., Robins, S.J., *et al.* (2006) Plasma phosphatidylcholine docosahexaenoic acid content and risk of dementia and Alzheimer disease: the Framingham Heart Study. *Archives of Neurology* 63, 1545–1550.

Schiffrin, E.J., Morley, J.E., Donnet-Hughes, A. and Guigoz, Y. (2010) The inflammatory status of the elderly: the intestinal contribution. *Mutation Research* 690, 50–56.

Schlatter, J., Ortuno, F. and Cervera-Enguix, S. (2004) Lymphocyte subsets and lymphokine production in patients with melancholic versus nonmelancholic depression. *Psychiatry Research* 128, 259–265.

Seidell, J.C. and Visscher, T.L. (2000) Body weight and weight change and their health implications for the elderly. *European Journal of Clinical Nutrition* 54 Suppl 3, S33–S39.

Senn, J.J., Klover, P.J., Nowak, I.A. and Mooney, R.A. (2002) Interleukin-6 induces cellular insulin resistance in hepatocytes. *Diabetes* 51, 3391–3399.

Shurin, G.V., Yurkovetsky, Z.R., Chatta, G.S., Tourkova, I.L., Shurin, M.R. *et al.* (2007) Dynamic alteration of soluble serum biomarkers in healthy aging. *Cytokine* 39, 123–129.

Solfrizzi, V., Frisardi, V., Capurso, C., D'introno, A., Colacicco, A.M., *et al.* (2010) Dietary fatty acids in dementia and predementia syndromes: epidemiological evidence and possible underlying mechanisms. *Ageing Research Reviews* 9, 184–199.

Steinberg, D., Parthasarathy, S., Carew, T.E., Khoo, J.C. and Witztum, J.L. (1989) Beyond cholesterol. Modifications of low-density lipoprotein that increase its atherogenicity. *New England Journal of Medicine* 320, 915–924.

Thies, F., Nebe-Von-Caron, G., Powell, J.R., Yaqoob, P., Newsholme, E.A., *et al.* (2001a) Dietary supplementation with eicosapentaenoic acid, but not with other long-chain n-3 or n-6 polyunsaturated fatty acids, decreases natural killer cell activity in healthy subjects aged >55 y. *American Journal of Clinical Nutrition* 73, 539–548.

Thies, F., Nebe-Von-Caron, G., Powell, J.R., Yaqoob, P., Newsholme, E.A., *et al.* (2001b) Dietary supplementation with gamma-linolenic acid or fish oil decreases T lymphocyte proliferation in healthy older humans. *Journal of Nutrition* 131, 1918–1927.

Thies, F., Miles, E.A., Nebe-Von-Caron, G., Powell, J.R., Hurst, T.L., *et al.* (2001c). Influence of dietary supplementation with long-chain n-3 or n-6 polyunsaturated fatty acids on blood inflammatory cell populations and functions and on plasma soluble adhesion molecules in healthy adults. *Lipids* 36, 1183–1193.

Tidball, J.G. (2005) Inflammatory processes in muscle injury and repair. *American Journal of Physiology and Regulatory Integrative Comparative Physiology* 288, R345–R353.

Tsitouras, P.D., Gucciardo, F., Salbe, A.D., Heward, C. and Harman, S.M. (2008) High omega-3 fat intake improves insulin sensitivity and reduces CRP and IL6, but does not affect other endocrine axes in healthy older adults. *Hormone and Metabolic Research* 40, 199–205.

Van De Rest, O., Geleijnse, J.M., Kok, F.J., Van Staveren, W.A., Dullemeijer, C., *et al.* (2008a) Effect of fish oil on cognitive performance in older subjects: a randomized, controlled trial. *Neurology* 71, 430–438.

Van De Rest, O., Geleijnse, J.M., Kok, F.J., Van Staveren, W.A., Hoefnagels, W.H., *et al.* (2008b) Effect of fish-oil supplementation on mental well-being in older subjects: a randomized, double-blind, placebo-controlled trial. *American Journal of Clinical Nutrition* 88, 706–713.

Walther, C., Mobius-Winkler, S., Linke, A., Bruegel, M., Thiery, J., *et al.* (2008) Regular exercise training compared with percutaneous intervention leads to a reduction of inflammatory markers and cardiovascular events in patients with coronary artery disease. *European Journal of Cardiovascular Prevention and Rehabiliation* 15, 107–112.

Wang, L., Xie, Y., Zhu, L.J., Chang, T.T., Mao, Y.Q. *et al.* (2010) An association between immunosenescence and CD4(+)CD25(+) regulatory T cells: a systematic review. *Biomedical and Environmental Sciences* 23, 327–332.

Wannamethee, S.G., Lowe, G.D., Rumley, A., Bruckdorfer, K.R. and Whincup, P.H. (2006) Associations of vitamin C status, fruit and vegetable intakes, and markers of inflammation and hemostasis. *American Journal of Clinical Nutrition* 83, 567–574.

Wannamethee, S.G., Lowe, G.D., Whincup, P.H., Rumley, A., Walker, M. *et al.* (2002) Physical activity and hemostatic and inflammatory variables in elderly men. *Circulation* 105, 1785–1790.

Witztum, J.L. (1994) The oxidation hypothesis of atherosclerosis. *Lancet* 344, 793–795.

Wood, J.G., Rogina, B., Lavu, S., Howitz, K., Helfand, S.L., *et al.* (2004) Sirtuin activators mimic caloric restriction and delay ageing in metazoans. *Nature* 430, 686–689.

World Cancer Research Fund / American Institute for Cancer Research (2007) *Food, Nutrition, Physical Activity, and the Prevention of Cancer: a Global Perspective.* AICR, Washington, DC.

Wu, D., Han, S.N., Meydani, M. and Meydani, S.N. (2004) Effect of concomitant consumption of fish oil and vitamin E on production of inflammatory cytokines in healthy elderly humans. *Annals of New York Acadamy of Sciences* 1031, 422–424.

Ye, J. and Keller, J.N. (2010) Regulation of energy metabolism by inflammation: a feedback response in obesity and calorie restriction. *Aging (Albany NY)* 2, 361–368.

20 Bone Health and Inflammation

M.C. Kruger*
Institute of Food, Nutrition and Human Health, Massey University, Palmerston North, New Zealand

Introduction

The most significant disease of the bone is osteoporosis. Osteoporosis is defined as a systemic skeletal disease characterized by low bone mass and micro-architectural deterioration of bone tissue with a consequent increase in bone fragility and susceptibility to fracture (Consensus Development Conference, 1993). About 10 million people in the USA are affected by osteoporosis, and more than 33 million people have low bone mass or osteopenia (reduced bone mineral density) and are therefore at risk of developing osteoporosis (NIH Consensus Statement, 2000). Most of the individuals with osteoporosis are females – a result of the withdrawal of oestrogen during menopause. Oestrogen therefore has the most

* Author, M.C.Kruger@Massey.ac.nz

significant effect on female bone loss with ageing (Weitzman and Pacific, 2006).

Inflammation has also been implicated in post-menopausal bone loss; several inflammatory diseases have been associated with bone resorption, including rheumatoid arthritis, systemic lupus and inflammatory bowel disease. The common denominators seem to be pro-inflammatory cytokines, which stimulate bone resorption via the osteoclast (OC) cells (Pacifici, 1996; Weitzman and Pacifici, 2006; Straub, 2007).

In this chapter we aim to clarify both the specific role of oestrogen withdrawal in accelerating bone loss and the contribution of inflammation by reviewing the role of the bone cells involved in bone formation and resorption, the involvement of the T cells, and the various cytokines and growth factors involved in these processes. We will also review the possible anti-inflammatory effects of certain foods, and the contribution of physical exercise to reducing inflammation and improving bone health.

Bone and Bone Cells

Bone is a dynamic tissue that constantly adapts during life in order to preserve skeleton size and integrity. The skeleton is continually being remodelled and this remodelling includes the various bone cells. The process of remodelling is tightly controlled, so that the various activities of the bone cellular compartment are coordinated and bone resorption and formation will occur at a specific location in the bone and skeleton in a specific sequence to ensure coupling and control of the events. This coupling is crucial to ensure maintenance of bone mass under normal physiological conditions. The various cells participating in bone turnover are the osteoblasts, osteoclasts and osteocytes.

Osteoblasts

Osteoblasts (OBs) are bone-forming cells and produce bone matrix protein and several factors that will affect and control the formation and activation of the osteoclast (OC). The OB originates from mesenchymal stem cells that have the potential to differentiate into adipocytes, myocytes, chondrocytes and OBs. The OB population includes both immature OB lineage cells (cells that are in the process of differentiating) and mature matrix-producing cells. This differentiation into the various cells is controlled by several transcription factors, including runt-related factor 2 (Runx2) or core-binding factor 1 (cbfa1) (Proff and Römer, 2009; Martin *et al.*, 2009; Kruger *et al.*, 2010; Raggatt and Partridge, 2010). Runx2, a member of the Runt family and expressed by mesenchymal cells at the beginning of skeletal development, is present in OBs throughout their differentiation. Recent work has shown that Runx2 can interact with several nuclear regulatory proteins that in turn can activate or repress genes controlling OB proliferation and differentiation (Marie, 2008; Proff and Römer, 2009; Kruger *et al.*, 2010).

Other transcription factors include:

- Osterix (Osx), which acts downstream from Runx/Cbfa1. Osx, a zinc finger transcription factor specifically expressed by OBs, is important for the differentiation of OBs (Marie, 2008; Martin *et al.*, 2009).
- The canonical Wnt signalling pathway is important in the control of bone formation and bone mass. The interaction of Wnt proteins with Frizzled and LRP5 co-receptors leads to the inhibition of β-catenin phosphorylation and results in the accumulation of β-catenin and translocation to the nucleus where it binds to transcription factors and activates downstream genes (Marie, 2008; Martin *et al.*, 2009; Kruger *et al.*, 2010).
- Proliferation-activated receptor γ2 (PPARγ2) is also involved in the OB differentiation pathway. Increased expression induces adipocyte differentiation (Fig. 20.1). PPARγ2 can also bind Runx2 and inhibit transcription.

The process of OB differentiation and activation is controlled by several hormones including parathyroid hormone (PTH), oestrogens, glucocorticoids and vitamin D, all of which control the expression of various transcription factors. Oestrogen has also been shown to activate Runx2 and increase OB survival via WNT and β-catenin (Marie, 2008; Proff and Römer, 2009; Kruger *et al.*, 2010).

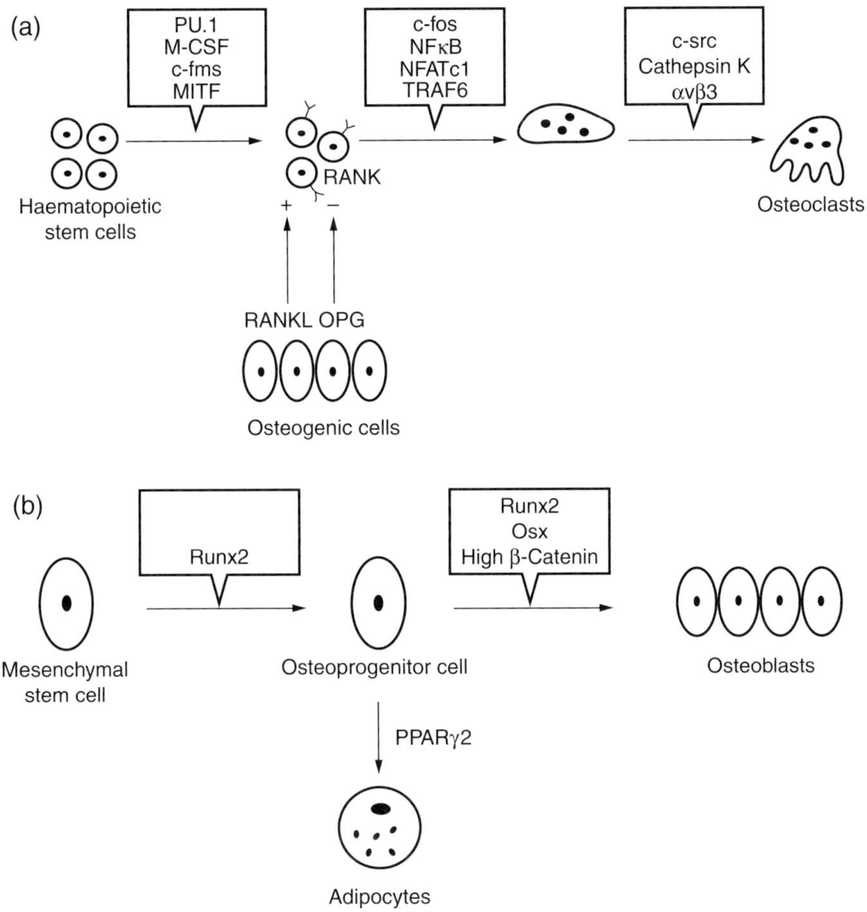

Fig. 20.1. A simplified diagram of the differentiation of (a) osteoclast precursors into osteoclasts and (b) osteoblast precursors into osteoblasts. PU.1, transcription factor PU.1; M-CSF, macrophage-colony stimulating factor; c-fms, c-fms genes; MITF, microphthalmia-associated transcription factor; c-fos, c-fos gene; NFκB nuclear factor κB; NFATc1, nuclear factor of activated T cells 1; TRAF6, tumour necrosis factor receptor-associated factor-6; c-src, cellular-sarcoma gene; αvβ3, αvβ3-integrin; RANKL, receptor activator of nuclear factor-κB-ligand; OPG, osteoprotegerin; Osx, osterix; PPARγ2, peroxisome proliferator activated receptor γ2. (From Kruger *et al.*, 2010, with permission from Elsevier Ltd.)

Osteocytes

As bone is being formed, osteoid, which is unmineralized, is deposited, engulfing some OBs that have differentiated to early osteocytes (Proff and Römer, 2009; Raggatt and Partridge, 2010). As bone mineralizes, these osteocytes are fixed into the matrix and form a network throughout the mineralized bone. The osteocytes, which possess long dendrite-like processes that extend throughout tunnels in the matrix, are sensitive to mechanical load, and communicate with other osteocytes in the matrix as well as with OBs on the surface of the bone (Turner and Pavalko, 1998).

Osteoclasts

OCs are multi-nucleated cells that break down osteoid through a process known as bone resorption (Marks and Hermey, 1996). OCs are derived from haematopoietic cells of the monocyte–macrophage lineage, and undergo a phase through which they can either become OCs or macrophages.

Osteoclastogenesis refers to the process of converting a macrophage to a mature OC (Boyle *et al.*, 2003). For the precursor macrophage to differentiate into the OC, there must be direct contact between the OB/stromal cell and the macrophage (Boyle *et al.*, 2003; Novack and Teitelbaum, 2008; Raggatt and Partridge, 2010). The OB expresses two essential ligands, receptor activator of nuclear factor-κB (NFκB) ligand (RANKL) and macrophage colony-stimulating factor (M-CSF). M-CSF is essential for inducing the differentiation of precursor cells into OCs. RANKL is a transmembrane protein that is expressed as both membrane-bound as well as secreted protein. RANKL expression, stimulated by the various factors stimulating OC formation and activity (Boyle *et al.*, 2003; Novack and Teitelbaum, 2007; Martin *et al.*, 2009), is expressed in inflamed joints by the synovial cells and secreted by activated T cells (Lorenzo, 2000). RANKL binds to the receptor activator of NFκB (RANK) located on the OC membrane, leading to a cascade of events that in turn lead to the differentiation and activation of the OC. RANK, a transmembrane protein on the OC, is responsible for increased NFκβ signalling (Boyle *et al.*, 2003; Kobayashi *et al.*, 2009; Kruger *et al.*, 2010).

Another ligand expressed by OB is osteoprotegerin (OPG), commonly called a 'decoy receptor', which also binds to RANKL thus preventing the conversion of the macrophage into the OC, and acting as negative regulator of osteoclastogenesis. In general the ratio between OPG and RANKL controls whether osteoclastogenesis is upregulated or not (Martin *et al.*, 2009; Proff and Römer, 2009).

Following the binding of RANK and RANKL, the tumour necrosis factor (TNF) receptor associated factor-6 (TRAF6) is recruited. TRAF6 binds to the binding sites in the intracellular domain of the RANK receptor, and then signals downstream involving NFκB, mitogen-activated (MAP) kinases, extracellular signal-regulated kinase (ERrk), Janus N-terminal kinase (JNK) and p38 (Sugatini *et al.*, 2003; Zaidi *et al.*, 2003). The factor that directly controls the differentiation process, however, is thought to be RANKL (Asagiri and Takayanagi, 2006). NFκB activation is among the very early molecular events induced by RANK. These proteins are usually found in the cytoplasm of non-stimulated cells but, on stimulation with RANKL, enter the nucleus.

In order to resorb bone, OCs must adhere to the bone surface with integrin proteins and form a tight seal with the bone matrix. Inside these sealed zones they form a ruffled border. The OCs then secrete hydrochloric acid and the proteolytic enzyme cathepsin K, which dissolves the mineral and degrades the bone matrix releasing calcium, phosphorus and fragments of type I collagen to the blood (Zaidi *et al.*, 2003; Kobayashi *et al.*, 2009).

Other cells involved with remodelling

The possible cross talk between skeletal and immune systems has been under-investigated for many years. It was thought that the immune cells were only involved when pathology was present that results in bone loss, but it has now become apparent that immune cells also participate in normal bone homeostasis. Studies in mice have shown that lack of either B or T cells results in bone loss (Lorenzo, 2000). Although the B cells are responsible for production of a significant amount of OPG, which is bone protective, the exact role of the T cells is less clear, but it is thought they may support the B cells in enhancing secretion of OPG.

Megakaryocytes have also been implicated in bone homeostasis, but their role is not clear. *In vitro* these cells express OPG and RANKL, and seem to be able to affect both resorption and formation (Raggatt and Partridge, 2010). The osteomacs, tissue macrophages that are found close to endosteal and periosteal surfaces, are important for homeostasis and repair. *In vitro*, osteomacs are required for differentiation and mineralization of the OBs. *In vivo*, the osteomacs can be found next to the matrix-producing OBs at the sites of remodelling, suggesting that these cells are needed to maintain mature OBs (Raggatt and Partridge, 2010).

Process of Bone Remodelling

The above sets of cells and factors therefore play an integral role in initiation and control of bone turnover. Bone remodelling, which occurs over weeks and months, takes place in units called 'basic multicellular units' (BMUs) (Fig. 20.2). The BMUs are covered by a set of cells, which results in the formation of a defined compartment (Hauge *et al.*, 2001) that generates a microenvironment to facilitate coupled osteoclast resorption and reduce minimal change in bone volume. There are several bone remodelling units active at the same time throughout the skeleton. The remodelling process comprises a few linked processes: OCs will be at the front resorbing bone, followed by reversal cells that prepare the exposed bone surface for the deposition of new bone. The OBs deposit unmineralized bone matrix, osteoid, which then becomes mineralized and mature bone. An abbreviated description of the process of remodelling follows (Fig. 20.2).

Activation and resorption

The process of remodelling is initiated at the level of the osteocyte, where either apoptosis of the osteocyte or microdamage of bone results in signals to surface cells to increase RANKL production. Signals from either the osteocytes or systemic hormones such as the parathyroid hormone (PTH) result in recruitment of the OB precursors to the area of remodelling. The OBs produce monocyte chemoattractant protein-1 (MCP-1), which attracts the OC precursors, the expression of colony stimulating factor-1 (CSF-1) and RANKL increase as the expression of OPG decreases. Both CSF-1 and RANKL will promote the proliferation and survival of the OCs, with RANKL in turn affecting the differentiation of OC precursors to mature OCs, as well as increasing resorption activity (Novack and Teitelbaum, 2007; Martin *et al.*, 2009;. Proff and Römer, 2009). Other factors from the OB include metalloproteinases (MMPs), which will degrade the unmineralized osteoid; and this in turn leads to the exposure of sites where the OC can adhere and start the resorption process. Once the OC adheres, the resorption zone is sealed off and the secretion of acid and proteolytic enzymes proceeds (Raggatt and Partridge, 2010b).

Reversal

The resorption area is cleaned of debris remaining from the collagen matrix, making the Howship's lacunae ready for bone formation (Raggatt and Partridge, 2010). A mononuclear cell, possibly from OB origin, possibly controlled by immune cells – osteomacs and macrophages (Raggatt and Partridge, 2010) – may be responsible for the cleaning-up process, whereas the osteomacs may be responsible for removal of debris. The coupling of bone resorption and formation has also been ascribed to the release of growth factors from the matrix that will stimulate bone formation. These include insulin-like growth factor (IGF-1), fibroblast growth factor (FGFs), transforming growth factor (TGF-β), bone morphogenic proteins (BMPs) and others. Of these, it was proposed that TGF-β can be released from the matrix and activated by the acidic environment, or by being cleaved by the OCs (Martin *et al.*, 2009). Another possible coupling factor, ephrinB2, is produced by the OC under the control of PTH and PTH-related peptide (PTH-rP). The receptor for ephrinB2 is located on the OB and is called EphB4. It is suggested that ephrinB2 is produced by the OC, which then binds to the receptor EphB4 inducing OB differentiation and bone formation. This pathway could be a local control located in the OB lineage (Martin *et al.*, 2009). The Wnt pathway, discussed above in relation to the OB, might also be defining for the reversal process, affecting the differentiation and activation of the OBs (Marie, 2008).

A more recent discovery of sclerostin indicated that this factor might also be part of the process of events that control bone formation. Sclerostin is produced by the osteocyte and its action is to inhibit Wnt signalling through binding to LRP5/6, thereby inhibiting bone formation. Mechanical strain and PTH signalling both inhibit the expression of sclerostin

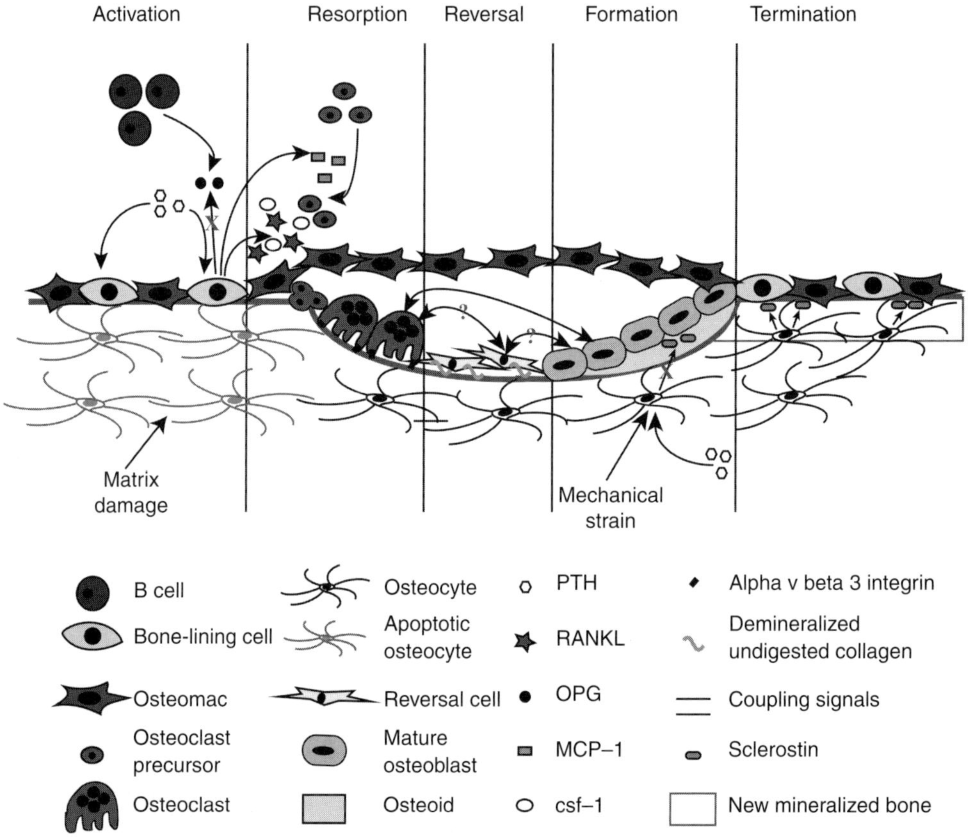

Fig. 20.2. Schematic representation of a basic multicellular unit and the associated bone-remodelling process. Prior to activation, the resting bone surface is covered with bone-lining cells, including pre-osteoblasts (pre-OBs) intercalated with osteomacs. B cells are present in the bone marrow and secrete osteoprotegerin (OPG), which suppresses osteoclastogenesis. Activation: the endocrine bone-remodelling signal PTH binds to the PTH receptor on pre-OBs. Damage to the mineralized bone matrix results in localized osteocyte apoptosis, reducing the local transforming growth factor (TGF)-β concentration and its inhibition of osteoclastogenesis. Resorption: in response to PTH signalling, monocyte chemoattractant protein-1 (MCP-1) is released from OBs and recruits pre-osteoclasts to the bone surface. Additionally, OB expression of OPG is decreased, and production of colony-stimulating factor (CSF)-1 and receptor activator of nuclear factor-κB-ligand (RANKL) is increased to promote proliferation of osteoclast precursors and differentiation of mature osteoclasts. Mature osteoclasts anchor to RGD-binding sites, creating a localized microenvironment (sealed zone) that facilitates degradation of the mineralized bone matrix. Reversal: reversal cells engulf and remove demineralized undigested collagen from the bone surface. Transition signals are generated that halt bone resorption and stimulate the bone formation process. Formation: formation signals and molecules arise from the degraded bone matrix, mature osteoclasts and, potentially, reversal cells. PTH and mechanical activation of osteocytes reduces sclerostin expression, allowing for Wnt-directed bone formation to occur. Termination: sclerostin expression probably returns, and bone formation ceases. The newly deposited osteoid is mineralized, the bone surfaces return to a resting state with bone-lining cells intercalated with osteomacs, and the remodelling cycle concludes. (From Raggatt and Partridge, 2010, with permission from The American Society for Biochemistry and Molecular Biology.)

by the osteocyte, which in turn will remove the inhibition of the Wnt signalling pathway leading to bone formation (Martin *et al.*, 2009; Raggatt and Partridge, 2010). Several of the mechanisms described above could therefore affect coupling/reversal.

Formation

The formation of bone is mediated via OB, which first fills the lacunae with osteoid (unmineralized bone) by secreting collagen type I; the osteoid later becomes mineralised (Novack and Teitelbaum, 2008). Other protein components secreted by the differentiated OBs include proteoglycans, Gla-containing proteins and lipids. After the laying down of the osteoid layer, mineralization takes place.

Termination

Once the damaged bone has been resorbed and replaced entirely by newly formed bone, the (re)modelling cycle is complete and terminated, though the signals that terminate the cycle have not yet been identified (Novack and Teitelbaum, 2008). Mature OBs can undergo apoptosis, or become embedded in the mineralized matrix, and separate into osteocytes (Novack and Teitelbaum, 2008; Raggatt and Partridge, 2010).

Bone and Inflammation

Several inflammatory diseases have been associated with bone resorption, including rheumatoid arthritis and periodontal disease, while osteoporosis has been found to be more prevalent in the presence of systemic lupus erythematosus, inflammatory bowel disease and chronic obstructive pulmonary disease. Several of the inflammatory cytokines have been implicated in the development of osteoporosis because they can mediate resorption (Hardy and Cooper, 2009). The cytokines play a role in the immune response and include interleukin (IL)-1, IL-6, IL-11, IL-15, IL-17 (Mundy, 2007; Latavica and De Farias, 2010) and tumour necrosis factor-α (TNF-α) (Lorenzo, 2000). *In vitro* and animal data suggest that these cytokines can promote bone loss through increasing OC differentiation, activation and survival, by increasing RANKL expression and by inhibiting OB survival. Research has indicated that localized and systemic increases in pro-inflammatory cytokines may lead to the uncoupling of bone remodelling and an increase in bone resorption (Hardy and Cooper, 2009).

The generation of these inflammatory cytokines is increased during oestrogen withdrawal at menopause, and *in vitro* cell culture work using the conditioned medium from cultures of peripheral blood mononuclear cells (PBMCs) from osteoporotic women showed increased generation of IL-1 and TNF-α (Lorenzo, 2000). The exact role of inflammation in the development of osteoporosis has not been proved in human intervention or observation studies, but a significant amount of work supports the putative role of the various cytokines in bone turnover and resorption (McLean, 2009).

Some epidemiological studies suggest that cytokines might be associated with decreased bone mass and increased fracture risk, but the evidence supporting a specific role for the cytokines in the development of osteoporosis is limited. A few studies have reported that production of IL-6 and TNF-α is increased in whole blood cultures from osteoporotic women (McLean, 2009; Lacativa and De Faria, 2010). In contrast, other studies reported no difference between the serum levels of IL-1α, IL-1β and IL-6 of normal and osteoporotic women, and no greater production of TNF-α by PBMCs in women with osteoporosis (Zarrabeita *et al.*, 1991). Similarly, there is little evidence that raised peripheral levels of cytokines are associated with lower bone density. Although one study, by Zheng *et al.* (1997), found a significant negative correlation between PBMC secretion of IL-1β, IL-6 and TNF-α and lumbar spine bone mineral density (BMD), another reported a similar negative correlation that was not significant (Papadopoulos *et al.*, 1997). Other studies in pre- as well as post-menopausal women have not reported any correlation between IL-1 production and plasma IL 6 levels with lumbar spine or femoral neck BMD. Cauley *et al.* (2007) measured IL-6, TNF-α, C-reactive protein (CRP) and several of the soluble receptors present in blood collected from 2985 men and women enrolled in the Health ABC study. This cohort was followed for 5 or more years, and incident fractures were confirmed in 268 subjects. Baseline inflammatory markers were higher among subjects who had a fracture, and the relative risk for fracture was significantly higher for the cohort with high serum CRP levels. Increased systemic CRP results in the lowering of bone density in healthy women (Chung *et al.*, 2009), whereas high CRP is related to increased fracture risk in elderly women (Pasco *et al.*, 2006).

There is some data to support the role of cytokines in bone loss. Work by Ding *et al.* (2008) showed that high serum IL-6 was associated with increased bone loss at the hip, spine and total body over 3 years, and raised TNF-α was linked to bone loss at the spine and total body.

Link between Inflammation and Oestrogen

Withdrawal of oestrogen is the main factor leading to the development of post-menopausal osteoporosis. With the loss of oestrogen, bone resorption increases significantly, owing to the increased activity of the OC. Oestrogen, however, does not stimulate the OC directly. The activated OC is present in stromal and other cells in the lineage, and these cells produce pro-inflammatory cytokines in the absence of oestrogen (Mundy, 2007). Studies in pre-menopausal women indicated that surgical menopause (OVX) resulted in a rise in IL-1 and TNF-α secretion by PBMCs, and in women treated with oestrogen after OVX, IL-1 and TNF-α levels increased for a short while but then returned to baseline levels after 4 weeks of oestrogen treatment (Mundy, 2007). Several studies in animals also point to the role of inflammation in the increased bone resorption observed after loss of oestrogen. OVX in rats was associated with an increased number of bone marrow cells producing IL-1 and TNF-α, and bone loss via augmentation of RANKL-induced osteoclastogenesis (Roggia *et al.*, 2001), whereas use of an IL-1 receptor antagonist and a TNF-binding protein after OVX significantly reduced the loss of bone and was comparable to replacement of oestrogen (Mundy, 2007). In mice, OVX enhanced T-cell production of TNF-α, which in turn, via the p55 receptor, as shown by Roggia *et al.* (2001), increased M-CSF- and RANKL-induced osteoclastogenesis (Cenci *et al.*, 2000); but bone resorption was absent in T-cell-deficient mice, indicating the importance of the T cells in oestrogen-deficiency-induced bone loss. This study of mice points to the importance of IL-6 and the relationship with oestrogen because IL-6-deficient mice did not lose bone after OVX and, in addition, OC production following OVX was reduced by antibodies against IL-6 or implanted oestrogen.

The pro-inflammatory cytokines effecting bone resorption during loss of oestrogen are secreted by the T cells. There is a shift with age in T-cell immunity that alters the systemic cytokine profiles from T helper 1 (Th1) to T helper 2 (Th2) type, and this change has been observed to be associated with bone-loss conditions. The T cells produce TNF as well as IL-1 and IL-6 and, with age, IL-6 aggravates systemic inflammation and increases hepatic CRP production (Chung *et al.*, 2009; Quinn and Saleh, 2009; Yun and Lee, 2004). Both bone marrow stromal cells and OC precursors express TNF-α receptors (Lacativa and De Farias, 2010). TNF enhances OC formation, and upregulates production of RANKL by bone marrow stromal cells, and increases the responsiveness of the OC to RANKL. TNF mediates these effects by interactions at the level of NFκB. TNF-α, together with RANKL, upregulates RANK expression in OC precursors. The resulting effect is increased activity of the OCs, and inhibition of osteoblastogenesis (Weitzmann and Pacifici, 2006). IL-1 supports the effects of TNF-α and acts synergistically by promoting RANKL expression by the stromal cells and by prolonging OC lifespan and increasing OC activity. IL-1 also stimulates OC activity by increasing production of M-CSF (Latavica and De Farias, 2010; Quinn and Saleh, 2009). Both TNF and IL-1 significantly reduce OC apoptosis, and prolong the lifespan of the OC (Novack and Teitelbaum, 2008; Quinn and Saleh, 2009).

T cells also produce interferon-α and -γ, both of which can partly limit RANKL-induced bone resorption by reducing NFκB and JNK signalling pathways. The net effect of the T cells on OC formation may be a balance between pro- and anti-osteoclastogenic

T-cell cytokine secretion (Yun and Lee, 2004). During inflammation and loss of oestrogen, however, the net effect is induced by the pro-osteoclastogenic cytokines (Straub, 2007). OVX upregulates T-cell TNF production by increasing the number of TNF-producing T cells (Cenci *et al.*, 2000; Weitzman and Pacifici, 2006). Loss of oestrogen upregulates INF-γ production by downregulating TGF-β. Oestrogen usually directly stimulates production of TGF-β via the TGF promoter, and TGF is a strong suppressor of T-cell activation, as well as its production of pro-inflammatory cytokines (Pacifici, 1996). Oestrogen also suppresses production of IL-7, thus regulating IFN-γ and TNF production (Weitzmann and Pacifici, 2006). The decrease in TGF-β, owing to loss of oestrogen, could increase IL-7 levels further and impact on the production of osteoclastogenic cytokines and bone loss. IL-7 also suppresses bone formation, contributing to the uncoupling of bone turnover (Cenci *et al.*, 2000; Roggia *et al.*, 2000; Straub, 2007).

Nutrition, Inflammation and Bone

Nutritional deficiencies co-exist with over-nutrition in developing countries, evident in the high incidence of central obesity and overweight. In developed countries, 20% of the population is obese, and this high incidence of obesity is a risk factor for both cardiovascular disease and osteoporosis. Kartikey *et al.* (2010) proposed that overweight initially comes with inflammation, hyperinsulinemia and central obesity, which is then followed by glucose intolerance, type 2 diabetes, hypertension and increased blood lipids (metabolic syndrome). A further complication of this widespread inflammation could be bone and joint diseases. All these diseases are associated with the production of thromboxane A2, leukotrienes, IL-1 and IL-6, TNF-α and CRP. Meydani *et al.* (2007) suggested that production of prostaglandins (PGs) is upregulated in these inflammatory diseases, especially the production of PGE_2 by the macrophages, which is due to increased expression of cyclooxygenase 2 (COX-2), the inducible form of COX and the rate-limiting enzyme for PG synthesis. PGE_2 is associated with increased bone resorption, probably via upregulation of RANKL (Coon *et al.*, 2007).

Certain foods and nutrients may reduce inflammation, modify the development of cardiovascular disease and be associated with reduced risk of fractures. A study by Renaud *et al.* (1995) investigated the associations between food consumption patterns and the omega-6/omega-3 fatty acid ratio of the diet. They investigated a population with hip fractures (n = 60) and compared them with control subjects (n = 95) over 50 years of age. Other measures investigated included physical activity and circulating cytokines. Fruit, vegetable and milk-product intakes were significantly lower and omega-6 intake higher in the patients with fractures. Blood levels of IL-6 and TNF-α were also associated with fractures.

Another nutritional compound that may modify inflammation is vitamin E. In mice, vitamin E reduced the increase in PG production caused by ageing, by inhibiting COX-2 (Meydani and Wu, 2007). A low-fat diet with high fish consumption also reduced inflammatory products, and lowered baseline PG production in the elderly (Meydani *et al.*, 1993). Clinical studies recently supported the significant role the omega-3 long-chain fatty acids (n-3 PUFAs) could play in inflammation. The n-3 PUFAs not only could affect blood lipids but could also affect cellular adhesion molecules, cytokines and inflammatory markers such as TNF-α and CRP (Gillies, 2007). The potent anti-inflammatory role of the n-3 PUFAs could partly be ascribed to the presence of derivatives of the omega-3 PUFA called resolvin E1 (RVE1), given that, by down-regulating NFκB activation, RVE1 can modify inflammation as well as bone resorption (Ordovas, 2007; Kruger *et al.*, 2010).

Another nutrient/hormone of interest in inflammation is vitamin D. Vitamin D is well known for its regulation of calcium homeostasis, but recent work points to its significant role in the immune system. Vitamin D contributes to the regulation of the proliferation, differentiation and function of immune cells. Both T and B cells have the enzyme required to convert 25-hydroxyvitamin D to 1,25-dihydroxyvitamin D, and macrophages have both the enzymes to form active 1,25-dihydroxyvitamin D. In addition, the vitamin D receptor is expressed in many types of immune cells in the body. The specific role of vitamin D in inflammation is reviewed by Guillot *et al.* (2010) (see also Chapter 5, this volume). Owing to its anti-inflammatory role, vitamin D could therefore also be implicated in the prevention of inflammation-induced bone loss. Although studies have reported a correlation between the degree of inflammation in diseases such as rheumatoid arthritis and inflammatory bowel disease and vitamin D sufficiency (Hardy and Cooper, 2009), there are, however, no intervention studies demonstrating a modulation of inflammation using vitamin D supplementation.

Phytoestrogens promote bone formation via the bone morphogenic proteins, specifically BMP-2, and a role for these compounds in control of bone turnover has been proved during the past few years (Mundy, 2006). BMP-2 stimulates the differentiation of mesenchymal cells into OBs and also activates intracellular signalling molecules Smad 1 and Smad 5. These signals then lead to the expression of Cbfa1 (Runx2), which results in the expression of several proteins crucial for bone formation (Mundy, 2006; Poulsen *et al.*, 2008). More recent work points to a possible role for polyphenols in bone turnover. Although there have been no long-term intervention studies of humans (except using the phytoestrogens) to investigate the role of the polyphenols, there is a whole body of evidence, using *in vitro* and animal models, that these compounds can affect bone formation and resorption.

The specific role of the omega-3 PUFAs and polyphenols in inflammation-induced bone turnover will be reviewed in the following sections of this chapter (Fig. 20.3).

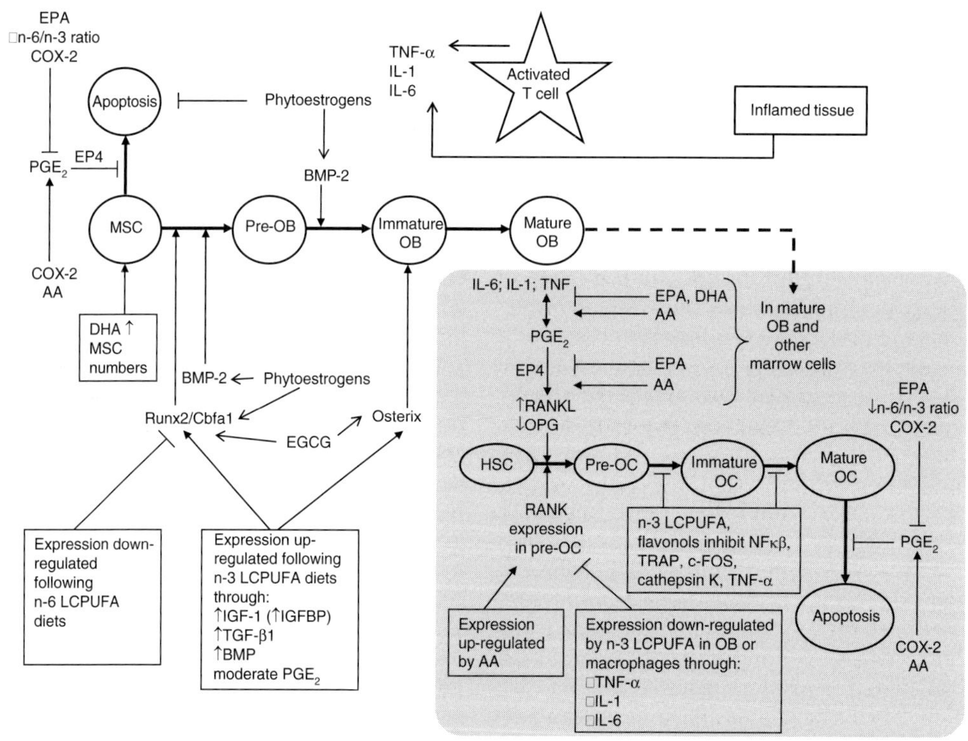

Fig. 20.3. Schematic model of postulated mechanisms by which dietary ingredients affect mesenchymal stem cell differentiation into mature osteoblasts with cross-talk to hematopoietic stem cell differentiation into mature osteoclasts. See text for abbreviations. (Modified from Kruger *et al.*, 2010.)

Phenolic phytochemicals, inflammation and bone

Phytonutrients, plant-based compounds present in the diet through fruit and vegetables, fruit juice, green or black tea, coffee, beans and grains, are classified as phenolics, carotenoids, phytosterols, alkaloids, terpenes and sulfur-containing compounds. Phytonutrients might offer beneficial effects for a range of chronic diseases, including osteoporosis.

The majority of work in this area has focused on the isoflavones, genistein and daidzein. These are also called phytoestrogens owing to their oestrogenic activity, and they are able to bind to both the oestrogen receptors α and β. Isoflavones are provided only by soybean-derived products and are present in these as glycosides. The intestinal microflora can then convert daidzein into several products, including equol.

Serum from women consuming a diet supplemented with phytoestrogens had significantly lower concentrations of IL-1 and TNF-α (Huang *et al.*, 2005), and serum levels of IL-1β and TNF-α were significantly decreased in the OVX rat when fed with genistein (Li and Yu, 2003). The isoflavones may have an anti-inflammatory effect because they are able to inhibit TNF-α-induced apoptosis (Poulsen *et al.*, 2008), and they can modulate the production of IL-6 and PGE_2 in MC3T3-E1 osteoblastic cells (Suh *et al.*, 2003; Poulsen *et al.*, 2008). Genistein, in turn, can stimulate the production of OPG by human trabecular OBs (Viereck *et al.*, 2002). A study with daidzein suggests that daidzein at 1nM can act anti-resorptively by regulating Runx2/Cbfa1 production, as well as stimulating OPG and RANKL secretion (De Wilde *et al.*, 2004). The phytoestrogens have been promoted as having anabolic effects that could be mediated by BMP-2. Both genistein and daidzein inhibit apoptosis of OCs and tyrosine kinase, activate tyrosine phosphorylase and change intracellular calcium levels, all of which can inhibit OC activity (Poulsen *et al.*, 2008).

The flavonol quercetin, present in onions, broccoli, apples and blueberries, has also been linked to bone metabolism. *In vitro* quercetin inhibits bone resorption by the OCs, at concentrations of 10 and 100 μM. The possible mechanism seems to be via inhibition of NFκB, whereas other work also suggests that quercetin can inhibit bone loss owing to suppression of inflammatory cytokines. Son *et al.* (2006) suggested that quercetin could both increase TNF-α-induced inhibition of OB growth, as well as apoptosis and suppress cytokines including IL-1, IL-6 and PGE_2, whereas Pang *et al.* (2006) indicated that quercetin inhibits RANK-L-induced formation of the mature OCs, as well as expression of RANK.

Green tea contains a mixture of polyphenols, specifically flavonols, which are present at 30% of the fresh leaf dry weight. Of these, a catechin, (-)-epigallocatechin-3-gallate (EGCG), seems to be the most bioactive for bone health (Chacko *et al.*, 2010). Chen *et al.* (2005), using a murine bone marrow mesenchymal stem cell line, D1, showed that EGCG increases the mRNA expressions of Cbfa1/Runx2, osterix and other markers of OB differentiation. Vali *et al.* (2007) showed increased Cbfa1/Runx expression in SaSO2-human OB-like cells, and Yun *et al.* (2007) showed that EGCG inhibits survival of the RAW 264.7 cells, a model for osteoclastogenesis, while inducing apoptosis possibly via activation of caspase-3. Recent work reports that EGCG suppresses OC differentiation by significantly inhibiting RANKL-induced NFκB transcriptional activity and nuclear translocation (Ko *et al.*, 2009; Lin *et al.*, 2009). The effect of green tea polyphenols (GTPs) was assessed *in vivo* using rat models of chronic inflammation, where lipopolysaccharide (LPS) was used to induce systemic inflammation (Shen *et al.*, 2010a,b, 2011). Rats receiving green tea as their drinking water had higher trabecular volume and bone formation compared with rats who received no green tea. GTP was able to suppress TNF-α expression in the tibia, suggesting an anti-inflammatory role, and also reduced mRNA expression of TNF-α and COX-2 in the spleens of OVX rats, as well as lypoxygenase and inducible nitric oxide synthase (Shen *et al.*, 2008, 2009).

Dried plums, which contain high amounts of vitamin K and boron, are also rich in flavonoids and coumarins, with significant levels of chlorogenic acid isomers. Dried plum has the highest oxygen radical absorbance capacity

(ORAC) ranking among the most commonly consumed fruits (Hooshmand and Arjmandi, 2009). This significant antioxidant capacity may contribute to its effects on bone metabolism. Earlier clinical studies indicated some bone sparing effect in post-menopausal women eating 100 g dried plums/day (Hooshmand and Arjmandi, 2009). Feeding rats between 5% and 25% (w/w) of prunes inhibited bone resorption by decreasing osteoclastogenesis both through a reduction in RANKL and by a stimulation of IGF-1 (Franklin *et al.*, 2006; Bu *et al.*, 2007). Using RAW 264.7 cells, Bu *et al.* (2008) then confirmed an anti-inflammatory effect by the plum polyphenols. Inflammation was induced in these cells using LPS, and the plum extract was able to downregulate COX expression as well as nitric oxide in the pre-OCs. TNF-α was suppressed in the presence of RANKL during osteoclastogensis and OC differentiation was also suppressed under inflammatory conditions by downregulating nuclear factor of activated T cells 1 (NFATc1) (Habuzit and Horcajada, 2008; Hooshmand and Arjmandi, 2009).

Oleuropein, a polyphenol found in olives, has an anti-inflammatory effect, and inhibits lypoxygenase activity and production of leukotriene B4 (De la Puerta *et al.*, 1999). Puel *et al.* (2004, 2006) investigated the bone-sparing effect of oleuropein in the OVX rat with and without induced inflammation. Interestingly, oleuropein only affected bone mass in the presence of inflammation. Other components from olives, tyrosol and hydroxytyrosol, were able to prevent bone loss in a rat model with induced granulomatosis inflammation (Puel *et al.*, 2008), possibly via suppression of COX-2. *In vitro* studies using these polyphenols indicated an effect on NFκB as well.

Long-chain polyunsaturated fatty acids, inflammation and bone

Cytokine secretion and expression

A large body of literature now points to the fact that the omega-6 fatty acid arachidonic acid (AA) increases adverse cytokine production while various omega-3 fatty acids can reverse this trend in bone cells (Poulsen *et al.*, 2007). *In vitro* exposure of OBs to various PUFAs has shown that AA (25–100 μM) stimulated expression of IL-1α, IL-1β, TNF-α and M-CSF. Eicosapentaenoic acid (EPA) and oleic acid (25–100 μM), on the other hand, had no stimulatory effects, but caused a significant inhibition of AA-induced cytokine mRNA expression (Priante *et al.*, 2002). In this system, results from inhibitor studies suggested that a protein-kinase-C-dependent mechanism could account for the effects of AA on cytokine production; the latter was confirmed by Bordin *et al.* (2003), who showed that AA increases IL-6 expression via protein kinase Cα activation.

Omega-3 PUFAs reduce TNF-α secretion by RAW 264.7 macrophages (Skuladottir *et al.*, 2007), and a study by Bhattacharya *et al.* (2007) showed that when ageing C57BL/6 mice were fed fish oil for 6 months they were shown to have higher bone density as well as a decreased activity of pro-inflammatory cytokines IL-6 and TNF-α in concanavalin-stimulated splenocytes. Downregulation of resorptive cytokines such as TNF-α and IL-6 by n-3 PUFA in OVX mice was also reported by other research groups (Zeitlin *et al.*, 2003). Thus, by increasing n-3 PUFA intake, dietary modulation could affect the generation of IL-1, IL-6 and TNF-α, which in turn could modulate bone health (Miggiano *et al.*, 2005). PGE_2 stimulates IL-6 production (Calder *et al.*, 2006) and there is *in vitro* evidence of cross-talk between the COX-2/PGE_2 and IL-6 systems (Liu *et al.*, 2005) in murine OB–OC co-cultures that results in increased osteoclastogenesis via effects on the RANK/RANKL/OPG system. Although PGE_2 and PGE_3 (derived from EPA) both stimulated IL-6 secretion in the pre-osteoclastic RAW 264.7 macrophage cell line, the effect of PGE_3 was significantly lower than PGE_2 in inducing IL-6 secretion in these cells (Bragga *et al.*, 2003).

Effects of PUFAs on osteoclastogenesis

Poulsen *et al.* (2008) showed that, while COX products from AA and gamma-linolenic acid (GLA) induce RANKL in mouse MC3T3-E1/4 cells, EPA and docosahexaenoic acid (DHA) did not affect RANKL. Coetzee *et al.* (2007) showed that, while AA inhibited the secretion of OPG by OBs, it also stimulated RANKL secretion in this system, thus decreasing the OPG/RANKL ratio, and upregulating osteoclastogenesis. Rahman *et al.* (2008) reported that n-3 PUFAs reduce NFκB expression and modulate RANKL signalling, while n-6 PUFAs such as AA increase NFκB expression leading to increased osteoclastogenesis.

Exposure of cell cultures from primary murine bone marrow cells and RAW 264.7 cells to EPA or DHA, or both, inhibited OC maturation (Rahman *et al.*, 2008), correlating with inhibition of TNF-α. Pretreatment of these cells with DHA caused reduced activation of NFκB compared with pretreatment with EPA. DHA may therefore be much more effective than EPA in alleviating RANKL-induced pro-inflammatory cytokine production; EPA did have a small effect, possibly via the E-series resolvins, because the topical application of RvE1 prevented osteoclast-mediated bone loss (Hasturk *et al.*, 2006).

Physical Activity, Inflammation and Bone

Weight-bearing exercise has beneficial effects on bone health over the lifetime. Physical exercise can increase bone mineral gain in children, and there is some evidence that physical activity in childhood can have benefits that are maintained into adulthood. For the adult person, physical activity helps maintain bone mass and could aid in slowing loss with ageing. There is, however, no strong evidence that physical activity could attenuate the menopause-related bone loss in females. Mechanical loading and forces will only have an osteogenic effect if the stress to the bone is unique and variable. Static loading does not result in an osteogenic response (Colbert *et al.*, 2004; Kohrt *et al.*, 2004).

The osteocytes are the main cells sensing the strain on the bone resulting from mechanical load, and these cells are located throughout the bone and can stretch as deformation takes place owing to strain. Pressure gradients are formed due to bending forces and these gradients result in extracellular fluid flow across the osteocytes. This flow creates fluid shear stress on the osteocyte as well as electric potentials owing to the streaming effect (Turner and Pavalko, 1998). The biochemical coupling can be via different pathways, one of which involves a mechanotransducer located in the cell membrane, which is linked to a G protein. Activation causes an increase in intracellular calcium through membrane ion channels or because of its release from stores. Activation of the G protein can also mediate the activity of isoforms of COX and NO synthase enzymes. Mechanical stimuli immediately activate these enzymes in the OBs and osteocytes resulting in production of PGs and NO; inositol triphosphate may also be involved (Klein-Nulend *et al.*, 1995; Johnson *et al.*, 1996). Another pathway involved in mechanotransduction is the integrin–cytoskeleton complex. The flow of fluid across the bone cells brings about the recruitment of integrins to focal adhesions, resulting in reorganization of the actin filaments into stress fibres. While this reorganization is taking place, there is a change in the expression of COX-2 (Forwood, 1996). The cell-to-cell communication between the osteocytes and bone-lining cells to the pre-OBs involves PGs and NO, which in turn cause recruitment and differentiation of OBs, inducing bone formation (Turner and Pavalko, 1998). The release of PGE_2 promotes the recruitment of the OB precursor cells, increasing the proliferation of the OBs, alkaline phosphatase activity and collagen synthesis (Ehrlich and Lanyon, 2002).

With ageing and with menopause, the skeleton fails to maintain sufficient bone architecture to withstand load and possible fracture. Although disorders of the endocrine system, lack of calcium and other nutrients, and genetic predisposition have been given as the reasons for loss of bone structure, failure of mechanical adaptation of bone to load is now also offered as a possible reason (Ehrlich and Lanyon, 2002). With ageing, the skeleton responds less to exercise, and loss of oestrogen with menopause results in failure of the bone cells to respond to mechanical stress, resulting in bone loss. Oestrogen deficiency has been shown to lead to preferential loss of bone in areas with low strain, whereas the PGE_2-related response to strain is reduced in isolated cells from osteoporotic patients (Sterck *et al.*, 1998; Joldersma *et al.*,

2001). As described above, loss of oestrogen also results in an inflammatory response that, together with the age-associated chronic inflammation, disrupts bone homeostasis (Chung *et al.*, 2009). The systemic cytokine profile changes, generating IL-4, IL-5 and IL-6, which, with age, aggravate systemic inflammation and increase hepatic CRP production; CRP has also been found to be related to increased fracture risk in elderly women (Pasco *et al.*, 2006). As described before, IL-6, together with IL-1 and TNF-α, stimulates OC differentiation and maturation as well as activation. The result is apoptosis of the OBs and bone loss. Because chronic inflammation can play a role in the aetiology of osteoporosis, therapies that reduce inflammation, such as non-steroidal anti-inflammatory drugs, NFκB antagonists and physical exercise, could reduce bone loss with age (Chung *et al.*, 2009).

Moderate regular physical activity has been associated with reduced levels of TNF-α, IL-6 and CRP in healthy older adults (Colbert *et al.*, 2004). More recent work indicates that aerobic exercise is associated with decreased serum levels of IL-6 and increased levels of IL-10, which is a potent anti-inflammatory cytokine (Beavers *et al.*, 2010). In addition, exercise increases the inflammatory modulator IL-1 receptor antagonist molecule (Pederson *et al.*, 2001; 2003). On the other hand, chronic high-intensity exercise subjects the athlete to hypoxia, metabolic acidosis, excessive oxidative stress and increased pro-inflammatory cytokines, and exercise results in catabolism (Beavers *et al.*, 2010). Ultra-distance running elevated IL-6 8000-fold in male runners, while bone markers were increased and bone mass reduced when compared with controls (Margeli *et al.*, 2005). Increased levels of IL-6 can result in PPARγ production and T-cell activation, which raise RANKL production and resultant bone resorption (McCormick, 2007). In overweight post-menopausal women, aerobic exercise in conjunction with a weight-loss programme increased BMD and the soluble receptor for TNF-α, sTNFR1, was significantly associated with the change in femoral neck BMD (Silverman *et al.*, 2009).

Several lines of evidence support the anabolic effect on bone of physical exercise via mechanotransduction, whereas the generation of anti-inflammatory cytokines through exercise can counteract the inflammation that results from loss of oestrogen and the ageing process. The mechanisms responsible for the anti-inflammatory effects of physical exercise may be related to reduction of adiposity, but as yet they are not fully understood and require further work.

Summary and Conclusions

Inflammation has been implicated in post-menopausal bone loss; several inflammatory diseases have been associated with bone resorption, including rheumatoid arthritis, systemic lupus and inflammatory bowel disease. The withdrawal of oestrogen during menopause also results in the generation of these cytokines. The common denominators seem to be pro-inflammatory cytokines and TNF-α, which stimulates bone resorption via OC cells (Pacifici, 1996; Weitzman and Pacifici, 2006; Straub, 2007). The cytokines can promote bone loss through increasing OC differentiation, activation and survival by increasing RANKL expression and by inhibiting osteoblast survival (Hardy and Cooper, 2009). The cytokines responsible for inducing bone resorption during menopause and loss of oestrogen are secreted by the T cells. The T cells produce TNF as well as IL-1 and IL-6, and, with age, IL-6 aggrevates systemic inflammation and increases hepatic CRP production (Yun and Lee, 2004; Chung *et al.*, 2009; Quinn and Saleh, 2009). T cells also produce interferon-α which can partly limit RANKL-induced bone resorption by inducing NFκB and JNK signalling pathways. The net effect of the T cells on OC formation may be between pro- and anti-osteoclastogenic T cell cytokine secretion (Yun and Lee, 2004).

Certain foods may reduce inflammation. In the preceding text the roles of phenolic phytochemicals and omega-3 fats were discussed. The phytoestrogens, genistein and daidzein, may reduce circulating levels of IL-1 and TNF-α in humans and at the level of the bone cells they can modulate production of IL-6 and PGE_2. The flavonol quercetin can suppress cytokines such as IL-1, IL-6 and PGE_2 as well as inhibit RANKL-induced formation of the mature OCs (Pang *et al.*, 2006). The bioactive component found in green tea, EGCG, suppresses OC differentiation by inhibiting RANKL-induced NFκB transcriptional activity. In an animal model of chronic inflammation, rats receiving green tea as drinking water had higher bone volume and formation, with inhibited expression of TNF-α in the tibia (Lin *et al.*, 2009; Shen *et al.*, 2010a,b, 2011). In pre-osteoclasts, a plum extract downregulated COX expression as well as nitric oxide (Bu *et al.*, 2008), whereas oleuropein from olives had an anti-inflammatory effect, inhibiting lypoxygenase activity while reducing production of leukotriene B4 (De La Puerta *et al.*, 1999).

There is ample evidence that n-3 long-chain PUFA diets are associated with higher bone mass. Key mechanisms relate to reduction in PGE_2 synthesis along with suppression of inflammatory cytokines. DHA or other n-3 PUFAs may enhance or preserve bone mass through enhanced expression of key transcriptional factors such as Cbfa1 or osterix. Mature osteoclasts and other bone marrow cells such as T cells enriched with n-3 long-chain PUFA release less RANKL and reduced OPG, resulting in reduced ligand for RANK on immature osteoclasts. The latter could be due to reduced synthesis of IL-6 and PGE_2 (Kruger *et al.*, 2010). Much of the research has emanated from animal models fed diets with n-3 long-chain PUFA far in excess of that in the human diet. None the less, randomized clinical trials and cohort studies support an important role for long-chain PUFAs in human bone health. Figure 20.3 summarizes possible effects of the phytochemicals and n-3 PUFAs on bone cells.

Moderate physical exercise is associated with reduced levels of TNF-α, IL-6 and CRP in healthy older adults (Colbert *et al.*, 2004), whereas aerobic exercise is associated with decreased levels of serum IL-6 and increased levels of IL-10, which is anti-inflammatory. Chronic high intensity exercise, however, results in a rise in pro-inflammatory cytokines (Beavers *et al.*, 2010).

There is ample evidence that certain nutrients can reduce inflammation and therefore affect menopause-induced bone loss or bone loss owing to inflammatory disease. There are however, little data to support a synergistic or combined effect of physical activity and dietary modification (excluding calcium) on inflammation and bone loss. Further work is required.

References

Asagiri, M. and Takayanagi, H. (2007) The molecular understanding of osteoclast differentiation. *Bone* 40, 251–264.

Beavers, K.M., Brinkley, T.E. and Nicklas, J. (2010) Effect of exercise training on chronic inflammation. *Chinica Chimica Acta* 411, 785–793.

Bhattacharya, A., Rahman, M., Sun, D. and Fernandes, G. (2007) Effect of fish oil on bone density in ageing C57BL/6 female mice. *Journal of Nutritional Biochemistry* 18, 372–379.

Bordin, L., Priante, G., Musacchio, E., Giunco, S., Tibaldi, E., *et al.* (2003) Arachidonic acid-induced IL-6 expression is mediated by PKC alpha activation in OBic cells. *Biochemistry* 42, 4485–4491.

Boyle, W.J., Simonet, S. and Lacey, D.L. (2003) Osteoclast differentiation and activation. *Nature* 423, 337–342.

Bragga, D.W.L., Farias-Eisner, R., Glaspy, J.A. and Reddy, S.T. (2003) Differential effects of prostaglandin derived ω-6 and ω-3 polyunsaturated fatty acids on COX-2 expression and IL-6 secretion. *Proceedings of the National Academy of Sciences* 100, 1751–1756.

Bu, S.Y., Lucas, E.A., Franklin, M., Marlow, D., Brackett, D., *et al.* (2007) Comparison of dried plum supplementation and intermittent PTH in restoring bone in osteopenic archidectomised rats. *Osteoporosis International* 18, 931–942.

Bu, S.Y., Lerner, M., Stoecker, B.J., Boldrin, E., Brackett, D.J., *et al.* (2008) Dried plum polyphenols inhibit osteoclastogenesis by downregulating NFATc1 and inflammatory mediators. *Calcified Tissue International* 82, 475–488.

Calder, P.C. (2006) n-3 Polyunsaturated fatty acids, inflammation, and inflammatory diseases. *American Journal of Clinical Nutrition* 83, 1505S–1519S.

Cauley, J.A., Danielson, M.E., Boudreau, R.M., Forrest, K.Y.Z., Zmuda, J.M., *et al.* (2007) Inflammatory markers and incident fracture risk in older men and women: The health aging and body composition study. *Journal of Bone and Mineral Research* 23, 1008–1094.

Cenci, S., Weitzmann, M.N., Roggia, C., Namba, N., Novack, D., *et al.* (2000). Oestrogen deficiency induces bone loss by enhancing T-cell production of TNF-α. *The Journal of Clinical Investigation* 106, 1229–1237.

Chacko, S.M., Thambi, P.T., Kuttan, R. and Nishigaki, I. (2010) Beneficial effects of green tea: A literature review. *Chinese Medicine* 5, 13–21.

Chen, C-H., Ho, M-L., Chang, J-K., Hung, S-H. and Wang, G-J. (2005) Green tea catechin enhances osteogenesis in a bone marrow mesenchymal stem cell line. *Osteoporosis International* 16, 2039–2045.

Chung, H.Y., Cesari, M., Anton, S., Marzetti, E., Giovannini, S., *et al.* (2009) Molecular inflammation: Underpinnings of aging and age-related diseases. *Ageing Research Reviews* 8, 18–30.

Coetzee, M., Haag, M. and Kruger, M.C. (2007) Effects of arachidonic acid, docosahexaenoic acid, prostaglandin E2 (PGE2) and parathyroid hormone on osteoprotegerin (OPG) and RANKL secretion by MC3T3-E1 OB-like cells. *Journal of Nutritional Biochemistry* 18, 54–63.

Colbert, L.H., Vissr, M., Simonsick, E.M., Tracy, R.P., Newman A.B., *et al.* (2004) Physical activity, exercise and inflammatory markers in older adults: findings from the Health Ageing and Body Composition Study. *Journal of the American Geriatric Association* 52, 1098–1104.

Consensus Development Conference: Diagnosis, prophylaxis, and treatment of osteoporosis (2003) *American Journal of Medicine* 94, 646–650.

Coon, D., Gulati, A., Cowan, C. and He, J. (2007) The role of cyclooxygenase-2 (COX-2) in inflammatory bone resorption. *Journal of Endodontics* 33, 432–436.

De La Puerta, R., Ruiz Gutierrez, V. and Hoult, J.R. (1999) Inhibition of leukocyte 5-lipoxygenase by phenolics from virgin olive oil. *Biochemistry and Pharmacology* 57, 445–449.

De Wilde, A., Colin, C. and Lacroix, A. (2001) In vivo and ex vivo effects of an isoflavone-rich diet on bone formation in growing pigs. *Annals of Nutrition and Metabolism* 45, 227 (Abstract).

Ding, C., Parameswaran, V., Udayan, R., Burgess, J. and Jones, G. (2008) Circulating levels of inflammatory markers predict change in bone mineral density and resorption in older adults: A longitudinal study. *Journal of Clinical Endocrinology and Metabolism* 93, 1952–1958.

Ehrlich P.J. and Lanyon, L.E. (2002) Mechanical strain and bone cell function: A review. *Osteoporosis International* 13, 688–700.

Forewood, M.R. (1996) Inducible cyclo-oxygenase (COX-2) mediates the induction of bone formation by mechanical loading in vivo. *Journal of Bone and Mineral Research* 11, 1688–1693.

Franklin, M., Bu, S.Y., Lerner, M.R., Lancaster, E.A., Bellmer, D., *et al.* (2006) Dried plum prevents bone loss in a male osteoporosis model via IGF-I and the RANK pathway. *Bone* 39, 1331–1342.

Guillot, X., Semerano, L., Saidenberg-Kermanac'h, N., Falgarone, G. and Boissier, M-C. (2010) Vitamin D and inflammation. *Joint Bone Spine* 77, 552–557.

Habauzit, V. and Horcajada, M-N. (2008) Phenolic phytochemicals and bone. *Phytochemical Reviews* 7, 313–344.

Hauge, E.M., Qvesel, D., Eriksen, E.F., Moselikde, L. and Melsen, F. (2001) Cancellous bone remodeling occurs in specialized compartments lined by cells expressing osteoblastic markers. *Journal of Bone and Mineral Research* 16, 1575–1582.

Johnson, D.L., McAllister, T.N. and Frangos, J.A. (1996) Fluid flow stimulates rapid and continuous release of nitric oxide in osteoblasts. *American Journal of Physiology* 271, E205–E208.

Gillies, P.J. (2007) Preemptive nutrition of pro-inflammatory states: A nutrigenomic model. *Nutrition Reviews* 65, S217–S220.

Hardy, R. and Cooper, M.S. (2009) Bone loss in inflammatory disorders. *Journal of Endocrinology* 201, 309–320.

Hasturk, H., Kantarci, A., Ohira, T., Arita, M., Ebrahimi, N., *et al.* (2006) RvE1 protects from local inflammation and osteoclast-mediated bone destruction in perionditis. *FASEB Journal* 20, 401–403.

Hooshmand, S. and Arjmandi, B.H. (2009) Viewpoint: Dried plum, an emerging functional food that may effectively improve bone health. *Ageing Research Reviews* 8, 122–127.

Huang, Y.F., Cao, S.M., Nagamani, M., Anderson, K.E., Grady, J.J. *et al.* (2005) Decreased circulating levels of tumour necrosis factor-alpha in postmenopausal women during consumption of soy-containing isoflavones. *Journal of Clinical Endocrinology and Metabolism* 90, 3956–3962.

Joldersma, M., Klein-Nuland, J., Oleksik, A.M., Heyligers, I.C. and Burger E.H. (2001) Oestrogen enhances mechanical stress-induced prostaglandin production by bone cells from elderly women. *American Journal of Endocrinology and Metabolism* 280, E436–E442.

Kartikey, K., Singh, G., Singh, R.B., Wilczynska, A. and De Meester, F. (2010) Inflammation, osteoporosis and atherosclerosis: The Tsimtsoum concept. *The Open Nutraceuticals Journal* 3, 174–178.

Klein-Nuland, J., Van der Plas, A., Semeins, C.M., Ajubi, N.E., Frangos, J.A., *et al.* (1995) Sensitivity of osteocytes to biomechanical stress in vitro. *FASEB Journal* 9, 441–445.

Ko, C.H., Lau, K.M., Choy, W.Y. and Leung, P.C. (2009) Effects of tea catechins, epigallocatechin, gallocatechin, and gallocatechin gallate, on bone metabolism. *Journal of Agricultural and Food Chemistry* 57, 7293–7297.

Kobayashi, Y., Udagawa, N. and Takahashi, N. (2009) Action of RANKL and OPG for osteoclastogenesis. *Critical Reviews in Eukaryotic Gene Expression* 19, 61–72.

Kohrt, W.M., Bloomfield, S.A., Little, K.D., Nelson, M.E. and Yingling, V.R. (2004) ACSM position stand: Physical activity and bone health. *Medicine & Science in Sports & Exercise* 36, 1985–1996.

Kruger, M.C., Coetzee, M., Haag, M. and Weiler, H. (2010) Long-chain polyunsaturated fatty acids: selected mechanisms of action on bone. *Progress in Lipid Research* 49, 438–449.

Lacativa, P.G.S. and de Farias, M.L.F. (2010) Osteoporosis and inflammation. *Arquivos Brasileiros de Endocrinologia* 54, 123–132.

Li, B.B. and Yu, S.F. (2003) Genistein prevents bone resorption diseases by inhibiting bone resorption and stimulating bone formation. *Biology and Pharmacology Bulletin* 26, 780–786.

Lin, R-W., Chen, C-H., Wang, Y-H., Ho, M-L., Hung, S-H., *et al.* (2009) (-)-Epigallocatechin gallate inhibition of osteoclastic differentiation via NF-κB. *Biochemical and Biophysical Research Communications* 379, 1033–1037.

Liu, X., Kirschenbaum, A., Yao, S. and Levine, A.C. (2005) Cross-talk between interleukin-6 and prostaglandin E2 signaling systems results in enhancement of osteoclastogenesis through effects on the osteoprotegerin/receptor activator of nuclear factor-κß (RANK) ligand/RANK system. *Endocrinology* 146, 1991–1998.

Lorenzo, J. (2000) Interactions between immune and bone cells: new insights with many remaining questions. *The Journal of Clinical Investigation* 106, 749–752.

Margeli, A., Skenderi, K., Tsironi, M., Hantzi, E., Matalas, A.L., *et al.* (2005) Dramatic elevations in interleukin-6 and acute-phase reactants in athletes participating in the ultradistance foot race "spartathlon": severe systemic inflammation ad lipid and lipoprotein changes in protracted exercise. *Journal of Clinical Endocrinology and Metabolism* 90, 3914–3918.

Marie, P.J. (2008) Transcription factors controlling osteoblastogenesis. *Archives of Biochemistry and Biophysics* 473, 98–105.

Marks, S.C. and Hermey, D.C. (1996) The structure and development of bone. In: Bilezikian, J.P., Raisz, L.G., Rodan, G.A. (eds) *Principles of Bone Biology*. Academic Press, San Diego, California, pp. 3–14.

Martin, T.J., Gooi, J.H. and Sims, N.A. (2009) Molecular mechanisms in coupling of bone formation to resorption. *Critical Reviews in Eukaryotic Gene Expression* 19, 73–88.

McCormick, K.R. (2007) Osteoporosis: Integrating biomarkers and other diagnostic correlates into the management of bone fragility. *Alternative Medicine Review* 12, 113–145.

McLean, R.R. (2009) Proinflammatory cytokines and osteoporosis. *Current Osteoporosis Reports* 7, 134–139.

Meydani, S.N. and Wu, D. (2007) Age-associated inflammatory changes: Role of nutritional intervention. *Nutrition Reviews* 65, S213–S216.

Meydanie, S.N., Lichtenstein, A.H., Cornwall, S., Meydani, M., Goldin, B.R., *et al.* (1993) Immunologic effects of national cholesterol education panel step-2 diets with and without fish-derived N-3 fatty acid enrichment. *Journal of Clinical Investigation* 92, 105–113.

Miggiano, G.A. and Gagliardi, L. (2005) Diet, nutrition and bone health. *Clinical Therapy* 156, 47–56.

Mundy, G.R. (2006) Nutritional modulators of bone remodelling during ageing. *American Journal of Clinical Nutrition* 83, 4275–4305.

Mundy, G.R. (2007) Osteoporosis and inflammation. *Nutrition Reviews* 65, S147–S151.

NIH. Osteoporosis prevention and therapy (2000) *NIH Consensus statement* 17, 1–36.

Novack, D.V. and Teitelbaum, S.L. (2008) The osteoclast: Friend or Foe? *Annual Reviews* 3, 457–484.

Ordovas, J. (2007) Diet/genetic interactions and their effects on inflammatory markers. *Nutrition Reviews* 65, S203–S207.

Pacifici, R. (1996) Oestrogen, cytokines, and pathogenesis of postmenopausal osteoporosis. *Journal of Bone and Mineral Research* 11, 1043–1051.

Pang, J.L., Ricupero, D.A., Huang, S., Fatma, N., Singh, D.P., *et al.* (2006) Differential activity of keampferol and quercetin in attenuating tumor necrosis factor receptor family signalling in bone cells. *Biochemistry and Pharmacology* 71, 818–826.

Papadopoulos, N.G., Georganas, K., Skoutella, V., Konstantellos, E. and Lyritis, G.P. (1997) Correlation of interleukin -6 serum levels with bonedensity in postmenopausal women. *Clinical Rheumatology* 16, 162–165.

Pasco, J.A., Kotowicz, M.A., Henry, M.J., Nicholson, G.C., Spilsbury, H.J., *et al.* (2006) High-sensitivity C-reactive protein and fracture risk in elderly women. *Journal of the American Medical Association* 296, 1353–1355.

Pederson, B.K., Sreenberg, A. and Scherling, P. (2001) Muscle-derived interleukin-6: possible biological effects. *Journal of Physiology* 536, 329–337.

Pedersen, B.K., Steensberg, A., Fischer, C., Keller, C., Keller, P., *et al.* (2003). Searching for the exercise factor-is IL-6 a candidate. *Journal of Muscle Research and Cell Motility* 24, 113–119.

Poulsen, R.C. and Kruger, M.C. (2008) Soy phytoestrogens: impact on postmenopausal bone loss and mechanisms of action. *Nutrition Reviews* 66, 359–374.

Poulsen, R.C., Moughan, P.J. and Kruger M.C. (2007) Long-chain polyunsaturated fatty acids and the regulation of bone metabolism. *Experimental Biology and Medicine* 232, 1275–1288.

Poulsen, R.C., Wolber, F., Moughan, P.J. and Kruger M.C. (2008) Long chain polyunsaturated fatty acids alter membrane bound RANK-L expression and osteoprotegerin secretion by MC3T3-E1 OB-like cells. *Prostaglandins and other Lipid Mediators* 85, 42–48.

Priante, G., Bordin, L., Musacchio, E., Clari, G. and Baggio, B. (2002) Fatty acids and cytokine mRNA expression in human osteoblastic cells: a specific effect of arachidonic acid. *Clinical Science* 102, 403–409.

Proff, P. and Römer, P. (2009) The molecular mechanism behind bone remodelling: a review. *Clinical Oral Investigations* 13, 355–362.

Puel, C., Quintin, A., Agalias, A., Mathey, J., Obled, C., *et al.* (2004) Olive oil and its main phenolic micronutrient (oleuropein) prevent inflammation-induced bone loss in the ovariectomised rat. *British Journal of Nutrition* 92, 119–127.

Puel, C., Mathey, J., Agalias, A., Kati-coulibaly, S., Mardon, J., *et al.* (2006) Dose-response study of effect of oleuropein, an olive oil polyphenols, in an ovariectomy/inflammation experimental model of bone loss in the rat. *Clinical Nutrition* 25, 859–868.

Quinn, J.M.W. and Saleh, H. (2009) Modulation of osteoclast function in bone by the immune system. *Molecular and Cellular Endocrinology* 310, 40–51.

Raggatt, L.J. and Partridge, N.C. (2010) Cellular and molecular mechanisms of bone remodeling. *The Journal of Biological Chemistry* 295, 25103–25108.

Rahman, M.D., Bhattacharya, A. and Fernandes, G. (2008) Docosahexaenoic acid is more potent inhibitor of osteoclast differentiation in RAW 264.7 cells that eicosapentaenoic acid. *Journal of Cellular Physiology* 214, 201–209.

Renaud, S., de Lorgeril, M., Delaye, J., Guidollet, J., Jacquard, F., *et al.* (1995) Cretan Meditiranean diet for prevention of coronary heart disease. *American Journal of Clinical Nutrition* 61, 1360S–1367S.

Roggia, C., Gao, Y., Cenci, S., Weitzmann, M.N., Toraldo, G., *et al.* (2001) Up-regulation of TNF-producing T cells in the bone marrow: A key mechanism by which oestrogen deficiency induces bone loss *in vivo.* *Proceedings of the National Academy of Sciences* 98, 13960–13965.

Shen, C.-L., Wang, P., Guerrieri, J., Yeh, J.K. and Wang, J.-S. (2008) Protective effect of green tea polyphenols on bone loss in middle-aged female rats. *Osteoporosis International* 19, 979–990.

Shen, C-L., Yeh, J.K., Cao, J. and Wang, J-S. (2009) Green tea and bone metabolism. *Nutrition Research* 29, 437–456.

Shen, C-L., Yeh, J.K., Cao, J.J., Tatum, O.L., Dagda, R.Y., *et al.* (2010a) Synergistic effects of green tea polyphenols and alphacalcidol on chronic inflammation-induced bone loss in female rats. *Osteoporosis International* 21, 1841–1852.

Shen, C-L., Yeh, J.K., Cao, J.J., Tatum, O.L., Dagda, R.Y., *et al.* (2010b) Green tea polyphenols mitigate bone loss of female rats in a chronic inflammation-induced bone loss model. *Journal of Nutritional Biochemistry* 21, 968–974.

Shen, C-L., Yeh, J.K., Samathanam, C., Cao, J.J., Stoecker, B.J., *et al.* (2011) Green tea polyphenols attenuate deterioration of bone microarchitecture in female rats with systemic chronic inflammation. *Osteoporosis International* 22, 327–337.

Silverman, N.E., Nicklas, B.J. and Ryan, A.S. (2009) Addition of aerobic exercise to a weight loss program increases BMD, with an associated reduction in inflammation in overweight menopausal women. *Calcified Tissue International,* 84, 257–265.

Skuladottir, I.H., Petursdottir, D.H. and Hardardottir, I. (2007) The effects of omega 3 polyunsaturated fatty acids on TNF-alpha and IL-10 secretion by murine peritoneal cells in vitro. *Lipids* 42, 699–706.

Son, Y.O., Kook, S.H., Choi, K.C., Jang, Y.S., Jeon, Y.M., *et al.* (2006) Quercetin, a bioflavonoid, accelerates TNF-alpha-induced growth inhibition and apoptosis in MC3T3-E1 osteoblastic cells. *European Journal of Pharmacology* 529, 24–32.

Streck, J.G., Klein-Nuland, L., Lips, P. and Burger, E.H. (1998) Response of normal and osteoporotic human bone cells to mechanical stress in vitro. *American Journal of Physiology* 274, E1113–E1120.

Straub, R.H. (2007) The complex role of oestrogens in inflammation. *Endocrine Reviews* 28, 521–574.

Suh, K.S., Koh, G., Park, C.Y., Woo, J.T., Kim, S.W., *et al.* (2003) Soybean isoflavones inhibit tumour-necrosis factor-alpha induced apoptosis and the production of interleukin-6 and prostaglandin E2 in osteoblastic cells. *Phytochemistry* 63, 209–215.

Sugatini, T., Alvarez, U.M. and Hruska, K.A. (2003) Activin stimulates Iκβ/NFκβ and RANK expression for osteoclast differentiation, but not AKT survival pathway in osteoclast precursors. *Journal of Cellular Biochemistry* 90, 59–67.

Turner, C.H. and Pavalko, F.M. (1998) Mechanotransduction and functional response of the skeleton to physical stress: The mechanisms and mechanics of bone adaptation. *Journal of Orthopaedic Science* 3, 346–355.

Vali, B., Rao, L.G. and El-Sohemy, A. (2007) Epigallocatechin-3-gallate increases the formation of mineralized bone nodules by human osteoblast-like cells. *Journal of Nutritional Biochemistry* 18, 341–347.

Viereck, V., Gründker, C., Blaschke, S., Siggelkow, H., Emons, G., *et al.* (2002) Phytoestrogen genistein stimulates the production of osteoprotegerin by human trabecular osteoblasts. *Journal of Cellular Biochemistry* 84, 725–735.

Weitzmann, M.N. and Pacifici, R. (2006) Oestrogen deficiency and bone loss: an inflammatory tale. *The Journal of Clinical Investigation* 116, 1186–1194.

Yun, A.J. and Lee, P.Y. (2004) Maldaptation of the link between inflammation and bone turnover may be a key determinant of osteoporosis. *Medical Hypotheses* 63, 532–537.

Yun, J-H., Kim, C-S., Cho, K-S., Chai, J-K., Kim, C-K. *et al.* (2007) (-)-Epigallocatechin gallate induces apoptosis, via caspase activation, in osteoclasts differentiated from RAW 264.7 cells. *Journal of Periodontal Research* 42, 212–218.

Zaidi, M., Blair, H.C., Moonga, B.S., Abe, E., Huang, C.L.H. (2003). Osteoclastogenesis, bone resorption and osteoclast-based therapeutics. *Journal of Bone and Mineral Research* 18, 599–609.

Zarabeitia, M.T., Riancho, J.A., Amado, J.A., Napal, J. and Gonzales-Macias, J. (1991) Cytokine production by peripheral blood cells in postmenopausal osteoporosis. *Bone and Mineral* 14, 161–167.

Zeitlin, L., Segev, E., Fried, A. and Wientroub, S. (2003) Effects of long-term administration of n-3 polyunsaturated fatty acids (PUFA) and selective oestrogen receptor modulator (SERM) derivatives in ovariectomized (OVX) mice. *Journal of Cellular Biochemistry* 90, 347–360.

Zheng, S.X., Vrindts, Y., Lopez, M., De Groote, D., Collette, J., *et al.* (1997) Increase in cytokine production (IL-1 beta, IL-6, TNF-alpha but not IFN-gamma, GM-CSF or LIF) by stimulated whole blood cell in postmenopausal osteoporosis. *Maturitas* 26, 63–71.

21 Eye Health and Inflammation

I. Jalbert,*[,1] B. Golebiowski,[1] F.J. Stapleton[1] and M.C. Madigan[1,2]
[1]*School of Optometry and Vision Science, University of New South Wales and* [2]*Save Sight Institute, Sydney Medical School, University of Sydney, Australia*

Introduction

Inflammation can affect any part of the eye or surrounding tissue including the eyelids, ocular surfaces – cornea, conjunctiva and sclera – intraocular structures including the iris, ciliary body and choroid and retina, extraocular muscles, lacrimal gland and optic nerve. The consequences of excessive inflammatory responses around and within the eye have significant morbidity. Specifically, inflammation can critically impact on vision, comfort and overall quality of life. In this chapter we review two of the eye conditions most commonly associated with inflammation: dry eye disease (DED) and age-related macular degeneration (AMD). Although these conditions affect different parts of the eye, similarities are seen in the chronic involvement of inflammation, the complex interactions between genes and environment, their increased incidence with ageing and the emerging use of nutritional interventions to ameliorate symptoms and to delay or even prevent disease progression.

* Corresponding author, i.jalbert@unsw.edu.au

Dry Eye Disease, Age-Related Macular Degeneration and Eye Health

Dry eye disease (DED)

Dry eye disease is a chronic symptomatic condition that affects the anterior surface of the eye. The ocular surface comprises the cornea, palpebral and bulbar conjunctivae, eyelids including the meibomian glands, which have openings along the upper and lower lid margins (Fig. 21.1), and the tear film constituents. Maintenance of the integrity of the ocular surface is a complex and dynamic process, the breakdown of which results in dry eye disease (DED). The International Dry Eye Workshop recently defined DED as 'a multifactorial disease of the tears and ocular surface that results in symptoms of discomfort, visual disturbance, and tear film instability with potential damage to the ocular surface. It is accompanied by increased osmolarity of the tear film and inflammation of the ocular surface' (International Dry Eye Workshop Report, 2007). The currently accepted scheme for DED involves classifying the condition into aqueous-deficient or evaporative DED on the basis of the major aetiology of each case. Causes of aqueous-deficient DED include autoimmune conditions such as Sjögren's Syndrome and extrinsic causes such as refractive surgery. Common causes of evaporative DED include meibomian gland dysfunction, environmental factors (e.g. computer use, air conditioning, office work) and contact lens wear (International Dry Eye Workshop Report, 2007). Estimates of the prevalence of DED from large epidemiological studies conducted worldwide range from 5% to as high as 35% (International Dry Eye Workshop Report, 2007). Clinically, damage to the ocular surface induced by DED is characterized with the use of vital stains such as fluorescein, rose bengal and lissamine green (Fig. 21.2a) and assessment of tear film quality and quantity.

Meibomian gland dysfunction is considered one of the most common causes of DED with a reported prevalence of up to 70% in people aged 40 and over (Schaumberg *et al.*, 2011). Meibomian gland dysfunction has recently been redefined by the International Workshop on Meibomian Gland Dysfunction as a 'chronic, diffuse abnormality of the meibomian glands, commonly characterized by

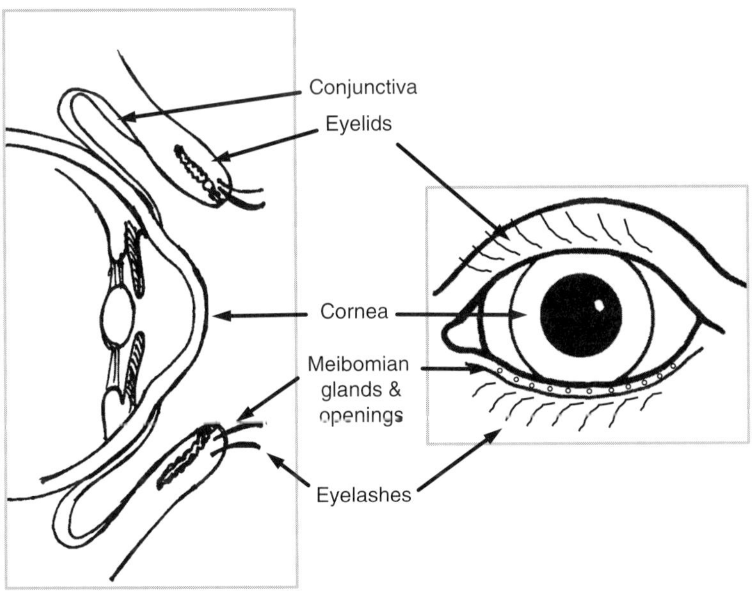

Fig. 21.1. Diagram showing the main features of the anterior eye, including eyelids, eyelashes, cornea and location of meibomian glands within the eyelids.

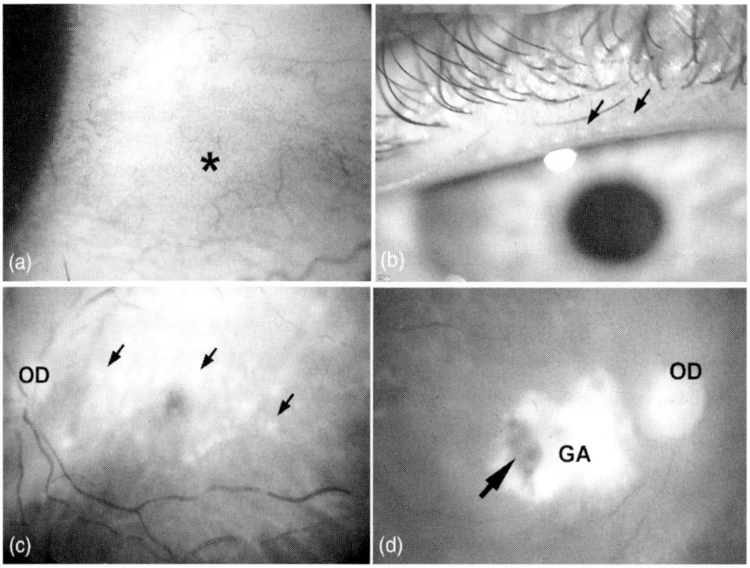

Fig. 21.2. Clinical appearance of common inflammatory conditions of the eye. (a) Surface damage to the conjunctiva is highlighted using lissamine green stain (*) in a sufferer of aqueous-deficient dry eye disease (DED). (b) Blocked meibomian gland openings (small arrows), lid margin hyperaemia, blood vessel telangectasia and oily eyelashes are characteristics of evaporative DED. (c) Numerous drusen (small arrows) and pigment changes are observed in the macula of an eye with moderate age-related macular degeneration (AMD). OD, optic disc. (d) Marked atrophy (GA) and pigment clumping (arrow) is observed in the macula of an eye with advanced AMD. OD, optic disc.

terminal duct obstruction and/or changes in the glandular secretion. This may result in alteration of the tear film, symptoms of eye irritation, clinically apparent inflammation and ocular surface disease' (Nelson *et al.*, 2011). There is clearly considerable overlap between the conditions of DED and meibomian gland dysfunction and the conditions are not mutually exclusive. Clinically, signs such as dilated blood vessels at the lid margin, plugging of the meibomian glands (Fig. 21.2b), and rapid evaporation (break-up) of the tear film layer will be noted whenever meibomian gland dysfunction is involved (Schaumberg *et al.*, 2011). Also of note is the recent focus on the potential role of the lid margin in the pathophysiology and diagnosis of DED (Yamaguchi *et al.*, 2006; Korb *et al.*, 2010; Knop *et al.*, 2011b; Jalbert *et al.*, unpublished observations).

Ocular symptoms are frequently associated with DED. The eye is acutely susceptible to changes in systemic health and to environmental challenges such as computer work, air conditioning or contact lens wear. For individuals, these circumstances manifest as increased ocular discomfort, reported as dryness most commonly but also irritation, burning, stinging, grittiness, tiredness, pain, itchiness and foreign body sensation (Bandeen-Roche *et al.*, 1997; Begley *et al.*, 2001; Johnson and Murphy, 2007). Discomfort is reported by 64% of non contact lens wearers and 79% of contact lens wearers in the general population (Begley *et al.*, 2001). More than 715,000 individuals in Australia currently wear contact lenses and 50% of those use artificial tears to alleviate symptoms of discomfort, while another 320,000 have discontinued contact lens wear owing to discomfort (Stapleton *et al.*, 2008). We recently conducted a survey at the University of New South Wales that confirmed these findings with 67% of a general sample of 1758 campus volunteer students and staff reporting sensation of ocular discomfort either sometimes, often or all the time (Jalbert *et al.*, 2011).

The burden of DED is often underestimated, yet quality-of-life studies show that patients with DED are about three times more likely to report problems with everyday activities, including reading, carrying out professional work, using a computer, watching television, driving during the day and at night, than those without dryness (Miljanovic *et al.*, 2007). The effects of ocular dryness can be substantial, leading to decreased productivity and reduced quality of life (Reddy *et al.*, 2004). DED has social as well as physical impacts in that it can affect the ability to wear contact lenses and use cosmetics (Reddy *et al.*, 2004; Miljanovic *et al.*, 2007). Utility assessment, a tool used widely in medicine to compare the effect of different diseases on quality of life, has also been applied to DED. Interestingly, the utility scores for DED were similar to those for moderate angina (Schiffman *et al.*, 2003).

Treatments available for DED involve frequent topical application of lubricating drops and ointments, plugging of tear drainage ducts and/or advice to avoid environmental triggers. More severe aqueous-deficient DED is managed with topical anti-inflammatory agents such as corticosteroids or T cell modulators such as cyclosporine (International Dry Eye Workshop Report, 2007). More recently, systemic therapies have been utilized including either tetracycline or macrolide antibiotics for the meibomian gland dysfunction component of DED and nutritional intervention.

Age-related macular degeneration (AMD)

AMD is a potentially blinding condition that affects the posterior eye. It is a progressive age-related degeneration affecting the central retina (macula), the region that provides our most acute vision, crucial in reading and tasks requiring resolution of fine detail. In Australia, AMD accounts for approximately 10% of visual loss and 50% of blindness in people aged over 40 years of age (~40,000 people in 2009) (Access Economics Pty Ltd, 2010). The prevalence of any AMD for people aged over 40 years in the USA between 2005 and 2008 was reported to be 6.5% (Klein *et al.*, 2011). Clinically, early AMD is characterized by abnormal accumulations or deposits of material (drusen) between the retinal pigmented epithelium (RPE) and the underlying Bruch's membrane in the macular region, associated with RPE changes (Fig. 21.2c). Advanced AMD is described as either 'dry' or atrophic AMD (Fig. 21.2d), with a slowly progressing chronic loss of retinal photoreceptors and RPE; or 'wet' or exudative AMD, where new vessels invade into the subretinal space and/or neural retina. In wet AMD, these leaky new vessels lead to macular oedema and consequently vision distortion; subretinal haemorrhage and sudden loss of vision generally occur followed by the formation of irreversible fibrovascular scarring in the macula. Dry AMD is more common, occurring in approximately 85% of those with intermediate and advanced AMD. Wet AMD however accounts for most of the vision loss in advanced AMD cases.

Therapeutic interventions for AMD have focused on delaying, stabilizing or recovering vision loss in patients with wet AMD. Numerous laboratory and clinical studies have investigated drugs and techniques that can inhibit new blood vessel growth. Photodynamic therapy was initially used; however, antibodies inhibiting vascular endothelial growth factor-A (VEGF) are now routine for patients with wet AMD (reviewed in Mitchell, 2011; Patel *et al.*, 2011). Clinical trials of anti-VEGF agents Lucentis and Avastin indicate stabilization of vision in about 90% of patients, with some improvement in vision for about 30% of treated patients. A novel anti-VEGF drug, VEGF Trap-Eye, that targets a broader range of VEGF isoforms plus other critical pro-angiogenic factors is currently being trialled and shows promise as a next generation therapy for wet AMD (Dixon *et al.*, 2009).

There are currently no therapies for patients with dry AMD, although a number of early phase clinical trials are investigating various drugs including complement pathway inhibitors (Fig. 21.3) (reviewed in Yehoshua *et al.*, 2011). Anti-inflammatories such as fluocinolone acetonide, antioxidants and other nutrients (from the Age-Related Eye Disease Study; AREDS) and neuroprotective agents are also being considered as potential therapies for slowing progression of dry AMD (reviewed in Yehoshua *et al.*, 2011).

Epidemiological, genetic and laboratory studies over the past 20 years have confirmed the importance of genetic predisposition, complement pathway malfunction and local

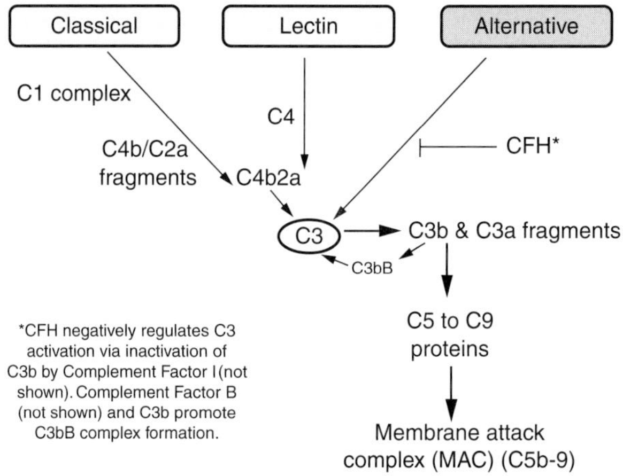

Fig. 21.3. Simplified schematic showing the main complement system pathways. Complement factor H (CFH) is the main inhibitor of the alternative pathway and normally regulates C3b activation. Genetic variants of complement system regulators and receptors are known to be associated with an increased risk for developing AMD, with consequences for local chronic inflammation in the neural retina and choroid/ Bruch's membrane/retinal pigmented epithelium complex.

chronic inflammation in the pathogenesis of AMD. These studies highlight complex interactions between genetics, ageing and external risk factors such as smoking, obesity and dietary intake of fats and antioxidants, levels of physical activity and light exposure in all phenotypes of AMD (reviewed in Hageman *et al.*, 2001; Penfold *et al.*, 2001; Klein *et al.*, 2004; Anderson *et al.*, 2010).

Role of Inflammation in Eye Health

DED and inflammation

As suggested by the currently accepted definition of DED, inflammation plays a major role in the pathogenesis of DED (International Dry Eye Workshop Report, 2007). The underlying pathogenesis of DED is complex and includes inflammatory processes, deficiencies in the production of tear lipids, as well as malfunction or destruction of the tissue components of the ocular surface, including a reduction in the number of conjunctival goblet cells. Decreased tear aqueous production, and subsequent tear hyperosmolarity are also implicated. Tear hyperosmolarity causes hyperosmolarity of the epithelial cells, stimulating the generation of cytokines (International Dry Eye Workshop Report, 2007). Numerous pro- and anti-inflammatory tear cytokines (interleukin (IL)-1β, IL-2, IL-4, IL-5, IL-6, IL-10, interferon-γ, tumour necrosis factor-α) and chemokines (IL-8) are upregulated in dry eye (Massingale *et al.*, 2009). Ocular surface corneal and conjunctival receptors (IL-1, IL-6, CCR2, CCR5) are also overexpressed in DED (Gulati *et al.*, 2006; Narayanan *et al.*, 2008). Human leucocyte antigen (HLA)DR expression is a marker of immune stimulation that is upregulated in early DED (Rolando *et al.*, 2005). Ocular mucins (e.g. MUC1, MUC4, MUC5AC, MUC7, MUC16) show reduced expression or altered glycosylation in dry eye, making the ocular surface less hydrophilic (Fig. 21.4) (Gipson *et al.*, 2004). Once inflammatory cells have been recruited to the ocular surface, they further potentiate damage to the structures involved (e.g. the lacrimal gland) perpetuating the hyperosmolarity of the milieu. A vicious circle therefore links the various structures of the ocular surface system in DED, which is the key to understanding the chronic nature of the disease.

Although meibomian gland dysfunction can often present as a subset of DED, expert consensus suggests that it involves both obstructive and inflammatory processes. Non-inflammatory processes such as hyperkeratinization and gland atrophy lead-

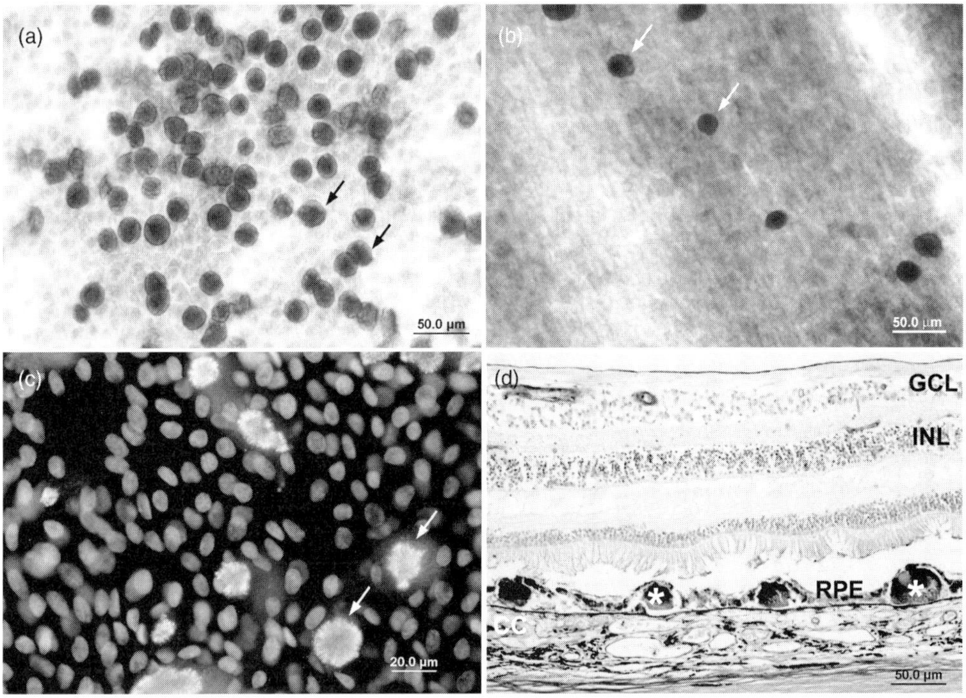

Fig. 21.4. Light microscopy of common inflammatory conditions of the eye. (a–b) Impression cytology samples from the conjunctiva of a normal patient (a) and a Sjögren's disease DED patient (b). Note the differences in the frequency of mucin-producing (PAS+) goblet cells (arrows) (Periodic acid Schiff's (PAS) reagent and haematoxylin). (c) Normal bulbar conjunctiva MUC5AC immunoreactive goblet cells (small arrows) visible amongst epithelial cell nuclei (counterstained with Hoechst). (d) Drusen (asterisk) can be seen between the retinal pigmented epithelium (RPE) and Bruch's membrane of a patient with early AMD (PAS and haematoxylin). GCL, ganglion cell layer; INL, inner nuclear layer; CC, choriocapillaris.

ing to obstructive disease are important factors in the pathogenesis of meibomian gland dysfunction (Knop *et al.*, 2011a). Such meibomian gland dysfunction, however, often leads to destabilization of the tear film through inadequate production of surface tear lipids. This instability in turn leads to increased evaporation and hyperosmolarity of the tear fluid, the recruitment of inflammatory cytokines and chemokines and subsequent inflammation of the ocular surface. Whether localized inflammatory processes are at play in the meibomian gland themselves is more uncertain. Although normally colonized by commensal bacteria, the skin of and around the eyelid can also be colonized by large numbers of opportunistic bacteria such as coagulase negative staphylococci (CNS), *Staphylococcus aureus* and *Propionibacterium acnes* (Dougherty and McCulley, 1986). The effect of the lipases released locally by these bacteria can alter the meibum obstructed at the openings of nearby keratinized meibomian glands, leading to the release of irritating pro-inflammatory toxic mediators into the tear film and onto the ocular surface (Dougherty and McCulley, 1986). The effectiveness of sub-therapeutic doses of oral antibiotics, tetracycline and doxycycline, in the treatment of meibomian gland dysfunction lends support to inflammatory processes being involved (Shine *et al.*, 2003).

AMD and inflammation

Inflammation is a major factor in the pathogenesis of AMD. Significant observations in epidemiological, genetic and laboratory studies confirm the major role of the immune system and inflammation in the pathogenesis of

AMD (reviewed by Penfold *et al.*, 2001; Gehrs *et al.*, 2010). In particular, variants of several major complement pathway regulatory genes have been found to be strongly associated with increased risk or susceptibility to developing AMD (reviewed by Gehrs *et al.*, 2010).

The complement system is normally involved in immune responses including cell defence against foreign entities (for example, bacteria, viruses and toxins), clearing damaged cells and immune complexes, and maintaining tissue homeostasis (Ricklin *et al.*, 2010). These responses are mediated via several complement pathways (Fig. 21.3): the classical pathway involving complement component 1 (C1) interactions with antigen–antibody complexes and non-immune cell debris, the lectin pathway activated by microbial carbohydrates, and the alternative pathway that involves hydrolysis of C3 and deposition of C3b fragments on target cells that are targeted and cleared by macrophages. These pathways converge on C3 as a common point of activation, with a downstream aggregation of complement proteins (C5 to C9) to form Membrane Attack Complexes (MACs), leading to cell lysis and death (Fig. 21.3). There is also an intrinsic complement pathway (not shown) that can activate the complement system via proteolytic enzymes released from damaged tissues.

Cumulative evidence shows that the molecular constituents of drusen, early markers of AMD, include lipids, complement pathway proteins, activators and regulatory proteins, and inflammation-related products (reviewed by Hageman *et al.*, 2001; Anderson *et al.*, 2010). Genetic studies have also found highly significant associations between AMD and variants of several complement-associated genes including complement factor H *(CFH)*, complement factor H-related 1 and 3 (*CFHR1* and *CFHR3*), complement factor B (*CFB*), *C2* and *C3*. The initial discovery of a strong association of *CFH* gene polymorphisms with increased susceptibility to developing AMD has been confirmed in many independent genetic studies (Edwards *et al.*, 2005, Haines *et al.*, 2005). The *CFH* variant *Y402H* accounts for approximately 60% of the attributable risk for AMD (Haines *et al.*, 2005; Jakobsdottir *et al.*, 2005; Gehrs *et al.*, 2010). Protective variants of *CFH* and other complement-pathway-associated genes have also been associated with AMD including *C2/CFB* (Gold *et al.*, 2006). More recently, multivariate analysis has found that the presence of several gene variants, *CFH, C3* and *CFB/C2* (complement-related genes), and *ARMS2* and *HTRA1* (non-complement related gene) could be highly predictive of advanced AMD development (Despriet *et al.*, 2008). Many questions remain to be explored in this area including why the macula is exquisitely susceptible to these immune-mediated pathways.

The local complement system in the choroid/Bruch's membrane/RPE membrane complex, and to a much lesser extent in the neural retina, have been studied in ageing and AMD eyes (detailed review by Anderson *et al.*, 2010). Interestingly, a rat retinal light damage model study recently showed that photoreceptor cell death was associated with significant changes in gene expression of various complement pathway regulators and receptors (Rutar *et al.*, 2011). Macrophages/microglia deposited C3 in the outer retina associated with photoreceptor damage/death, particularly at the edges of the retinal degeneration (Rutar *et al.*, 2011). Similar processes may underlie the insidious degeneration and loss of photoreceptors and RPE seen in patients with dry AMD.

Taken together, these findings highlight the importance of the complement system and chronic inflammation in the pathogenesis of AMD, particularly for those with genetic susceptibility conferred by variants of complement and non-complement related genes, and exposed to known external risk factors. Therapeutic interventions that target the complement system, particularly alternative pathway proteins, are increasingly a focus of AMD research, especially for patients with dry AMD (reviewed in Gehrs *et al.*, 2010; Yehoshua *et al.*, 2011).

Nutritional Interventions, Inflammation and Eye Health

DED and nutritional interventions

Seminal work conducted by Dr Sommers and his colleagues in the 1970s established the link between childhood malnutrition and a blinding form of ocular surface disease called keratomalacia and demonstrated the effectiveness of vitamin A supplementation in preventing blindness and childhood mortality (Sommer *et al.*, 1975). The suggestion of a role for nutrition in the management of more moderate forms of DED arose out of research published in 2005. In a large population study conducted in the USA, the odds of self-report of DED in women aged 45 to 85 years with an omega-6 to omega-3 ratio of more than 15 were increased 2.5-fold when compared with those with a ratio of less than 4 (Miljanovic *et al.*, 2005). Those consuming more than 5 servings per week of tuna fish also had significantly lower odds of developing DED than those consuming less than 1 serving of tuna per week (Miljanovic *et al.*, 2005). Fish oils contain the omega-3 polyunsaturated fatty acids eicosapentaenoic (EPA) and docosahexaenoic acid (DHA). These dietary fatty acids are thought to swing the balance of EPA–arachidonic acid metabolism away from pro-inflammatory prostaglandins and leukotrienes towards those that have an overall anti-inflammatory effect, such as prostaglandins of 3- and 1-series. A higher intake of omega-3 fatty acids, supplemented vitamin B6 and unsupplemented vitamin D have been shown to be associated with a different fatty acid profile of meibomian gland secretions than those with lower intakes of these nutrients (Sullivan *et al.*, 2002).

The findings above support a role for dietary intervention and supplementation in the management of DED. The proposed mechanism of action involves these foods or supplements shifting the metabolism of omega-3 and omega-6 fatty acids towards more anti-inflammatory mediators downstream. A number of studies have since attempted to test the effects of fatty-acid-based dietary nutraceuticals on ocular surface health (Table 21.1).

Early trials have assessed the effectiveness of omega-6 fatty acid based supplementation (e.g. evening primrose oil) based on the previous findings of prostaglandin-1 being able to stimulate lacrimal gland tear secretion (Pholpramool, 1979). An increased concentration of tear prostaglandin E1 and reduced ocular symptoms and ocular surface damage were found in Sjögren's women after 1-month supplementation using omega-6 fatty acid supplements (Aragona *et al.*, 2005). Six months of oral omega-6 fatty acid supplementation was associated with an increase in the comfort and volume of tears in contact lens wearing females (Kokke *et al.*, 2008). More recent trials have looked at combination formulations. An omega-3 and -6 fatty acid oral supplement was associated with reduced HLA-DR expression at the ocular surface in a recent trial (Brignole-Baudouin *et al.*, 2011). It is not clear from these studies what mechanisms are involved, nor are we sure which of the major fatty acids, at what dosage and for how long would have the most potent effect on the ocular surface. Although they do not convincingly demonstrate improvement in any one specific component of DED, most of the placebo-controlled blinded studies do show an improvement in subjective discomfort in patients ingesting fatty acid supplements. It is possible that the benefits of a lifelong (40 years +) ingestion of omega-3 fatty acid rich foods may never be fully replicated by the short-term ingestion of dietary nutraceuticals. There is a clear need for more research to confirm these promising findings using a large multi-centre properly conducted randomized clinical trial.

AMD and nutritional interventions

Nutritional supplements including antioxidants and omega-3 fatty acids are increasingly being advocated as interventions to inhibit or slow the progression of various stages of AMD (reviewed in Krishnadev *et al.*, 2010). The lack of any effective therapeutic interventions for dry AMD, the recognition that anti-VEGF therapies alone do not 'cure' wet AMD, and a better understanding of the complex interactions of genetics, inflammation and external factors, such as diet in AMD, provide a background for these studies.

The Age-Related Eye Disease Study (AREDS), a major randomized controlled clinical trial, investigated the effects of nutritional supplements for AMD (Table 21.1). A beneficial effect was reported following nutritional supplementation with antioxidants plus zinc, with a 25% reduced risk of progression to advanced AMD in patients with intermediate

Table 21.1. Some of the key clinical studies investigating nutrition and eye health.

Study	Nutritional supplements	Primary outcomes
Vitamin E, Cataract and Age-related Maculopathy Trial (VECAT) (Australia) (Taylor *et al.*, 2002)	Vitamin E	Daily vitamin E supplement did not prevent the development or progression of early or later stages of AMD
Carotenoids and Age-Related Eye Disease (CAREDS) (USA) (Moeller *et al.*, 2006)	Lutein, zeaxanthin, β-carotene	Diets rich in lutein plus zeaxanthin may protect against intermediate AMD in healthy women < 75 years
The Age-Related Eye Disease Study (AREDS) (USA) (Age-Related Eye Disease Study Research Group, 2001)	Vitamin C, Vitamin E, β-carotene, zinc, copper	For those with intermediate AMD or advanced AMD in one eye, high levels of antioxidants and zinc significantly reduced the risk of advanced AMD and associated vision loss. No apparent benefit for those with either no AMD or early AMD
The Age-Related Eye Disease Study II (AREDS2) (USA) (http://www.areds2.org/)	Lutein and zeaxanthin, omega-3 (DHA and EPA), reduced zinc, no β-carotene	In progress
Subset of Women's Health Study (WHS) (USA) (Miljanovic *et al.*, 2005)	Assessed dietary intake of omega-3 and -6 and dry eye symptoms	Higher dietary intake of omega-3 fatty acids associated with decreased incidence of dry eye symptoms in women
Aragona *et al.*, 2005	Omega-6 fatty acids	Supplementation with omega-6 fatty acids for 1 month increased levels of anti-inflammatory tear prostaglandin E1 and reduced symptoms of ocular discomfort and ocular surface staining in women with the autoimmune disease Sjögren's syndrome
Kokke *et al.*, 2008	Evening primrose oil (EPO)	Supplementation with omega-6 fatty acids (EPO) in women contact lens wearers for 6 months may help reduce symptoms of discomfort and slightly increase tear volume
Brignole-Baudouin *et al.*, 2011	Omega-3 and -6 fatty acids, vitamins and zinc	Supplementation with omega-3 and omega-6 fatty acids may help with dry eye symptoms; reduced expression of conjunctival inflammatory marker (human leukocyte antigen (HLA))-DR

AMD or with advanced AMD in one eye at 5 years follow-up (Age-Related Eye Disease Study Research Group, 2001). The formulations used in AREDS comprised combinations of vitamin C (500 mg), vitamin E (400 IU) and β-carotene (15 mg), zinc (80 mg) and copper (2 mg) (Table 21.1). At this stage, the use of antioxidants and vitamin supplements by the general population to prevent or delay the onset of AMD is not supported by the available evidence (Evans, 2008).

As discussed above, omega-3 fatty acids may down-regulate inflammatory and immune processes, suggesting potential application in slowing the onset or progression of AMD. Omega-3 fatty acids can form anti-inflammatory lipid factors such as resolvins and neuroprotectins, which are implicated in down-modulating retinal inflammatory responses (Mukherjee *et al.*, 2004; Tian *et al.*, 2009). Macular carotenoids, the yellow pigments observed clinically within the macula, have been implicated in AMD. Several studies suggest that increased macula pigment optical density can reduce the risk of AMD, perhaps related to potential antioxidant effects and by reducing blue-light-associated retinal damage (Snodderly, 1995; Krinsky, 2002; Moeller *et al.*, 2006). Various studies have reported benefits from increased dietary intake of omega-3 fatty acids and macular carotenoids (lutein and zeaxanthin), associated with a lower risk for AMD (San Giovanni *et al.* 2007, 2008; Chong *et al.*, 2008; Leung, 2008; Parisi *et al.*, 2008; Querques *et al.*, 2009). A large multicentre prospective study, including AREDS participants with bilateral drusen at baseline, also reported that increased dietary intake of omega-3 fatty acids and fish was associated with a decreased risk of progression from bilateral drusen to dry AMD over approximately 6 years (SanGiovanni *et al.*, 2008). Similar findings were found recently in a large-scale cohort study of women without AMD at baseline, where the relationship of dietary intake of omega-3 fatty acids and fish with AMD during 10 years follow-up was assessed (Christen *et al.*, 2011). This study also found that the ratio of omega-6 to omega-3 fatty acids was a strong predictor of early AMD; earlier studies reported similar observations for advanced AMD (Seddon *et al.*, 2003; SanGiovanni and Chew, 2005).

Following on from AREDS and many other studies using combinations of nutrients (Table 21.1), including omega-3 fatty acids and antioxidants for various stages of AMD, the Age-Related Eye Disease Study II (AREDS2) is now prospectively studying additional nutritional interventions for AMD as well as the original AREDS formula (http://www.areds2.org/). AREDS2 includes a randomized controlled clinical trial of the effects of the dietary macular carotenoids (lutein and zeaxanthin) and/or omega-3 fatty acids (DHA and EPA) on reducing the risk for AMD and on the rate of progression to advanced AMD. In light of the increased risk for lung cancer in current smokers taking β-carotene and the increased zinc-associated urinary tract problems seen in AREDS, the effect of eliminating β-carotene and reducing zinc from the original AREDS formulation is currently being assessed in AREDS2 (Table 21.1). The first outcomes from AREDS2 are expected in 2013 and are anticipated widely by the eye-health professions. More recently, a role for antioxidants as adjunct therapy in diabetic retinopathy, specifically for new vessel-related complications, has been advocated (Kowluru and Zhong, 2011).

Physical Activity Interventions, Inflammation and Eye Health

Exercise and physical activity are generally considered to regulate immune function, and may reduce inflammatory markers; our understanding of the molecular mechanisms involved in these processes continues to evolve (Ford, 2002; Warburton *et al.*, 2006). The effects of physical activity on eye health and the possible benefits for inflammation-associated eye disease are largely unexplored. There are no studies to date, as far as we are aware, that suggest physical activity as either a risk factor or possible intervention for DED. There is, however, an emerging interest in associations between physical activity and AMD.

The potential role of physical activity as a risk factor for AMD progression is increasingly included in epidemiological and observational studies. The rationale for this inclusion can be considered in light of risk factors identified as important in pathogenesis of AMD: complement pathway malfunction, oxidative stress, inflammation and cardiovascular-disease-associated factors. Interestingly, moderate level exercise was recently reported to have anti-inflammatory effects mediated by the complement system, with decreased complement factor B expression, and increased CFH (Yang *et al.*, 2010). The importance of the complement pathway in the pathogenesis of AMD (discussed above) is consistent with a role for exercise in preventing macular degeneration (and vascular disease) (Yang *et al.*, 2010).

Several studies indicate that physical activity can potentially reduce the risk of AMD development or progression (The Eye Disease Case-Control Study Group, 1992; Age-Related Eye Disease Study Research Group, 2001; Seddon *et al.*, 2003; Knudtson *et al.*, 2006; Williams, 2009; Mares *et al.*, 2011). Seddon *et al.* (2003) reported that, compared with no vigorous physical activity, three sessions per week of vigorous activity was associated with a 25% reduction in the progression to dry or wet AMD over approximately 5 years, for patients with early or intermediate AMD. Furthermore, the Beaver Dam Eye Study found that levels of activity (walking several city blocks each day, or three or more times/week of sweat-inducing physical activity) reduced the risk for wet AMD by 30% and 70%, respectively, over 15 years (Knudtson *et al.*, 2006). The level of physical activity in this study did not, however, relate to either early AMD or dry AMD. Participants in the National Runners' Health Study were also assessed at 7.7 years after baseline in regard to development of AMD (Williams, 2009). This analysis found that more vigorous physical activity was associated with a lower age-adjusted risk for AMD. Most recently, Mares *et al.* (2011) considered how various lifestyle factors, including physical activity, related to the subsequent development of AMD, as part of the Carotenoids in Age-Related Eye Disease Study. An inverse relationship between levels of physical activity and signs of early AMD was observed. Most importantly, this study emphasized the effect of a combination of healthy lifestyles (including physical activity, healthy diets and not smoking) in significantly reducing the prevalence of early AMD, on average 6 years later, in post-menopausal women (Mares *et al.*, 2011). These authors proposed several pathways by which healthy lifestyles may reduce the risks for early AMD including reducing inflammation, oxidative stress and blood pressure, and a healthy diet-associated increase in macular pigment density (macular carotenoids lutein and zeaxanthin) (Mares *et al.*, 2011).

Physical activity can also reduce the incidence of cardiovascular disease, a risk factor for AMD, and might benefit other cardiovascular disease risk factors reported to be associated with AMD such as adiposity and blood pressure (reviewed in Klein *et al.*, 2004). Indirect indicators of physical activity are also reported to be risk factors for AMD. For example, higher body mass index (BMI) has been reported to increase the risk for progression to advanced AMD (Seddon *et al.*, 2003). Evidence suggests that regular physical activity generally benefits health by reducing BMI, weight, blood pressure, systemic inflammation and endothelial dysfunction, and improving serum lipoprotein profiles (Warburton *et al.*, 2006). Recent studies of healthy lifestyles have found that lowering the risk for AMD had a greater impact on patients with genotypes associated with a higher attributable risk for AMD, particularly *CFH Y402H* (Schaumberg *et al.*, 2007; Seddon *et al.*, 2009). Whether physical activity alone can reduce the risk for AMD for people with high risk genotypes such as the *CFH* variant *Y402H* remains to be investigated.

Summary and Conclusions

DED and AMD are common inflammation-associated eye diseases that affect an increasing proportion of ageing populations in our community. The impact of these conditions on ocular comfort, functional vision and capacity to perform everyday life tasks is significant. The potential for nutritional interventions and physical activity to ameliorate symptoms and reduce disease progression in these conditions is increasingly recognized, based on our improved understanding of the pathogenesis of the conditions and the molecular mechanisms involved. Future long-term population-based studies with a broader inclusion of different ethnic backgrounds and prospective clinical trials are needed to substantiate the role of nutritional interventions in DED and AMD.

Disclosures

Research funding by Blackmores Limited and the Sydney Foundation for Medical Research (MCM).

References

Access Economics Pty Ltd (2010) Clear focus - The Economic Impact of Vision Loss in Australia in 2009. Vision 2020, Melbourne, Australia.

Age-Related Eye Disease Study Research Group (2001) A randomized, placebo-controlled, clinical trial of high-dose supplementation with vitamins C and E, beta-carotene, and zinc for age-related macular degeneration and vision loss. *Archives of Ophthalmology* 119, 1417–1436.

Anderson, D.H., Radeke, M.J., Gallo, N.B., Chapin, E.A., Johnson, P.T., *et al.* (2010) The pivotal role of the complement system in aging and age-related macular degeneration: hypothesis re-visited. *Progress in Retinal and Eye Research* 29, 95–112.

Aragona, P., Bucolo, C., Spinella, R., Giuffrida, S. and Ferreri, G. (2005) Systemic omega-6 essential fatty acid treatment and PGE1 tear content in Sjogren's Syndrome patients. *Investigative Ophthalmology and Visual Science* 46, 4474–4479.

Bandeen-Roche, K., Munoz, B., Tielsch, J.M., West, S.K. and Schein, O.D. (1997) Self-reported assessment of dry eye in a population-based setting. *Investigative Ophthalmology and Visual Science* 38, 2469–2475.

Begley, C.G., Chalmers, R.L., Mitchell, G.L., Nichols, K.K., Caffery, B., *et al.* (2001) Characterization of ocular surface symptoms from optometric practices in North America. *Cornea* 20, 610–618.

Brignole-Baudouin, F., Baudouin, C., Aragona, P., Rolando, M., Labetoulle, M., *et al.* (2011) A multicentre, double-masked, randomized, controlled trial assessing the effect of oral supplementation of omega-3 and omega-6 fatty acids on a conjunctival inflammatory marker in dry eye patients. *Acta Ophthalmologica* 89, e591–e597.

Christen, W.G., Schaumberg, D.A., Glynn, R.J. and Buring, J.E. (2011) Dietary omega-3 fatty acid and fish intake and incident age-related macular degeneration in women. *Archives of Ophthalmology* 129, 921–929.

Despriet, D.D., Van Duijn, C.M., De Jong, P.T., Vingerling, J.R., Bergen, A.a.B., *et al.* (2008) Genetic diagnosis of age-related macular Degeneration: The Role of molecular genetics in the Identification of high risk eyes. *Investigative Ophthalmology and Vision Science [ARVO Meeting Abstract]* 49, 1769.

Dixon, J.A., Oliver, S.C., Olson, J.L. and Mandava, N. (2009) VEGF Trap-Eye for the treatment of neovascular age-related macular degeneration. *Expert Opinion on Investigational Drugs* 18, 1573–1580.

Dougherty, J.M. and Mcculley, J.P. (1986) Bacterial lipases and chronic blepharitis. *Investigative Ophthalmology and Visual Science* 27, 486–491.

Edwards, A.O., Ritter, R., 3rd, Abel, K.J., Manning, A., Panhuysen, C. *et al.* (2005) Complement factor H polymorphism and age-related macular degeneration. *Science* 308, 421–424.

Evans, J. (2008) Antioxidant supplements to prevent or slow down the progression of AMD: a systematic review and meta-analysis. *Eye* 22, 751–760.

Ford, E.S. (2002) Does exercise reduce inflammation? Physical activity and C-reactive protein among U.S. adults. *Epidemiology* 13, 561–568.

Gehrs, K.M., Jackson, J.R., Brown, E.N., Allikmets, R. and Hageman, G.S. (2010) Complement, age-related macular degeneration and a vision of the future. *Archives of Ophthalmology* 128, 349–358.

Gipson, I.K., Hori, Y. and Argueso, P. (2004) Character of ocular surface mucins and their alteration in dry eye disease. *Ocular Surface* 2, 131–148.

Gold, B., Merriam, J.E., Zernant, J., Hancox, L.S., Taiber, A.J., *et al.* (2006) Variation in factor B (BF) and complement component 2 (C2) genes is associated with age-related macular degeneration. *Nature Genetics* 38, 458–462.

Gulati, A., Sacchetti, M., Bonini, S. and Dana, R. (2006) Chemokine receptor CCR5 expression in conjunctival epithelium of patients with dry eye syndrome. *Archives of Ophthalmology* 124, 710–716.

Hageman, G.S., Luthert, P.J., Victor Chong, N.H., Johnson, L.V., Anderson, D.H. *et al.* (2001) An integrated hypothesis that considers drusen as biomarkers of immune-mediated processes at the RPE-Bruch's membrane interface in aging and age-related macular degeneration. *Progress in Retinal and Eye Research* 20, 705–732.

Haines, J.L., Hauser, M.A., Schmidt, S., Scott, W.K., Olson, L.M., *et al.* (2005) Complement factor H variant increases the risk of age-related macular degeneration. *Science* 308, 419–421.

International Dry Eye Workshop Report (2007) *Ocular Surface* 5, 65–204.

Jakobsdottir, J., Conley, Y.P., Weeks, D.E., Mah, T.S., Ferrell, R.E., *et al.* (2005) Susceptibility genes for age-related maculopathy on chromosome 10q26. *American Journal of Human Genetics* 77, 389–407.

Jalbert, I., Yusop, S. and Stapleton, F. (2011) Dry eye in a university campus population. *Optometry Vision Science [AAO Abstract]* 88 (in press).

Johnson, M.E. and Murphy, P.J. (2007) Measurement of ocular surface irritation on a linear interval scale with the ocular comfort index. *Investigative Ophthalmology and Visual Science* 48, 4451–4458.

Klein, R., Peto, T., Bird, A. and Vannewkirk, M.R. (2004) The epidemiology of age-related macular degeneration. *American Journal of Ophthalmology* 137, 486–495.

Klein, R., Chou, C.-F., Klein, B.E.K., Zhang, X., Meuer, S.M. *et al.* (2011) Prevalence of age-related macular degeneration in the US population. *Archives of Ophthalmology* 129, 75–80.

Knop, E., Knop, N., Millar, T., Obata, H. and Sullivan, D.A. (2011a) The International Workshop on Meibomian Gland Dysfunction: Report of the Subcommittee on Anatomy, Physiology, and Pathophysiology of the Meibomian Gland. *Investigative Ophthalmology and Visual Science* 52, 1938–1978.

Knop, E., Knop, N., Zhivov, A., Kraak, R., Korb, D.R., *et al.* (2011b) The lid wiper and muco-cutaneous junction anatomy of the human eyelid margins: an in vivo confocal and histological study. *Journal of Anatomy* 218, 449–461.

Knudtson, M.D., Klein, R. and Klein, B.E. (2006) Physical activity and the 15-year cumulative incidence of age-related macular degeneration: the Beaver Dam Eye Study. *British Journal of Ophthalmology* 90, 1461–1463.

Kokke, K.H., Morris, J.A. and Lawrenson, J.G. (2008) Oral omega-6 essential fatty acid treatment in contact lens associated dry eye. *Contact Lens and Anterior Eye* 31, 141–146.

Korb, D.R., Herman, J., Blackie, C.A., Scaffidi, R., Greiner, J., *et al.* (2010) Prevalence of lid wiper epitheliopathy in subjects with dry eye signs and symptoms. *Cornea* 29, 377–383.

Kowluru, R.A. and Zhong, Q. (2011) Beyond AREDS: Is There a Place for Antioxidant Therapy in the Prevention/Treatment of Eye Disease? *Investigative Ophthalmology and Visual Science* 52, 8665–8671.

Krinsky, N. (2002) Possible biologic mechanisms for a protective role of xanthophylls. *The Journal of Nutrition* 132, 540S–542S.

Krishnadev, N., Meleth, A.D. and Chew, E.Y. (2010) Nutritional supplements for age-related macular degeneration. *Current Opinion in Ophthalmology* 21, 184–189.

Mares, J.A., Voland, R.P., Sondel, S.A., Millen, A.E., Larowe, T., *et al.* (2011) Healthy lifestyles related to subsequent prevalence of age-related macular degeneration. *Archives of Ophthalmology* 129, 470–480.

Massingale, M.L., Li, X., Vallabhajosyula, M., Chen, D., Wei, Y. *et al.* (2009) Analysis of inflammatory cytokines in the tears of dry eye patients. *Cornea* 28, 1023–1027.

Miljanovic, B., Trivedi, K.A., Dana, M.R., Gilbard, J.P., Buring, J.E., *et al.* (2005) Relation between dietary n-3 and n-6 fatty acids and clinically diagnosed dry eye syndrome in women. *The American Journal of Clinical Nutrition* 82, 887–893.

Miljanovic, B., Dana, R., Sullivan, D.A. and Schaumberg, D.A. (2007) Impact of dry eye syndrome on vision-related quality of life. *American Journal of Ophthalmology* 143, 409–415.e2.

Mitchell, P. (2011) A systematic review of the efficacy and safety outcomes of anti-VEGF agents used for treating neovascular age-related macular degeneration: comparison of ranibizumab and bevacizumab. *Current Medical Research and Opinion* 27, 1465–1475.

Moeller, S., Parekh, N., Tinker, L., Ritengaugh, C., Blodi, B., *et al.* (2006) Associations between intermediate age-related macular degeneration and lutein and zeaxanthin in the Carotenoids in Age-related Eye Disease Study (CAREDS): ancillary study of the Women's Health Initiative. *Archives of Ophthalmology* 124, 1151–1162.

Mukherjee, P.K., Marcheselli, V.L., Serhan, C.N. and Bazan, N.G. (2004) Neuroprotectin D1: a docosahexaenoic acid-derived docosatriene protects human retinal pigment epithelial cells from oxidative stress. *Proceedings of the National Academy of Sciences USA* 101, 8491–8496.

Narayanan, S., Corrales, R.M., Farley, W., Mcdermott, A.M. and Pflugfelder, S.C. (2008) Interleukin-1 receptor-1-deficient mice show attenuated production of ocular inflammatory cytokines in experimental dry eye. *Cornea* 27, 811–817.

Nelson, J.D., Shimazaki, J., Benitez-Del-Castillo, J.M., Craig, J.P., Mcculley, J.P., *et al.* (2011) The International Workshop on Meibomian Gland Dysfunction: Report of the Definition and Classification Subcommittee. *Investigative Ophthalmology and Visual Science* 52, 1930–1937.

Patel, R.D., Momi, R.S. and Hariprasad, S.M. (2011) Review of Ranibizumab Trials for Neovascular Age-Related Macular Degeneration. *Seminars in Ophthalmology* 26, 372–379.

Penfold, P.L., Madigan, M.C., Gillies, M.C. and Provis, J.M. (2001) Immunological and aetiological aspects of macular degeneration. *Progress in Retinal and Eye Research* 20, 385–414.

Pholpramool, C. (1979) Secretory effect of prostaglandins on the rabbit lacrimal gland in vivo. *Prostaglandins and Medicine* 3, 185–192.

Reddy, P., Grad, O. and Rajagopalan, K. (2004) The economic burden of dry eye: a conceptual framework and preliminary assessment. *Cornea* 23, 751–761.

Ricklin, D., Hajishengallis, G., Yang, K. and Lambris, J.D. (2010) Complement: a key system for immune surveillance and homeostasis. *Nature Immunology* 11, 785–797.

Rolando, M., Barabino, S., Mingari, C., Moretti, S., Giuffrida, S. *et al.* (2005) Distribution of conjunctival HLA-DR expression and the pathogenesis of damage in early dry eyes. *Cornea* 24, 951–954.

Rutar, M., Natoli, R., Kozulin, P., Valter, K., Gatenby, P., *et al.* (2011) Analysis of complement expression in light-induced retinal degeneration: synthesis and deposition of C3 by microglia/macrophages is associated with focal photoreceptor degeneration. *Investigative Ophthalmology and Visual Science* 52, 5347–5358.

Sangiovanni, J.P. and Chew, E.Y. (2005) The role of omega-3 long-chain polyunsaturated fatty acids in health and disease of the retina. *Progress in Retinal and Eye Research,* 24, 87–138.

Sangiovanni, J.P., Chew, E.Y., Agron, E., Clemons, T.E., Ferris, F.L., 3rd, *et al.* (2008) The relationship of dietary omega-3 long-chain polyunsaturated fatty acid intake with incident age-related macular degeneration: AREDS report no. 23. *Archives of Ophthalmology* 126, 1274–1279.

Schaumberg, D.A., Hankinson, S.E., Guo, Q., Rimm, E. and Hunter, D.J. (2007) A prospective study of 2 major age-related macular degeneration susceptibility alleles and interactions with modifiable risk factors. *Archives of Ophthalmology* 125, 55–62.

Schaumberg, D.A., Nichols, J.J., Papas, E.B., Tong, L., Uchino, M., *et al.* (2011) The International Workshop on Meibomian Gland Dysfunction: Report of the Subcommittee on the Epidemiology of, and Associated Risk Factors for, MGD. *Investigative Ophthalmology and Visual Science* 52, 1994–2005.

Schiffman, R.M., Walt, J.G., Jacobsen, G., Doyle, J.J., Lebovics, G., *et al.* (2003) Utility assessment among patients with dry eye disease. *Ophthalmology* 110, 1412–1419.

Seddon, J.M., Cote, J. and Rosner, B. (2003) Progression of age-related macular degeneration: association with dietary fat, transunsaturated fat, nuts, and fish intake. *Archives of Ophthalmology* 121, 1728–1737.

Seddon, J.M., Reynolds, R., Maller, J., Fagerness, J.A., Daly, M.J., *et al.* (2009) Prediction model for prevalence and incidence of advanced age-related macular degeneration based on genetic, demographic, and environmental variables. *Investigative Ophthalmology and Visual Science* 50, 2044–2053.

Shine, W., Mcculley, J. and Pandya, A. (2003) Minocycline effect on meibomian gland lipids in meibomianitis patients. *Experimental Eye Research* 76, 417–420.

Snodderly, D. (1995) Evidence for protection against age-related macular degeneration by carotenoids and antioxidant vitamins. *The American Journal of Clinical Nutrition* 62, 1448S–1461S.

Sommer, A., Faich, G. and Quesada, J. (1975) Mass distribution of vitamin A and the prevention of keratomalacia. *American Journal of Ophthalmology* 80, 1073–1080.

Stapleton, F., Keay, L., Edwards, K., Naduvilath, T., Dart, J.K.G., *et al.* (2008) The incidence of contact lens-related microbial keratitis in Australia. *Ophthalmology* 115, 1655–1662.

Sullivan, B., Cermak, J., Sullivan, R., Papas, A., Evans, J., *et al.* (2002) Correlations between nutrient intake and the polar lipid profiles of meibomian gland secretions in women with Sjogren's syndrome. *Advances in Experimental Medicine and Biology,* 506, 441–447.

Taylor, H., Tikellis, G., Robman, L., Ca, M. and Jj, M. (2002) Vitamin E supplementation and macular degeneration: randomised controlled trial. *British Medical Journal* 325, 11.

The Eye Disease Case-Control Study Group (1992) Risk factors for neovascular age-related macular degeneration. *Archives of Ophthalmology* 110, 1701–1708.

Tian, H., Lu, Y., Sherwood, A.M., Hongqian, D. and Hong, S. (2009) Resolvins E1 and D1 in choroid-retinal endothelial cells and leukocytes: biosynthesis and mechanisms of anti-inflammatory actions. *Investigative Ophthalmology and Visual Science* 50, 3613–3620.

Warburton, D.E., Nicol, C.W. and Bredin, S.S. (2006) Health benefits of physical activity: the evidence. *Canadian Medical Association Journal Journal de l'Association Medicale Canadienne* 174, 801–809.

Williams, P.T. (2009) Prospective study of incident age-related macular degeneration in relation to vigorous physical activity during a 7-year follow-up. *Investigative Ophthalmology and Visual Science* 50, 101–106.

Yamaguchi, M., Kutsuna, M., Uno, T., Zheng, X., Kodama, T. *et al.* (2006) Marx line: fluorescein staining line on the inner lid as indicator of meibomian gland function. *American Journal of Ophthalmology* 141, 669–675.

Yang, K.D., Chang, W.C., Chuang, H., Wang, P.W., Liu, R.T. *et al.* (2010) Increased complement factor H with decreased factor B determined by proteomic differential displays as a biomarker of tai chi chuan exercise. *Clinical Chemistry* 56, 127–131.

Yehoshua, Z., Rosenfeld, P.J. and Albini, T.A. (2011) Current clinical trials in dry AMD and the definition of appropriate clinical outcome measures. *Seminars in Ophthalmology* 26, 167–180.

Index